Radiology Department
Children's Hospital National Medical Center
111 Michigan Avenue N.W.
Washington, DC 20010

THE CIBA COLLECTION OF MEDICAL ILLUSTRATIONS

Volume 1

Nervous System

Part II
Neurologic and
Neuromuscular Disorders

A compilation of paintings depicting
pathophysiology, pathology,
and clinical features and management

Prepared by

Frank H. Netter, M.D.

H. Royden Jones, Jr., M.D.
Guest Editor

Regina V. Dingle
Managing Editor

Commissioned and published by

C I B A

Other published volumes of
THE CIBA COLLECTION OF MEDICAL ILLUSTRATIONS
prepared by
Frank H. Netter, M.D.

Nervous System, Part I: Anatomy and Physiology
Reproductive System
Digestive System, Part I: Upper Digestive Tract
Digestive System, Part II: Lower Digestive Tract
Digestive System, Part III: Liver, Biliary Tract and Pancreas
Endocrine System and Selected Metabolic Diseases
Heart
Kidneys, Ureters, and Urinary Bladder
Respiratory System

First Printing

ISBN 0-914168-11-8
Library of Congress Catalog No: 53-2151

Printed in U.S.A.

Book printed offset by Wetzel Brothers, Inc.
Laser-scanned color separations by R.R. Donnelley & Sons Company
Layout design by Pierre J. Lair
Mechanical art by Cesareo Studio
Text photocomposed in Mergenthaler Garamond No. 3 by Arrow Typographers, Inc.
Contents printed on Cameo dull text, basis 80, by S.D. Warren Company
Smyth-sewn case binding by R.R. Donnelley & Sons Company
End papers: White Flannel text, basis 80, by Curtis Paper Division, James River Corporation
Cover material: Buckram linen cloth by Joanna Western Mills
Front and spine cover design by Philip Grushkin
Index by Steele/Katigbak Indexers

Introduction

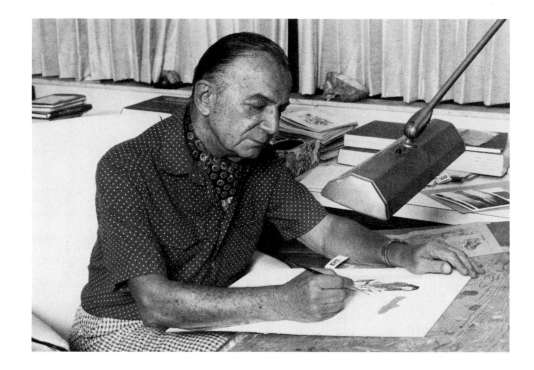

In the introduction to Part I of this volume on the nervous system, I wrote of why, after almost 35 years of widespread acceptance, it was necessary to revise and update the original atlas, Volume 1 of THE CIBA COLLECTION of MEDICAL ILLUSTRATIONS. I also told there of how, as I progressed with the revision, the amount of material to be included grew to such a magnitude that it was decided to publish it in two parts. Part I, published in 1983, contained a depiction of what may be called the "basic science" of the nervous system, that is, the bony encasements, the gross anatomy, and the vasculature of the brain and spinal cord, the autonomic nervous system, the cranial nerves, the nerve plexuses and peripheral nerves, the embryology, and the physiology and functional neuroanatomy of the nervous system. Part II, presented herewith, is devoted to portraying the disorders and diseases of the nervous system. But once again, to my dismay, as I progressed with picturing the pathology and clinical aspects of those multitudinous ailments, the volume of material grew to such an extent that I was hard put to confine it to the limits of one book. Furthermore, the fantastic progress which was being made in the field even as I worked added to the difficulty of space limitation. Accordingly, I tried to place emphasis on those disorders most threatening to mankind because of incidence or severity, with due consideration for timeliness, diagnostic difficulty, and potential for beneficial management.

I believe that, in studying many of the conditions portrayed in this book, the reader will find it most helpful to refer repeatedly to Part I of this volume for an understanding of the basic science aspects underlying the disorder. For example, study of stroke in this book may be enhanced by reference to the arterial supply and functional subdivisions of the brain, as covered in Part I. Likewise, study of the peripheral neuropathies may call for a review of nerve conduction as well as of the course and distribution of the peripheral nerves.

But the nervous system is not an isolated entity. It is intimately involved with the function of every other system of the body as portrayed in other volumes of the CIBA COLLECTION. The association is, however, most marked with the musculoskeletal system. Indeed, there is great overlap between the fields of neurology and neurosurgery with the field of orthopedics, both diagnostically and therapeutically. Cerebral palsy and poliomyelitis are, of course, basically neurologic diseases, and they are so presented in this volume.

Introduction

But the after-care, corrective surgery, and rehabilitation of such patients are usually in the hands of the orthopedists. Accordingly, those aspects of these diseases will be covered in the forthcoming atlases on the musculoskeletal system, on which I am now at work. Intervertebral disc herniation and spinal stenosis likewise fall into both fields of practice, and thus, while presented herein, their management will be amplified in the musculoskeletal volume. The neuromuscular diseases are among many other examples of overlap between the two disciplines.

The trials and tribulations of the production of this atlas were far outweighed by the pleasure and stimulation I received from working on it. This was largely due to those wonderful people, my consultants and collaborators, who helped me, taught me, advised me, and supplied me with pertinent reference material as a basis for many of my illustrations. They are all listed separately herein and I thank them, each and every one, for the knowledge they imparted to me and for the time they so graciously gave me.

I was especially fortunate to have had the guidance and counsel of that delightful personality, Dr. H. Royden Jones, Jr. ("Roy" to me), of the Lahey Clinic. The many long hours we spent together planning and organizing the material to be included were not only informative and productive, but exceedingly pleasurable as well. I was constantly impressed by his broad knowledge, his unique ability to define the essence of each subject we dealt with, and his ability to call upon knowledgeable consultants for special topics, yet maintaining an overall perspective of the project in relation to the total field of medical practice and of neurology in particular. Our collaboration thus developed into a lasting friendship which I cherish highly.

I express here also my appreciation for the help and encouragement which I received from Dr. William (Bill) Fields, professor and chairman of the department of neuro-oncology at the M.D. Anderson Hospital and Tumor Institute, Houston. He was not only a definitive collaborator for some specific subjects, but readily gave me much practical advice and counsel throughout the undertaking. I thank Mr. Philip Flagler, director of Medical Education for the CIBA Company, and Dr. Milton Donin, a relative newcomer to our team, for their continuous efforts in coordinating the varied aspects of the undertaking, to keep it moving along and to insure that each person involved understood and felt happy in their contribution to it. My accolades go also to Ms. Gina Dingle for her diverse editorial activities, for her untiring and patient attention to frustrating details, for her great organizing accomplishments, and especially for her ever-present personality. Finally, I express once more my appreciation of the CIBA Pharmaceutical Company and its executives for their understanding of the significance of this project and for the free hand they have given me in its creation.

Frank H. Netter, M.D.

· Preface

Frank Netter, MD: need anything more be said? Probably not, especially if one has a love for both medicine and art. It has been a unique privilege and professional opportunity to collaborate as guest editor with this very intuitive physician, superlative teacher and renowned artist.

When, as a freshman medical student, I first encountered the complexity of the nervous system, Dr. Netter's first volume of THE CIBA COLLECTION OF MEDICAL ILLUSTRATIONS provided me with a concise means of learning. Not only did he present many essentials of the basic neurologic sciences, but his vivid pictures of patients provided an added stimulus to the anticipated clinical years.

The contributors hope that this atlas will provide an introduction and formulation for many future students, becoming an impetus for a more in-depth study. The broad concepts of neurologic disease presented in this volume will make it useful to the family physician, internist, pediatrician, orthopedic surgeon and any other physician who initially sees the 10% to 20% of our population eventually confronted with a neurologic disorder.

It is difficult to highlight all the important advances which have taken place in the 33 years since the publication of Volume 1.

Despite a significant decrease in incidence in the past two decades, cerebrovascular disease is still the third most common cause of death in Western countries. Trauma to the brain and spine continues to be a major frustration to patient, family and physician, especially as it is often preventable. Pediatric neurology was nonexistent as a subspecialty in 1953. In 1986, an entire section of the revised book is devoted to this field alone.

Technological advances have provided pathophysiologic data not conceived possible at the inception of Volume 1. Computers have led to the development of CT scanning, digital subtraction angiography and magnetic resonance imaging. Our neuroradiologists depend on these techniques in up to 85% of all studies performed.

Early diagnosis using CT scanning and the development of the operating microscope have made removal of benign central nervous system tumors an exceedingly low-risk procedure, particularly for those lesions involving the pituitary and cerebellopontine angle areas. It is hoped that more efficacious therapy will be developed for primary and metastatic malignancies of the brain.

Recent developments in the understanding of the illnesses affecting higher cortical function have emphasized the fact that Alzheimer's disease is the primary cause of dementia. One has to carefully exclude the treatable causes of dementia, which are now well defined. Because of the breakthroughs in neurochemistry that occurred in the 1960s, a more effective treatment of Parkinson's disease is now available.

Some of the enigmas of psychiatry, particularly depression, have also yielded to the inquiry of the neurochemists. Empiric utilization of psychotropic agents, such as those used in schizophrenia, has allowed for widespread deinstitutionalization of many individuals previously committed for life. Dr. Netter's vivid portrayals of these subjects, although rendered almost four decades ago, were immediately classified by our consultant psychiatrist.

Infectious diseases of the central nervous system are less common, especially bacterial meningitis and brain abscess. Poliomyelitis has been conquered in societies providing adequate immunization. In the third world, leprosy continues to be the most common cause of peripheral neuropathy. In some patients, their immunosuppressed states have provided a basis for opportunistic infections to cause serious neurologic infections. Concepts of transmissible

Preface

slow virus illnesses, such as kuru and Creutzfeldt-Jakob disease, were introduced less than two decades ago. These may provide a model leading to an understanding of common, albeit now idiopathic, neurologic illnesses.

Immunologic advances have important implications in the appreciation of some neurologic disorders. These advances are best illustrated by the discovery that myasthenia gravis is an autoimmune disease. Other rare diseases possibly having an immunologic basis, such as acute disseminated encephalomyelitis, may provide clues to some common neurologic disorders, such as multiple sclerosis.

Electromyography and nerve conduction testing provide a pathophysiologic classification of neuropathies. These studies also have therapeutic implications, as illustrated by the very common carpal tunnel syndrome. New histologic techniques have further broadened the pathophysiologic conceptualization of diseases of the peripheral motor-sensory units. However, multiple challenges remain. The motor neuron diseases, various neuropathies and dystrophies are still undefined in terms of etiology and therapy.

Finally, my thanks to all those who helped in the evolution of this project. The decision to produce this book in the middle of other commitments by CIBA and the dedication to its completion were greatly aided by Mrs. Gina Dingle and the members of her editorial team. Also, my family's encouragement is much appreciated. Most importantly, thanks to Frank Netter, MD, a teacher and hero to me when I was a medical student and now a dear and gracious friend with whom it has been a distinct pleasure to work on the various aspects of this volume.

H. ROYDEN JONES, JR., M.D.
GUEST EDITOR

Acknowledgments

Pierre Lair was Design and Production Manager of this series for almost twelve years. Schooled both in his native France and in the United States, Pierre brought to the publications of CIBA-GEIGY's Medical Education Division a wealth of technical knowledge, a finely developed sense of design, and a keen understanding of the color reproduction process. His commitment to the making of fine books is evident in this volume, *Nervous System, Parts I and II*, the design for which he completed before his untimely death. His colleagues dedicate this book to his memory.

Acknowledging and thanking all of the contributors to a book of this size and complexity is a formidable task; it involves a large number of talented people and interactions that have taken place over an extended period of time. Dr. Netter, of course, is the primary focus of our thanks, as he has clearly been the lifeblood of the project. It is his book and we are proud to be associated with it.

Dr. Netter is widely recognized as the premier medical illustrator in the world. This derives in part from his broad background in medicine and his highly developed technical skills as an artist. Most important, though, is his extraordinary ability to graphically present complex medical concepts, stripping away all that is superfluous while highlighting the essential details. This is not a spontaneous process. Rather, Dr. Netter carefully researches the literature and consults experts in the field. He may visit an operating room to observe a procedure or return to the dissection table. When he has finally seen in his mind's eye how he wishes to portray the subject, he produces a series of pencil sketches and reviews them with the collaborating author. Only then does he begin to paint. The illustration may show anatomy, pathology, or function in a way that no human has ever seen it; but it conveys a sense of reality and helps the physician or student clarify the subject in his own mind. Therein lies the core of Frank Netter as a Renaissance man—physician, artist, and teacher.

There are others, of course, who have contributed greatly to the complex process of pulling such a book together and they, too, must be acknowledged and profusely thanked. First are the contributors and consultants—the extent of their contributions is staggering and full recitation of the details would fill another book. We thank them for their meticulous care in writing the texts and for their cooperation throughout all the stages of editorial preparation. Likewise, we must thank Dr. H. Royden Jones, Jr, our guest editor who, in addition to being a contributor, was also a consummate organizer, talent scout and cheerleader. Finally, there is a host of others whose contributions help make the difference between a good presentation and one that excels.

Among these we particularly wish to acknowledge the guidance and assistance of Dr. William S. Fields, who has been involved with the revision since it was first considered in 1970. We are also most grateful to Dr. Marc A. Flitter for his advice and help during the early stages of the revision process.

Our very sincere appreciation to Dr. Richard A. Baker, who meticulously reviewed almost all the radiologic images in the book, and also supplied the images used in the majority of the illustrations.

We are also indebted to Dr. Ana Sotrel for reviewing and supplying the histologic materials used in the illustrations dealing with motor neuron disease, with the exception of some examples that were provided by Dr. E. Tessa Hedley-Whyte and Dr. Haruo Okazaki.

Dr. Netter wishes to thank Dr. James Grotta and Doralene Vital, RN, for demonstrating the techniques of noninvasive tests for carotid artery blood

Acknowledgments

flow, depicted in Section III, Plates 20–21. Dr. Charles Hufnagel's advice on the subject of endarterectomy was most valuable in the preparation of Plate 25 in Section III. Dr. Jules Hardy is thanked for his guidance and for supplying materials on the transsphenoidal approach for the removal of pituitary tumors, illustrated in Section V, Plate 8. Dr. Robert Terry and Dr. Alex Comfort are thanked for supplying valuable reference material and for their discussions of Alzheimer's disease, Section VII, Plates 1–2. Dr. Carl Sadowsky and Mr. Robert Alexander are thanked for demonstrating the techniques of evoked response testing, Section IX, Plates 2–3.

We are also grateful to the following consultants for contributing materials used in these illustrations:

Section I, Plate 23: Dr. Roy Strand and Dr. James Wallman–CT scan on Sturge-Weber disease. Plate 24: Dr. Barbara Westmoreland–EEG tracing.

Section III, Plate 29: Dr. James Wallman, Dr. Gerald O'Riley and Dr. Samuel Wolpert–some of the radiologic images.

Section VIII, Plates 5 and 12: Dr. William S. Fields–histology slides. Plate 13: Dr. E. Tessa Hedley-Whyte–histology slide.

Section IX, Plate 5: Dr. David Norman–radiologic images on acute disseminated encephalomyelitis.

Section XI, Plate 12: Dr. James Kelly–x-ray film. Plate 19: Dr. Paul W. Brand–biopsy specimen slide of median nerve.

Within the CIBA organization, we are especially grateful to the publication team which worked with dedication to bring this book to completion. As head of that team, Ms. Gina Dingle deserves special kudos for coordinating all the varied aspects of this multifaceted project, from interaction with contributors, editors and author to terminology and typesetting; she truly "saw the project through" from beginning to end. Ms. Sally Chichester, Ms. Nicole Friedman and Ms. Jeffie Lemons contributed to the project those extra efforts that bring about the smooth functioning of the myriad behind-the-scenes activities, from maintaining schedules with outside suppliers to proofreading all texts and illustrations. Ms. Mary Earl McKinsey is thankfully acknowledged for her manuscript editing. Mr. Don Canter, Mr. Geoffrey Wooding and Mr. Clark Carroll, of our production and design department, are thanked for preparing the book materials for the printing and manufacturing phases.

This new atlas contains 150 new plates, in addition to 57 from the earlier edition and CIBA CLINICAL SYMPOSIA issues. The accompanying texts have been prepared by distinguished consultants who are experts in their fields. Whether there is universal agreement about the theoretical aspect of a text or whether, in some cases, there may be scientific controversy, the view expressed by Dr. Netter in the preface to the volume still pertains: "Clinical significance has been the guiding principle."

In all, it has been a stimulating project, one we are delighted to bring to a conclusion, but one we will also miss because of the warm camaraderie that has been built amongst the many participants.

MILTON N. DONIN, PH.D.
EDITORIAL DIRECTOR

PHILIP B. FLAGLER
DIRECTOR,
MEDICAL EDUCATION DIVISION

Contributors
and Consultants

The artist, editors and publishers express their appreciation for the dedicated collaboration of these contributing authors:

J. Paul Badami, M.D.
Diagnostic Neuroradiologist,
Lahey Clinic Medical Center,
Burlington, Massachusetts

Ann Sullivan Baker, M.D.
Assistant Professor of Medicine, Harvard Medical School;
Consultant in Infectious Disease, Massachusetts Eye and Ear Infirmary;
Associate Physician, Infectious Disease Unit,
Massachusetts General Hospital,
Boston, Massachusetts

Richard A. Baker, M.D.
Assistant Clinical Professor of Radiology, Harvard Medical School;
Clinical Instructor in Radiology, Tufts University School of Medicine;
Diagnostic Neuroradiologist,
Lahey Clinic Medical Center,
Burlington, Massachusetts

Michael Brant-Zawadzki, M.D.
Associate Professor of Radiology, Neurology and Neurosurgery;
Co-Director of Magnetic Resonance Imaging,
Neuroradiology Section, Department of Radiology,
University of California School of Medicine at San Francisco,
San Francisco, California

Michael J. Bresnan, M.D.
Associate Professor of Neurology, Harvard Medical School;
Associate Chief of Clinical Services, Department of Neurology,
The Children's Hospital,
Boston, Massachusetts

Louis R. Caplan, M.D.
Neurologist-in-Chief, New England Medical Center Hospitals;
Professor and Chairman, Department of Neurology,
Tufts University School of Medicine,
Boston, Massachusetts

Roger C. Duvoisin, M.D.
Professor and Chairman, Department of Neurology,
University of Medicine and Dentistry of New Jersey,
Rutgers Medical School,
New Brunswick, New Jersey

William S. Fields, M.D.
Formerly Professor and Chairman, Department of Neurology,
University of Texas Medical School at Houston;
Professor and Chairman, Department of Neuro-Oncology,
University of Texas System Cancer Center,
M.D. Anderson Hospital and Tumor Institute,
Houston, Texas

Marc A. Flitter, M.D.
Associate Attending Physician, Department of Neurosurgery,
Mt. Sinai Medical Center;
Consultant, Department of Neurosurgery, Miami Heart Institute;
Chief, Department of Neurosurgery, St. Francis Hospital,
Miami Beach, Florida

Stephen R. Freidberg, M.D.
Chairman, Department of Neurosurgery,
Lahey Clinic Medical Center,
Burlington, Massachusetts

Contributors and Consultants

William A. Friedman, M.D.
Assistant Professor, Departments of Neurological Surgery and Neuroscience,
University of Florida College of Medicine,
Gainesville, Florida

Paul T. Gross, M.D.
Associate Professor of Neurology,
University of Massachusetts Medical School;
Clinical Instructor in Neurology, Harvard Medical School;
Department of Neurology,
Lahey Clinic Medical Center,
Burlington, Massachusetts

Jose A. Gutrecht, M.D., M.Sc.
Department of Neurology,
Lahey Clinic Medical Center,
Burlington, Massachusetts

John R. Hayes, M.D.
Assistant Professor of Psychiatry and Medicine,
and Director, Consultation/Liaison Psychiatry,
Indiana University School of Medicine,
Indianapolis, Indiana

Martin S. Hirsch, M.D.
Associate Professor of Medicine, Harvard Medical School;
Associate Physician, Infectious Disease Unit,
Massachusetts General Hospital,
Boston, Massachusetts

Charles A. Hufnagel, M.D.
Professor of Surgery Emeritus, Georgetown University School of Medicine;
Clinical Professor of Surgery, George Washington University
School of Medicine and Health Sciences,
Washington, District of Columbia

Roger L. Hybels, M.D.
Clinical Assistant Professor of Otolaryngology,
Boston University School of Medicine;
Department of Otolaryngology–Head and Neck Surgery,
Lahey Clinic Medical Center,
Burlington, Massachusetts

H. Royden Jones, Jr., M.D.
Assistant Neurologist, The Children's Hospital;
Assistant Clinical Professor of Neurology, Harvard Medical School;
Department of Neurology, and Chairman, Department of Education,
Lahey Clinic Medical Center,
Burlington, Massachusetts

Hugo A. Keim, M.D.
Associate Professor of Clinical Orthopaedics,
Columbia-Presbyterian Medical Center,
New York, New York

Thomas L. Kemper, M.D.
Consultant in Neurology and Neuropathology, Harvard Medical School;
Professor of Neurology and Anatomy, Boston University School of Medicine;
Director, Neuropathology,
Boston City Hospital,
Boston, Massachusetts

Contributors and Consultants

H. Stephen Kott, M.D.
Chairman, Department of Neurology,
Lahey Clinic Medical Center,
Burlington, Massachusetts

Irma M. Lessell, M.D.
Clinical Instructor in Neurology, Harvard Medical School;
Department of Neurology,
Lahey Clinic Medical Center,
Burlington, Massachusetts

Michael J. Moore, M.D.
Fellow, Royal College of Physicians (Canada) in Neurology;
Consultant Neurologist, Massachusetts Multiple Sclerosis Society;
Associate Professor of Neurology,
Boston University School of Medicine,
Boston, Massachusetts

Albert B. Sabin, M.D.
Emeritus Distinguished Professor of Research Pediatrics,
University of Cincinnati;
Emeritus Distinguished Research Professor of Biomedicine,
Medical University of South Carolina College of Medicine;
Senior Expert Consultant, Fogarty International Center for
Advanced Study in Health Sciences,
National Institutes of Health,
Bethesda, Maryland

Thomas D. Sabin, M.D.
Professor of Neurology and Psychiatry, Boston University School of Medicine;
Lecturer in Neurology, Harvard Medical School;
Lecturer in Neurology, Tufts University School of Medicine;
Director, Neurological Unit,
Boston City Hospital,
Boston, Massachusetts

R. Michael Scott, M.D.
Professor of Neurosurgery, Tufts University School of Medicine;
Senior Neurosurgeon,
New England Medical Center Hospitals,
Boston, Massachusetts

Ana Sotrel, M.D.
Assistant Professor of Neuropathology, Harvard Medical School;
Neuropathologist,
The Children's Hospital,
Boston, Massachusetts

Vincent P. Sweeney, M.D.
Professor of Medicine, Division of Neurology, University of
British Columbia Faculty of Medicine;
Consulting Neurologist,
Vancouver General Hospital,
Vancouver, British Columbia, Canada

Edward Tarlov, M.D.
Department of Neurosurgery,
Lahey Clinic Medical Center,
Burlington, Massachusetts

Barbara F. Westmoreland, M.D.
Professor of Neurology, Mayo Medical School;
Section of Electroencephalography, Department of Neurology, Mayo Clinic,
Rochester, Minnesota

Contents

Some of the illustrations in this volume originally appeared in CIBA CLINICAL SYMPOSIA issues. We wish to acknowledge the original authors' contribution in the development of these illustrations.

Section	Plates	Adapted from Volume:
II	1-4	33/2, Headaches
III	3, 6-7,	26/4, Aortocranial Occlusive
	10	Vascular Disease (Stroke)
	30-36	29/4, Congenital Traumatic Aneurysms
IV	1-2, 5,	35/4, Head Injuries
	8-9, 11,	
	15-16	
	3, 12-13	18/3, The Pathophysiology of Head Injuries
	4, 7	19/1, The Treatment of Head Injuries

Section	Plates	Adapted from Volume:
IV	14	29/4, Congenital Traumatic Aneurysms
	17, 21,	34/2, Comprehensive Management of
	25	Spinal Cord Injury
	18-20,	32/1, Acute Cervical Spine Injury
	22-23,	
VI	1-6	9/5, Treatment of the Office Neurotic
X	1-2	34/2, Comprehensive Management of
		Spinal Cord Injury
	5, 14-17	32/6, Low Back Pain

Section I

Primary Neurologic Disorders in Infancy and Childhood

Frank H. Netter, M.D.

in collaboration with

Michael J. Bresnan, M.D.   *Plates 1–5, 10, 12, 16, 23*

Michael J. Bresnan, M.D. and H. Royden Jones, Jr., M.D.   *Plates 11, 18*

Marc A. Flitter, M.D.   *Plates 6–9*

H. Royden Jones, Jr., M.D.   *Plates 13–15, 17*

Thomas L. Kemper, M.D.   *Plates 19–20*

Irma M. Lessell, M.D.   *Plate 24*

R. Michael Scott, M.D.   *Plates 21–22*

Craniosynostoses

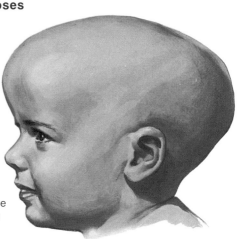

Acrocephaly: premature closure of coronal and lambdoid sutures

Scaphocephaly: premature closure of sagittal suture

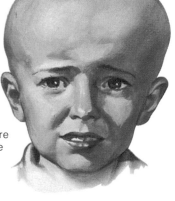

Brachycephalia: bilateral premature closure of coronal suture

Craniosynostoses

Craniosynostosis implies a premature closure of one or more cranial sutures. This abnormality occurs in one of every 2,000 infants, with a predominance in males. Normally, the metopic, or frontal, suture closes before birth; the posterior fontanelle, at the union of the lambdoid and sagittal sutures, by 3 months; and the anterior fontanelle, at the junction of the coronal, sagittal and metopic sutures, by 18 months. After a suture is fused, growth occurs parallel to that suture; ie, growth is inhibited at 90° to the suture. The fusion itself is felt as a ridge. Cranial sutures cannot be separated by increased intracranial pressure after 12 years of age.

The most common premature closure occurs in the *sagittal suture*, which leads to *scaphocephaly, dolichocephaly,* or elongated head. The next most common premature closure is in the *coronal suture,* which may be either unilateral or bilateral. If unilateral, it causes a unilateral ridge, with a pulling up of the orbit and a flattening of the frontal area on the affected side (anterior plagiocephaly), which produces a quizzical expression. If premature closure is bilateral, *brachycephalia,* manifested by an abnormally broad skull, is the result.

Closure of *all sutures*, with the associated facial anomalies of hypertelorism, proptosis and choanal atresia, is known as *craniofacial dysostosis*, or Crouzon's disease. This condition is inherited as an autosomal dominant trait, with variable expression. Intelligence is normal, but these premature total closures can interfere with brain growth, as well as with drainage of cerebrospinal fluid (CSF), which causes hydrocephalus.

In *acrocephalosyndactyly*, or Apert's syndrome, the head is elongated, the result of premature closure of all sutures; the orbits are shallow, causing exophthalmos; and either syndactyly or polydactyly is present. Inheritance is autosomal dominant, the first case usually representing a

Acrocephalosyndactyly (Apert's syndrome)

Microcephaly

spontaneous mutation, ie, the risk that the unaffected parents will have another affected child is negligible, while the risk that an affected person will pass on the defect is 50%. Saethre-Chotzen, Pfeiffer and Carpenter have also identified syndromes of acrocephalosyndactyly that include various combinations of synostosis, syndactyly and other anomalies.

Conditions that can be confused with craniosynostosis include *microcephaly*, secondary to decreased brain growth, and *plagiocephaly* (irregular skull shape). The latter is most often caused by a baby's being inactive and lying on one occipital area, which flattens (posterior plagiocephaly). A corresponding frontal predominance is usually

present. Both microcephaly and plagiocephaly may lead to secondary synostosis.

The diagnosis of these various conditions is confirmed by appropriate radiographic examinations.

Treatment for multiple synostoses is surgical, to prevent interference with brain growth and the possible development of increased intracranial pressure. Since single premature suture closures cause only cosmetic abnormalities, surgical correction is less urgent. However, the associated morbidity and mortality are so low, that surgical procedure is justified in most instances. The osteotomy must be extensive. Morcellation of the adjoining bones assures that the neural mass will mold the cranium into a normal shape. □

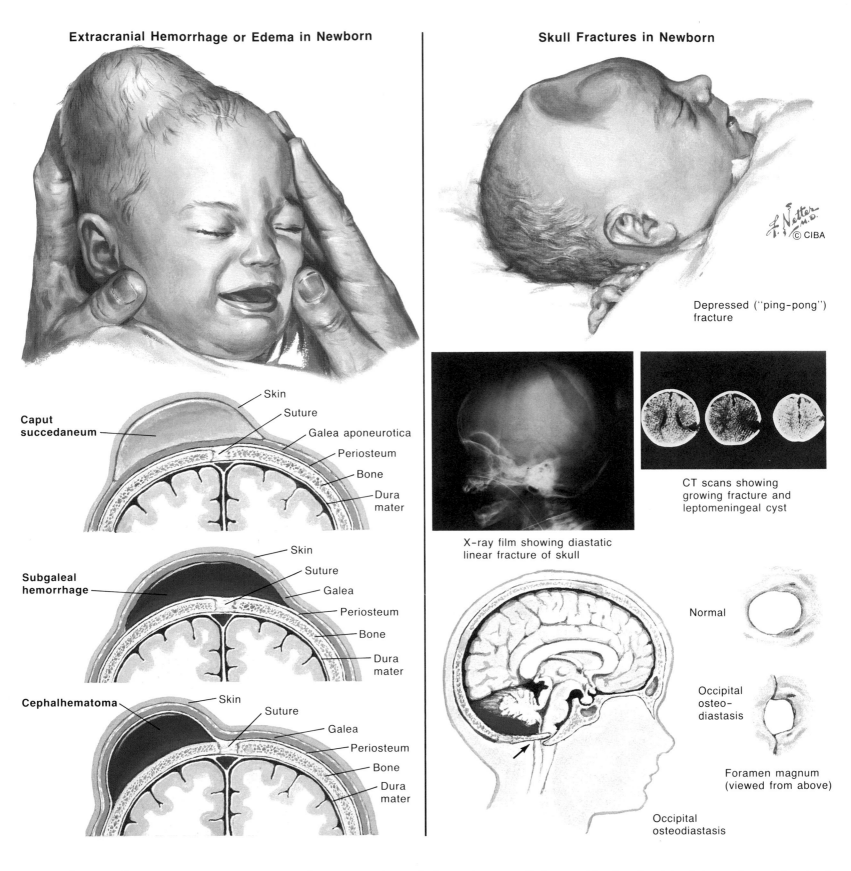

Extracranial Hemorrhage or Edema in Newborn

Caput succedaneum

- Skin
- Suture
- Galea aponeurotica
- Periosteum
- Bone
- Dura mater

Subgaleal hemorrhage

- Skin
- Suture
- Galea
- Periosteum
- Bone
- Dura mater

Cephalhematoma

- Skin
- Suture
- Galea
- Periosteum
- Bone
- Dura mater

Skull Fractures in Newborn

Depressed ("ping-pong") fracture

X-ray film showing diastatic linear fracture of skull

CT scans showing growing fracture and leptomeningeal cyst

Normal

Occipital osteo-diastasis

Foramen magnum (viewed from above)

Occipital osteodiastasis

SECTION I PLATE 2   *Slide 3305*

Extracranial Hemorrhage and Skull Fractures in Newborn

Modern obstetric practice has decreased the incidence of trauma to the neonate that is clearly associated with primiparity, large infant size, difficult or breech delivery and use of forceps.

Caput succedaneum, an edematous swelling that may be hemorrhagic, is seen in vaginal deliveries. It may transilluminate, is soft, pits, is usually at the vertex over suture lines, and resolves rapidly.

Subgaleal hemorrhage, which usually results from shearing forces tearing veins, occurs between the galea aponeurotica and the periosteum of the skull. It spreads widely, crosses suture lines, may dissect over the forehead and even into an orbit, and may take weeks to resolve. Blood loss may necessitate transfusion.

Cephalhematoma is a subperiosteal hemorrhage associated with a linear skull fracture in about 5% of cases. It may result from the use of forceps, can also be related to mechanical factors in the pelvis and the shearing forces of active labor, and palpates like a depressed fracture.

Skull Fractures. Neonatal skull fractures may be classified as linear, depressed or occipital osteodiastasis. *Linear fracture* may be associated with cephalhematoma or, in traumatic deliveries, with epidural and subdural hemorrhage. Most heal without complication. Rarely, they become diastatic and are associated with a leptomeningeal cyst due to associated dural and meningeal tears.

Depressed ("ping-pong") fractures are of little clinical significance. Most are associated with the use of forceps, but some are related to intrauterine trauma against pelvic prominences in automobile accidents and falls, and also in active labor. Treatment includes digital pressure, use of a vacuum extractor, or surgical elevation.

Occipital osteodiastasis is seen in breech deliveries. The associated dural sinuses may be ruptured, causing a subdural hemorrhage of the posterior fossa. Surgical drainage may be possible. □

Intracranial Hemorrhage in Newborn

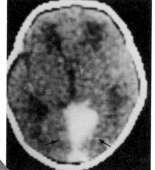

CT scan showing subdural hematoma due to tentorial tear

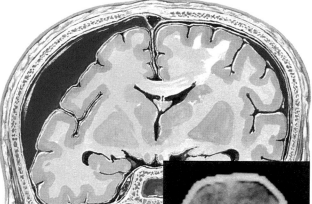

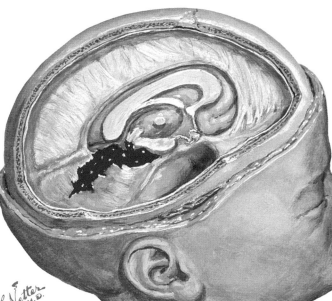

Tear of tentorium and great cerebral vein (of Galen), with massive subdural hemorrhage in posterior fossa

Large subdural hemorrhage over convexity of right cerebral hemisphere; subarachnoid hemorrhage on left side

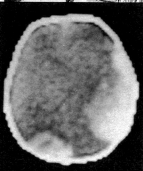

CT scan: subdural and subarachnoid hemorrhage

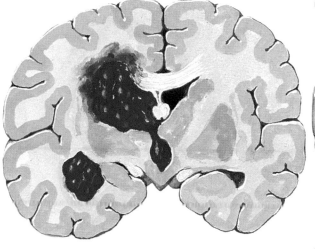

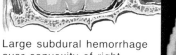

Periventricular-intraventricular hemorrhage filling and distending lateral and 3rd ventricles, passing through cerebral aqueduct (of Sylvius) into 4th ventricle, then via lateral and median apertures into cerebellomedullary cistern of posterior fossa

Unilateral periventricular-intraventricular hemorrhage originating in germinal center over head of caudate nucleus, distending frontal and temporal horns of lateral ventricle and passing through interventricular foramen (of Monro) into 3rd ventricle

Intracerebellar hemorrhage ruptured into 4th ventricle

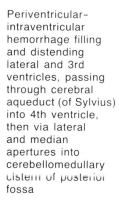

CT scan showing periventricular-intraventricular hemorrhage

SECTION I   PLATE 3   *Slide 3306*

Intracranial Hemorrhage in Newborn

Intracranial hemorrhage in the neonate is classified by location and in order of frequency as (1) periventricular-intraventricular, (2) subarachnoid, (3) subdural, or (4) posterior fossa hemorrhage.

Periventricular-intraventricular hemorrhage originates in the germinal matrix and occurs in up to 50% of infants born before 34 weeks' gestation. Other etiologic factors include asphyxia, endothelial factors, and the loose cellular structure and fibrinolytic activity of the matrix. Massive bleeding precipitates a bulging fontanelle, respiratory difficulties, tonic posturing, seizures, anemia and, ultimately, multisystem failure. Survival is possible if minor bleeding occurs, but hydrocephalus is a significant early problem and often requires shunting. Long-term structural deficits are common. In full-term babies, intraventricular hemorrhage can occur from the choroid plexus, with potential hydrocephalus.

Subarachnoid hemorrhage may be caused by asphyxia or by forces of normal delivery. In premature newborns, it is overshadowed by intraventricular hemorrhage. In full-term infants, it may be asymptomatic or associated with focal or generalized seizures, with no interictal symptoms.

Subdural hemorrhage results from tears in the falx cerebri and tentorium, rupture of bridging veins over the hemispheres, or occipital osteodiastasis in breech delivery. Causes include excessive molding forces during delivery, the infant's size and difficult extractions. Symptoms are acute or subacute hemiparesis, focal seizures and ipsilateral pupillary abnormalities. Surgical drainage is the appropriate treatment.

Posterior fossa hemorrhage can result from tentorial trauma or occipital osteodiastasis. Relatively minor bleeding causes brainstem compression, acute hydrocephalus, respiratory difficulties and seizures. Surgical drainage is occasionally possible. □

Brain Malformations

When neurologic maldevelopment is observed in an infant or child who has a normal postnatal history, knowledge of possible prenatal abnormalities and their cause is important. In prenatal encephalopathies, the time of onset predicts the type of maldevelopment. Injury during the first trimester interferes with the formation of the neural tube; during the second trimester, with neuronal proliferation and migration; and during the final trimester, with neuronal organization and myelination.

Defective Neural Tube Formation

The central nervous system (CNS) begins as a groove on the dorsal aspect of the embryo at 3 to 4 weeks. Interference with cranial closure results in either anencephaly or an encephalocele, and defective caudal closure, in meningomyelocele.

Onset of *anencephaly*, a fatal maldevelopment, is by the twenty-fourth day. The skull vault is absent, and the brain is a vascular mass. Ultrasound examination and an elevated α-fetoprotein level in maternal blood and amniotic fluid indicate the diagnosis prenatally. Risk of recurrence is 5%.

Although *encephalocele* usually occurs in the occipital region, it can develop frontally or in the nasal passages (Plate 4). The herniated brain tissue is connected through a narrow isthmus. There may be associated abnormalities of the cerebellum and midbrain. The Meckel-Gruber syndrome includes a posterior encephalocele, microcephaly, microphthalmus, cleft lip and palate, polydactyly and polycystic kidneys. This syndrome is inherited in an autosomal recessive manner, while for parents of a child with simple encephalocele, the risk of recurrence is 5%.

Computed tomography (CT) is particularly valuable in delineating the structural abnormality. All affected infants require neurosurgical intervention. The prognosis depends on the degree of CNS involvement, which may be difficult to assess in the neonate.

Meningomyelocele results from failure of caudal closure of the neural tube, with an 80% incidence in the lumbar region.

Ventral induction processes occur during the fifth and sixth weeks of gestation, and maldevelopments may also involve facial structures. The prosencephalon is cleaved to produce two hemispheres, ventricles and basal ganglia, as well as paired optic vesicles and olfactory tracts. The most common CNS malformation is *holoprosencephaly* (arrhinencephalia), characterized by a single ventricle, an absent olfactory system, hypoplastic optic nerves or even a single optic system. The corpus callosum is absent, and the cortex is malformed. Potential facial anomalies include a single eye (cyclops) and a single nasal protuberance (proboscis), but in less severe cases, defects include ocular hypotelorism, microphthalmus, a flat nose, and a median cleft lip and palate.

Ultrasound examination indicates the prenatal diagnosis, and CT scans can delineate the extent of the defects. Early death is predictable.

Chromosomal abnormalities (trisomy 13–15, trisomy 18) are present in 50% of cases, and genetic counseling is important.

Neuronal Proliferation and Migration

All neurons are derived from the subependymal regions of the developing CNS. Proliferation of neurons occurs between the second and fourth months, while migration peaks in the third through fifth months. By 26 weeks, the final complement of neurons is in place.

Defective Proliferation. A *decrease* in neuronal number may lead to *microcephaly* (microencephaly vera), whereas an *increase* may result in *megalencephaly*.

Prenatal influences, including familial factors, are paramount in each abnormality, especially in the latter. Microcephaly may be caused by irradiation or exposure to toxins, while megalencephaly may be associated with neurofibromatosis, achondroplasia or cerebral gigantism. Familial megalencephaly is the most common and most benign form and is usually inherited through the father. Excessive postnatal growth also occurs often, suggesting hydrocephalus. Measurements of the parental head circumference and CT scans showing normal ventricles aid in diagnosis. Approximately 70% of infants with microcephaly and 30% of those with megalencephaly have developmental defects.

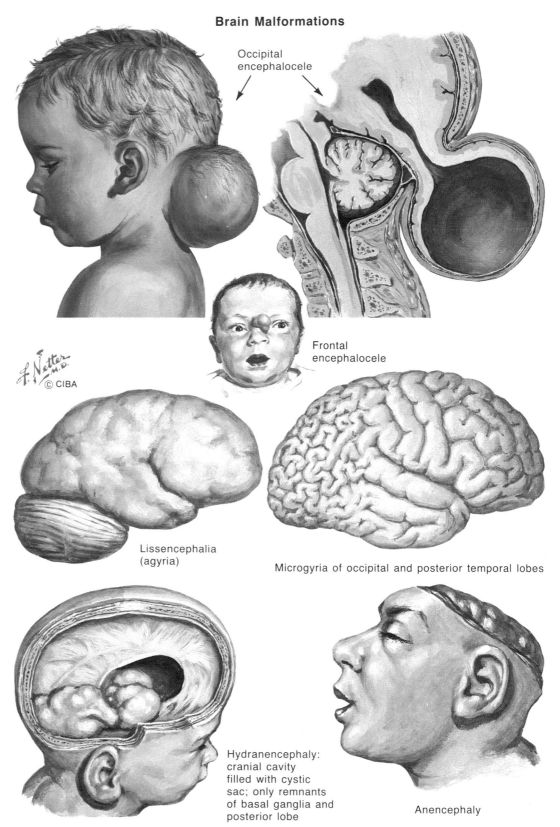

Brain Malformations

Occipital encephalocele

Frontal encephalocele

Lissencephalia (agyria)

Microgyria of occipital and posterior temporal lobes

Hydranencephaly: cranial cavity filled with cystic sac; only remnants of basal ganglia and posterior lobe

Anencephaly

Brain Malformations
(Continued)

Defective Migration. After proliferation in the subependymal region, neurons migrate to the cortex. The neurons appear to follow radial glial cells like raindrops on telephone wires. Early migrations form the deepest cortical layers, and later migrations, the more superficial layers, ultimately forming a six-layer cortex.

The cellular complement is greatest in the outer cortical layers, leading to an increased surface area, with buckling causing gyri to begin to appear between 26 and 28 weeks, and become increasingly complex in the final trimester. If the normal complement of neurons is absent, gyral formation does not take place, and *lissencephalia* (smooth brain, agyria) results.

An abnormally thick gyral formation is known as *pachygyria*. In this anomaly, the cortex lacks the six-layer configuration.

The presence of multiple small gyri having no resemblance to a normal gyral pattern, along with deranged lamination of the cortical mantle, is called *polymicrogyria*.

Schizencephaly is characterized by an abnormal cleft that joins the cortex and the ventricles. It is usually bilateral but can be unilateral. Malformed gyri (polymicrogyria) are aligned radially around the cleft.

Agenesis of the corpus callosum, partial or complete, is often accompanied by disorders stemming from defective neuronal migration. This results in developmental defects, seizures, mental retardation and occasional hydrocephalus (Plate 5). The diagnosis may be suggested by ocular hypertelorism, an antimongoloid slant to the eyes, and other midline facial defects. Aicardi's syndrome, a sporadically occurring abnormality seen in female infants, is associated with retinal defects that suggest chorioretinitis, infantile spasms, hypsarrhythmia and severe psychomotor retardation. Agenesis is one of the most common anomalies diagnosed by CT in "idiopathic" psychomotor retardation.

Cerebral *heterotopias* appear to result from defective neuronal migration and subsequent accumulation of aberrant neurons anywhere between the ependyma and cortex. Significant numbers of such heterotopias occurring in isolation are likely to result in some degree of mental retardation. Most of the disorders of migration discussed previously have associated heterotopias.

A "normal" CT scan does not rule out localized gyral malformations or, most important, significant defects of the cortical layers and heterotopias of neurons.

Defective Neuronal Organization

After the neurons have arrived in the cortex, they are aligned and oriented; interneuronal contacts (dendritic and axonal) are elaborated, synapses proliferate, and the glial support system develops. This process begins at 6 months' gestation and continues into the second decade or later.

Although circumstances of birth, especially premature birth, and the neonatal period can interfere with this organizational process, it is also

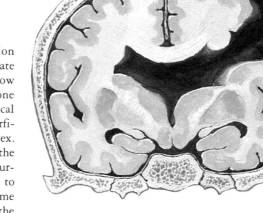

Porencephaly, with absence of septum pellucidum and thinning of overlying skull

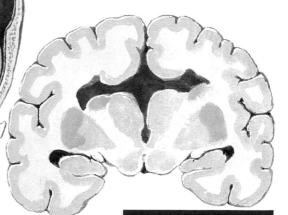

Agenesis of corpus callosum: ventricles may communicate with longitudinal fissure

CT scan showing agenesis of corpus callosum

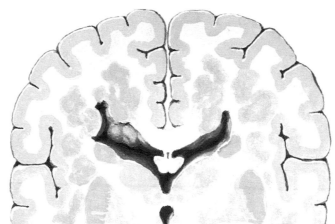

Heterotopic gray matter: islands of gray matter within white matter in centrum ovale; in subependymal area, with projections into ventricles; and in insular regions

Perinatal telencephalic leukoencephalopathy: scarcity of white matter, with resultant enlargement of ventricles

likely that intrauterine influences during the last trimester, some known (rubella, trisomy 21, phenylketonuria and inadequate nutrition) but most unknown, can result in a nonspecific syndrome of mental retardation with or without seizures. Disorders of synaptogenesis are defined only with the aid of microscopic studies using Golgi techniques. No in vivo tests are diagnostic.

In the rare disorder *hydranencephaly*, the cerebral hemispheres are replaced by membranous sacs filled with cerebrospinal fluid (CSF). The occipital and temporal lobes and basal ganglia are relatively preserved, although abnormal. The most probable cause, bilateral interference with carotid blood flow, is always an intrauterine event.

Affected infants may look remarkably normal at birth. Transillumination is dramatic, and CT scans confirm the diagnosis. Hydrocephalus may be superimposed, and is usually secondary to aqueductal stenosis.

Porencephaly is characterized by cystic spaces in brain parenchyma that can communicate with a ventricle or the subarachnoid space. They are most common in the distribution of the middle cerebral artery. The cysts are caused by intrauterine vascular accidents or perinatal events, and produce hemiplegia with or without seizures. A bulge in the skull and an area of transillumination may be present. Rarely, surgical drainage is required. □

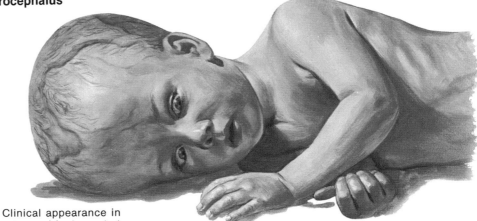

Clinical appearance in
advanced hydrocephalus

Hydrocephalus

Hydrocephalus, characterized by enlarged ventricles of the brain, can result either from increased production or decreased absorption of cerebrospinal fluid (CSF) or from blockage of one of the normal outflow pathways of the ventricular system. The most common forms of hydrocephalus occur in infants. Because cranial sutures are not yet fused, head size increases progressively; thus, periodic measurement of the skull's circumference to detect such enlargement is important in neonatal and infant care (Plate 7).

Most cases of hydrocephalus result from congenital stenosis of the cerebral aqueduct (of Sylvius), which obstructs CSF drainage from the lateral and third ventricles—*obstructive hydrocephalus*. A brainstem tumor or a posterior fossa tumor encroaching on the fourth ventricle and obstructing the lateral aperture (of Luschka) or the median aperture (of Magendie) can produce the same situation. Another type of hydrocephalus may occur after intraventricular hemorrhage in premature infants. In these patients, the presence of blood breakdown products in the CSF interferes with the normal rate of CSF absorption, producing a form of *communicating hydrocephalus*.

In advanced infantile hydrocephalus, scalp veins are distended because venous drainage from the scalp is impaired as a result of elevated intracranial pressure. The downward deviation of the eyes, referred to as "sunset eyes," probably results from pressure transmitted to the midbrain by the dilatation of the posterior part of the third ventricle, which produces the paralysis of upward gaze, or *Parinaud's syndrome*, seen with lesions affecting the region at the superior colliculi. An affected infant appears emaciated, characterizing the poor feeding and recurrent vomiting that accompanies elevated intracranial pressure.

The coronal brain section shown in the illustration indicates that the hydrocephalus in this instance is caused either by obstruction of an outflow pathway distal to the third ventricle or is a form of communicating hydrocephalus, in which case the fourth ventricle would also be dilated. Differential diagnosis is made by computed tomography (CT).

Obstructive hydrocephalus frequently occurs in adults with brain tumors that impinge on the ventricular structures discussed above. In addition, communicating hydrocephalus with elevated intracranial pressure may follow an intracranial hemorrhage or an infection that causes blockage of CSF absorption pathways, as is

**Potential lesion sites in
obstructive hydrocephalus**

1 Interventricular foramina (of Monro)
2 Cerebral aqueduct (of Sylvius)
3 Lateral apertures (of Luschka)
4 Median aperture (of Magendie)

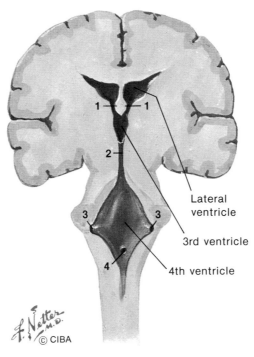

Lateral ventricle
3rd ventricle
4th ventricle

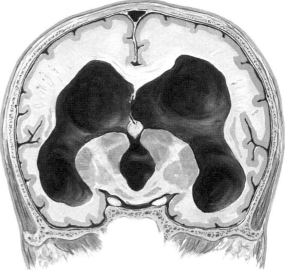

Section through brain showing marked
dilatation of lateral and 3rd ventricles

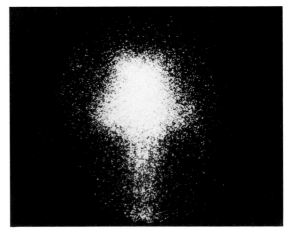

Cisternogram: 48-hour scan demonstrating
persistent ventricular penetration of isotope

the case in infants. Clinically, patients with obstructive hydrocephalus are somnolent and have headache and other features of elevated intracranial pressure (see Section IV, Plate 10).

Normal-pressure hydrocephalus is a well-described syndrome in adults that is not associated with an obvious increase in intracranial pressure. Initial symptoms are progressive dementia, gait disorders and urinary incontinence. The CT scan shows ventricular dilatation, and the condition must be differentiated from ventricular dilatation secondary to brain atrophy, which does not respond to treatment by CSF shunting.

To trace the CSF circulation within the ventricular system, an isotope cisternogram is carried out. After a suitable isotope has been injected into the subarachnoid space via a lumbar puncture, serial brain scans are made over 2 to 3 days to monitor the flow of the labeled CSF. Normally, the CSF ascends in the spinal canal, diffuses from the basilar cisterns over the convexities of the cerebral hemispheres, and is absorbed by the arachnoid granulations. In patients with normal-pressure hydrocephalus, the isotope is retained within the ventricular system, and absorption of that component of the isotope that circulates over the convexities is delayed. In many of these patients, symptoms have improved or reversed following the insertion of a CSF shunt (Plate 7). □

Slide 3310

Shunt Procedure for Hydrocephalus

Shunt Procedure for Hydrocephalus

Cannula inserted into anterior horn of lateral ventricle through trephine hole in skull

Reservoir at end of cannula implanted beneath galea permits transcutaneous needle puncture for withdrawal of CSF or introduction of antibiotic medication or dye to test patency of shunt

One-way, pressure-regulated valve placed subcutaneously to prevent reflux of blood or peritoneal fluid and control CSF pressure

Drainage tube may be introduced into internal jugular vein and thence into right atrium via neck incision, or may be continued subcutaneously to abdomen

Drainage tube is most often introduced into peritoneal cavity, with extra length to allow for growth of child

Head measurement is of value in diagnosis, especially in early cases, and serial measurements will indicate progression or arrest of hydrocephalus

The treatment of hydrocephalus depends on the cause of the ventricular dilatation. When hydrocephalus is caused by an overproduction of cerebrospinal fluid (CSF), such as from a choroid plexus papilloma or secondary to a tumor blocking CSF outflow pathways, removal of the tumor may suffice. However, a significant number of patients with communicating or obstructive hydrocephalus require a diversionary, or shunt, procedure to compensate for the underlying deficit. Successful shunting operations can halt progressive ventricular dilatation and the consequent elevation of intracranial pressure, and can frequently lead to a reversal of the patient's neurologic deficit.

For *communicating hydrocephalus*, the shunt device can originate anywhere in the subarachnoid space or ventricular system, because diversion of fluid from either cavity decompresses all the remaining central nervous system (CNS) regions containing CSF. For *obstructive hydrocephalus*, the origin of the shunt depends on the location of the obstructing lesion. Most shunting operations involve placing a tube or ventricular catheter in the anterior horn of the lateral ventricle. The intraventricular catheter is connected via a subcutaneous tube to either the right atrium of the heart or to the peritoneal cavity.

Both atrial and peritoneal shunts share several basic design characteristics. The tubing is constructed from inert Silastic material, and the various connecting parts are made of nonreactive metal. To control the rate of CSF drainage, the system has a pressure-regulating valve, which is usually located underneath the scalp or in the subcutaneous portion of the shunt just behind and below the ear. (If the CSF flow rate is not regulated, the ventricle could collapse, which would lead to an enlargement of the subdural spaces and dangerous traction on the bridging veins to the dural sinuses. Eventually, these veins would tear, producing subdural hematomas.) In addition, the valve permits flow in one direction only, to prevent reflux of blood or CSF into the ventricular system.

Occasionally, it is necessary to obtain CSF from the ventricle of a patient who is fitted with a shunt or to inject antibiotics into the ventricular system; therefore, most shunt systems now include a reservoir located proximal to the pressure-regulating valve. If necessary, contrast material may also be injected via this route to outline a malfunctioning shunt.

The long-term success of a shunt used to control a hydrocephalic condition depends on the continuing patency of the distal portion of the shunt, namely, the atrial or peritoneal catheter; thus, correct placement of these catheters is essential. Access to the right atrium is gained by introducing the distal catheter into the facial vein as it joins the internal jugular vein in the neck, beneath the angle of the jaw. The appropriate length of catheter to be threaded into the atrium can be determined by radiographic guidance.

Since a ventricular-atrial shunt terminates in the bloodstream, it is important to realize that it is exposed to any transient bacteremia and septicemia and is a potential source of infection.

The peritoneal catheter drains the CSF into the peritoneal cavity, from where it is subsequently absorbed into the vascular system. Use of this type of shunt substantially reduces the risk of blood-borne infections. In addition, several excess centimeters of catheter can be placed in the peritoneal cavity at the time of surgery, permitting gradual withdrawal of the tubing during growth periods in infants and children. This type of shunt decreases or completely obviates the need for elective or emergency shunt revisions. □

Spina bifida occulta

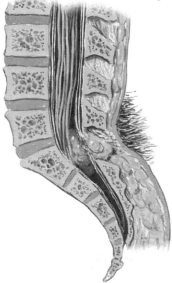

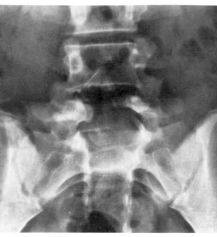

X-ray film showing deficit of lamina of sacrum (spina bifida occulta)

Dermal sinus

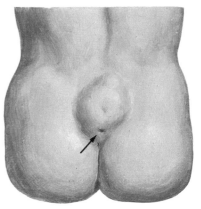

Dural sac

Cauda equina

Sinus with squamous plug

Fat pad overlying spina bifida occulta. Tuft of hair or only skin dimple may be present, or there may be no external manifestation. Dermal sinus also present in this case (arrow)

Types of spina bifida aperta with protrusion of spinal contents

Meningocele

Meningomyelocele

Spina bifida with central cicatrix

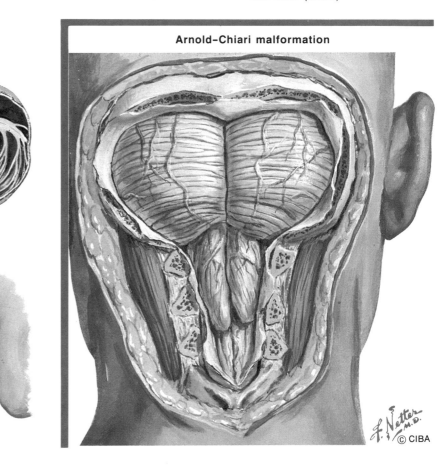

Arnold-Chiari malformation

f. Netter M.D. © CIBA

Slide 3311

Spinal Dysraphism

Several clinical conditions characterized by congenital failure of fusion of the midline structures of the spinal column are grouped under the general classification "spinal dysraphism." These various manifestations of the dysraphic state span a clinical continuum from asymptomatic and unseen bony abnormalities (spina bifida occulta), through cutaneous lesions of little more than cosmetic importance (subcutaneous lipomas or angiomas), to the most severe and disabling congenital malformations of the spinal structures (meningomyelocele). Frequently, a patient may have more than one of these related congenital anomalies. In such a case, the physician who is aware of the various manifestations of spinal dysraphism can reach a timely diagnosis and may prevent permanent damage.

Spina Bifida Occulta

The more benign forms of spinal dysraphism include occult bony abnormalities unaccompanied by any displacement of spinal canal contents and with or without cutaneous stigmata. In these cases, there is failure of bony fusion between the two laminae of the involved vertebra (Plate 8).

Spina bifida occulta is of no clinical significance when it occurs alone, although its serendipitous detection on x-ray films of the spine should alert the physician to the possibility of coexisting and potentially harmful conditions.

If spina bifida occulta occurs in conjunction with a dermal sinus (an epithelium-lined tract linking the dural sac with the skin surface), there is a potential for communication between the skin and intraspinal contents. Accordingly, sinus tracts located anywhere along the posterior midline should not be probed because of the danger of provoking meningitis. Dermal sinuses located above the sacrococcygeal region should be removed surgically. Cutaneous stigmata of spina bifida occulta may be absent or may include subcutaneous lipomas, tufts of hair or angiomas.

Spinal Dysraphism (continued)

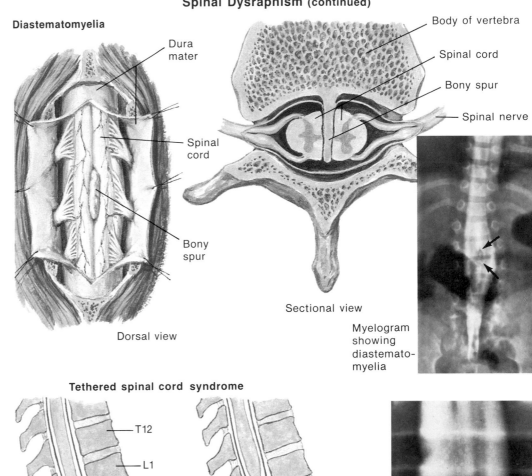

Diastematomyelia

Dura mater

Spinal cord

Bony spur

Dorsal view

Body of vertebra

Spinal cord

Bony spur

Spinal nerve

Sectional view

Myelogram showing diastematomyelia

Spinal Dysraphism

(Continued)

Spina Bifida Aperta

Dysraphic conditions in which there are overt manifestations of the underlying bony defect are referred to as "spina bifida aperta" (Plate 8). Within this group, the progression of neurologic sequelae is defined to a large extent by the degree to which the contents of the spinal canal are displaced from their normal location. In the case of a *meningocele*, the most benign form of spina bifida aperta, a meningeal cyst free of neural elements constitutes the extruded tissue. Often, a meningocele can be completely removed surgically and the defect closed by a dural graft, followed by closure of fascia and skin.

A far more devastating variant of spina bifida aperta is *meningomyelocele*, in which the spinal cord or nerve roots, or both, protrude through the posterior bony and cutaneous defects. These meningomyeloceles exact a neurologic toll based in large measure on their location along the spinal canal. Dysfunction is increasingly severe with lesions occurring progressively superior to the level of the sacrum. The neonate with this obvious congenital anomaly, which consists of a posterior midline mass with a thin cicatricial membrane covering the neural structures, requires prolonged and extensive multidisciplinary support.

Lesions in the lumbosacral region and higher produce paraplegia, with loss of bowel and bladder control. In addition, hydrocephalus develops in approximately 90% of these infants, necessitating the insertion and maintenance of a shunt device (Plate 7). The hydrocephalus is related to the presence of an accompanying congenital deformity of the hindbrain, referred to as the *Arnold-Chiari malformation*, in which the posterior fossa structures are displaced into the cervical spinal canal and interfere with the pathways of cerebrospinal fluid (CSF) circulation and absorption.

Other Dysraphic Conditions

Two other conditions related to the dysraphic state merit particular attention because they may be undetected for one or more decades until insidious but progressive neurologic dysfunction leads to their discovery. Both diastematomyelia and the tethered spinal cord syndrome may occur

Tethered spinal cord syndrome

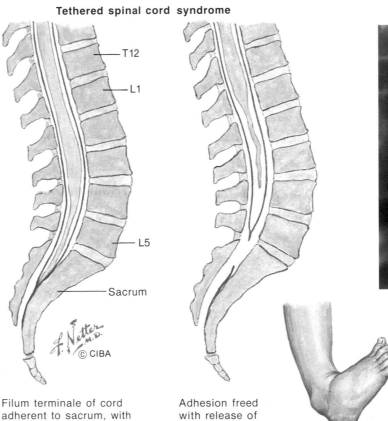

T12

L1

L5

Sacrum

Filum terminale of cord adherent to sacrum, with tension on spinal cord

Adhesion freed with release of cord tension

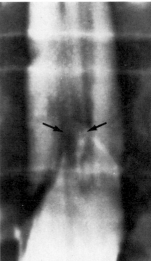

Myelogram showing tethered spinal cord

Clinical manifestations of spinal dysraphism may include foot deformity or progressive sphincter disturbances

in patients who may or may not have cutaneous or radiographic signs of dysraphism.

Diastematomyelia is a congenital malformation in which the spinal cord is split into two sections, or hemicords (Plate 9). Frequently, a bony or cartilaginous septum separates the divided sections. Although this anomaly can be asymptomatic, associated scoliosis or progressive myelopathy characterized by an unusual gait disorder and bowel and bladder dysfunction may develop. Surgical excision of the midline septum can halt the deteriorating condition and, in some cases, lead to restored function.

The *tethered spinal cord syndrome* occurs when a hypertrophied filum terminale adheres to the

sacrum, causing progressive traction and inferior displacement of the conus medullaris as the spine grows. This traction can produce progressive ischemia in the conus medullaris and, in previously normal individuals, lead to symptoms of gait disorders, sphincter dysfunction or torsion deformities of the feet. The tethered spinal cord syndrome can be diagnosed by myelographic demonstration of an abnormally low conus medullaris. Surgical section of the filum terminale allows immediate ascent of the conus medullaris toward a more normal location within the spinal canal, which in turn leads to improved perfusion of the neural tissue, and often, to a relief of the symptoms. □

Cerebral Palsy

The term "cerebral palsy" has been used historically to describe a static, nonprogressive motor disability present from birth and possibly caused by perinatal cerebral injuries of both hypoxic and traumatic origin. Currently, this term is often used more broadly to include other nonprogressive motor disabilities acquired in infancy and early childhood. Cerebral palsy is more accurately a descriptive and administrative diagnosis than an etiologic diagnosis, and is a useful term for par-

ents to whom "static encephalopathy" has little meaning. Although the disease may be manifested by either motor or mental defects, both disorders are frequently present. Included in the spectrum of associated handicaps are epilepsy, visual and hearing difficulties and progressive orthopedic deformities.

Many cases of cerebral palsy are related to birth trauma (Plates 2–3), but a much more significant number can be described as hypoxic-ischemic encephalopathy. This combination of low oxygen and low blood flow is particularly damaging to the brain, which has high energy requirements and low energy reserves.

The Apgar score in infants affected with hypoxic-ischemic encephalopathy, both full-term and premature, is frequently low, and resuscitation to overcome asphyxia is often necessary. With successful resuscitation, there may be a brief (12-hour) period of stupor and hypotonia before seizures and apnea supervene. The infant must be placed in a neonatal intensive care unit, so that acidosis, hypoxia, other organ failure, cerebral edema and seizures can be monitored and treated.

Cerebral Lesions

Five major cerebral lesions result from hypoxic-ischemic encephalopathy: (1) neuronal necrosis, (2) status marmoratus, (3) watershed infarcts, (4) periventricular telencephalic leukoencephalopathy, and (5) focal ischemic lesions. While these lesions describe the neuropathologic findings in the neonate, some of them (particularly neuronal necrosis and watershed infarcts) may underlie damage to the central nervous system (CNS) in the first few months of life that is secondary to infection, trauma or vascular diseases.

The various dysgeneses and migrational disorders of the developing brain also cause CNS damage and are an important cause of cerebral palsy.

Neuronal Necrosis. Hypoxia damages neurons in the cortex, hippocampus, cerebellum, thalamus, basal ganglia and brainstem. The long-term sequelae are spastic hemiplegia or quadriplegia, with associated mental retardation and seizures.

Status Marmoratus. This lesion affects the basal ganglia (caudate nucleus, putamen, globus pallidus and the thalamus), which are shrunken and have a whitish, marblelike appearance representing foci of nerve cell loss and gliosis, with abnormal condensation of myelinated fibers. Affected infants are most often full-term. Clinical features of status marmoratus include initial hypotonia of the "central" type (Plate 12), with subsequent development of rigidity (spastic quadriparesis) and choreoathetosis.

Watershed Infarcts. In the presence of hypotension, regions most distant from the heart receive the least amount of blood; therefore, watershed infarcts begin at the confluence of the middle, anterior and posterior cerebral arteries in the posterior parietooccipital area and spread anteriorly and posteriorly in a bucket-handle fashion. Lesions can be unilateral or bilaterally symmetric or asymmetric, probably secondary to asymmetries in the circle of Willis and related to available collateral vessels. Watershed infarcts are most common in full-term infants. The clinical result can be diplegia or hemiplegia.

Perinatal Telencephalic Leukoencephalopathy. This lesion is most common in premature infants and is most easily seen close to the lateral

angles of the ventricles in the centrum ovale, where it can interrupt nerve fibers supplying the leg and also the acoustic and optic radiations. Minor lesions may lead to a paucity of white matter, visible as "atrophy," while more severe lesions appear as cystic spaces on computed tomography (CT). Minor lesions could be the source of learning disabilities, while more severe lesions may cause diplegia.

Focal Ischemic Lesions. These lesions are rather large and occur in the beds of specific blood vessels, most often the middle cerebral artery. Probable causes are hypoxic-ischemic events, emboli and thromboses. Typically, focal ischemic lesions cause hemiplegia, with the arm more affected than the leg or face. Seizures may also occur. The large area of damage is likely to become cavitated and develop into a porencephalic cyst, which may or may not communicate with the ventricle. Occasionally, a noncommunicating cyst enlarges and causes a mass effect that requires surgical drainage.

Clinical Manifestations

Hemiplegia. This condition is rarely diagnosed at birth. When the parents note that the infant has a hand preference at about 3 months of age, a brachial plexus injury may be suspected because the limb is hypotonic and deep tendon reflexes may not be brisk. Careful neurologic examination, however, reveals similar, more subtle difficulties in the leg and face. Subsequently, the development of spasticity, with persistent fisting and flexion deformity of the upper extremity, and a tendency toward talipes equinovarus become more evident. Cortical sensory loss (astereognosis, or inability to recognize the size, texture or shape of objects) and hemianopsia may be present.

Quadriplegia. The form of cerebral palsy characterized by quadriplegia is the most severe from the aspect of associated defects, ie, pseudobulbar palsy, mental retardation and epilepsy. Although spasticity is usually evident early in the course, occasionally, hypotonia is present initially, with subsequent development of spasticity. When hypoxic or traumatic perinatal cerebral injuries have not occurred, this clinical picture may result from developmental abnormalities of the brain, either gross (agenesis of the corpus callosum, lissencephalia, pachygyria, schizencephaly) or microscopic (disorders of cortical lamination).

Diplegia. In a child with this condition, the legs are dramatically more affected than the arms. The legs are usually spastic, but hypotonia is seen occasionally. When spasticity is present, the legs are stiff and scissoring. Instead of stepping when supported, the child may "bunny hop" with both legs. He may stand early and "too well" when supported. Typically, paraplegia is present, and orthopedic procedures, crutches and braces are necessary to enable the child to walk. The prognosis is better in the atonic than in the spastic type of diplegia. The child with atonia often has good function of the trunk and upper extremities, but is reluctant to bear weight. In both types, deep tendon reflexes are brisk and bilateral Babinski responses are present.

Ataxia. Cerebral palsy characterized by ataxia is the rarest form of the disease. Either hypotonia (floppy baby syndrome) or mild spasticity may be associated clinical findings, depending on the other systems involved. Other causes of ataxia in

Cerebral Palsy

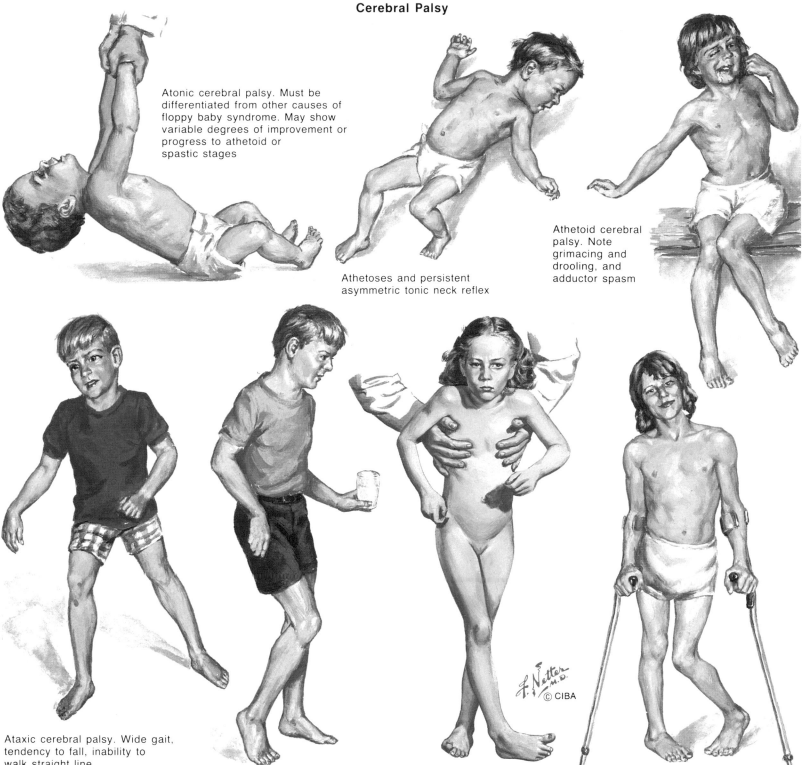

Atonic cerebral palsy. Must be differentiated from other causes of floppy baby syndrome. May show variable degrees of improvement or progress to athetoid or spastic stages

Athetoses and persistent asymmetric tonic neck reflex

Athetoid cerebral palsy. Note grimacing and drooling, and adductor spasm

Ataxic cerebral palsy. Wide gait, tendency to fall, inability to walk straight line

Hemiplegia on right side. Hip and knee contractures and talipes equinus. Astereognosis may be present

Spastic quadriplegia. Characteristic "scissors" position of lower limbs due to adductor spasm

Diplegia (lower limbs more affected). Contractures of hips and knees and talipes equinovarus (clubfoot)

infancy and childhood, including hydrocephalus, neoplasms and degenerative disorders, should be ruled out before cerebral palsy (nonprogressive encephalopathy) is diagnosed.

Athetosis. With the current treatment of Rh and ABO incompatibility, the incidence of cerebral palsy characterized by athetosis has markedly decreased. However, cases are still seen as a result of hypoxic-ischemic encephalopathy (asphyxia). The affected infant is initially hypotonic, but a tendency toward arching and opisthotonus (dystonia) is noted, and obligatory tonic neck reflexes are present. These primitive motor patterns preclude orderly motor development such as reaching, rolling and sitting.

Toward the end of the first year, involuntary movements become more consistent with the full-blown picture of choreoathetoid cerebral palsy. A degree of spasticity is often present. Speech may be markedly delayed, even when receptive skills and mentation are normally preserved. The child must be carefully examined for the presence of deafness, and means of nonverbal communication must be explored.

Treatment

Although nonprogressive in the sense of deterioration, cerebral palsy is clearly not static in its evolution. In any single child, several different types of the condition may be present. Thus,

evaluation and treatment of all the ramifications of cerebral palsy demand a multidisciplinary approach, with participation of the pediatrician, neurologist, physical therapist, orthopedist, speech therapist and psychologist.

The most important treatment is intensive physical therapy directed toward correcting the abnormal postures. Various orthopedic procedures to correct the musculoskeletal deformities caused by the spastic components of the disease are also important.

(A comprehensive discussion of the treatment and management of cerebral palsy will appear in the CIBA COLLECTION, Volume 8/II, "Musculoskeletal System," to be published.) □

Hypotonia

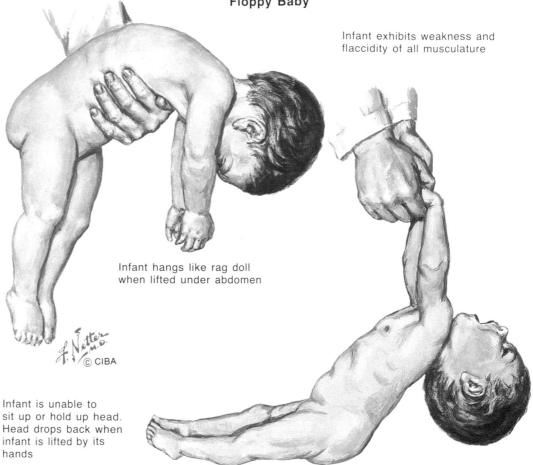

Floppy Baby

Infant exhibits weakness and flaccidity of all musculature

Infant hangs like rag doll when lifted under abdomen

Infant is unable to sit up or hold up head. Head drops back when infant is lifted by its hands

Hypotonia, a clinical sign of neurologic problems in the infant, is manifested by hyperextensibility and abnormal postures of the joints, poor fixation of the upper extremities and head lag on traction; an inverted U position on ventral suspension; and absence of positive supporting, stepping or placing reactions (Plate 11).

Fundamental to the diagnosis of the underlying disorder is whether or not muscle weakness coexists with hypotonia. Muscle weakness implies an involvement of the peripheral nervous system. Although the presence of brisk reflexes and a positive Babinski sign clearly indicate an involvement of the central nervous system (CNS), the absence of reflexes is much less specific.

In the older child, the absence of reflexes is invariably diagnostic of anterior horn cell or peripheral nerve disease, but in the infant, myopathies and CNS diseases can be associated with an absence of reflexes. Fasciculations in the tongue and a tremor of the fingers may be equally important indications of anterior horn cell disease. Facial nerve palsy or oculomotor nerve palsy suggests neuromuscular disease, including congenital myotonic dystrophy, centronuclear myopathy, infantile facioscapulohumeral muscular dystrophy, congenital muscular dystrophy, congenital myasthenia gravis or mitochondrial myopathies, although many CNS abnormalities are associated with esotropia or exotropia.

Neurodiagnostic techniques such as electromyography and nerve conduction velocity studies, muscle biopsy, electroencephalography, and computed tomography (CT), used in conjunction with general metabolic studies, have allowed a more accurate classification of the etiologic factors involved in hypotonia. The modern clinical and laboratory approach to the hypotonic infant emphasizes localization of the lesion by every available means. The many anatomic sites that can be involved in hypotonia, the causative disorders at each site, and the probable clinical signs are shown in Plate 12.

Causative Disorders

Central Nervous System Disorders. Damage to a normally formed brain, eg, *hypoxic-ischemic encephalopathy*, is the cause of the majority of cases of atonic cerebral palsy (Plate 10).

Malformations of the brain (dysgenesis) that occur during the first trimester, eg, agenesis of the corpus callosum, cause easily recognizable defects (Plate 5). Malformations occurring in the second trimester are more subtle and include lissencephalia, or areas with no cortical gyral formation, and associated abnormalities of cortical

---

Muscle biopsy specimens in different cases

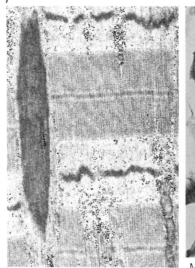

Electron micrograph showing nemaline body continuous with Z band (× 30,000)

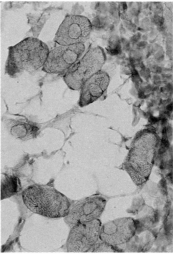

Muscle fibers with well–defined "cores." Muscle is largely replaced by adipose tissue (PAS stain)

Large number of small fibers with abnormally located central nuclei (trichrome stain)

---

lamination (Plate 4). Chromosomal anomalies such as trisomy 13 or Down's syndrome (trisomy 21) can be present.

Degenerative disorders may become apparent after a period of normal development. Abnormalities of both gray and white matter (the latter especially if peripheral myelin is affected) can cause initial hypotonia, as seen in Tay-Sachs disease (GM$_2$) and Krabbe's disease, respectively.

Spinal Cord Disorders. *Transection* of the spinal cord, most often associated with breech delivery, leaves an infant hypotonic for a long period. Spinal shock can initially be involved, but early injury that interferes with the development of systems causing spasticity is a more probable cause.

In spinal cord *maldevelopment*, such as occult spinal dysraphic defects, hypotonia is usually limited to the trunk and lower extremities. Vertebral anomalies are always associated with these disorders.

Anterior Horn Cell Disease. Infants affected with *Werdnig-Hoffmann disease* (infantile spinal muscular atrophy) are areflexic and hypotonic, have fasciculating tongues, but are obviously bright and intelligent. The degree of motor deficit and survival vary with age of onset (see page 16 for a detailed discussion).

Glycogenosis type II (Pompe's disease) also affects anterior horn cells and muscle and produces hypotonia.

Hypotonia
(Continued)

Neuropathies. Along with disorders that cause demyelination in both the peripheral nervous system and the CNS, such as metachromatic leukodystrophy and Krabbe's disease, other conditions resulting in myelin and axonal degeneration and producing hypotonia are *hypertrophic neuropathies* (Déjerine-Sottas disease), hypomyelinative neuropathies, *familial dysautonomia* (Riley-Day syndrome), and *infantile neuroaxonal dystrophy*. Rarely, *polyneuritis* (Guillain-Barré syndrome) affects infants, causing hypotonia.

Neuromuscular Disorders. Botulism is an important acquired cause of hypotonia and *muscle weakness* in infants less than 6 months of age. Toxin absorbed from *Clostridium botulinum* in the gastrointestinal tract blocks the presynaptic release of acetylcholine at the neuromuscular junction (see Section XI, Plate 34). A similar syndrome can be seen in the neonate secondary to hypermagnesemia or administration of aminoglycoside antibiotics.

Transient *neonatal myasthenia gravis*, which causes a floppy baby syndrome and is secondary to transplacental transfer of acetylcholine receptor antibodies, occurs in 10% to 15% of infants born to mothers with myasthenia. The rare *congenital myasthenia gravis* resembles acquired childhood myasthenia, and probably results from abnormally formed postsynaptic membranes. (See Section XI, Plates 20–22 for a detailed discussion of myasthenia gravis.)

Congenital Myopathies. The conditions must be considered in the differential diagnosis of hypotonia. With the exception of myotonic dystrophy, which is an autosomal dominant trait, most of these disorders are of autosomal recessive inheritance. In addition to congenital muscular dystrophy, structural myopathies such as centronuclear myopathy, nemaline myopathy and central core disease must be considered. Muscle biopsy is essential to the diagnosis.

The syndrome of *arthrogryposis multiplex congenita*, or multiple contractures of joints at birth, results from intrauterine hypotonia and lack of movement.

Benign Congenital Hypotonia. The diagnosis of benign congenital hypotonia is usually retrospective, and is indicated not only by a positive family history of delayed walking, but also by a significant laxity of the ligaments. The many systemic illnesses that can cause hypotonia in infancy, such as hypothyroidism, amino acid abnormalities, malabsorption disease and congenital heart disease, must be considered. The Prader-Willi syndrome, which is characterized by striking hypotonia and also by hypogonadism, obesity and mild mental retardation, should also be excluded. This disorder has been associated with an abnormality of chromosome 15.

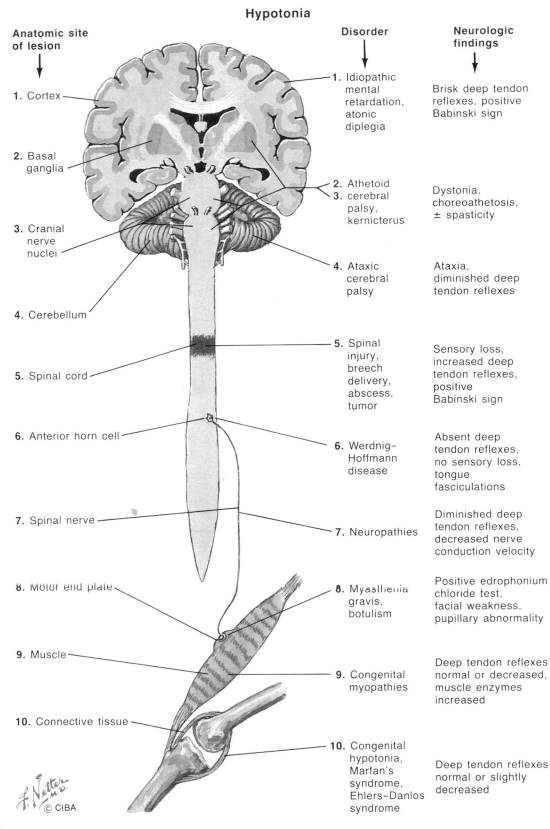

Hypotonia

Anatomic site of lesion	Disorder	Neurologic findings
1. Cortex	1. Idiopathic mental retardation, atonic diplegia	Brisk deep tendon reflexes, positive Babinski sign
2. Basal ganglia	2. Athetoid 3. cerebral palsy, kernicterus	Dystonia, choreoathetosis, ± spasticity
3. Cranial nerve nuclei		
4. Cerebellum	4. Ataxic cerebral palsy	Ataxia, diminished deep tendon reflexes
5. Spinal cord	5. Spinal injury, breech delivery, abscess, tumor	Sensory loss, increased deep tendon reflexes, positive Babinski sign
6. Anterior horn cell	6. Werdnig-Hoffmann disease	Absent deep tendon reflexes, no sensory loss, tongue fasciculations
7. Spinal nerve	7. Neuropathies	Diminished deep tendon reflexes, decreased nerve conduction velocity
8. Motor end plate	8. Myasthenia gravis, botulism	Positive edrophonium chloride test, facial weakness, pupillary abnormality
9. Muscle	9. Congenital myopathies	Deep tendon reflexes normal or decreased, muscle enzymes increased
10. Connective tissue	10. Congenital hypotonia, Marfan's syndrome, Ehlers-Danlos syndrome	Deep tendon reflexes normal or slightly decreased

Diagnosis

The workup of the patient must be tailored to either a CNS or a peripheral nervous system disorder. In 80% of children referred to a pediatric neurologist, a CNS abnormality is present. CT, electroencephalography, lumbar puncture, determination of muscle enzymes, electromyography, nerve conduction velocity studies, and carefully performed muscle biopsy may all be necessary to establish the diagnosis.

Many of these conditions are of genetic origin, and a specific diagnosis is therefore important, not only for appropriate management but also for family counseling.

Treatment

Treatment of the floppy baby depends on the underlying disorder. Abnormalities of the CNS are treated in the same manner as cerebral palsy (Plate 10). Neuromuscular disorders require a multidisciplinary approach that involves the neurologist, orthopedist and physical therapist. Particular attention must be paid to the hips, feet and spine.

The prognosis for the floppy baby is directly related to the cause of the hypotonia and can vary greatly. Time is the most important factor, allowing the medical team and parents to assess the child's development and plan future care. □

Werdnig-Hoffmann Disease

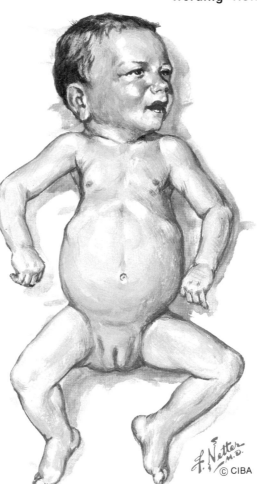

Infant with typical bell–shaped thorax, frog–leg posture, and "jug-handle" position of upper limbs

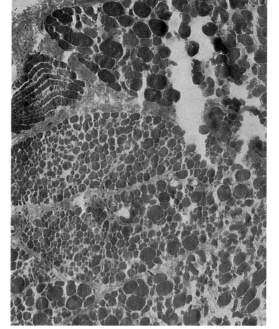

Muscle biopsy specimen showing groups of small atrophic muscle fibers and areas of normal or enlarged fibers (group atrophy). (Trichrome stain)

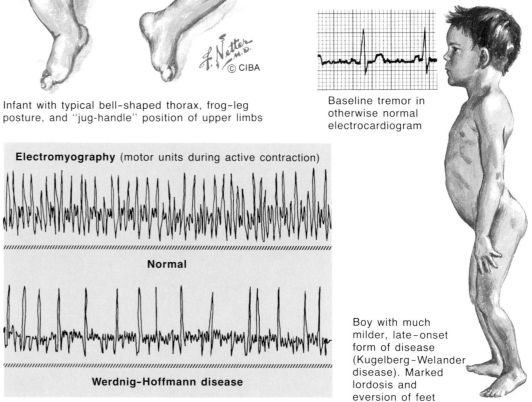

Electromyography (motor units during active contraction)

Normal

Werdnig-Hoffmann disease

Baseline tremor in otherwise normal electrocardiogram

Boy with much milder, late–onset form of disease (Kugelberg–Welander disease). Marked lordosis and eversion of feet

In the normal newborn, the purposeless movements of the extremities are associated with a well-defined muscular tone, despite the lack of motor skills. In addition, the newborn has a well-developed ability to suck and swallow. Occasionally, an infant is born with a limp body and no evidence of significant skeletal muscle activity. In retrospect, the mother may recall that the fetus was much less active than expected, and that she was not aware of the usual fist pounding and kicking during the pregnancy. These newborns are often unable to swallow appropriately, which may lead to aspiration and frequent episodes of pneumonia. At other times, the baby may appear normal at birth, but normal motor developmental milestones, such as holding up the head, rolling over or sitting up, are not reached during the first 3 to 6 months. This combination of symptoms eventually leads to referral to a pediatric neurologist for diagnostic evaluation.

Werdnig-Hoffmann disease, or infantile spinal muscular atrophy, is a hereditary illness, most often of autosomal recessive inheritance. Affected infants have a limp, frog-leg posture, and evidence paradoxical respiration and absence of deep tendon reflexes. However, they are bright and attentive, with full extraocular movements. Careful evaluation of the tongue may show the almost pathognomonic fasciculations. In contrast to motor neuron disease in the adult, fasciculations in the extremities are concealed by subcutaneous fat. Electromyography demonstrates active and chronic neurogenic changes, with a dropout in the number of motor units firing and abnormalities on needle insertion, with fibrillation potentials. Examination of a muscle biopsy specimen shows findings typical of neurogenic atrophy.

Other lesions in the motor unit can mimic Werdnig-Hoffmann disease, but as a rule can be differentiated by clinical and electromyographic findings and examination of muscle biopsy specimens. Family history is important. Similar illness

in other siblings may immediately indicate another type of motor-sensory unit dysfunction. Similarly, maternal illnesses, such as myasthenia gravis or myotonic dystrophy, may predispose to a floppy baby.

Onset of primary diseases of the peripheral nerves is rarely in the neonatal period. Diseases of the neuromuscular junction, such as transient *neonatal myasthenia gravis* and *infantile botulism*, should be considered in the differential diagnosis. A number of *hereditary congenital myopathies* may also become evident in the neonatal period, including disorders such as nemaline, central core and centronuclear myopathies (Plate 15). These conditions have been identified by histologic

techniques, including increasing use of muscle biopsy specimens in recent years.

Until the underlying pathophysiologic mechanism is identified, the treatment for Werdnig-Hoffmann disease is supportive.

The prognosis is generally poor, especially if onset is in the neonatal period. Many of these infants do not survive until their first birthday. A variety of other infantile motor neuron diseases, some with late infantile onset, have a less malignant course than Werdnig-Hoffmann disease, particularly when appropriate respiratory care is administered. A few infants with such disorders live much longer, some into adolescence or beyond. □

Hereditary Motor-Sensory Neuropathy Type III and Type IV

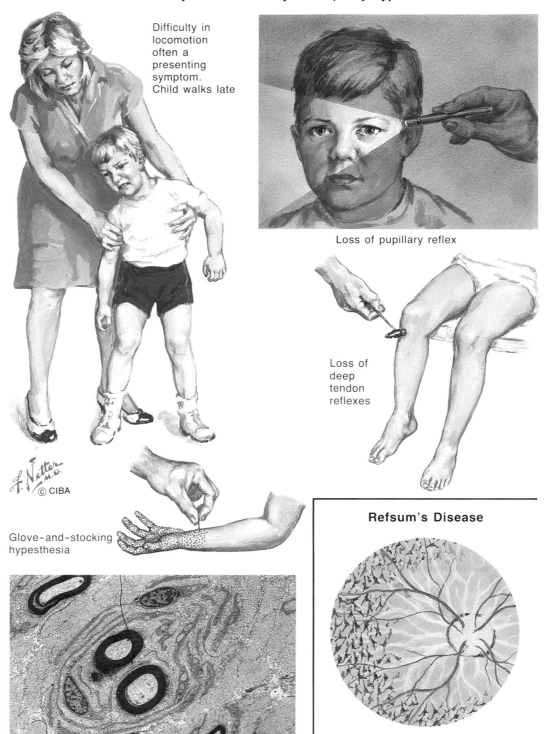

Difficulty in locomotion often a presenting symptom. Child walks late

Loss of pupillary reflex

Loss of deep tendon reflexes

Glove-and-stocking hypesthesia

Onion bulb with two myelinated fibers in center surrounded by attenuated Schwann cell processes

Refsum's Disease

Retinitis pigmentosa is characteristic feature of Refsum's disease, which may clinically resemble Déjerine-Sottas disease or Friedreich's ataxia

Hereditary Motor-Sensory Neuropathy Type III (HMSN III). Also known as Déjerine-Sottas disease, HMSN III is a rather rare peripheral neuropathy of autosomal recessive inheritance, with onset between infancy and childhood. Rarely, it manifests in infancy as a floppy baby. Typically, motor developmental milestones are delayed in affected children. They walk later than their unaffected siblings, some not until 4 years of age. Most acquire other motor skills slowly. The course may be insidiously progressive, although in some children, it is remitting and relapsing, with relatively acute relapses.

The distal atrophy may not be obvious in early childhood because of subcutaneous baby fat. Although weakness of the distal musculature is noted mainly in the feet and legs early in the disease, it later is evident in the upper extremities and is manifested by the child's inability to perform fine tasks such as coloring, drawing, manipulating small objects, or using simple tools. The deep tendon reflexes are absent. When the child is old enough to answer questions and react reliably, detailed sensory examination demonstrates a loss of sensation in the extremities that predominantly affects touch, pressure and vibration. Miotic pupils unresponsive to light stimuli have been noted in some patients. As in HMSN I, skeletal abnormalities such as pes cavus or kyphoscoliosis develop in many patients (see Section XI, Plate 16). Careful examination shows that peripheral nerves are thickened.

Cerebrospinal fluid (CSF) protein is significantly increased. Studies of nerve conduction velocity may show absent sensory potentials and marked slowing of motor conduction velocity, with values in the range of 5 to 20 m/sec. Nerve biopsy studies demonstrate a characteristic histologic picture of concentric myelin lamination, which produces the classic onion bulb appearance.

No specific pathophysiologic mechanism has been identified, although an underlying biochemical disorder has been suggested. The course of this illness is relentlessly progressive, and by their teenage years, most patients usually require significant assistance, including some need for a wheelchair.

Hereditary Motor-Sensory Neuropathy Type IV (HMSN IV). Also known as Refsum's disease, this peripheral neuropathy of autosomal recessive inheritance is exceedingly rare and is seen mainly in northern Europe, particularly in Norway, in children of consanguineous marriages. A specific biochemical disorder appears to be responsible for the neurologic lesion. All these patients have an inborn error of metabolism causing dysfunction of fatty acid oxidation. This is demonstrated in laboratory tests by elevated levels of serum phytanic acid.

Refsum's disease usually begins in adolescence with a slowly evolving peripheral neuropathy, although it has a remitting, relapsing course in

some patients. The vast majority have retinitis pigmentosa characterized by night blindness. Associated pupillary changes, nerve deafness, ataxia, cardiomyopathy and ichthyosis may also be seen. In some patients, ataxia mimicking Friedreich's ataxia is the initial complaint.

CSF findings and results of nerve conduction velocity studies are similar to those in Déjerine-Sottas disease. Although phytanic acid is a relatively ubiquitous compound found in many foods, a carefully controlled diet that excludes whole milk, all vegetables except potatoes, fat meats, chocolate and nuts may prevent further relapses and possibly improve the patient's clinical condition. □

Congenital Myopathies

In the past, muscle biopsy specimens from patients who had a weakness of proximal and sometimes of facial muscles typical of a myopathy failed to show any pathologic changes when stained with standard hematoxylin and eosin preparations. However, current histologic, histochemical and electron microscopy techniques, as well as the multiple stains now available, have revealed specific and stereotyped ultrastructural abnormalities of the muscle cell in many subgroups of patients. These abnormalities suggest a congenital and often a genetic defect in muscle development.

In contrast to the muscular dystrophies, many congenital myopathies are not associated with significantly progressive deterioration; rather, the course is static and demonstrates limited muscle reserve. These abnormalities may be manifested in newborns by the floppy baby syndrome (Plate 11) and, in children, by delay in reaching developmental milestones for motor activities such as walking, running and riding a bicycle. Occasionally, clinical symptoms do not develop until later in life. Serum levels of muscle enzymes are usually normal or only slightly increased. Results of nerve conduction velocity studies are also within normal limits. In general, needle electromyography demonstrates nonspecific myopathic changes, but no significant abnormalities on needle insertion.

Although no specific treatment is available for myopathic illnesses, various forms of supportive treatment often prove useful. For example, with meticulous respiratory care, many affected newborns can survive the critical period when pneumonia may well be life-threatening.

Nemaline Myopathy. One of the better-known congenital myopathies, this disease derives its name from the numerous subsarcolemmal nemaline (threadlike) inclusions found in affected muscle. Newborns afflicted with nemaline myopathy demonstrate the same weakness as the floppy baby. Because the inheritance pattern may be either autosomal recessive or autosomal dominant, the family history may not always be helpful. If the feeding and respiratory status can be vigorously supported, these children gradually begin to show some reasonable motor development. However, they may never be able to run or compete in a number of athletic endeavors.

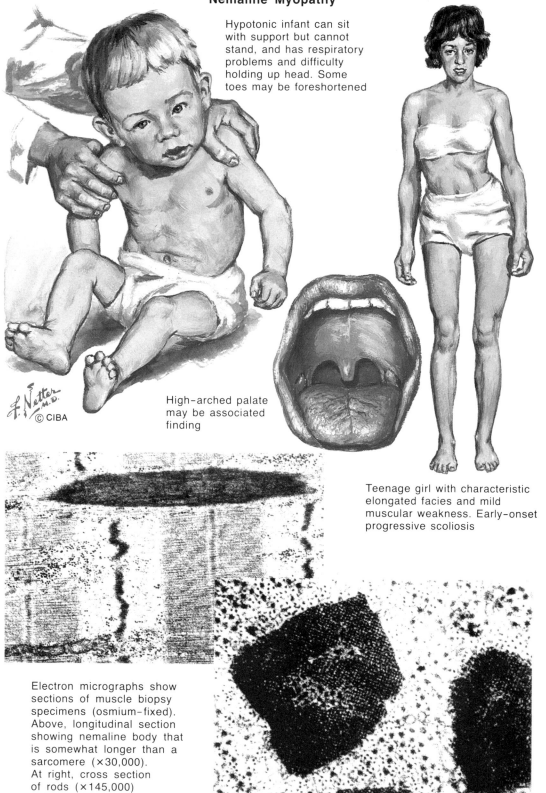

Nemaline Myopathy

Hypotonic infant can sit with support but cannot stand, and has respiratory problems and difficulty holding up head. Some toes may be foreshortened

High-arched palate may be associated finding

Teenage girl with characteristic elongated facies and mild muscular weakness. Early-onset progressive scoliosis

Electron micrographs show sections of muscle biopsy specimens (osmium-fixed). Above, longitudinal section showing nemaline body that is somewhat longer than a sarcomere (×30,000). At right, cross section of rods (×145,000)

Examination may reveal fairly diffuse muscle weakness, usually more severe in the proximal muscles, but often with a significant distal component. As in many of the congenital myopathies, the facial musculature is usually affected. Ptosis and, less commonly, a degree of ophthalmoparesis may be seen. The facies is drawn and dysmorphic, almost "birdlike" at times, as seen in myotonic dystrophy. The voice often has a nasal quality. Because the muscles are so hypoplastic, these patients have a particularly asthenic appearance. Skeletal abnormalities, such as a high-arched palate, pes cavus, foreshortening of some of the toes, and kyphoscoliosis, are another hallmark of this syndrome.

Central Core Disease. In this congenital myopathy, the majority of the muscle fibers have central cores that are devoid of mitochondria and oxidative enzymes. In general, patients with central core disease are not as severely affected as those with nemaline myopathy.

Myotubular (Centronuclear) Myopathy. Muscle biopsy specimens from patients with this disease show central nuclei surrounded by a halo that is devoid of myofibrils but contains organelles. These fibers resemble embryonic myotubules. Clinically, the early predominance of ptosis and ophthalmoparesis is more pronounced, and the course may be more progressive in myotubular myopathy than in the other myopathies. □

Brachial Plexus and/or Cervical Nerve Root Injuries at Birth

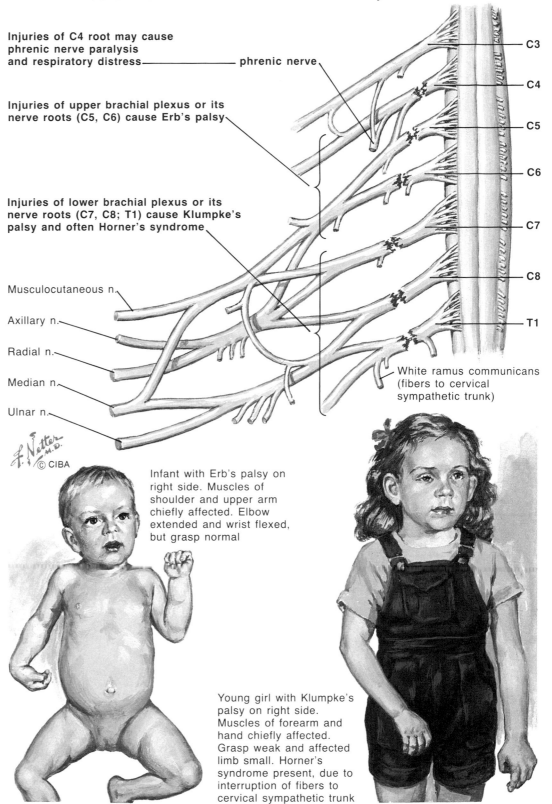

Injuries of C4 root may cause phrenic nerve paralysis and respiratory distress———— phrenic nerve

Injuries of upper brachial plexus or its nerve roots (C5, C6) cause Erb's palsy

Injuries of lower brachial plexus or its nerve roots (C7, C8; T1) cause Klumpke's palsy and often Horner's syndrome

Musculocutaneous n.

Axillary n.

Radial n.

Median n.

Ulnar n.

C3
C4
C5
C6
C7
C8
T1

White ramus communicans (fibers to cervical sympathetic trunk)

Infant with Erb's palsy on right side. Muscles of shoulder and upper arm chiefly affected. Elbow extended and wrist flexed, but grasp normal

Young girl with Klumpke's palsy on right side. Muscles of forearm and hand chiefly affected. Grasp weak and affected limb small. Horner's syndrome present, due to interruption of fibers to cervical sympathetic trunk

Brachial plexus injuries in the newborn now occur much less commonly than formerly, although the incidence is still approximately one in 1,000 live births. The injury results from traction forces in delivering the shoulder in vertex deliveries and delivering the head in breech deliveries. The associated obstetric factors are occipitoposterior or transverse presentation, the use of oxytocin, shoulder dystocia, and large babies (weighing over 3,500 g) with low Apgar scores.

Brachial birth palsy is believed to be secondary to a stretching of the plexus by traction, with the nerve roots being anchored by the spinal column and cord. In less severe lesions, only the myelin sheath may be damaged, which is evidenced by swelling and edema that may in turn damage the myelin. If only a small segment of the axon is affected or if it is stretched but not ruptured, quick repair and recovery are likely. However, if the axon is interrupted, repair can take a very long time, considering that the rate of axonal growth is believed to be 1 mm/day. If the axon is completely ruptured, recovery is unlikely. Bilateral brachial injuries almost always indicate spinal involvement, and avulsion of the nerve roots may be evident on a rarely performed myelogram. Upper brachial plexus injuries involve the junction of C5 and C6 roots (Erb's point), and lower injuries involve the junction of C8 and T1 roots.

Upper Brachial Plexus Injury (Erb's Palsy). This is the most common of the brachial plexus injuries, affecting muscles supplied by C5 and C6 and accounting for 90% of the total incidence. An *asymmetric Moro response* is usually the first indication of the injury. The upper extremity assumes the "waiter's tip" position: the shoulder is adducted and internally rotated; the elbow is extended, and the forearm is pronated, with the hand in flexion. A mild sensory loss may develop over the lateral aspect of the shoulder and arm, but is rather difficult to distinguish. Associated fractures of the clavicle or humerus must be ruled

but, and fluoroscopic examination should be carried out to exclude the rare diaphragmatic paralysis caused mainly by a C4 lesion.

Lower Brachial Plexus Injury (Klumpke's Palsy). A pure lower brachial plexus injury is quite uncommon, and most cases of Klumpke's palsy involve the more proximal muscles supplied by C7 or C6. An *absent grasp reflex* is the most prominent clinical feature. Involvement of sympathetic fibers from T1 causes Horner's syndrome (ptosis, miosis, anhidrosis). A significant sensory deficit is usually present. Infants and children may sometimes traumatize their fingers unwittingly, with occasionally severe results such as loss of a fingertip. Prognosis for full recovery in

these infants is poor. The upper extremity often remains small and distally foreshortened.

Treatment. In all cases of brachial plexus injury, treatment is conservative. No surgical procedure is likely to improve the immediate situation or the prognosis. The limb should be placed in its best functional position, ie, across the chest, not abducted and flexed. Gentle, passive, range-of-motion exercise should be initiated within 7 to 10 days of birth. Hand and wrist splints can be constructed later as necessary. Electromyography, while of diagnostic value in determining the extent of the injury, is of little value in management. After the child is 5 to 6 years of age, muscle transfers may be helpful. □

Metachromatic Leukodystrophy

Metachromatic leukodystrophy, also known as sulfatide lipidosis, is an inborn error of metabolism of autosomal recessive inheritance that causes demyelination of both the central and the peripheral nervous systems. Age at onset determines three fairly distinct clinical syndromes: late infantile, juvenile and adult variants.

The common metabolic defect in each type is a deficiency of the enzyme arylsulfatase A, which normally effects the degradation of sulfatides (sulfated lipids) to cerebroside. Deficiency of this enzyme allows accumulation of sulfatides in the white and gray matter, producing the clinical picture of one of the more common leukodystrophies.

Late Infantile Variant. Affected infants typically develop normally during the first 1 to 4 years of life. Further maturation of motor skills then fails, and difficulty in walking eventually develops. A wide, ataxic gait becomes increasingly apparent. Neurologic examination shows positive Babinski signs and absence of deep tendon reflexes. Later in the course of the disease, signs of intellectual deterioration appear. The disease progresses inexorably over the next 1 to 3 years, resulting in lack of comprehension and speech, quadriplegia, and associated decorticate or decerebrate posturing, or both.

The cerebrospinal fluid (CSF) protein is usually increased to 100 to 150 mg/100 ml. Nerve conduction studies, after appropriate age correction, show evidence of a demyelinating neuropathy, with moderate to marked slowing in motor and sensory nerve conduction velocity. Sensory compound action potentials may not be recordable. Because this is primarily a demyelinating disease, needle electromyography does not always show denervation, although the number of motor units firing may be moderately to markedly reduced.

Few other diseases occurring in this age group produce the combination of demyelinating peripheral neuropathy and corticospinal tract dysfunction. Déjerine-Sottas disease or other forms of chronic inflammatory polyneuropathy may develop at the same age, but there is no evidence that central nervous system (CNS) dysfunction affects either the corticospinal tracts or mental function. In infancy, Cockayne's syndrome and Krabbe's disease, which are characterized by motor retardation spasticity, seizures and optic atrophy, may be associated with the demyelinating forms of peripheral neuropathy.

Although the clinical picture and results of nerve conduction velocity studies may suggest metachromatic leukodystrophy, ultimate diagnosis depends on the demonstration of abnormalities in sulfatide metabolism. When tissues containing

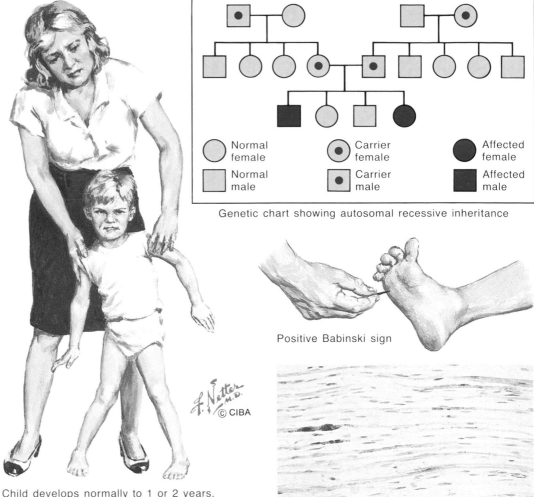

Metachromatic Leukodystrophy

Normal female	Carrier female	Affected female
Normal male	Carrier male	Affected male

Genetic chart showing autosomal recessive inheritance

Positive Babinski sign

Child develops normally to 1 or 2 years, then becomes progressively ataxic. Intellectual deterioration soon appears

Section of peripheral nerve with metachromatically (brown) staining granules (modified cresyl violet stain)

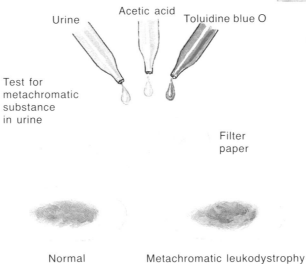

Urine   Acetic acid   Toluidine blue O

Test for metachromatic substance in urine

Filter paper

Normal   Metachromatic leukodystrophy

Section of hemispheric white matter showing myelin degeneration and PAS–positive macrophages

highly polar anionic groups are stained with cationic aniline dyes, a metachromatic reaction results. The sulfatides produce a spectral shift (metachromasia) in transmitted light, so that tissue that normally stains purple may appear orange or brown. The abnormal sulfatides are excreted in the urine, and the amount excreted can be precisely measured. Similarly, a nerve biopsy specimen demonstrates metachromasia from the sulfatide deposits. Decreased amounts or absence of arylsulfatase A in the urine can also be demonstrated.

Juvenile Variant. This less common form of metachromatic leukodystrophy develops between 6 and 14 years of age. Personality or intellectual changes, or both, may be the first clinical sign. Gait difficulties develop, and nerve conduction studies may demonstrate a demyelinating disorder. This variant is thought to result from a different genetic mutation. In some patients, the level of arylsulfatase A is only minimally to modestly diminished, and the defect appears to be in the process by which the enzyme is activated or in transport of the sulfatide to the enzyme site.

Adult Variant. This is the rarest form of metachromatic leukodystrophy. Onset is usually in early adulthood. A psychosis or dementia, or both, is commonly the first sign of the disease. Corticospinal and cerebellar dysfunction may become evident later in the course. ☐

Friedreich's Ataxia

Friedreich's ataxia is the most common of the spinocerebellar degenerations. It is inherited in an autosomal recessive fashion and has a reasonably specific set of symptoms and signs. Its biochemical basis is unknown.

The pathologic changes in Friedreich's ataxia include degeneration of the sensory nerves, ganglion cells and posterior nerve roots. Associated findings in the posterior columns affect position and vibration sense, and degeneration in the spinocerebellar tracts causes ataxia. The corticospinal tract is also affected, producing distal weakness and a positive Babinski sign.

Clinical Manifestations. Onset is usually in the first or early in the second decade, with ataxia initially manifested as general clumsiness. Occasionally, scoliosis is the first sign, and ataxia and clumsiness become evident only after surgical correction of the scoliosis. Pes cavus is an early and frequent orthopedic finding. The ataxia is further complicated by loss of position sense, with a positive Romberg sign. Areflexia becomes universal.

The combination of cerebellar ataxia, loss of kinesthetic sensation, and corticospinal weakness eventually leads to a nonambulatory state. This may develop as early as the end of the second decade in severe cases, and virtually all patients are wheelchair-bound by the fourth decade. A scanning dysarthria makes communication difficult, but mentation does not appear to be affected. Nystagmus is a frequent finding and may be further complicated by "sticky" eye movements.

Diabetes mellitus, which requires management with insulin, occurs in about 20% of patients, often with onset in the third decade. Neurologic complications cause further deterioration.

Cardiomegaly is evident on x-ray films, and electrocardiography and echocardiography confirm the presence of cardiomyopathy, which may ultimately lead to cardiac failure and arrhythmias.

Motor nerve conduction velocities are only mildly reduced, consistent with an axonal neuropathy. Sensory nerve action potentials, however, are markedly reduced.

Differential Diagnosis. Hereditary motor-sensory neuropathy type I (peroneal muscular atrophy) may be associated with a significant tremor (Roussy-Lévy disease) that could be confused with Friedreich's ataxia, except that there is no nystagmus, toe responses are flexor, and motor nerve conduction velocities are markedly delayed. Disorders that should be considered are structural lesions such as a *posterior fossa brain tumor* or *Arnold-Chiari malformation*; metabolic disorders, including *ataxia-telangiectasia, abetalipoproteinemia; Refsum's disease; Wilson's disease*; the *Chédiak-Higashi syndrome; chronic liver disease*; and malabsorption syndromes, including *cystic fibrosis.*

Ataxia-telangiectasia is a disorder of autosomal recessive inheritance, and is characterized by onset of progressive cerebellar ataxia in infancy or early childhood. It may be labeled "ataxic cerebral palsy." Subsequently, reflexes begin to disappear

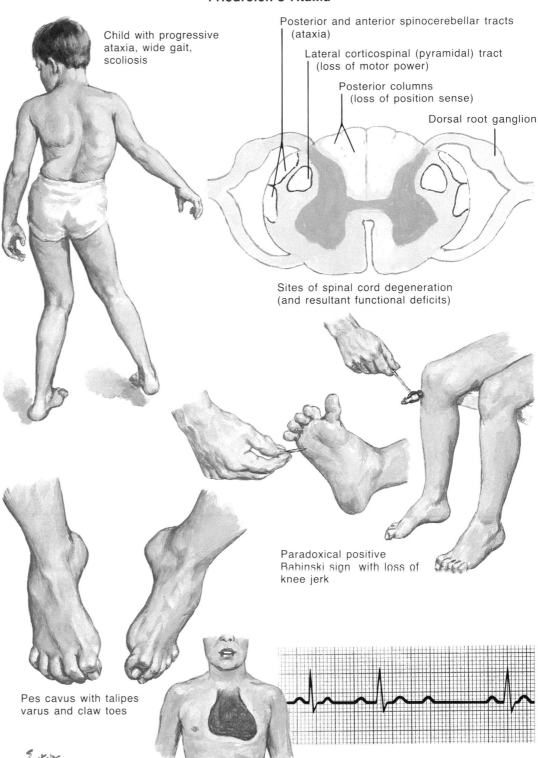

Child with progressive ataxia, wide gait, scoliosis

Posterior and anterior spinocerebellar tracts (ataxia)

Lateral corticospinal (pyramidal) tract (loss of motor power)

Posterior columns (loss of position sense)

Dorsal root ganglion

Sites of spinal cord degeneration (and resultant functional deficits)

Paradoxical positive Babinski sign with loss of knee jerk

Pes cavus with talipes varus and claw toes

f. Netter M.D.
© CIBA

Death often caused by cardiac abnormalities (interstitial myocarditis, fibrosis, enlargement, arrhythmias, murmurs, heart block)

and the ataxia worsens. Telangiectases develop on the conjunctiva, usually after age 3 or 4. In the first decade, the course is progressively downhill, with an evolving spinocerebellar syndrome, and most patients are wheelchair-bound by 10 to 12 years of age. Supranuclear third cranial nerve palsy, immobile facies, and severe dysarthria develop, along with a variable degree of sinopulmonary infection. Biochemical abnormalities include deficient immunoglobulins and abnormal cellular immunity consistent with a thymic defect, and an accompanying elevation of α-fetoprotein. Lymphoreticular malignancies are also likely. Infection or malignancy usually causes death when the patient is in the teens or 20s.

Abetalipoproteinemia (Bassen-Kornzweig syndrome) is an autosomal recessive disorder that begins as a spruelike malabsorption syndrome in early childhood, with a subsequent development of spinocerebellar degeneration and retinitis pigmentosa. Acanthocytes are seen in thick blood smears. Cholesterol and triglycerides are low, and the diagnosis is confirmed by demonstrating an absence of beta-lipoproteins. Treatment with vitamin E may halt progression.

Physical therapy, orthopedic procedures and use of adaptive equipment such as wheelchairs are the principal methods of treatment in Friedreich's ataxia, with appropriate management of symptomatic cardiomyopathy and diabetes. □

Developmental Dyslexia

Developmental Dyslexia

Developmental dyslexia, or developmental reading disorder, is defined as a significant impairment in the development of reading skills that cannot be attributed to chronologic age, mental age or inadequate schooling. This disorder frequently occurs in association with other specific learning disabilities, such as disturbances in auditory comprehension, expressive language, articulation and visual discrimination. Although its exact incidence is unknown, it is common, is more frequent in boys than in girls, and is often present in siblings and other family members.

Since the primary deficit in developmental dyslexia is in reading and writing, the abnormality is usually not noted until the first few years of grade school, and most parents are not aware of any disorder in their child before this time. Because it is common and affects skills recently acquired by man, developmental dyslexia may have had certain advantages in preliterate societies, since dyslexic persons often have enhanced visual-spatial and artistic skills.

Etiologic Theories. Early writers postulated that developmental dyslexia was caused by a lesion in the left angular gyrus, an area of the brain in which a lesion in adults produces word blindness. Later, Orton (1925) felt that the disorder was caused by equipotential visual association areas in the two cerebral hemispheres actively competing with each other, with one side seeing a mirror image of the other. Orton was particularly impressed with reversals of letters and letter sequences in words, the inconsistency of these errors, and the ability of some dyslexic students to read better with the aid of a mirror. Emotional problems and improper instruction were also thought to cause dyslexia.

Recent investigations, including computed tomography (CT), computed evoked electroencephalographic studies, and postmortem studies of the brain, have all provided evidence of a structural basis for dyslexia. In the first brain study, Drake (1968) noted *abnormally formed gyri* in the parietal region and *ectopic neurons* in the white matter, arrested during their migration to the cerebral cortex.

Galaburda and Kemper (1979), examining a second brain, also noted cerebral cortical abnormalities, with *microgyria* and *microsulci* centered on the sensory speech area (Wernicke's area) and two types of widely scattered smaller malformations confined to the language-dominant left cerebral hemisphere. One of these was *focal dysplasia*, with abnormally large neurons that extended from the cerebral cortex into the subcortical white matter. The other malformation was *verrucose dysplasia*, which varied from abnormal ectopic accumulations of neurons in layer I of the cerebral cortex to wartlike accumulations of abnormally placed cortical neurons.

The third brain examined showed only verrucose dysplasia almost exclusively confined to the left cerebral hemisphere (Kemper, 1984). Thus,

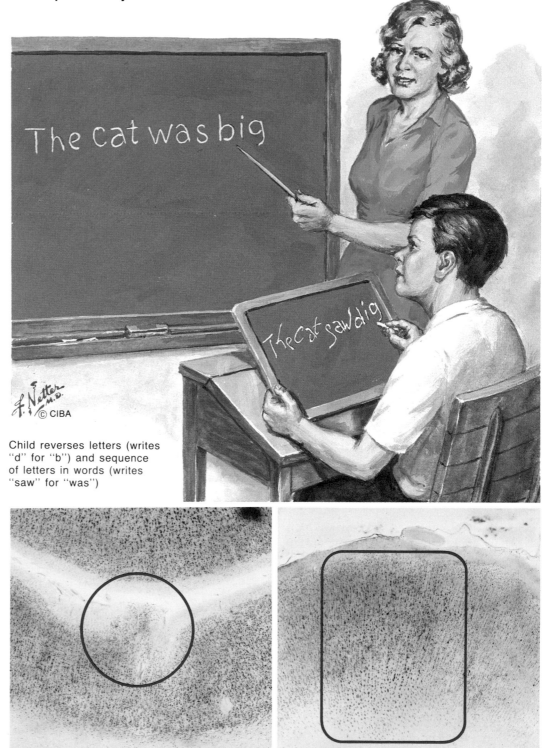

Child reverses letters (writes "d" for "b") and sequence of letters in words (writes "saw" for "was")

Verrucose dysplasia, with focal accumulation of neurons in layer I of cerebral cortex

Focal dysplasia, with abnormally large neurons extending into white matter of brain

examination of all three brains has demonstrated minor malformations.

Analysis of human malformations and animal models indicates that the microgyria, microsulci and verrucose dysplasia probably arise during the later stages of neuronal migration to the cerebral cortex, and appear to result from the migration of neurons into focal areas of cortical destruction. In man, neuronal migration to the cerebral cortex occurs from the eighth to approximately the sixteenth week of gestation. Consistent with this timing is the presence of ectopic neurons in the white matter in two of the three brains examined. The nature of this postulated destructive process is unknown. Recently, however, Geschwind and

Behan (1982) have noted a significant clustering of dyslexia, left-handedness, autoimmune disease and migraine in persons related to each other, indicating an association between these disorders.

Treatment. Early identification of dyslexia, together with appropriate testing to identify the areas of deficit, is essential for proper treatment. Although virtually all dyslexic persons respond to educational programs geared to their specific difficulties, many have significant residual disabilities as adults. Treatment should be aimed at enabling the affected person to overcome deficits where possible and to learn strategies to circumvent and compensate for difficulties that cannot be overcome. □

Infantile Autism

Infantile Autism

Early infantile autism was first described by Kanner in 1943. It is a behaviorally defined syndrome of unknown cause, with onset before 30 months of age, and occurs in 2 to 4 of every 10,000 infants. A genetic component is suggested by a male-to-female ratio of 3:1 and by an incidence 50 times greater than expected in siblings of autistic patients.

Clinical Manifestations. The essential features of autism are a lack of responsiveness to others, grossly impaired communication skills, and bizarre or catastrophic reactions to minor changes in the environment. Additional features include repetitive and stereotypic behavior, poor eye contact, an obsessive insistence on sameness and, often, striking islands of rote memory. These characteristics all contrast with a normal physical appearance and normal or nearly normal early motor development.

Affected infants may show indifference to affection or physical contact, with no desire for cuddling, and lack of eye contact and facial expression. In early childhood, autistic children fail to develop cooperative play or friendships, although at later ages, some attachment to parents or other family members may develop. Only 1 in 6 autistic persons is able to do some type of regular work in adulthood, and virtually all require special educational facilities.

Verbal and nonverbal communication is often totally impaired, and when speech is present, it is characterized by immature grammar and frequent repetition of what has been said by others. Intelligence is also impaired, with 40% of the children having an IQ below 50. In intelligence tests, the poorest responses are to tests of verbal skills and to tests requiring symbolic or abstract thinking. Surprising islands of rote memory are evidenced by a knowledge of dates, detailed schedules, or exact words of songs. Striking examples of this characteristic are so-called idiot savants, the majority of whom are autistic. These persons are able, for example, to provide the day of the week for any past date.

Etiologic Theories. The older literature suggests that infantile autism should be considered a psychiatric disorder resulting from abnormal maternal-infant interaction. However, abnormal electroencephalograms, seizures, abnormalities on neurologic examination, and the demonstration of abnormal processing of auditory information by the brainstem all suggest structural abnormalities.

The only postmortem study on the brain of an autistic person to date provides support for the latter theory. Abnormalities were found in the forebrain and cerebellum. Those seen in the forebrain were confined to the hippocampal complex and three areas directly related to it, the entorhinal cortex, mamillary body and septum, and to several nuclei of the amygdala. In these areas, the nerve cells were unusually small and more densely distributed than normal, resembling the configuration usually seen at earlier stages of development. These involved areas are key components of the limbic system, a system of neuronal intercon-

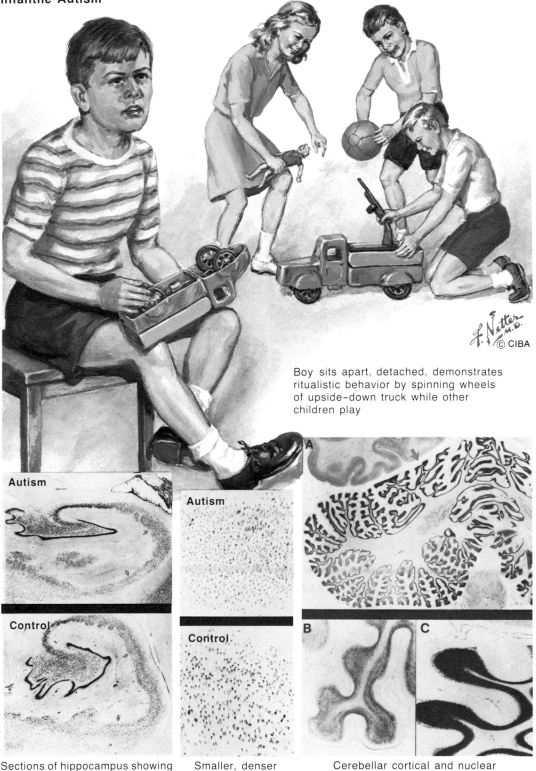

Boy sits apart, detached, demonstrates ritualistic behavior by spinning wheels of upside-down truck while other children play

Sections of hippocampus showing impaired development in autistic brain compared with normal (control) brain

Smaller, denser neurons in autistic hippocampus

Cerebellar cortical and nuclear atrophy in autistic brain. Arrows indicate areas of sections **B** and **C**

nections thought to be essential to the normal functioning of memory, behavior and emotion.

In adult animals, experimentally induced lesions in these areas have reproduced many of the symptoms of infantile autism. The most convincing evidence that autistic behavior is related to lesions in the hippocampus and amygdala has been provided by studies conducted by Mishkin and Bachevalier of the National Institutes of Health. These investigators have noted striking autisticlike behavior following bilateral lesions in these areas in neonatal monkeys.

The only other abnormality noted in the brain examined was atrophy of the lateral lobes of the cerebellum, with a loss of Purkinje and granule

cells and a marked decrease in the number and size of neurons in the cerebellar roof nuclei. The relationship of these lesions to autistic behavior is less certain.

Treatment. Early diagnosis of autism is critical. Appropriate treatment to prevent the development of secondary behavioral problems must be instituted and family members must be reassured that the child's abnormal behavior is not the result of their relationship with the child. The most successful treatment is behavior modification to facilitate the development of the child's skills and ability to communicate. Virtually all autistic persons need some degree of protection and supervision. □

Brain Tumors in Children

Medulloblastoma

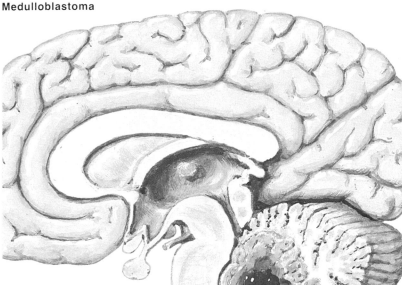

Medulloblastoma arising from vermis of cerebellum, filling 4th ventricle and protruding into cisterna magna

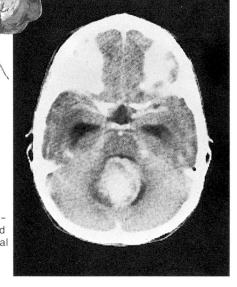

CT scan showing enhancing medulloblastoma in region of 4th ventricle. Obstructive hydrocephalus indicated by dilated temporal horns

Postoperative lumbar metrizamide myelogram showing lumbar seeding of tumor evidenced by nonfilling of S1 root on right side (arrow)

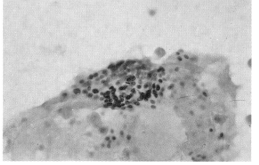

Positive CSF cytologic findings in patient with medulloblastoma. Malignant tumor cells clumped on Millipore filter

Brain Tumors in Children

Brain tumors in the pediatric age group are most commonly found in the posterior fossa. These tumors obstruct cerebrospinal fluid (CSF) pathways, particularly in the fourth ventricle, and the patient's initial complaints of headache, nausea and vomiting are often related to increased intracranial pressure secondary to hydrocephalus. Because the more common *astrocytomas* and *medulloblastomas* arise from the parenchyma of the cerebellum (Plate 21), cerebellar dysfunction (typically truncal and appendicular ataxia) is usually superimposed on these symptoms.

Ependymomas, which grow from the ependymal cells lining the ventricular system, also produce early symptoms of hydrocephalus as the fourth ventricle becomes blocked by tumor. However, in addition, they cause intrinsic brainstem dysfunction as the brainstem is invaded or cerebellar signs as the overlying cerebellum is compressed.

Brainstem *gliomas* grow in the substance of the brainstem, enlarging and distorting it (Plate 22), and cause hydrocephalus only late in their course. Headache is therefore less common in a child with a brainstem glioma, but cranial nerve palsies involving extraocular and facial muscles develop, and damage to motor and sensory pathways leads to hemiparesis, hyperreflexia and positive Babinski signs.

Diagnostic Studies

The diagnosis in all cases is confirmed by computed tomography (CT). Arteriography is also used in selected patients to delineate the vascular supply to the tumor and to plan the surgical approach. Children with posterior fossa tumors occasionally complain of stiff neck, presumably because of meningeal irritation and pressure in the region of the foramen magnum from the downward-displaced cerebellar tonsils. However, lumbar puncture must not be included in the diagnostic workup because of the danger of further downward herniation of the swollen cerebellum into the foramen magnum as CSF is withdrawn from below. This can cause fatal brainstem compression.

Treatment

As soon as the diagnosis is made, high-dose steroid therapy should be started to reduce edema around the tumor. Although the response to steroid therapy may be dramatic, emergency ventricular shunting may be necessary to relieve the symptoms of acute intracranial pressure prior to a definitive surgical procedure. In a child with a tumor in the pineal region and acute hydrocephalus secondary to compression of the aqueduct, ventricular shunting also provides safe access to ventricular CSF, which can be assayed for hormonal markers produced by these neoplasms and for cytologic investigation.

The definitive treatment for all posterior fossa tumors in children is *surgical exploration*, with attempted total removal of the lesion. Cystic cerebellar astrocytomas and some medulloblastomas and ependymomas can be completely excised, and recent statistics indicate that survival figures in all types of posterior fossa tumors are improved if

Brain Tumors in Children
(Continued)

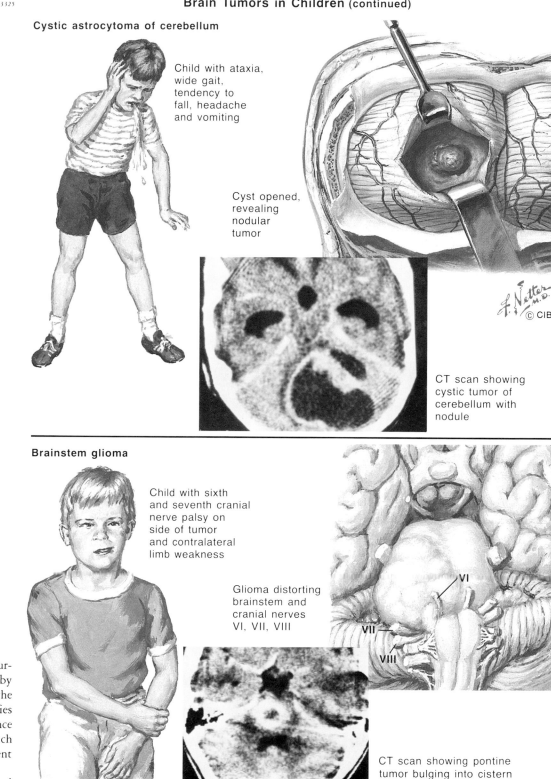

Cystic astrocytoma of cerebellum

Child with ataxia, wide gait, tendency to fall, headache and vomiting

Cyst opened, revealing nodular tumor

CT scan showing cystic tumor of cerebellum with nodule

Brainstem glioma

Child with sixth and seventh cranial nerve palsy on side of tumor and contralateral limb weakness

Glioma distorting brainstem and cranial nerves VI, VII, VIII

CT scan showing pontine tumor bulging into cistern anteriorly and into 4th ventricle posteriorly

radical excision can be carried out. The neurosurgeon has been aided in achieving this goal by several recent technologic advances, including the Cavitron ultrasonic aspirator, which emulsifies and aspirates tumor tissue with little disturbance of adjacent brain matter, and the laser, which permits vaporization of tumor fragments adherent to the brainstem and other vital structures.

The role of adjuvant radiation therapy and chemotherapy for posterior fossa neoplasms in children has been firmly established in only a few tumor types. The cystic astrocytoma does not require additional therapy of any type, because total excision usually eradicates the tumor. Unquestionably, *postoperative irradiation* in medulloblastoma has considerably lengthened survival time. When surgery is combined with craniospinal irradiation, 10-year survival has been 40% to 50% in some reported series. Medulloblastoma can seed the subarachnoid spaces, and postoperative cytologic examination of CSF and total myelography are now frequently used to stage the disease and plan the postoperative radiation therapy course.

The effectiveness of adjuvant *chemotherapy* in the initial treatment of posterior fossa tumors remains uncertain at present. Several protocols combining

radiation therapy with chemotherapy in the treatment of medulloblastoma, for example, have failed to demonstrate a convincing benefit from such combined treatment. In general, chemotherapy in the treatment of posterior fossa tumors has been helpful only in the management of recurrent disease. Continuing efforts in this direction should be pursued, however, since long-term harmful effects of craniospinal irradiation on both mental and physical maturation, particularly in the younger child, are becoming evident as these children survive longer and the initial tumor is cured.

The prognosis of the patient with a brainstem glioma remains bleak. A major advance in the

treatment of these tumors has been an aggressive approach to diagnosis, with biopsy and partial excision whenever feasible with use of the laser, ultrasound aspirator and other sophisticated microsurgical tools. Treatable neoplasms, infectious processes and vascular lesions can masquerade as intrinsic gliomas and carry a more favorable prognosis if diagnosis and treatment are carried out in a timely fashion. *Magnetic resonance imaging (MRI)* can provide better visualization of this area of the nervous system than any other diagnostic technique currently in use, and this scanning technique will greatly aid physicians in the difficult management of children with this type of tumor. □

Tuberous Sclerosis

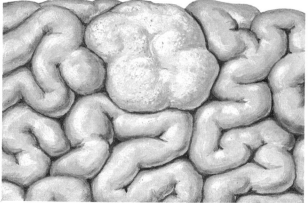

Tuber of cerebral cortex consisting of many astrocytes, scanty nerve cells, some abnormal cells

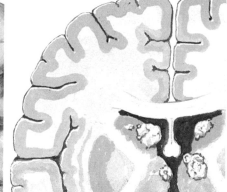

Multiple small tumors of caudate nucleus and thalamus projecting into ventricles

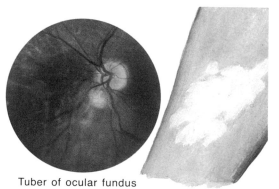

Tuber of ocular fundus

Depigmented skin area

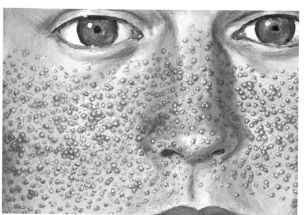

Adenoma sebaceum over both cheeks and bridge of nose

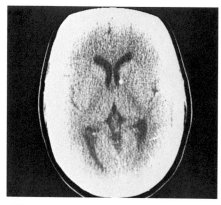

CT scan showing one of many calcified lesions in periventricular area

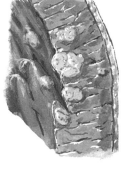

Rhabdomyomas of heart muscle

Multiple small tumors in kidney

Sturge-Weber Disease

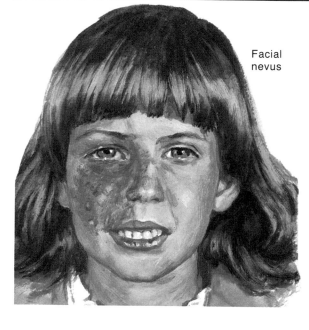

Facial nevus

CT scans showing calcifications and atrophy in temporoparietal area

Calcific deposits and hypervascularity in leptomeninges and gray matter of brain

X-ray film showing "railroad" calcification

f. Netter
©CIBA

SECTION I   PLATE 23   *Slide 3326*

Neurocutaneous Syndromes

Tuberous Sclerosis. This disease is an important cause of epilepsy with a genetic implication. In *infancy*, it presents with infantile spasms, hypsarrhythmia and depigmented nevi.

In early *childhood*, the first clinical signs are epilepsy and mental retardation. In addition to the depigmented nevi, adenoma sebaceum is present and increases with age. A shagreen patch in the lumbar area and subungual fibromas are seen in older children. Retinoscopy may reveal a retinal tuber. Periventricular calcification increases with age and, if located close to the interventricular foramen, may cause ventricular obstruction. Tubers in the cortex, the cause of the seizures and mental retardation, calcify less often and may be seen on computed tomography (CT) as areas of decreased density. Rhabdomyomas of the heart, renal cysts and angiomyolipomas coexist.

Although this disease is inherited as an autosomal dominant trait, many sporadic cases occur (60% to 80%). Up to 33% of patients have normal intelligence and may not have seizures. Parents of an affected child should be screened with an ultraviolet light, a fundoscopic examination and CT of the head.

Sturge-Weber Disease. This disease occurs sporadically and is evident from birth. The characteristic port-wine nevus always involves the forehead and upper lid and, usually, parts of the cheek and nose. It is most often unilateral, but can be bilateral. The ipsilateral eye may be glaucomatous. In the infant, cerebral involvement may be difficult to prove in the absence of hemiparesis, hemianopsia or seizures. CT initially shows an area of decreased density. Later, calcification appears in the cortex (laminar necrosis).

The course is progressive, with increasing seizures and hemiparesis, hemianopsia and, possibly, mental retardation.

In addition to medical treatment of seizures, a surgical approach must be carefully considered in all patients. □

Reye's Syndrome

In 1963, Reye et al described a clinical syndrome consisting of acute encephalopathy associated with fatty degeneration of the viscera. The illness occurs primarily in children less than 18 years of age. The cause is unknown, but the syndrome characteristically follows a recent or resolving viral infection, especially varicella or influenza A or B. It is one of the most common acute neurologic disorders of childhood, with an annual incidence of 1 to 2 per 100,000 persons younger than age 18. The mortality has varied roughly from 22% to 42% in recent years.

Reye's syndrome has been divided into clinical stages to aid in assessment and prognosis. *Stage I* begins with prodromal symptoms of vomiting, lethargy and sleepiness, which develop *after* the child has begun to recuperate from the preceding viral disease. Results of laboratory studies and liver function tests are abnormal and the electroencephalogram (EEG) shows predominantly theta activity. Although children tested have had abnormal liver biopsy specimens, a large number have not progressed to coma; prognosis for survival without sequelae is excellent.

Stage II is heralded by disorientation and combativeness, progressing to delirium, associated with hyperventilation and hyperreactive reflexes. Liver dysfunction continues, and the EEG shows progressive abnormalities, with more delta activity.

Obtundation and coma supervene in *stage III*, with continued hyperventilation, decortication and liver dysfunction. The EEG shows diffuse high-voltage rhythmic or arrhythmic activity.

Stage IV is characterized by deepening coma, decerebrate activity and a rostral-caudal progression of brain dysfunction. Hepatic dysfunction is only minimally abnormal, but the EEG is diffusely abnormal, showing mostly low-voltage delta or burst-suppression activity.

Seizures usher in *stage V*, associated with loss of deep and superficial reflexes and respiratory arrest. The liver dysfunction is now corrected, but the EEG is nearly isoelectric.

Diagnostic Studies. Characteristic abnormal results of laboratory studies include mild to moderate hypoglycemia, elevated serum aspartate aminotransferase and serum alanine aminotransferase, elevated serum ammonia levels, and prolonged prothrombin time. The presence of these abnormalities confirms the diagnosis, and spinal tap should not be done because of the risks with brain edema.

The cerebrospinal fluid (CSF) is generally normal other than showing increased pressure. Computed tomography (CT) may show diffuse edema and is nonspecific. A liver biopsy specimen reveals an almost pathognomonic pattern of microvesicular fat in a panlobular distribution, and deranged mitochondria ultrastructurally.

Prognosis. The prothrombin time and serum ammonia levels at the time of the patient's admission determine the prognosis. An ammonia level greater than 300 µg/ml, or 5 times the normal level, indicates a very poor prognosis, as does

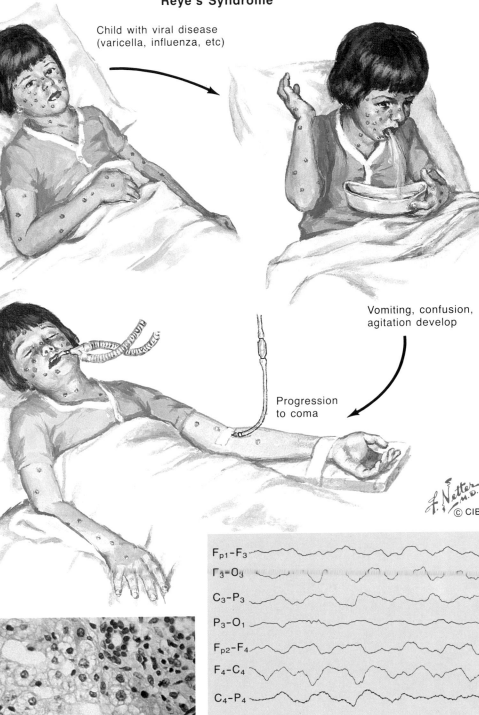

Child with viral disease (varicella, influenza, etc)

Vomiting, confusion, agitation develop

Progression to coma

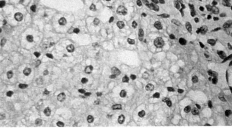

Liver biopsy specimen: panlobular distribution of microvesicular fat (H and E stain)

EEG in comatose 12-year-old boy who had viral illness 1 week previously and persistent vomiting 2 days previously

prothrombin time in excess of 3 seconds beyond control. Ammonia levels of twice normal predict progression into deeper coma.

Treatment. In stage I, treatment consists of intravenous glucose, fluid and electrolyte therapy and supportive measures. As intracranial pressure increases and coma deepens, monitoring of intracranial pressure is initiated. The patient is intubated to maintain a partial pressure of carbon dioxide greater than 20 mm Hg, and pH is regulated. Vitamin K is given and the ammonemia is treated with neomycin given in enemas or by gastric tube. Vigorous antiedema therapy is started with fluid restriction and use of dexamethasone, glycerol and mannitol. Seizure

therapy is instituted as required. This vigorous intensive care therapy has reduced mortality.

Surprisingly, many of the children who survive even deep coma remain remarkably intact. However, in those with the most severe form of Reye's syndrome or in the very young, motor disorders of voice and speech have been noted and deficits in neurologic function, intellectual capacity and emotional behavior have been well documented.

The role of aspirin in the etiology of Reye's syndrome is controversial. Although a firm decision regarding warning labels and contraindications has not been made, it is probably unwise to use aspirin to treat varicella or influenza in a child less than 18 years of age. □

Section II

Common Problems in Neurology

Frank H. Netter, M.D.

in collaboration with

Louis R. Caplan, M.D. *Plates 1–7, 15*

Paul T. Gross, M.D. *Plate 8*

Barbara F. Westmoreland, M.D. *Plates 9–14*

Migraine

Aura

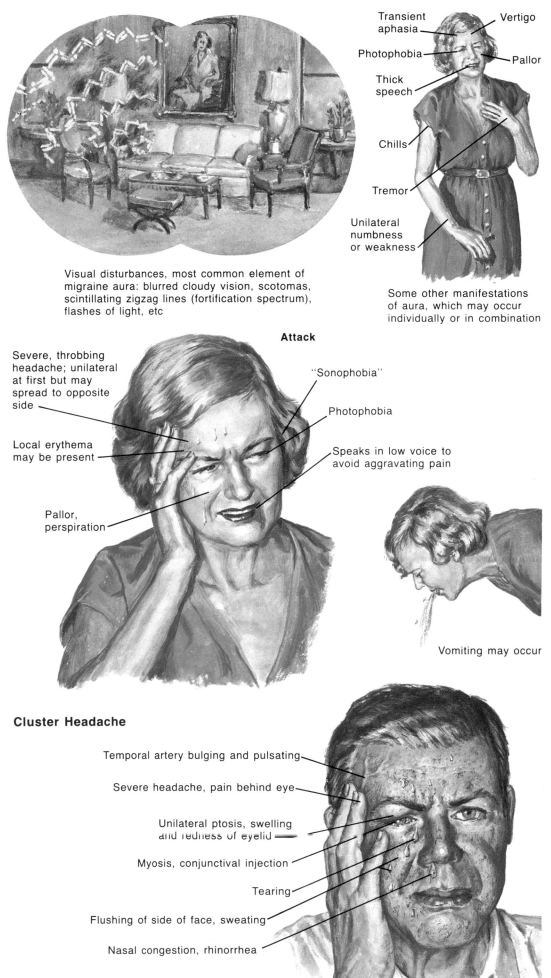

Visual disturbances, most common element of migraine aura: blurred cloudy vision, scotomas, scintillating zigzag lines (fortification spectrum), flashes of light, etc

Transient aphasia · Vertigo · Photophobia · Pallor · Thick speech · Chills · Tremor · Unilateral numbness or weakness

Some other manifestations of aura, which may occur individually or in combination

Attack

Severe, throbbing headache; unilateral at first but may spread to opposite side · "Sonophobia" · Photophobia · Local erythema may be present · Speaks in low voice to avoid aggravating pain · Pallor, perspiration

Vomiting may occur

Cluster Headache

Temporal artery bulging and pulsating · Severe headache, pain behind eye · Unilateral ptosis, swelling and redness of eyelid · Myosis, conjunctival injection · Tearing · Flushing of side of face, sweating · Nasal congestion, rhinorrhea

Headache

A physician treating a patient for the common complaint of headache must first decide whether the headache indicates serious cranial or intracranial disease or is one of a group of benign, usually recurrent headache syndromes (vascular headache or muscle contraction headache and their variants).

The brain itself is insensitive to pain, but the vessels on the surface of the brain, the meninges, and bone are pain-sensitive. Headache is usually caused by conditions that produce traction or pressure on vessels or by meningeal irritation. Pain is referred to the forehead in lesions of the anterior cranial fossa; to the temple or face in middle fossa lesions; and to the occiput, posterior neck and shoulders in posterior fossa lesions. Convexity tumors often produce parietal or frontal headache on the side of the lesion. Space-occupying lesions nearly always give rise to signs and symptoms of a neurologic disorder, or to seizures.

Diagnosis depends on a thorough history and results of neurologic examination. If the patient's history is typical of a common vascular or muscle contraction syndrome and there are no indications of neurologic dysfunction, extensive laboratory evaluation is unnecessary; prudent observation for the appearance of neurologic symptoms is sufficient.

In a typical headache, especially in one of recent onset, computed tomography (CT), electroencephalography, skull radiographs and lumbar puncture may be necessary for diagnosis. It is crucial to detect small subarachnoid hemorrhages, so-called sentinel leaks, from intracranial aneurysms because they can warn of an impending large, often fatal hemorrhage. When headache develops abruptly, lasts more than 24 hours, and prevents normal activities in a patient who does not have a history of recurrent headache, lumbar puncture is indicated to exclude subarachnoid hemorrhage or infection.

Migraine

The most common recurrent headache syndrome is migraine (vascular headache), which affects as much as 25% of the population at some period of life. Onset of migraine is most often in childhood (especially near puberty) or during the first 3 decades of life. This hereditary disorder is characterized by recurrent, transient neurologic disturbances, headache, and postheadache disorders such as polyuria. The presence of neurologic dysfunction in *classic migraine* differentiates this syndrome from *common migraine*, which is probably at least 5 times more frequent but has no associated neurologic deficit.

Muscle Contraction Headache

Intermittent, recurrent or constant head pain, often in forehead, temples, or back of head and neck. Commonly described as "bandlike," "tightness" or "viselike"

Soreness of scalp; pain on combing hair

Occipital tension

Bandlike constriction

Temporal tightness or pressure

Pressure on contracted muscle may augment pain

Rigidity of neck

Sleep disturbances common. Diurnal incidence: headache occurs most often between 4 and 8 AM and 4 and 8 PM

Psychogenic factors: emotional conflict and depression often seen in chronic headache

Headache
(Continued)

Neurologic Symptoms. In classic migraine, neurologic symptoms most often precede headache, although they may occur with or without headache and usually last 20 to 30 minutes. Cerebral blood flow studies during this ischemic, or *aura*, phase usually show regions of decreased intracerebral perfusion. The most common symptoms are visual (Plate 1). Bright, shining, often scintillating, small white or colored shapes appear in the visual field. Sometimes described as dots, stars, angles or "heat waves," the shapes move gradually across the visual field, leaving in their wake areas of decreased vision, or scotomas. The shimmering brightness of these shapes and their slow movement across the visual field are important features that are unusual in amaurosis fugax caused by occlusive vascular disease, which must be considered in the differential diagnosis.

The visual symptoms in migraine last from 5 to 60 minutes, with an average duration of 20 minutes. After the visual symptoms clear, somatosensory symptoms, especially paresthesias, develop in some patients. Tingling may begin in a small region such as the fingers and usually spreads gradually on one side of the body to the hand, arm and face. The leg and trunk are rarely affected. Paresthesias may spread in unusual anatomic patterns, such as from one side of the face to the other. As the wave of paresthesias advances, numbness remains. Paresthesias, as well as visual symptoms, may occur alone or the symptoms may be complex, with one sensory modality affected after another has cleared. Confusion, aphasia, vertigo, blindness and even hemiparesis can also occur.

Headache. The pain of classic migraine usually begins in the temple or forehead. It typically is hemicranial, often spreading from one side to the other, but may be generalized. Usually described as pulsing, pounding or throbbing, it also can be steady, reaching crescendo within 10 minutes to 1 hour. Photophobia, nausea and vomiting frequently accompany the headache, which commonly lasts for hours and disappears after a nap or nocturnal sleep. After the headache subsides, elation, polyuria and diarrhea can occur.

Important variants of classic migraine are *basilar migraine*, in which vertigo, ataxia, diplopia and dysarthria mimic occlusive disease of the posterior cerebral circulation, and *ophthalmoplegic migraine*, in which paralysis of the extraocular muscles develops during the headache and may persist for days afterward.

Most often cited precipitating factors of headache include ingestion of alcohol and food substances such as chocolates, sharp cheese, processed meats and hot dogs; exercise and intercourse; sudden shift from hot to cold external temperatures, or vice versa; high altitude; use of reserpine, nitroglycerin or other vasodilating drugs; hypertension; hunger; nasal congestion; and withdrawal from caffeine or ergot compounds. Headaches usually begin in the morning on arising and seem to occur often on a Saturday or following a prolonged or intense period of work or study.

Frequency varies, but may be seasonal or cluster for weeks or months. In women, headaches may cluster around the menses and are usually affected by pregnancy, worsening in the first and third trimesters and puerperium and relenting in the second trimester. Occasionally, headache is dramatically improved during pregnancy.

Diagnosis. The diagnosis of migraine depends on the characteristics of the headache, previous identification of any single attack of classic migraine, a positive family history, presence of common precipitants of headache, alleviation of headache by pressure exerted by the examiner on the ipsilateral carotid artery or preauricular artery, and response to appropriate therapeutic agents.

Treatment. Anticonvulsants, ergot compounds, beta-adrenergic blocking agents, calcium channel blocking agents, as well as antiserotonin

Giant-Cell (Temporal) Arteritis, Polymyalgia Rheumatica

Headache
(Continued)

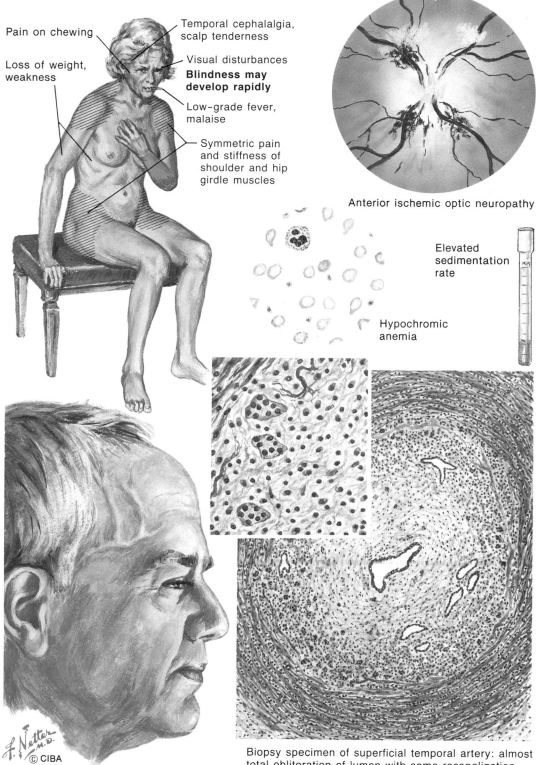

Pain on chewing

Temporal cephalalgia, scalp tenderness

Loss of weight, weakness

Visual disturbances
Blindness may develop rapidly

Low-grade fever, malaise

Symmetric pain and stiffness of shoulder and hip girdle muscles

Anterior ischemic optic neuropathy

Elevated sedimentation rate

Hypochromic anemia

Rigid, tender, nonpulsating temporal arteries may be visible or palpable

Biopsy specimen of superficial temporal artery: almost total obliteration of lumen with some recanalization. High-power insert shows infiltration with lymphocytes, plasma cells and giant cells; fragmentation of elastica

compounds all are effective to a variable degree in individual patients. Overuse of ergot compounds must be avoided in patients with peripheral vascular disease because of the danger of gangrene.

Cluster Headache

A variety of migraine, cluster headache occurs primarily in men 35 to 50 years of age. The pain begins abruptly behind or around one eye and spreads over the affected side, rapidly reaching crescendo and becoming severe, sharp and excruciating. It is usually brief, lasting 20 to 60 minutes. In an individual cluster attack, the pain is limited to one side of the face but may occur on the other side in subsequent clusters. Associated symptoms include unilateral facial flushing and warmth, oculosympathetic paralysis, tearing and redness of the eye, and rhinorrhea (Plate 1).

Headache most often awakens the patient at night several hours after he has retired, and can recur during the day, especially after a nap. Alcohol almost invariably precipitates a headache. Headaches cluster, occurring at least daily for a period of 4 to 12 weeks (average, 6 weeks), and then may disappear for years. They sometimes recur repeatedly at the same time of the year.

Treatment. Ergot compounds, corticosteroids and some migraine remedies are effective. Indomethacin dramatically relieves chronic paroxysmal hemicrania, a similar type of head pain that occurs daily but does not cluster.

Muscle Contraction Headache

Usually caused by emotional tension or depression, muscle contraction headaches occur most frequently in adulthood. However, these headaches can be caused by arthritis of the cervical spine, prolonged fixed posture of the head and neck, or soft-tissue neck injury or strain. They may also follow or complicate migraine, when a patient keeps his head taut in an effort to reduce the pain.

Constant contraction of the temporal, pericranial, occipital and nuchal muscles creates traction on the pain-sensitive cranium and gives rise to local metabolites that cause pain. The pain is bilateral, constant and nonpulsatile and is concentrated in the forehead, occipital or nuchal area. Patients describe the discomfort as a dull pressure, as though a cap, band or vise were around the head (Plate 2).

Muscle contraction headaches usually begin during the day and gradually increase in intensity as the day and evening progress. Alcohol or exercise may relieve or reduce the pain rather than exacerbating the headache, as in migraine. Headaches usually occur daily during a stressful period and may persist for days, weeks or months without respite. Light-headedness, dizziness and giddiness are frequent associated symptoms, and most patients say the headaches discourage and prevent them from performing their usual activities.

Treatment. Muscle contraction headaches are usually treated symptomatically with local heat, massage, muscle relaxants, tranquilizers or anti-

depressants. However, if severe emotional problems are the basis for the headaches, psychiatric counseling may be indicated.

Temporal (Giant-Cell) Arteritis

An inflammatory disease that occurs in late life, temporal (giant-cell) arteritis affects the temporal branches of the external carotid artery. It causes steady, aching pain in the temples and occiput, usually accompanied by malaise, fever and apathy. The temporal and occipital vessels are usually firm, tender and pulseless, and sausage-shaped thickenings can be palpated along the vessel wall (Plate 3). Occasionally, intracranial vessels are affected, especially the infraclinoid internal

Headache
(Continued)

carotid artery at the carotid siphon and the vertebral artery just before it pierces the dura. The erythrocyte sedimentation rate is usually elevated, and arteriography or biopsy documents the thickened granulomatous arteritis.

The patient rarely feels entirely well, and may note tenderness of the forehead and scalp, especially when combing the hair. Joint and muscle pain may be prominent; jaw claudication and tongue ulceration occur infrequently. Sudden monocular blindness or development of scotomas is a feared complication. Visual loss is seldom reversible, and usually affects both eyes if the disease is not quickly treated.

Treatment. Prompt treatment is mandatory in patients with headache of recent onset, a sedimentation rate over 50 mm, and impending blindness. Prednisone administered orally in a dosage of 40 to 60 mg/day almost immediately relieves the symptoms and generally protects the patient from later blindness. Corticosteroids should be continued for at least 6 months.

Trigeminal Neuralgia and Facial Pain

Sharp jabs or jolts of severe, momentary lancinating pain, often occurring in flurries or machine gun-like volleys, are the hallmark of trigeminal neuralgia (tic douloureux). Pain may affect any division of the trigeminal (V) nerve (Plate 4), but is most common in the maxillary division (nasal crease, cheek, zygomatic bone, upper lip, teeth, gums and palate) and in the mandibular division (lower teeth, lip, gums and jaw, and the skin below the oral cavity).

The pain can be elicited by touching sensitive "trigger" zones in the skin and oral cavity, and is often worse during eating, talking, chewing, shaving and exposure of the sensitive areas to cold. There are no symptoms or signs of fifth cranial nerve dysfunction, such as facial numbness or paresthesias; loss of facial sensibility to touch, pin or temperature; weakness of jaw or masticatory muscles; or loss of corneal reflex. Function of adjacent cranial nerves (especially the sixth, seventh and eighth) is preserved. Although radiographic procedures fail to reveal the cause of trigeminal neuralgia, exploration usually shows a loop of one of the cerebellar arteries impinging on the trigeminal nerve root.

This disorder characteristically affects persons in their sixth decade or older. Remission of months or years may follow weeks of severe pain, but the disease eventually recurs.

Differential Diagnosis. It is important to differentiate trigeminal neuralgia from disorders producing similar signs and symptoms. For example, *symptomatic tic* is most often caused by tumors of the fifth or eighth cranial nerve or cerebellopontine angle and metastatic spread of nasopharyngeal tumors to the skull base. In contrast

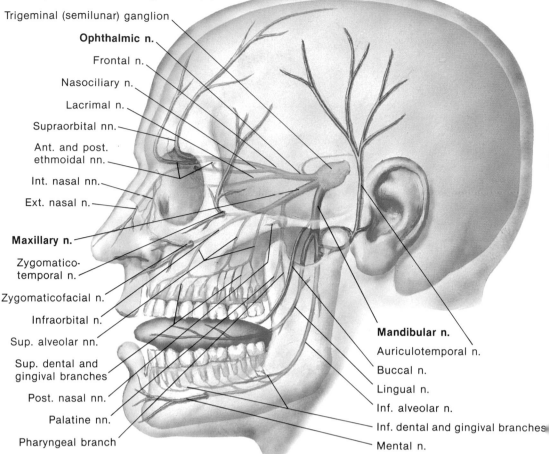

Trigeminal Neuralgia

Sensory distribution of trigeminal (V) nerve

- Trigeminal (semilunar) ganglion
- **Ophthalmic n.**
- Frontal n.
- Nasociliary n.
- Lacrimal n.
- Supraorbital nn.
- Ant. and post. ethmoidal nn.
- Int. nasal nn.
- Ext. nasal n.
- **Maxillary n.**
- Zygomatico-temporal n.
- Zygomaticofacial n.
- Infraorbital n.
- Sup. alveolar nn.
- Sup. dental and gingival branches
- Post. nasal nn.
- Palatine nn.
- Pharyngeal branch
- **Mandibular n.**
- Auriculotemporal n.
- Buccal n.
- Lingual n.
- Inf. alveolar n.
- Inf. dental and gingival branches
- Mental n.

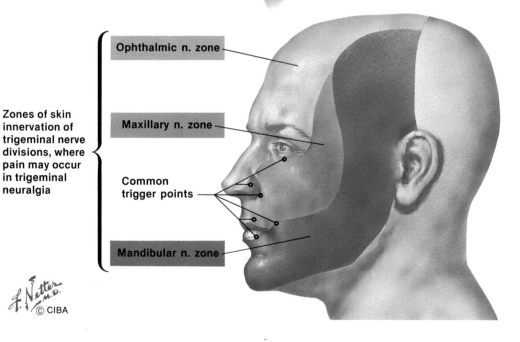

Zones of skin innervation of trigeminal nerve divisions, where pain may occur in trigeminal neuralgia

- Ophthalmic n. zone
- Maxillary n. zone
- Common trigger points
- Mandibular n. zone

to trigeminal neuralgia, these tumors produce steady pain and are associated with signs and symptoms of dysfunction of the trigeminal and the adjacent cranial nerves.

Trigeminal neuralgia, as well as temporal arteritis and cluster headache, must also be differentiated from diseases affecting the eye, nose and paranasal sinuses, oral cavity, salivary glands, as well as the facial and jaw bones, joints and musculature. Acute closed-angle *glaucoma* usually causes a red, painful eye and blurred vision. The pain is steady, often worse in a dark room, and not intermittent as in cluster headache or trigeminal neuralgia. *Acute sinusitis* produces steady pain and tenderness in the maxillary and frontal regions,

and radiographs show clouding of the antrum or frontal sinuses. *Dentalgia* is characterized by severe local pain and tooth tenderness. In *temporomandibular joint dysfunction*, the pain is steady and usually chronic; involves the jaw, zygomatic bone and temples; and is worse on opening the jaw or biting.

Treatment. Carbamazepine in a dosage of 1,200 mg/day is helpful in more than 50% of patients with trigeminal neuralgia. Numerous surgical procedures have also been used in conditions refractory to medical treatment, including radio frequency lesions, alcohol or other chemical injections, and decompression of the nerve by displacement of compressive vascular loops. □

Causes of Vertigo

The word "dizziness" is used by different people to describe a variety of feelings. To some, it refers to giddiness or abnormal cephalic sensations, as in confusion, intoxification, depression or dementia. Others describe faintness or near syncope as dizziness, and still others restrict use of the term to a description of vertigo, a sensation of motion of the environment. Patients commonly describe vertigo as spinning, turning, rotating, and a feeling that they or their environment is moving, so that they must "hang on" to avoid falling.

Vertigo may be caused by dysfunction of any of the structures that detect or relay vestibular input to the brain: labyrinthine receptors within the inner ear; the vestibular part of the vestibulocochlear (VIII) nerve; vestibular nuclei in the tegmental region of the medulla and pons; the flocculonodular lobes of the cerebellum; the lateral thalami, way stations for afferent vestibular input; and the medial temporal lobes, which ultimately receive vestibular information and make us consciously aware of rotation (see CIBA COLLECTION, Volume 1/I, pages 176–180, 182, 190–191). In order to diagnose accurately and treat a patient with vertigo, it is essential first to localize the disorder to one of these regions.

Useful clues to localization include an analysis of the following.

1. *Effect of movement or change of position.* Patients with labyrinthine lesions are very sensitive to motion. They are more comfortable when they are stationary, because dizziness increases with movement. In one particular vestibular disorder, "benign positional vertigo," nystagmus and a sensation of spinning are precipitated by turning, especially when the patient first reclines or arises.

2. *Character of the dizziness.* The more peripheral the lesion, the more likely are patients to describe the sensation as spinning, turning or revolving; central nervous system (CNS) lesions produce a feeling of rocking, wavering or instability. The patient who has cerebellar disease often localizes the disability to the legs and denies a cephalic sensation of dizziness.

3. *Abnormal symptoms or signs referable to dysfunction of adjacent structures.* Ear pain, tinnitus and decreased hearing point to disease of the ear or eighth cranial nerve, although tumors of the eighth cranial nerve usually do not cause episodic vertigo. The brainstem tegmentum near the vestibular nuclei is packed with important structures, so that brainstem disease that causes vertigo is usually accompanied by facial pain, numbness or tingling; limb weakness or ataxia; loss of sensation on the body or trunk; dysphagia; dysarthria; hoarseness; or Horner's syndrome. Headache is also common. Vertigo that is not associated with other signs or symptoms is almost always due to peripheral vestibular disease.

4. *Prior attacks.* Many patients who have peripheral vestibular disease have recurrent attacks of spinning dizziness for years, whereas brainstem ischemia usually causes dizziness and

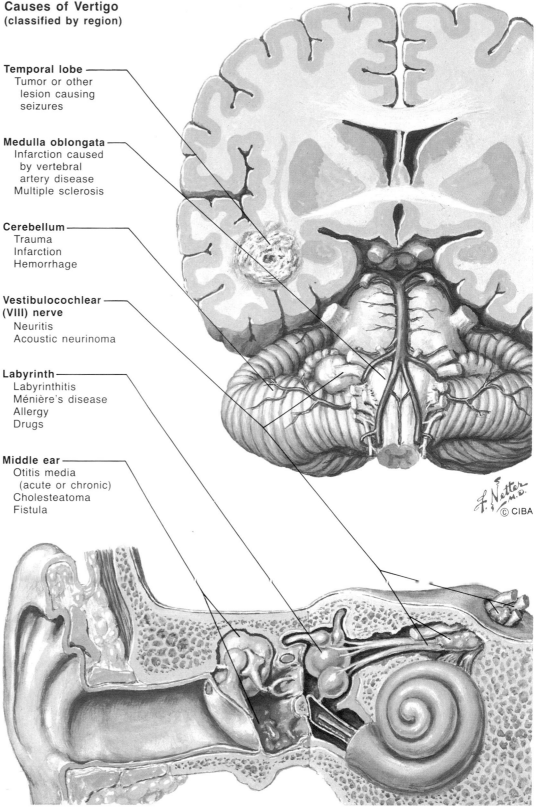

Causes of Vertigo
(classified by region)

Temporal lobe
Tumor or other lesion causing seizures

Medulla oblongata
Infarction caused by vertebral artery disease
Multiple sclerosis

Cerebellum
Trauma
Infarction
Hemorrhage

Vestibulocochlear (VIII) nerve
Neuritis
Acoustic neurinoma

Labyrinth
Labyrinthitis
Ménière's disease
Allergy
Drugs

Middle ear
Otitis media (acute or chronic)
Cholesteatoma
Fistula

other symptoms during a period limited to weeks or a few months.

5. *Nystagmus.* In peripheral vestibular disease, subjective vertigo equals or exceeds nystagmus, whereas in CNS disease, nystagmus may predominate, with minimal dizziness. Vertical nystagmus usually indicates brainstem disease.

6. *Laboratory tests.* Electroencephalography, audiometry, caloric stimulation and computed tomography (CT) are often helpful in localizing the lesions.

Loss of hearing and decreased response to caloric stimulation in addition to vertigo suggest an *acoustic neurinoma*, which can be documented by contrast-enhanced CT. The most common brain-stem lesions that cause vertigo are ischemia secondary to *vertebral artery disease* and *multiple sclerosis*. *Ischemic thalamic lesions* are usually associated with sensory loss and ataxia. *Temporal lobe tumors* or *trauma* can produce vertiginous epilepsy, and can be determined by CT or electroencephalography.

Peripheral labyrinthine disease is usually benign but unpleasant, and can be caused by viral infection, allergy, trauma, migraine or drugs, or may be attributable to Ménière's disease. Reassuring the patient that the problem is ear-related and not brain-related is important. Treatment is symptomatic, primarily with antimotion sickness medications. □

Alcoholism

Alcoholism leads to dysfunction at nearly all levels of the nervous system. The effects of alcohol itself are often difficult to differentiate from effects of the poor nutrition, frequent trauma, infection, and occasional ingestion of toxic alcohol substitutes that are associated with the patient's life-style.

Acute alcohol intoxication is manifested by poor judgment, slowed reaction time, sleepiness, dysarthria and ataxia. Twenty-four to 48 hours after consuming excessive amounts of alcohol, a person may have a grand mal seizure or a series of seizures, known as "rum fits" in the alcoholic community. These seizures are generalized and self-limited, and occur only on or after alcohol withdrawal.

Electroencephalography shows low-voltage fast activity, absence of epileptic discharges and also photosensitive myoclonus. Hypomagnesemia and alkalosis accompany the seizures. Standard anticonvulsants do not affect the course of these seizures and thus have no place in their treatment, either in acute situations or prophylactically.

Three to 5 days after alcohol withdrawal, delirium tremens (DTs), characterized by tachycardia, dilated pupils, agitation, hyperactivity, fever and auditory and visual hallucinations can occur. Adequate hydration, sedation, and a search for intercurrent disease such as pancreatitis or infection should be instituted.

Computed tomography (CT) has shown that alcoholism can lead to *cerebral atrophy and dementia.* In some persons, mentation and atrophic changes found on CT scans improve after prolonged abstinence. However, in some chronic alcoholics, the white matter in and near the corpus callosum degenerates, causing a condition referred to as *Marchiafava-Bignami disease.* Symptoms and signs relate to frontal lobe dysfunction and include apathy, apraxia, incontinence, gait abnormalities and forced reflex grasping.

The best known and most important and severe brain affliction caused by alcoholism is the Wernicke-Korsakoff syndrome. This disorder is caused by thiamine deficiency, and also occurs in nonalcoholics with hyperemesis gravidarum or uremia and in persons subsisting on "tea and toast." Nerve cells on the floor of the fourth ventricle, and nerve cells surrounding the cerebral aqueduct (of Sylvius) and third ventricle depend especially on cocarboxylase and transketolase (two coenzymes synthesized from thiamine) for survival and function. Thiamine deprivation leads to acute neuronal dysfunction and breakdown of capillaries and blood vessels in these selected regions. Clinical manifestations include (1) *confusion and poor memory,* evidenced by confabulation and inability to remember recent events; (2) *extraocular movement abnormalities,* commonly nystagmus, sixth nerve and conjugate gaze paresis; (3) *ataxia and abnormal voice control,* caused by degeneration of the anterior cerebellar vermis; and (4) *peripheral neuropathy,*

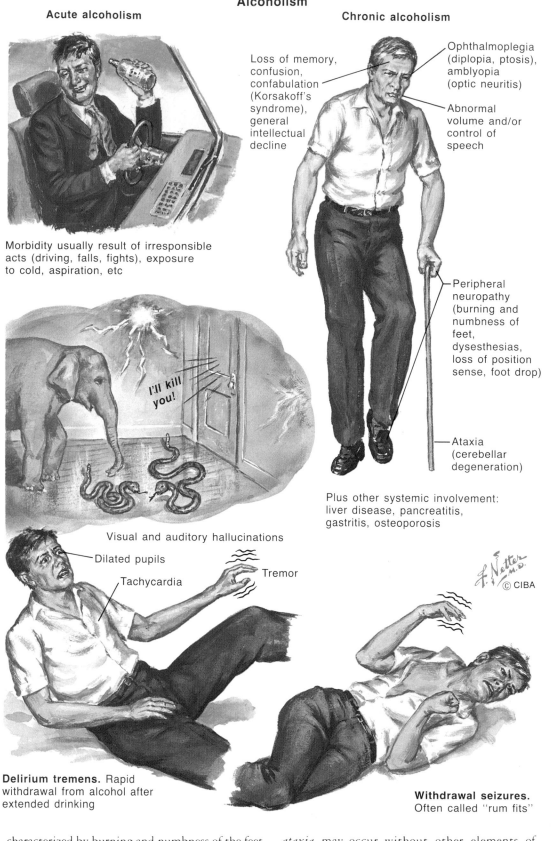

Alcoholism

Acute alcoholism

Morbidity usually result of irresponsible acts (driving, falls, fights), exposure to cold, aspiration, etc

I'll kill you!

Visual and auditory hallucinations

Dilated pupils

Tachycardia

Tremor

Delirium tremens. Rapid withdrawal from alcohol after extended drinking

Chronic alcoholism

Loss of memory, confusion, confabulation (Korsakoff's syndrome), general intellectual decline

Ophthalmoplegia (diplopia, ptosis), amblyopia (optic neuritis)

Abnormal volume and/or control of speech

Peripheral neuropathy (burning and numbness of feet, dysesthesias, loss of position sense, foot drop)

Ataxia (cerebellar degeneration)

Plus other systemic involvement: liver disease, pancreatitis, gastritis, osteoporosis

Withdrawal seizures. Often called "rum fits"

characterized by burning and numbness of the feet and absent ankle jerks, with limb paralysis in the presence of severe nutritional deprivation. Tachycardia, postural hypotension and sudden death are also common in patients with Wernicke's syndrome.

Immediate treatment with thiamine is imperative. Although treatment often quickly reverses ophthalmoplegia, the mental changes and neuropathy do not improve after thiamine. In fact, the neuropathy usually worsens gradually despite treatment, but improves if the patient remains abstinent and eats well.

Amblyopia, often bilateral and with sudden visual loss, may develop in alcoholism. *Cerebellar ataxia* may occur without other elements of Wernicke's syndrome, predominantly affecting the lower limbs and gait and fluctuating with alcohol intake. *Peripheral neuropathy* also often occurs alone. Alcohol and the electrolyte abnormalities accompanying its use can cause muscle dysfunction, often referred to as *alcoholic myopathy.* In some persons with severe protein malnutrition and alcoholism, a *spastic ataxic syndrome* develops as a result of damage to the long tracts in the thoracic spinal cord. These nervous system disorders must be carefully differentiated from subdural hematoma, hepatic encephalopathy, cerebral embolism secondary to alcoholic cardiomyopathy, and central nervous system (CNS) infection. □

Amnesia

The term "amnesia" is used generally to describe impairment or loss of memory, manifested by inability to recall past experiences. Memory is a complex process comprising three different functions: (1) registration of information, (2) storage by reinforcement, and (3) retrieval.

Registration of information. If information is not registered initially, it obviously will not be remembered later. Failure to register is the explanation for absentmindedness, probably the most common abnormality of memory.

Storage by reinforcement. Repetition of information to be remembered or relating such information to other factors or events enhances later recall.

Retrieval. To recall the information, a person must search the "memory bank," where it has been stored. Inability to recall information on request could result from a defect in any of the three aspects of memory function.

The key anatomic regions for registration and storage of memory traces are in an area often referred to as the Papez circuit, in which the fornix connects the hippocampus to the mamillary bodies, which in turn are connected to the anterior nuclei of the thalamus by the mamillothalamic tract. The anterior thalamic nuclei project to the cingulate gyri, which then connect with the hippocampus, completing the circuit. The memory system is primarily cholinergic. The left medial temporal lobe is most concerned with verbal memory, and the right temporal lobe, with visual recall.

The prototype of amnesic disorders is *Korsakoff's syndrome*, seen in chronic alcoholism and other states of vitamin B deficiency. This syndrome affects the medial thalamus and mamillary bodies, and is characterized by an inability to record new memories and recall events of the recent past. Some patients confabulate to fill in gaps in their memory. Any bilateral destructive lesion of the thalami and medial temporal lobes can cause a similar syndrome. Such lesions include gliomas that spread bilaterally over the fornix and splenium of the corpus callosum (see Section V, Plate 3); bilateral posterior cerebral artery infarctions, often caused by embolism of the top of the basilar artery (see Section III, Plate 15); and herpes simplex encephalitis, a viral disease with predilection for temporal lobe damage (see Section VIII, Plate 12). Lesions within the Papez circuit affect the "memory bank." The patient is unable to recall items despite being given cues or being asked to select the correct item to be recalled from a group of alternatives. Unilateral lesions of the left medial temporal lobe and thalamus can produce amnesia that may last up to 6 months.

In disorders that chiefly affect the frontal lobes, such as frontal lobe tumor, Pick's disease or

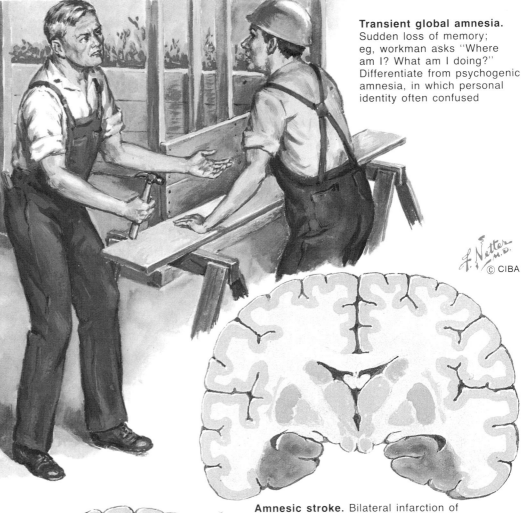

Transient global amnesia. Sudden loss of memory; eg, workman asks "Where am I? What am I doing?" Differentiate from psychogenic amnesia, in which personal identity often confused

Amnesic stroke. Bilateral infarction of hippocampus and medial temporal lobes

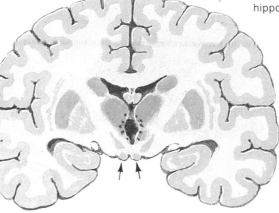

Korsakoff's syndrome. Small hemorrhages around enlarged 3rd ventricle and shrunken mamillary bodies (arrows). Clinical features include memory loss, confabulation, confusion, peripheral neuritis, nystagmus and ophthalmoplegia

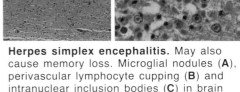

Herpes simplex encephalitis. May also cause memory loss. Microglial nodules (**A**), perivascular lymphocyte cupping (**B**) and intranuclear inclusion bodies (**C**) in brain

Alzheimer's disease (see Section VII, Plates 1–2), the major deficit is in the retrieval of memory traces. Although unable to recall items on request, the patient can select the proper items from a list or after cues are given.

Head trauma often disrupts functions of memory. The hallmark of concussion is *retrograde amnesia*, an inability to recall events from the very recent past, or *posttraumatic amnesia* (often called *anterograde amnesia*), an inability to learn new information after the injury despite recovery of alertness.

Transient global amnesia is a particularly common memory disorder. In this benign syndrome, the patient seems bewildered and asks repetitive questions about the environment and activities, and, despite accurate replies, asks the same questions moments later. The patient cannot form new memories and is often unable to recall events of the past days, months and even years. Speech, reading, writing, calculations, drawing and copying are normal, as are the results of the rest of the neurologic examination. This transient amnesia may occur after a swim in the ocean, a hot shower, a ride in a car or sexual intercourse. Behavior and memory usually return to normal within 24 hours, but the patient is never able to recall events during the period of amnesia. Such attacks may recur, but the cause of the syndrome remains obscure. □

Sleep Disorders

When a patient is concerned about being sleepy during the day, the physician should first consider the nature of the symptoms. Mental fatigue, weariness and depression should not be confused with sleepiness, which is characterized by a pressing need for sleep that cannot always be resisted. The most common cause of excessive sleepiness is insufficient sleep. Sleep requirements vary significantly among individuals. Rarely, adequate daytime alertness can be maintained with as little as 2 to 3 hours of sleep per night. However, most people need 6 to 9 hours of sleep in a 24-hour period. If less sleep is obtained, daytime sleepiness is probably secondary to insufficient sleep.

True excessive daytime sleepiness usually results either from impaired central nervous system (CNS) control of wakefulness and the sleep/wake cycle or from disturbed nocturnal sleep. In order to understand these disorders, it is necessary to have some understanding of sleep physiology.

Sleep is an active process during which many body functions fluctuate, including respiration, temperature, body tone and hormone secretion. A specialized type of sleep, rapid eye movement (REM) sleep, occurs at intervals throughout the night, the first episode usually occurring at about 90 minutes into sleep. REM sleep is associated with dreaming, fleeting eye movements, muscle twitching, a generalized decrease in body tone, and irregular respiration, heartbeat and blood pressure.

Narcolepsy

The most notable disorder resulting from impaired CNS control of wakefulness and the sleep/wake cycle is narcolepsy. This disorder is characterized by the intrusion of REM sleep into the waking state or into the transition periods between waking and sleep. Many narcoleptics are sleepy during most or all of the day, especially during times when normal people may become sleepy, eg, after the noon or evening meal or when watching television. Patients with narcolepsy are subject to narcoleptic sleep attacks, cataplexy, sleep paralysis and hypnagogic hallucinations; however, an individual patient may not have all these symptoms.

The *sleep attacks* may occur at any time of day and in embarrassing or dangerous situations, such as while talking with others, while climbing a ladder, or while driving. Attacks may be preceded by an overwhelming desire to sleep. The attacks are brief, lasting minutes, and the victim usually awakens feeling refreshed.

Cataplexy is characterized by loss of body tone without loss of consciousness. These attacks are also brief, lasting only seconds. The face and head may droop or all the muscles may become limp, resulting in the patient's fall to the floor. Cataplectic attacks occur during periods of sudden excitement and emotional change such as with laughter, anger or fear. Recognizing this, many patients with the narcolepsy syndrome shelter themselves by avoiding situations that may result in emotional change.

Sleep paralysis, which occurs just after awakening or when relaxing before sleep, may be a part of the narcolepsy syndrome or occur as an isolated symptom. Although consciousness is maintained, body tone is lost, resulting in a frightening paralysis lasting seconds to minutes.

Hypnagogic hallucinations also occur in the transition between awakening and sleep. These are vivid, often frightening, images, usually of a strange person or creature in the room.

Other features of narcolepsy include *disrupted nocturnal sleep* and periods of *automatic behavior*.

The narcolepsy syndrome usually starts in the second or third decade and may be lifelong. The cause is generally unknown, although a minority of patients manifest parts of the syndrome following encephalitis, severe head injury or, rarely, a brain tumor.

Sleep Apnea

As noted previously, excessive daytime sleepiness may be associated with disruptions of nocturnal sleep such as those secondary to a respiratory disturbance, or sleep apnea. A notable feature of sleep apnea is that, although sleep may be momentarily disrupted hundreds of times during the night, the patient usually reports sound and uninterrupted sleep. Daytime naps are often not refreshing because the sleep disturbance occurs during the naps as well.

The sleep apnea syndrome results when control of respiration is impaired during sleep. The apnea may be *central*, in which CNS stimulation to the muscles of respiration ceases, or *peripheral*, referring to intermittent obstruction of the oropharyngeal airway. This latter form of sleep apnea is also called *obstructive*, since the relaxed tongue and pharyngeal wall obstruct passage of air through the oropharynx. The terms "central" and "obstructive" do not represent a strict dichotomy, since CNS control of oropharyngeal muscles may be impaired in obstructive sleep apnea and episodes of obstructive sleep apnea are often preceded by central apnea. In such cases, the entire episode is called *mixed apnea*.

Monitoring of nasal, oral, chest and abdominal respiration helps to determine the type of apnea. Cessation of all respiratory activity suggests central apnea, while cessation of airflow through the nose and mouth, with respiratory effort continuing in the chest or abdomen, suggests obstructive apnea. Occasional brief episodes of apnea are a normal phenomenon, especially in the transition periods of sleep and in elderly persons. For some patients, however, the apnea is prolonged, lasts more than a minute, and occurs frequently. Monitoring shows that oxygen saturation falls, and an arrhythmia may also occur during apnea. Episodes of apnea may occur hundreds of times during the night, disrupting the flow of sleep and often associated with brief periods of arousal, as recorded on the electroencephalogram (EEG).

The consequences of sleep apnea may be life-threatening and include pulmonary and systemic hypertension and cardiac arrhythmia. In addition, the severe excessive daytime sleepiness is a frequent cause of automobile accidents, as exemplified by one patient's description of "catnapping on the straightaways and waking up for the curves."

In obstructive sleep apnea, which is often more severe than the central type, there is usually no daytime respiratory disturbance. This type of apnea occurs in thin as well as in obese patients. Unusually *loud snoring* is such a typical feature of obstructive sleep apnea that the physician, on hearing of this symptom, should seriously consider sleep apnea. Commonly, the noise prevents anyone else from sleeping in the same room as the patient, and the snoring can easily be heard throughout the house. The obstruction is typically worse when a person is sleeping in the supine position and during REM sleep, in which muscle relaxation is generalized and respiration is irregular. Obstructive sleep apnea may be present in childhood or at any time of adult life, and is 30 times more common in men than in women.

Nocturnal Movement Disorders

Another cause of excessive daytime sleepiness associated with disturbed nocturnal sleep is *nocturnal myoclonus*. This is a disorder of unknown cause, characterized by repeated movements in an extremity, usually including slow tonic dorsiflexion of the foot. These 1- to 10-second slow movements are often followed by a disruption of sleep and show a brief arousal pattern on the EEG. Sleep may be interrupted several hundred times during the night, although, as in sleep apnea, patients usually report uninterrupted sleep. Patients are usually unaware of the nocturnal movements. If the movements are vigorous, the patient's bed partner will be disturbed.

Nocturnal myoclonus should be differentiated from brief, generalized myoclonic jerks, which may occur at the onset of sleep. This is a normal phenomenon, especially in children.

Another nocturnal movement disorder, the *restless legs syndrome*, may delay the onset of sleep sufficiently to lead to excessive daytime sleepiness. Patients with this syndrome experience nagging, itchy, roving dysesthesias in the legs. The sensation is often brought on by reclining, and relieved by standing or walking. The syndrome may be associated with neuropathy or vascular insufficiency, but often the cause is obscure.

Less Common Sleep Disorders

Idiopathic CNS hypersomnolence, a poorly understood disorder, may result from poor brain control of waking, and is sometimes seen following a CNS insult. As in narcolepsy, this disorder is characterized by episodes of irresistible sleep, but the naps tend to be longer than in narcolepsy and are not refreshing. Other frequent symptoms are constant daytime sleepiness, as well as prolonged nocturnal sleep, and "sleep drunkenness," an inability to fully awaken during the several hours following nighttime sleep. Cataplexy and the other types of attacks associated with narcolepsy do not occur in idiopathic CNS hypersomnolence.

The *Kleine-Levin syndrome*, another cause of excessive sleepiness, is characterized by episodes of hypersomnolence lasting several weeks. During an episode, there are brief periods of wakefulness, during which behavioral changes and bulimia may be present.

Sleep Disorders
(Continued)

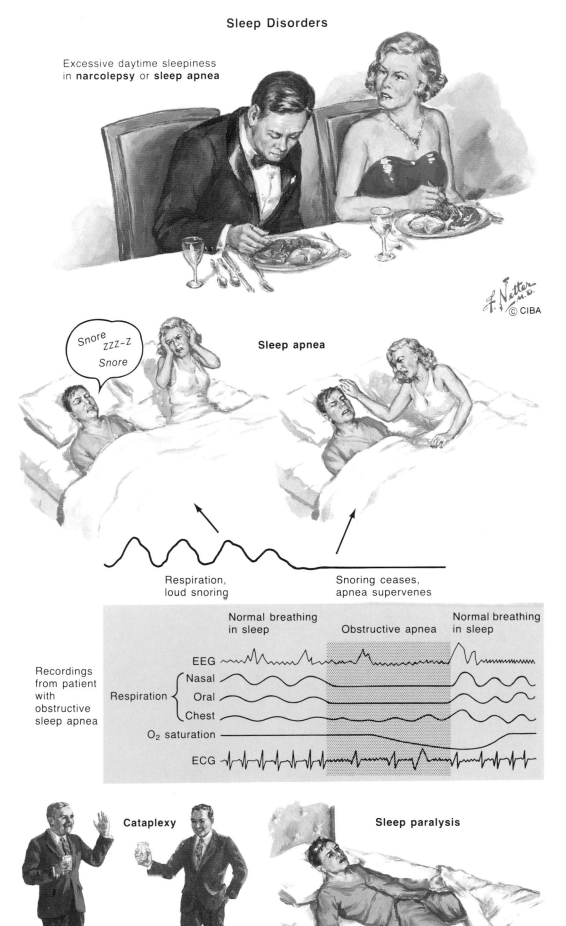

Sleep Disorders

Excessive daytime sleepiness
in **narcolepsy** or **sleep apnea**

Snore
ZZZ–Z
Snore

Sleep apnea

Respiration,
loud snoring

Snoring ceases,
apnea supervenes

Recordings
from patient
with
obstructive
sleep apnea

Respiration

	Normal breathing in sleep	Obstructive apnea	Normal breathing in sleep
EEG			
Nasal			
Oral			
Chest			
O₂ saturation			
ECG			

Cataplexy

Sudden loss of muscular–postural
tone with laughter or fright

Sleep paralysis

Momentary paralysis on awakening
lasts seconds to minutes

Prolonged states of hypersomnolence linked with the *menstrual cycle* have also been reported. Excessive sleepiness, especially in the morning, may be due to *delayed sleep phase insomnia*, a disorder in which the circadian cycle is altered so that the daily sleep period cannot begin before the early morning hours.

Diagnosis and Treatment

A carefully elicited history from the patient and the patient's bed partner, with specific inquiries about the symptoms mentioned above, either indicates the diagnosis or limits the diagnostic possibilities. Results of physical examination are often normal in these disorders but may provide information about associated brain lesions, airway obstruction, vascular insufficiency or neuropathy. Monitoring in the sleep laboratory may be done to determine the degree and type of daytime sleepiness and to diagnose and quantify nocturnal events.

Therapeutic modalities in this field are rapidly changing. CNS stimulants may be given for narcolepsy and respiratory stimulants for sleep apnea. Some patients with obstructive sleep apnea are helped by surgical procedures, such as palatopharyngoplasty or tracheostomy. □

Electroencephalography

The electroencephalogram (EEG) is a record of the electrical activity of the nerve cells of the brain. To record an EEG, small metal disc electrodes are attached to the scalp. The electrodes are then connected to the electroencephalograph, which amplifies the brain activity a million times and records the activity on a moving strip of paper.

Brain Wave Activity. The brain wave activity consists of rhythmic or arrhythmic wave forms, or both, that vary in polarity, shape and frequency, and usually range in voltage from 20 to 60 μV. The activity is divided into four main types, based on the frequency or number of wave forms per second (Hz). *Beta activity* is low-amplitude fast activity with a frequency of more than 13 Hz, and is usually present over the anterior head regions. *Alpha activity* ranges between 8 and 13 Hz. The alpha rhythm is present over the posterior head regions and is the characteristic background frequency of a normal awake person. It occurs when the eyes are closed and is attenuated when the eyes are open. *Theta activity* ranges from 4 to 7 Hz. *Delta activity* is the slowest activity, occurring at a frequency of less than 4 Hz.

The EEG of an awake person consists of alpha activity and some low-amplitude beta activity. During light to moderate levels of non-rapid eye movement (NREM) sleep, the EEG shows spindle activity (10 to 14 Hz sinusoidal activity) and V waves (vertex waves, high-amplitude sharp waves). During deeper levels of NREM sleep, high-voltage delta frequency slow waves are present. During rapid eye movement (REM) sleep (dream stage), the EEG consists of a low-amplitude background with rapid eye movements.

The EEG shows different patterns at different ages. For example, in an infant, the EEG shows amorphous delta activity, whereas in a young child, it shows moderate-amplitude activity in the theta and alpha range, with a progressive increase in background frequencies as the child gets older. In young and middle-aged adults, the EEG shows moderate-amplitude alpha activity, and in older adults, lower-amplitude alpha activity, with slower background frequencies and some scattered theta and delta wave forms.

The main types of abnormalities that may be seen in the EEG are slowing, epileptiform activity and suppression of activity.

Slow-wave abnormalities range from slowing of the background frequencies to slowing in the delta frequency range. The slower the frequency, the more severe is the abnormality.

Epileptiform activity consists of sharp waves, spikes and spike-and-wave discharges, which are associated with the presence of a seizure disorder.

Suppression of activity represents an attenuation or absence of cerebral activity.

Indications for EEG. The main indications for obtaining an EEG are seizure disorders, transient spells (see Section III, Plate 4), intracranial disease processes (see Section V), coma (Plate 15) and brain death (see Section III, Plate 37).

Electroencephalography

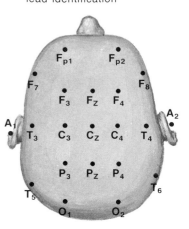

Electrode placement and lead identification

Odd numbers, left side
Even numbers, right side
Z locations, midline

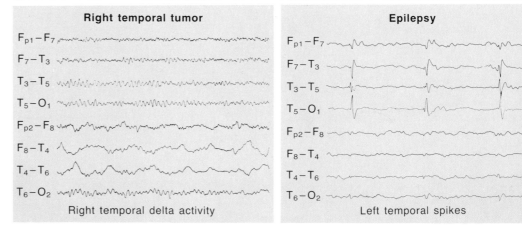

EEG in normal awake person, eyes closed

$F_{p1}-F_3$ Beta
F_3-C_3
C_3-P_3
P_3-O_1 Alpha
$F_{p2}-F_4$ Beta
F_4-C_4
C_4-P_4
P_4-O_2 Alpha

Normal sleep

F_3-A_1
F_4-A_2
C_3-A_1
C_4-A_2
P_3-A_1
P_4-A_2
O_1-A_1
O_2-A_2

Sleep spindles

Right temporal tumor

$F_{p1}-F_7$
F_7-T_3
T_3-T_5
T_5-O_1
$F_{p2}-F_8$
F_8-T_4
T_4-T_6
T_6-O_2

Right temporal delta activity

Epilepsy

$F_{p1}-F_7$
F_7-T_3
T_3-T_5
T_5-O_1
$F_{p2}-F_8$
F_8-T_4
T_4-T_6
T_6-O_2

Left temporal spikes

The greatest usefulness of the EEG is in the diagnosis of a *seizure disorder*. Depending on the type and location of the discharge, the EEG often can indicate the type of seizure disorder present.

The EEG is also helpful in the evaluation of *transient spells* such as transient ischemic attacks, syncope or hysterical episodes.

In intracranial disease processes, the EEG is helpful in detecting or confirming the presence of *focal cerebral abnormalities* such as focal mass lesions (tumors or abscesses) or focal vascular lesions involving the cerebral hemispheres.

Generalized slowing in the EEG indicates a *diffuse disturbance of cerebral function*, which can result from a metabolic disorder, encephalitis or a degenerative process. In certain disease processes, the EEG shows specific diagnostic patterns, such as generalized periodic sharp waves in Jakob-Creutzfeldt disease.

The EEG is particularly useful in the evaluation of *comatose patients*. The tracing may show a distinctive pattern that can confirm the diagnosis of the underlying condition, such as triphasic waves in hepatic coma, spike discharges in status epilepticus, and excessive beta activity in a drug overdose.

Finally, the EEG can be used to confirm *brain death* in patients in whom electroencephalographic activity has ceased and the clinical criteria for brain death are present. □

Causes of Seizures

The sudden, excessive, paroxysmal discharge of neurons that causes a seizure can occur as a result of: (1) a primary intrinsic disturbance affecting the neurons, (2) an alteration in neuronal membrane function or structure, (3) an increase in excitatory synaptic input, (4) a decrease in inhibitory mechanisms, or (5) extraneuronal or extrinsic influences such as metabolic, biochemical or toxic derangements, which in turn affect neuronal function.

Seizures can be classified as primary or secondary, and each type may result from one of a variety of causes.

Primary seizures, formerly called idiopathic or cryptogenic seizures, are thought to result from a constitutional or genetic predisposition in which the threshold for seizures is lower than normal. Most primary seizures are generalized from onset and consist of either absence (petit mal) or generalized tonic-clonic (grand mal) seizures.

Secondary seizures result from a known pathologic lesion or disease process, which may be either intracranial or extracranial. Secondary seizures may be either focal or generalized, depending on whether the precipitating cause is a focal lesion affecting the brain or a diffuse process causing a widespread disturbance of brain function.

Intracranial Causes. The most common types of intracranial lesions causing seizures are tumors, vascular lesions, head trauma, infectious diseases, congenital defects, and biochemical or degenerative disease processes affecting the brain.

Brain tumor is an important cause of seizures, particularly in the adult patient, becoming an increasingly likely cause after the second decade of life and one of the main causes in the fourth and fifth decades. Until proved otherwise, a brain tumor should be suspected in any person who has onset of seizures, especially focal seizures, after age 20.

Vascular disease is one of the most common causes of seizures in older persons, particularly after age 50. Seizures can occur transiently after an acute stroke (thrombotic, embolic or hemorrhagic) or may develop later as a sequela of cerebrovascular disease. Although uncommon, arteriovenous malformations are frequently associated with seizures. Other vascular causes include subdural hematomas, venous thrombosis and hypertensive encephalopathy.

Head trauma is another common cause of seizures, which may occur shortly after the head injury or, more often, several months to several

Causes of Seizures

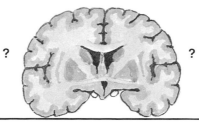

Primary

?   ?   Unknown (genetic or biochemical predisposition)

Intracranial

Tumor

Vascular (infarct or hemorrhage)

Arteriovenous malformation

Trauma (depressed fracture, penetrating wound)

Infection (abscess, encephalitis)

Congenital and hereditary diseases (tuberous sclerosis)

Extracranial

Metabolic

Electrolyte

Biochemical

Inborn errors of metabolism

Anoxia

Hypoglycemia

Drugs

Drug withdrawal

Alcohol withdrawal

years later. Factors that increase the chance of development of posttraumatic seizures are a penetrating head injury, severe damage to the brain, prolonged periods of unconsciousness, posttraumatic amnesia, complications of wound healing, and a persistent neurologic deficit.

Seizures may occur with any *acute infection* of the nervous system or as a complication of damage to the nervous system by the inflammatory process. Patients with *cerebral abscesses* have a high incidence of seizures, and *encephalitis* and *meningoencephalitis* may be associated with either focal or generalized seizures.

Extracranial Causes. Disease processes or disorders that can cause seizures include various

types of metabolic, electrolyte and biochemical disturbances, anoxia; hypoglycemia; toxic processes; drugs; or abrupt withdrawal from drugs or alcohol. Various conditions such as fever, fatigue, sleep deprivation, flashing lights, sound or emotional factors may also precipitate seizures in susceptible individuals.

Other Causes. Congenital and developmental anomalies and heredofamilial biochemical and degenerative diseases of the brain can also cause seizures. Such conditions include tuberous sclerosis, Tay-Sachs disease, phenylketonuria, maple syrup urine disease, homocystinuria, myoclonic epilepsy (Unverricht-Lundborg disease) and other degenerative processes. ☐

Generalized Tonic-Clonic Seizures

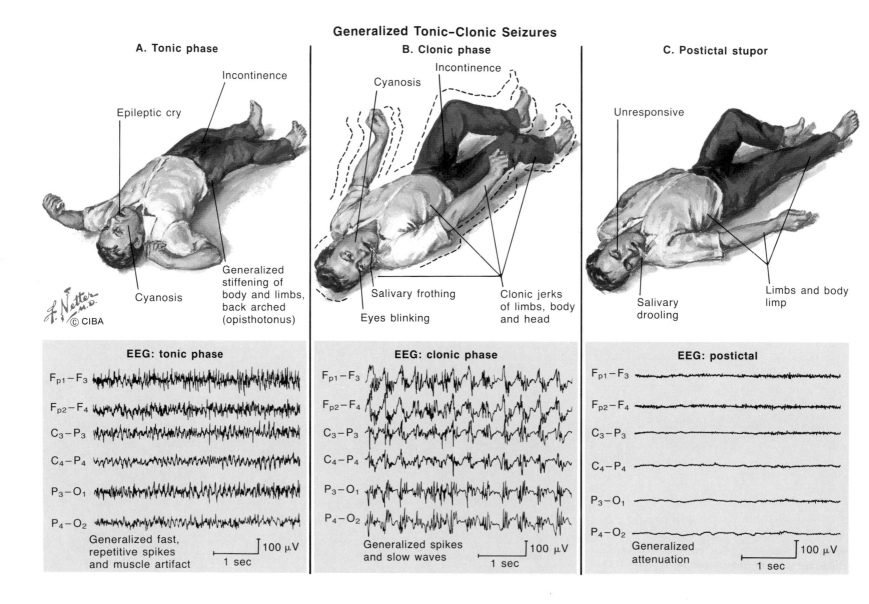

A. Tonic phase

Epileptic cry

Incontinence

Cyanosis

Generalized stiffening of body and limbs, back arched (opisthotonus)

B. Clonic phase

Incontinence

Cyanosis

Salivary frothing

Eyes blinking

Clonic jerks of limbs, body and head

C. Postictal stupor

Unresponsive

Salivary drooling

Limbs and body limp

EEG: tonic phase

Fp1–F3

Fp2–F4

C3–P3

C4–P4

P3–O1

P4–O2

Generalized fast, repetitive spikes and muscle artifact

100 μV

1 sec

EEG: clonic phase

Fp1–F3

Fp2–F4

C3–P3

C4–P4

P3–O1

P4–O2

Generalized spikes and slow waves

100 μV

1 sec

EEG: postictal

Fp1–F3

Fp2–F4

C3–P3

C4–P4

P3–O1

P4–O2

Generalized attenuation

100 μV

1 sec

SECTION II PLATE 11

Slide 3338

Generalized Tonic-Clonic Seizures

A seizure is a transient disturbance of cerebral function resulting from an excessive abnormal discharge of a group of neurons.

The clinical manifestations and type of seizure depend on the site of origin and area of the brain involved by the seizure discharge. Seizures are divided into two main categories: generalized and partial, or focal. A *generalized seizure* involves widespread, bilateral areas of the cerebral hemispheres, including the cerebral cortex, the thalamus and the thalamocortical radiations. A *partial, or focal, seizure* involves a localized area of the cerebral cortex. Generalized seizures include absence (petit mal), generalized tonic-clonic (grand mal), myoclonic, tonic, clonic and atonic (akinetic) seizures and infantile spasms.

A generalized tonic-clonic, or grand mal, seizure is the most severe type of seizure. It starts with a sudden loss of consciousness and generalized tonic stiffening and extension of the body secondary to a widespread contraction of the muscles. The patient utters a piercing epileptic cry resulting from forced expiration of air from the lungs through closed vocal cords. Cessation of respirations, with associated cyanosis, is secondary to the tonic muscle contractions that prevent normal respiratory movements. The patient often bites his tongue during this phase of the seizure. Salivation and frothing at the mouth occur because the patient cannot swallow during the seizure. In addition, urinary incontinence is often present.

The initial *tonic phase* of the seizure is succeeded by fine quivering movements of the muscles and diffuse trembling of the body, which last for several seconds. This period is followed by the *clonic phase*, in which generalized bilaterally synchronous clonic jerks of the body alternate with brief periods of relaxation. As the periods of relaxation become more prolonged, the clonic movements gradually decrease and finally cease.

During the *postictal period* following the seizure, the patient is limp, obtunded and unresponsive. The actual seizure may last about 1 to 2 minutes, while the postictal phase may last from 5 to 20 minutes. Afterward, the patient may arouse but remains confused, and, if left undisturbed, may sleep for an hour or so and awaken with a headache and generalized muscle soreness.

Generalized tonic-clonic seizures may occur at any age. They may be primary generalized seizures, which are generalized from onset, or secondary generalized seizures, which start as focal seizures and then become generalized as the seizure activity progresses to involve widespread areas of the brain.

Electroencephalographic Findings. The EEG of a generalized tonic-clonic seizure shows various types of seizure activity, which correspond to the different phases of the seizure. During the tonic phase, the EEG shows fast, repetitive, generalized spike discharges. During the clonic phase, the EEG shows spike-and-wave discharges, with the spike corresponding to the clonic jerks and the slow wave to the period of relaxation. The spikes gradually slow in frequency during the trembling phase. Finally, during the postictal phase, the EEG shows generalized attenuation followed by slow-wave activity, which gradually decreases as the patient recovers from the seizure.

Treatment. The drugs of choice for treatment of generalized tonic-clonic seizures are phenobarbital, phenytoin and carbamazepine. □

Absence (Petit Mal) and Other Generalized Seizures

Absence (Petit Mal) Seizures. One of the mildest forms of generalized seizure disorders, absence seizures, occur predominantly in children. They usually consist of simple absence episodes lasting 5 to 10 seconds, during which time the patient loses awareness of what is going on around him and shows a decrease in responsiveness and an interruption or cessation of motor activity. During the seizure, the patient has a blank stare, which may be accompanied by minor motor movements such as upward deviation of the eyes and mild twitching of the eyes, eyelids, face or limbs.

Sometimes, absence seizures are more complex and are accompanied by clonic movements of the face and extremities; apparently automatic behavior; chewing; lip smacking or mouthing movements; or a change or loss in postural tone, during which the patient may sway or stumble. The patient is often unaware that he has had a seizure, but usually recognizes that he has had a "blank" period.

In the untreated patient, absence seizures can occur quite frequently during the day. They sometimes occur in groups, particularly when the child is tired or drowsy. Hyperventilation can easily provoke absence seizures, and hypoglycemia and emotional stress can also potentiate attacks. Absence seizures are usually a relatively benign type of seizure disorder and often resolve after adolescence.

The electroencephalogram (EEG) in absence seizures shows a characteristic and diagnostic pattern of repetitive and stereotyped 3/second spike-and-wave discharges occurring in a generalized and bisynchronous fashion over the two hemispheres. Having the patient hyperventilate during the EEG recording helps to precipitate an absence seizure and the spike-and-wave pattern on the EEG.

The two drugs that are most widely used for the treatment of absence seizures are ethosuximide and valproic acid.

Other Generalized Seizures. Myoclonic seizures are abrupt, brief, involuntary jerks or contractions of the body, extremities or face, or of all these areas, and are associated with a generalized spike or spike-and-wave discharge on the EEG.

Tonic seizures, which consist of abrupt extension movements of the limbs, are associated with rapid serial spike discharges on the EEG.

Clonic seizures, which are characterized by repetitive jerks or twitching movements of the limbs, body or facial muscles, or of all of these

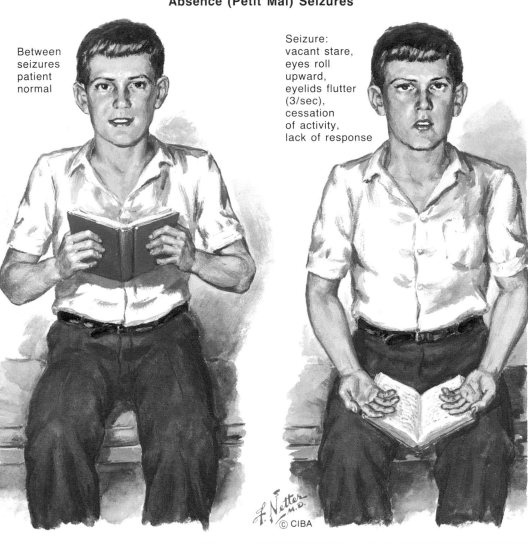

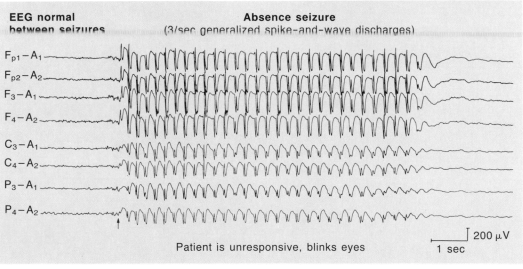

muscle groups, are accompanied by spike or spike-and-wave discharges on the EEG.

Atonic (akinetic) seizures are manifested by sudden loss of muscle tone, or a sudden fall to the ground. The EEG shows generalized spike-and-wave complexes.

Drugs used in the treatment of generalized seizures include clonazepam, diazepam and valproic acid.

Infantile spasms are brief episodes of tonic flexor or extensor movements, or both, of the body and limbs. These spasms are seen in infants and young children up to 4 years of age, and usually result from a severe cerebral insult before, at, or shortly following birth, or from an insult or disease process occurring within the first few months to

1 year following birth. One of the most common types of infantile spasm is characterized by forward flexion of the head and body with the arms flung forward and outward. The EEG in infantile spasms shows a characteristic pattern called hypsarrhythmia, consisting of high-amplitude multifocal spikes and slow waves. During the spasm, the EEG shows an abrupt generalized decrement in the amplitude of the ongoing activity.

Infantile spasms are often treated with adrenocorticotropic hormone (ACTH) or corticosteroids. Clonazepam has been used occasionally, and in some refractory conditions, a ketogenic diet may be helpful in controlling the seizures. □

Simple and Complex Partial Seizures

Partial, or focal, seizures originate from a seizure focus in a localized area of the cerebral cortex. Clinical manifestations depend on the site of origin and area of the brain involved by the seizure focus. Partial seizures are divided into two main types: *simple partial seizures*, in which there is no loss of consciousness, and *complex partial seizures*, in which consciousness is impaired.

Simple Partial Seizures

Focal motor, focal sensory and autonomic are the three classifications of simple partial seizures.

Focal motor seizures often originate in the frontal cortex. Seizures involving the motor strip area (precentral gyrus) are characterized by tonic-clonic movements of the opposite side of the body.

The tonic-clonic activity can occur in the face, extremities or body as discrete focal seizures, or these can spread sequentially to various parts of the body as a Jacksonian march or seizure. Named after John Hughlings Jackson, a Jacksonian seizure consists of tonic-clonic movements that begin in one part of the body, usually the face or hand, and progressively spread to involve other areas of the body in a sequential manner reflecting the somatotopic representation of the body in the motor strip area. The seizures may remain localized to one side of the body or may become secondarily generalized. Occasionally, a focal motor seizure may be followed by a transient weakness (Todd's paralysis) of the affected area of the body that may last for several minutes or hours.

Seizures arising from the supplementary motor area of the cortex (in the mesial portion of the frontal lobe anterior to the motor strip area) are associated with a characteristic posturing of the head and arm, in which the contralateral arm is abducted and elevated and the head and eyes are deviated toward the elevated arm. In addition, the patient may have other symptoms, including vocalization with repetitive utterances of words or sounds, speech and motor arrest, visceral sensations such as a rising epigastric aura, or autonomic symptoms.

Seizures arising in other parts of the frontal lobe may begin with deviation of the head and eyes either away from the side of the seizure focus (contraversive seizures) or to the side of the focus (ipsiversive seizures).

Focal sensory seizures can arise from any of the sensory areas of the cerebral hemispheres.

Somatosensory seizures arise from the sensory strip or postcentral gyrus of the parietal lobe, and are usually manifested as tingling sensation or a "pins and needles" feeling on the contralateral side of the body. The symptoms may involve a part of the body, face or limbs, or they may progress with a march of symptoms similar to that in a Jacksonian seizure.

Visual seizures arise from a focus in the occipital or posterior temporal lobe, and are manifested by formed or unformed visual hallucinations in the opposite visual field. Formed visual hallucinations, which represent actual scenes or pictures, usually arise from a focus in the posterior temporal lobe. *Unformed* visual hallucinations, consisting of flashing lights, scintillating scotomas or dimming of vision, usually arise from a seizure focus in the occipital lobe.

Auditory seizures arise from the superior temporal lobe and are characterized by buzzing, ringing or hissing noises or varying intensities of sound. Sometimes, the patient may hear actual recognizable sounds like music or ringing of bells.

Autonomic seizures are characterized by autonomic changes such as flushing, pallor, sweating, piloerection, epigastric sensations and various vasomotor changes. These usually occur as a result of a focus in the temporal, frontal or peri-insular area.

The electroencephalographic findings in simple partial seizures consist of focal spikes, sharp waves or spike-and-wave discharges over the involved area in the interictal (between seizures) period. During a seizure, the EEG shows repetitive or rhythmic epileptiform discharges.

Drugs that are most useful in the treatment of simple partial seizures are phenobarbital and phenytoin.

Complex Partial Seizures

When consciousness is altered during a focal seizure, the seizure is classified as a complex partial seizure. Most often, complex partial seizures originate from the temporal lobe, but occasionally arise from other locations, such as the frontal lobe. Based on symptomatology, complex partial seizures can be associated with: (1) impaired consciousness only, (2) psychomotor phenomena, (3) psychosensory phenomena, (4) cognitive disturbances, (5) affective symptoms, or (6) speech disturbances.

In complex partial seizures with *impaired consciousness only*, the patient is transiently confused and unaware of what is going on around him but has no other signs or symptoms of seizure activity.

Psychomotor phenomena seen in these seizures include automatisms and masticatory movements. During automatisms, the patient displays some type of automatic movement, such as rubbing his hands or clothes or brushing his hair without being aware of what he is doing. Masticatory movements include such actions as continuous chewing, swallowing, lip smacking, etc.

Psychosensory phenomena consist of illusions or hallucinations. An *illusion* is a distortion of a sensory experience, such as perceiving an object as being smaller or larger, nearer or farther away than it actually is, whereas a *hallucination* is a sensory perception in the absence of an external stimulus. Hallucinations may involve any type of sensory experience and may be either formed (recognizable scenes or sounds) or unformed (flashing lights or buzzing noises).

Olfactory hallucinations often consist of a disagreeable odor and are associated with a discharge in the uncus, which is located in the anterior mesial part of the temporal lobe. This type of seizure is often referred to as an *uncinate seizure*. *Gustatory seizures*, manifested by abnormal taste, occur with a discharge in the peri-insular area. *Visceral sensations* include such symptoms as nausea, a weak feeling in the stomach, a rising epigastric sensation, or a sense of fullness or pressure in the head. These sensations can occur with a discharge in either the temporal or frontal lobes.

Cognitive symptoms reflect a disturbance of thought or perception.

Déjà vu is a feeling of familiarity in an unfamiliar environment, whereas *jamais vu* is a feeling of unfamiliarity in a familiar environment. Time perception may be distorted, or a dreamy state or a feeling of unreality or depersonalization may be present.

Affective symptoms consist of various types of emotions such as fear, anxiety, pleasure or happiness. *Speech disturbances* are manifested by speech automatisms, vocalizations and dysphasia or speech apraxia if the dominant side of the brain is involved.

The interictal EEG shows focal spike or sharp wave discharges over the involved region. Drowsiness and sleep may enhance the presence of epileptiform activity, and a sleep EEG is often helpful in a patient with suspected complex partial seizures. During a seizure, the EEG may show rhythmic sharp waves, slow waves or sinusoidal rhythmic activity over the involved area.

Drugs that are helpful in treating complex partial seizures include carbamazepine, phenytoin and primidone. □

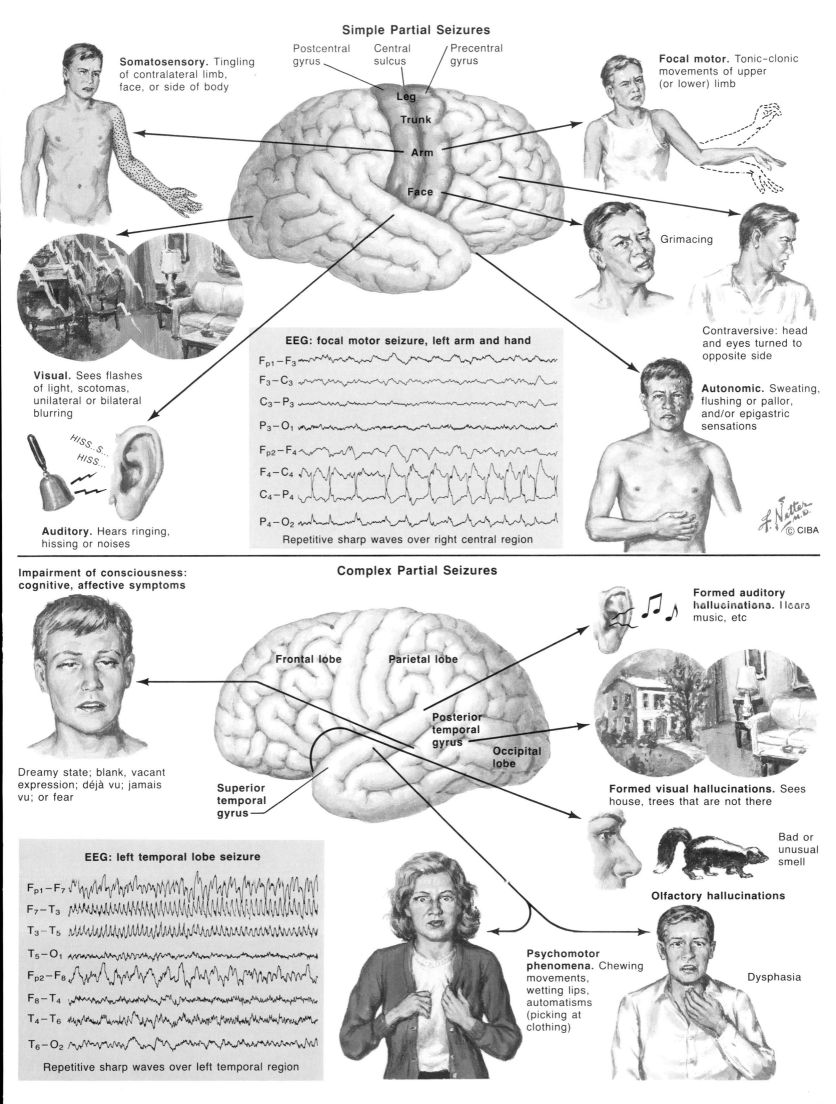

Simple Partial Seizures

Somatosensory. Tingling of contralateral limb, face, or side of body

Postcentral gyrus   Central sulcus   Precentral gyrus

Leg
Trunk
Arm
Face

Focal motor. Tonic-clonic movements of upper (or lower) limb

Grimacing

Contraversive: head and eyes turned to opposite side

Visual. Sees flashes of light, scotomas, unilateral or bilateral blurring

HISS..S...
HISS...

Auditory. Hears ringing, hissing or noises

EEG: focal motor seizure, left arm and hand

$F_{p1}-F_3$
F_3-C_3
C_3-P_3
P_3-O_1
$F_{p2}-F_4$
F_4-C_4
C_4-P_4
P_4-O_2

Repetitive sharp waves over right central region

Autonomic. Sweating, flushing or pallor, and/or epigastric sensations

Complex Partial Seizures

Impairment of consciousness: cognitive, affective symptoms

Dreamy state; blank, vacant expression; déjà vu; jamais vu; or fear

Frontal lobe   Parietal lobe

Posterior temporal gyrus

Occipital lobe

Superior temporal gyrus

Formed auditory hallucinations. Hears music, etc

Formed visual hallucinations. Sees house, trees that are not there

Bad or unusual smell

Olfactory hallucinations

EEG: left temporal lobe seizure

$F_{p1}-F_7$
F_7-T_3
T_3-T_5
T_5-O_1
$F_{p2}-F_8$
F_8-T_4
T_4-T_6
T_6-O_2

Repetitive sharp waves over left temporal region

Psychomotor phenomena. Chewing movements, wetting lips, automatisms (picking at clothing)

Dysphasia

Status Epilepticus

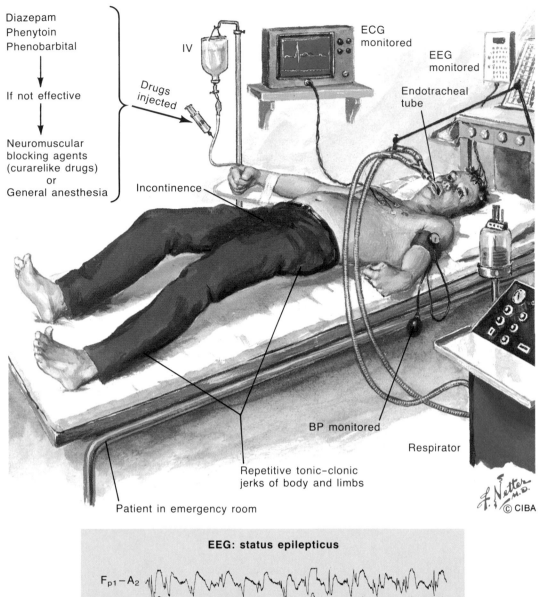

Diazepam
Phenytoin
Phenobarbital

↓

If not effective

↓

Neuromuscular
blocking agents
(curarelike drugs)
or
General anesthesia

Drugs
injected

IV

ECG
monitored

EEG
monitored

Endotracheal
tube

Incontinence

Repetitive tonic–clonic
jerks of body and limbs

BP monitored

Respirator

Patient in emergency room

Status epilepticus refers to a seizure disorder in which the patient has recurrent or continuous major motor seizures with little or no recovery between the attacks.

Generalized Tonic-Clonic (Grand Mal) Status. Repetitive, generalized tonic-clonic seizures without recovery of consciousness between seizures are the hallmark of grand mal status. The electroencephalogram (EEG) shows continuous, repetitive, generalized spike or spike-and-wave discharges in association with the seizures. Generalized tonic-clonic seizures can be caused by sudden withdrawal of anticonvulsant drugs in a patient with chronic epilepsy, inflammatory processes, metabolic or electrolyte derangements, alcohol, drugs, cerebral anoxia, head injury, tumor and vascular insults. Grand mal status is a real neurologic emergency, requiring immediate treatment. It is the most severe and potentially life-threatening of all seizure disorders, because associated anoxia and cardiovascular collapse can cause severe brain damage or death if the seizures are not quickly controlled.

An airway should be immediately provided and maintained. Cardiorespiratory status and other vital functions should be assessed and prompt support given if necessary. Blood samples should be drawn for analysis, and an intravenous infusion of normal saline should be started. Anticonvulsant medication is then given intravenously. The most commonly used drugs for status epilepticus are diazepam, phenytoin and phenobarbital. If the seizures are still uncontrolled, general anesthesia or neuromuscular blocking agents may be necessary to stop the seizure activity.

Absence (Petit Mal) Status. This type of status is characterized by prolonged or recurrent episodes of absence seizures, during which time

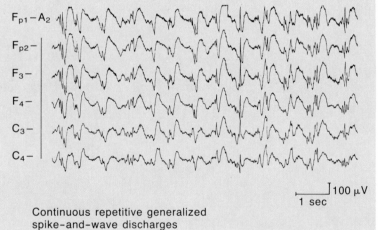

EEG: status epilepticus

$F_{p1}-A_2$

$F_{p2}-$

F_3-

F_4-

C_3-

C_4-

100 μV

1 sec

Continuous repetitive generalized
spike-and-wave discharges

the patient is somnolent, lethargic or confused. He may carry out various types of automatic activity without being aware of what he is doing. The EEG shows continuous, generalized spike-and-wave discharges during this time.

The treatment of choice for absence status is intravenously administered diazepam, followed by oral doses of ethosuximide or valproic acid.

Complex Partial Seizure Status. Prolonged periods of confusion with cognitive disturbances and automatic behavior are manifestations of complex partial seizure status. Following these attacks, the patient is usually amnestic for a period of time. The EEG usually shows repetitive epileptiform activity over the temporal or frontal

lobe, which at times may become secondarily generalized.

Treatment includes use of diazepam, phenytoin, carbamazepine and phenobarbital.

Focal Motor Status. Repetitive or continuous motor movements of various parts of the body are characteristic of focal motor status. In *epilepsia partialis continua*, continuous or recurrent focal motor contractions or clonic movements of the muscles of the face, limbs or part of the body may continue for days or weeks. The EEG shows repetitive or periodic spike or sharp wave discharges over the involved area.

Focal motor status may be treated with phenytoin or phenobarbital. □

Differential Diagnosis of Coma

Consciousness is maintained by each cerebral hemisphere with constant prodding from the reticular activating system within the central core of the brainstem tegmentum. Disruption of the reticular activating system or extensive damage to both cerebral hemispheres impairs consciousness. The five basic physiologic explanations for loss of consciousness are as follows:

1. *Bilateral cerebral hemisphere disease.* The cerebrum is particularly sensitive to chemical changes in the body; thus, toxic and metabolic disorders are the most common cause of coma resulting from hemispheric dysfunction. Encephalitis or hemorrhage or infection in the meninges and subarachnoid space can also adversely affect hemispheric function. Although infarcts, hemorrhages, tumors or abscesses can involve both hemispheres, the neurologic deficit becomes bilateral only sequentially.

2. *Unilateral cerebral hemisphere lesion with compression of the brainstem.* Any space-occupying lesion such as subdural hematoma, infarction, hemorrhage or tumor may compress the rostral brainstem and cause coma.

3. *Primary brainstem lesion.* An intrinsic brainstem lesion can cause coma by compromising the function of the medial tegmental structures bilaterally. The cause is usually stroke, either pontine hemorrhage or infarction resulting from occlusive disease of the basilar artery. Head trauma can also directly injure the brainstem.

4. *Cerebellar lesion with secondary brainstem compression.* A space-occupying lesion giving rise to cerebral dysfunction can also occur in the cerebellum and lead to posterior brainstem compression.

5. *Nonorganic or feigned stupor.* Swooning, or "hysterical" stupor, is difficult to diagnose unless the clinician is alert to this possibility.

Emergency Treatment. In most illnesses, treatment follows accurate diagnosis. Coma, however, is an emergency that the physician must treat before pursuing a diagnosis. Diminished consciousness, no matter what the cause, can lead to inadequate ventilation and hypotension, each with the potential to augment brain damage.

An adequate airway must be assured, and an intravenous line should be placed. If the patient is hypoventilating, intubation with assisted respiration should be considered. Vasopressors may be needed to treat hypotension. Blood should be drawn for determination of electrolytes, glucose and arterial blood gases and for toxicology screening. Serum is saved for further study if necessary. A bolus of glucose should be administered intravenously. If narcotic abuse is suspected or if the patient does not respond to these measures, naloxone can also be given.

History. After the necessary emergency treatment has been instituted, appropriate steps should be taken to determine the cause of coma. The patient's family, friends or physician can supply useful diagnostic information. Inquiries may elicit a history of diabetes; previous renal, hepatic or cardiac disease; severe depression; or drug use or abuse. It is important to know what medications have been prescribed and whether the patient had experienced any prodromal symptoms such as headache, unilateral weakness and ataxia, or previous episodes of stupor.

When the history is as complete as possible, the physician should conduct a careful physical and neurologic examination.

Neurologic Examination. It is important first to determine which of the five categories of coma is present. Further definitive tests then can be selected as dictated by the category of coma. Evaluation of the patient's spontaneous limb and bulbar movements, pupillary reactions, eye movements, and response to painful stimuli usually indicates the type of coma. If the patient is able to blink, yawn, lick and swallow, which are complex brainstem reflexes, lower brainstem function is preserved.

Pupillary size depends on the balance between sympathetic function (descending sympathetic fibers course in the lateral brainstem tegmentum) and parasympathetic function (parasympathetic fibers egress with the oculomotor [III] nerve in the midbrain). *Pupillary reaction* depends on the afferent light stimulus reaching the superior colliculus, as well as efferent transmission through the oculomotor nerve. This light reflex arc is located in the diencephalon and midbrain. *Eye movements* in the comatose patient can be observed by retracting the upper eyelids and observing spontaneous eye movements. When the head is rotated to one side, the eyes should move fully and conjugately in the opposite direction if the appropriate brainstem oculomotor and vestibular centers are preserved (doll's head phenomenon, or oculocephalogyric reflex). When the head is moved to the right, the eyes move conjugately to the left; when the head is moved downward, the eyes should roll upward. Ice water introduced into one ear canal should evoke conjugate eye movements toward the side of the stimulation (vestibuloocular reflex).

Horizontal reflex eye movements are controlled by the oculomotor, trochlear (IV) and abducens (VI) nerves and their nuclei; the medial longitudinal fasciculus, the parapontine reticular formation (pontine lateral gaze center); and the vestibular nuclei and nerves. All these structures are located within the pontine tegmentum. Vertical movements are controlled by centers in the rostral midbrain and caudal diencephalon. Spontaneous limb movements, as well as responses to pinching the limbs or chest, should be observed.

Differential Diagnosis. When coma is caused by *bilateral cerebral hemisphere disease*, swallowing, yawning and respirations are normal. The eyes rove spontaneously from side to side, and the limbs move symmetrically to pinch. Pupillary and oculomotor reflexes are preserved.

Primary *diencephalic brainstem lesions* cause small, poorly reactive pupils and poor vertical gaze. The eyes may rest downward and inward, and one eye may be lower than the other.

In *midbrain lesions*, the pupils are dilated or in midposition, and bilateral third cranial nerve palsy occurs. The eyes rest downward and outward and do not adduct or move vertically. Decerebrate posturing of the limbs is present.

Pontine lesions cause small, reactive pupils, failure of horizontal eye movements, preservation of vertical eye movements (sometimes with spontaneous bobbing), and decerebrate posturing. *Medullary lesions* may compromise vasomotor control and respiration.

When a *hemispheric lesion* has compressed the brainstem, the patient usually experiences premonitory signs or symptoms of hemisphere dysfunction, such as hemiparesis. As the lesion enlarges, intracranial pressure rises, and headache, vomiting, decreased alertness and papilledema develop. Signs of rostral brainstem diencephalic dysfunction follow. The midbrain and pons are disrupted sequentially, and signs of lower brainstem failure are added to dysfunction of rostral structures.

In contrast, when an *intrinsic brainstem lesion* is present, eg, a pontine infarct or hematoma, brainstem function rostral to the lesion is preserved. Toxic disorders often affect the brainstem and cerebral hemispheres at multiple levels, causing signs inconsistent with any single anatomic locus of disease. *Cerebellar space-occupying lesions* cause ataxia and vomiting, often followed by sixth cranial nerve or lateral gaze palsy to the side of the lesion. Signs of lower brainstem dysfunction, in the pons or medulla, then develop. Patients who feign unresponsiveness often lie stiff and motionless.

Treatment. If a cerebral or cerebellar lesion compresses the brainstem (categories 2 and 4), the situation is grave and must be handled on an urgent basis to avoid irreversible injury to the brainstem. Neuroradiographic investigations are critical in determining the nature of the space-occupying lesion. Treatment with corticosteroids, osmotic diuretics and forced hyperventilation, as well as computed tomography (CT) or magnetic resonance imaging (MRI), should be carried out immediately. Emergency neurologic or neurosurgical consultation should be obtained. Surgery may be necessary to save the patient's life.

Bilateral cerebral hemisphere disease causing coma (category 1) is usually treated medically rather than surgically. The most frequent cause of this type of coma is metabolic encephalopathy caused by *exogenous intoxication*, eg, drug overdose, alcohol intoxication or overmedication; *endogenous intoxication* caused by organ failure (carbon dioxide narcosis, liver failure, uremia), hyperglycemia, hypercalcemia or hypernatremia; or *insufficiency of endogenous or exogenous substances*, eg, hypoglycemia, hypothyroidism, hypocalcemia or hyponatremia.

High fever and severe pain, as in a fractured hip, can cause a similar clinical picture of metabolic encephalopathy with delirium. Less often, encephalitis, meningitis or subarachnoid hemorrhage causes bilateral hemisphere coma. Investigation usually includes a careful search for a metabolic cause. If fever or stiff neck is present, lumbar puncture is required, usually after CT. Treatment is determined by the underlying etiologic factors.

In coma caused by primary brainstem lesions (category 3), CT scans are usually needed to separate hemorrhage from infarction. Appropriate treatment then depends on the cause of the brainstem lesion.

Feigned coma (category 5) can usually be interrupted by suggestion, and most frequently is recognized some time after the patient's hospital admission. □

Differential Diagnosis of Coma

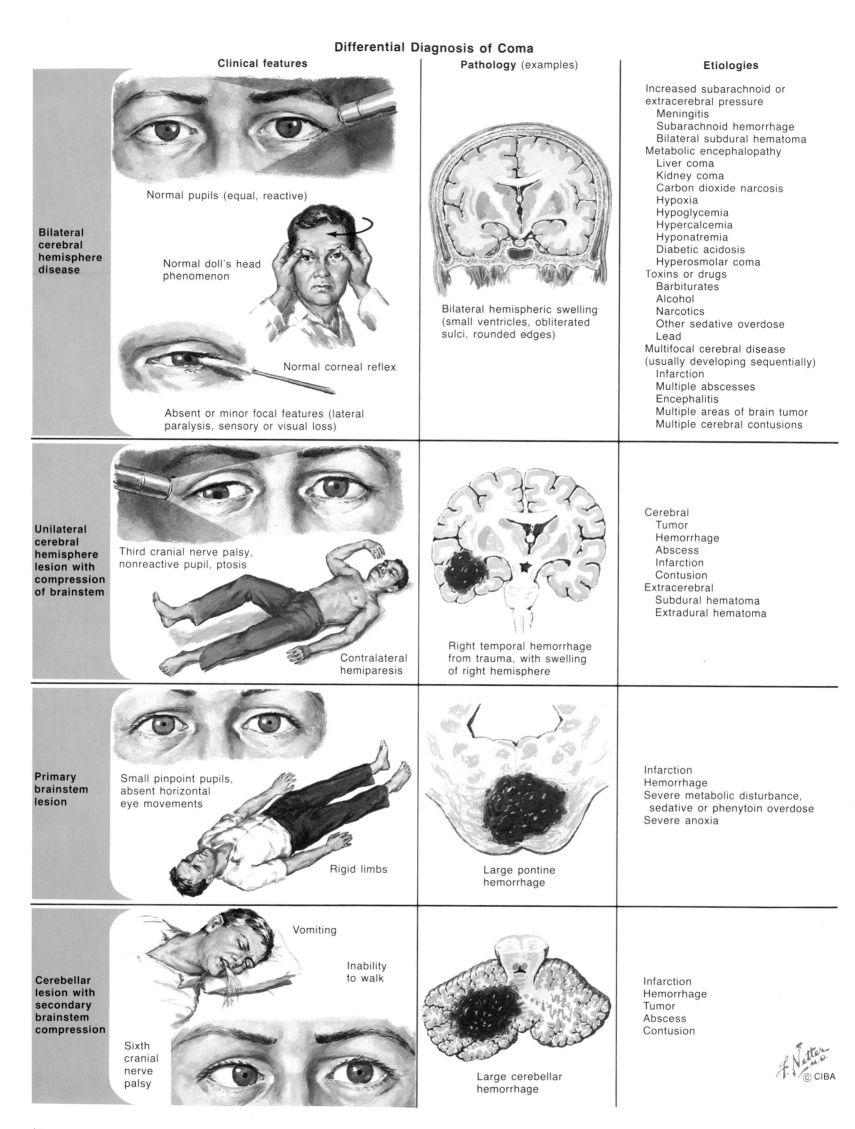

Clinical features	Pathology (examples)	Etiologies

Bilateral cerebral hemisphere disease

Normal pupils (equal, reactive)

Normal doll's head phenomenon

Normal corneal reflex

Absent or minor focal features (lateral paralysis, sensory or visual loss)

Bilateral hemispheric swelling (small ventricles, obliterated sulci, rounded edges)

Increased subarachnoid or extracerebral pressure
  Meningitis
  Subarachnoid hemorrhage
  Bilateral subdural hematoma
Metabolic encephalopathy
  Liver coma
  Kidney coma
  Carbon dioxide narcosis
  Hypoxia
  Hypoglycemia
  Hypercalcemia
  Hyponatremia
  Diabetic acidosis
  Hyperosmolar coma
Toxins or drugs
  Barbiturates
  Alcohol
  Narcotics
  Other sedative overdose
  Lead
Multifocal cerebral disease (usually developing sequentially)
  Infarction
  Multiple abscesses
  Encephalitis
  Multiple areas of brain tumor
  Multiple cerebral contusions

Unilateral cerebral hemisphere lesion with compression of brainstem

Third cranial nerve palsy, nonreactive pupil, ptosis

Contralateral hemiparesis

Right temporal hemorrhage from trauma, with swelling of right hemisphere

Cerebral
  Tumor
  Hemorrhage
  Abscess
  Infarction
  Contusion
Extracerebral
  Subdural hematoma
  Extradural hematoma

Primary brainstem lesion

Small pinpoint pupils, absent horizontal eye movements

Rigid limbs

Large pontine hemorrhage

Infarction
Hemorrhage
Severe metabolic disturbance, sedative or phenytoin overdose
Severe anoxia

Cerebellar lesion with secondary brainstem compression

Vomiting

Inability to walk

Sixth cranial nerve palsy

Large cerebellar hemorrhage

Infarction
Hemorrhage
Tumor
Abscess
Contusion

Section III

Cerebrovascular Disease

Frank H. Netter, M.D.

in collaboration with

Richard A. Baker, M.D.   *Plates 18–19, 22–23, 29*

Louis R. Caplan, M.D.   *Plates 1, 5, 8–9, 11–15, 26–27, 37*

Louis R. Caplan, M.D. and Richard A. Baker, M.D.   *Plate 28*

William S. Fields, M.D.   *Plates 2–3, 6–7, 10, 20–21*

William A. Friedman, M.D.   *Plates 30–36*

H. Royden Jones, Jr., M.D.   *Plates 4, 16–17, 24*

Edward Tarlov, M.D. and Charles A. Hufnagel, M.D.   *Plate 25*

Ischemic ◄———— Stroke ————► Hemorrhagic

Diagnosis of Stroke

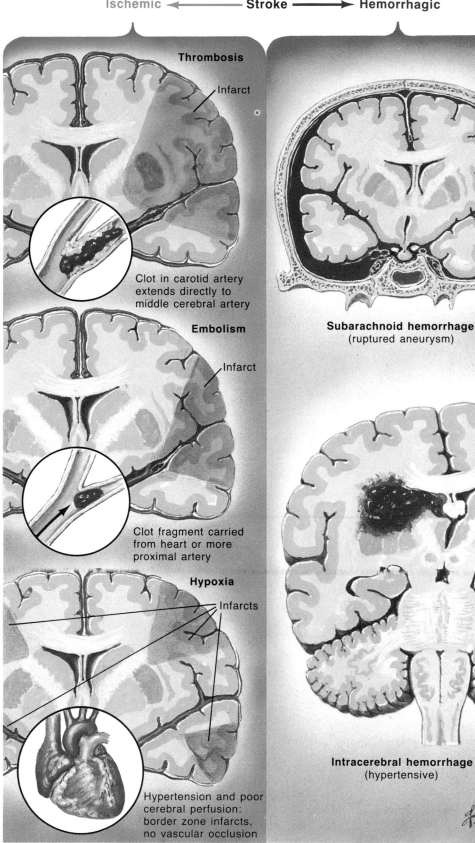

Thrombosis

Infarct

Clot in carotid artery extends directly to middle cerebral artery

Embolism

Infarct

Clot fragment carried from heart or more proximal artery

Hypoxia

Infarcts

Hypertension and poor cerebral perfusion: border zone infarcts, no vascular occlusion

Subarachnoid hemorrhage
(ruptured aneurysm)

Intracerebral hemorrhage
(hypertensive)

The term "stroke" is used to describe a heterogeneous group of disorders in which brain injury is caused by a vascular mechanism. In order to effectively treat a stroke patient, the physician must first determine the type and mechanism of the stroke.

The two major categories of stroke are *ischemic*, in which inadequate blood flow causes a circumscribed area of cerebral infarction, and *hemorrhagic*, in which bleeding in the brain parenchyma or subarachnoid space injures and displaces brain structures.

Ischemic Stroke. Thrombotic or embolic vascular occlusion or systemic reduction in blood flow can cause ischemic stroke. *Thrombosis*, the formation of a blood clot superimposed on an atherosclerotic plaque, may cause severe stenosis of large extracranial vessels such as the internal carotid or vertebral arteries, or affect minute, deep, penetrating intracerebral vessels. Increased red blood cell and platelet counts and blood hypercoagulability may contribute to clotting and sludged blood flow.

Embolism results in stroke when a clot, plaque or agglutinated platelets (material that originally formed in the heart or in the proximal arterial tree) are discharged into the circulation and subsequently block a distal artery.

Systemic reduction in flow, as in cardiac arrest or shock, also decreases cerebral blood flow and leads to ischemia, especially in the vulnerable border zones between major cerebral blood vessels such as the middle and posterior cerebral arteries.

Hemorrhagic Stroke. *Subarachnoid hemorrhage* causing stroke usually indicates rupture of a cerebral aneurysm, most commonly in an artery at the base of the brain. Bleeding quickly disseminates throughout the subarachnoid space and leads to a sudden increase in intracranial pressure. Symptoms of subarachnoid hemorrhage include headache, vomiting and interruption of behavior or consciousness.

Intracerebral hemorrhage, or bleeding into the brain parenchyma, is usually caused by hypertension. Blood is released into the brain under arteriolar or capillary pressure and causes dysfunction

of a localized area. If the hematoma is large, headache and altered states of consciousness ensue.

Differential Diagnosis. Certain characteristics of stroke and known predisposing factors should be considered in differentiating its various types.

Knowledge of the patient's *medical history* is particularly helpful. A history of angina or claudication indicates the presence of atherosclerosis, which predisposes to thrombosis of extracranial vessels. Known cardiac valvular disease or atrial fibrillation predisposes to embolism, and severe hypertension is a precursor of intracranial hemorrhage.

Onset and development of neurologic deficit provide additional clues to diagnosis. Thrombosis usually occurs in the morning, after sleep, and often has a stepwise or fluctuating clinical course. Embolism develops suddenly, often while the patient is awake, and intracerebral hemorrhage develops quickly but gradually, usually while the patient is active.

Associated symptoms are also important considerations. Sudden headache and vomiting without paralysis suggest subarachnoid hemorrhage, whereas headache preceding paralysis by days or weeks points toward thrombosis. □

Role of Platelets in Arterial Thrombosis

Role of Platelets in Arterial Thrombosis

Platelets circulating in blood contain thromboxane A$_2$, a substance that promotes their aggregation, while vascular endothelium secretes prostacyclin, an aggregation inhibitor that balances this effect. These products are synthesized after conversion of arachidonic acid into intermediate endoperoxides by cyclooxygenase enzymes

If endothelial continuity is interrupted by trauma, atherosclerosis, etc, subsurface collagen is exposed to blood and stimulates adhesion of platelets to vessel wall. Platelets then discharge thromboxane A$_2$, causing aggregation of adjacent platelets

Masses of platelets are produced by multinuclear megakaryocytes in the bone marrow and released into the peripheral blood, where they circulate for approximately 10 days. While circulating, these nonnuclear disc-shaped cells do not adhere to each other or to the vessel wall. If the integrity of the endothelium is breached, specific properties of the platelets are activated, which leads to thrombosis, a pathologic process that ultimately results in an occluding thrombus.

Ulceration or even minor loss of continuity in the endothelial surface initiates the development of a thrombus within the arterial lumen. When endothelial damage occurs as a result of trauma or disease, the blood is exposed to subendothelial collagen. The normally discoid circulating platelets are activated, undergo a shape change, form pseudopodia, and adhere to the vessel wall. These activated platelets release adenosine diphosphate (ADP), which causes adjacent platelets to adhere to them (aggregation). The platelet aggregate retracts, and coagulation factors consolidate it by producing a network of fibrin. Red blood cells may also become enmeshed in the platelet-fibrin aggregate and produce a more fully formed red thrombus. Thus, three elements are important in the formation of a thrombus: (1) platelets, (2) coagulation factors, and (3) vessel wall.

Collagen, which induces ADP release, also activates prostaglandin synthesis. Thromboxane A$_2$, a potent aggregator and vasoconstrictor, is produced by platelets. Prostacyclin (PGI$_2$), the most powerful aggregation inhibitor and vasodilator, is synthesized by the vascular endothelium. The balance between the two, all other factors being equal, presumably plays a key role in maintaining normal hemostasis and in preventing thrombus formation. Aspirin inhibits synthesis of these prostaglandins, and is therefore an important antithrombotic agent. □

As more platelets aggregate, fibrin network develops and stabilizes mass into "white thrombus," which then retracts into vascular wall. In some cases, endothelium may later heal over with or without narrowing of lumen

If thrombus develops further, red blood cells become enmeshed in platelet-fibrin aggregate to form "red thrombus," which may grow and block vessel lumen. Either platelet-fibrin aggregates or more fully formed clots may break off, with embolization into distal arterial branches

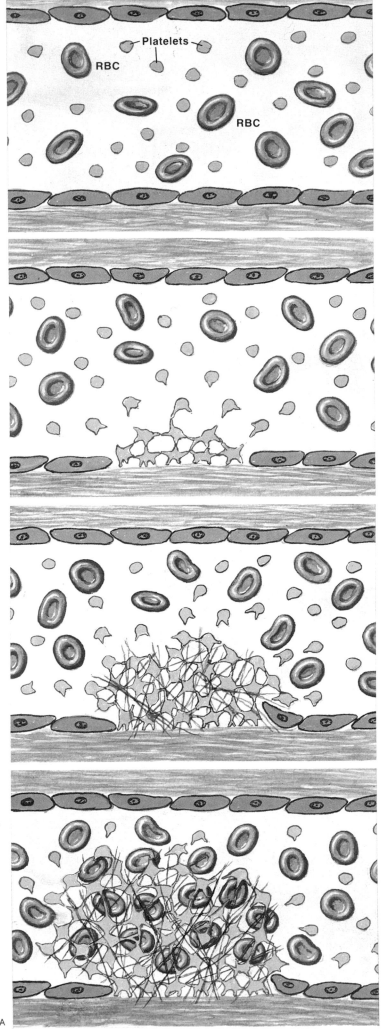

Atherosclerosis, Thrombosis and Embolism

A. Atherosclerotic plaque at arterial bifurcation

B. Loss of intimal continuity (ulcer formation)

C. Aggregation of platelets and fibrin on roughened surface. Platelet-fibrin emboli may occur

D. Thrombus formation superimposed

E. Embolization of contents of plaque (cholesterol) and/or platelet-fibrin. Occlusion of blood vessels distally in arterial tree

F. Thrombus causes total arterial occlusion

Atherosclerosis is characterized by the presence of nodular, irregularly distributed, yellow, fatty plaques involving the intima of large and medium-sized arteries. The initial pathologic finding, called the *fatty streak*, begins as an abnormal infiltration of lipids into the endothelial cells.

The fatty streak may regress, may remain static, or may progress to a *fibrous plaque*. In turn, the fibrous plaque may regress, may remain static, or may develop into a *complicated atheromatous lesion*, which is characterized by the occurrence of one or more events: hemorrhage into the plaque, subintimal necrosis, loss of intimal continuity, ulcer formation or calcification. Loss of intimal continuity may lead to the development of a thrombus within the lumen of the artery, which may progress to occlusive thrombosis or may fragment to produce thrombotic embolization.

Complicated atheromatous lesions are those most frequently associated with marked stenosis of the arterial lumen. For instance, hemorrhage into the subintima from vasa vasorum adjacent to the plaque may increase the size of the lesion and thereby narrow the lumen, or the plaque may ulcerate in association with subintimal hemorrhage or necrosis. The contents of the plaque are often discharged into the bloodstream, and embolization occurs in the distal intracranial branches.

The atherosclerotic process is variable and unpredictable. Even if a vessel is completely occluded, a number of factors influence the ultimate outcome. Depending on the adequacy of the *collateral circulation*, marked stenosis of an extracranial artery may cause ischemia within the territory supplied by the artery, or may have no effect. In turn, depending on the duration of the ischemic episode, there may be frank infarction or no tissue damage at all. Similarly, depending on size and location, an infarct may have no clinical manifestations or may produce permanent neurologic deficits.

Discharge of atherosclerotic debris and platelet-fibrin complexes into the bloodstream as the result of ulceration of a plaque in the extracranial vessels, or the occurrence of thromboembolism, produces neurologic disturbances of varying duration. Thus, the clinical course of patients with occlusive cerebrovascular disease is extremely difficult to predict. □

Temporal Profile in Cerebrovascular Disease

The clinical evolution of focal cerebral ischemic events follows various temporal profiles that serve as useful prognostic warnings to both physicians and patients. Although the prognosis for sustaining a second cerebral ischemic episode may be the same no matter what the temporal profile of the first event, the remediable potential before the development of a possible permanent deficit makes clinical classification of neurologic deficits important. The terms "transient ischemic attacks (TIAs)," "residual ischemic neurologic deficit (RIND)," and "completed infarction (CI)" are not all-encompassing. The anatomic and pathophysiologic subcategories of each disorder are of even greater importance. Clinically, the deficits implied by these terms are usually divided into the *carotid system* (anterior circulation) and the *vertebrobasilar system* (posterior circulation) TIAs.

Transient Ischemic Attacks. An acute focal neurologic deficit evidenced by transient loss of function in the territory of a specific intracerebral vessel and resolving usually within a few minutes or, at most, 24 hours is classified as a TIA. *Carotid system* TIAs may be manifested by symptoms stemming from the ophthalmic artery (Plate 6) or the middle cerebral artery territory (Plate 8). Amaurosis fugax (transient monocular blindness), the common symptom of *ophthalmic artery* ischemia, should be carefully differentiated from giant-cell arteritis (see Section II, Plate 3) or migrainous scotoma. *Middle cerebral artery* TIAs are manifested by transient numbness and/or weakness of the hand and arm, the lower face and, sometimes, the leg. If the dominant hemisphere is affected, aphasia may occur. TIAs of the *anterior cerebral artery* are quite uncommon.

Vertebrobasilar artery TIAs usually produce a combination of symptoms, including dysarthria, dysphagia, ataxia of gait or extremity, vertigo, facial paresthesias, contralateral or bilateral extremity weakness and/or paresthesias, diplopia and unilateral or bilateral homonymous hemianopsia.

The importance of recognizing a TIA has been repeatedly emphasized by the high rate of subsequent cerebral infarctions. Some persons may have multiple TIAs; others may have only one TIA preceding a devastating stroke. The risk appears greatest in the first year following a TIA, particularly in the first few months. A TIA is a neurologic emergency requiring hospitalization.

Residual Ischemic Neurologic Deficit. An acute focal neurologic dysfunction similar to a TIA but persisting more than 24 hours and usually totally resolving within 3 weeks is classified as a RIND. Such lesions may represent a period of persistent ischemia without actual infarction, but this hypothesis has not been pathologically or metabolically confirmed. As in TIAs, functional recovery in RIND is essentially total; the risk of subsequent completed infarction is increased to about 6 times that in normal age-controlled populations.

Evaluation of the patient who has had a RIND should be similar to that of the patient who has had a TIA.

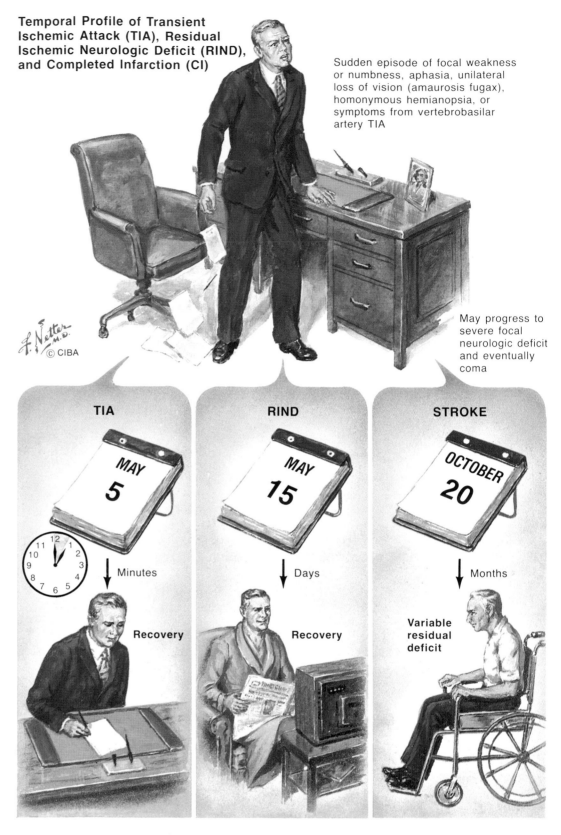

Completed Infarction. A persistent, severe neurologic deficit secondary to an acute focal cerebrovascular lesion in which improvement is not complete in at least 3 weeks is classified as a CI.

Progressive Stroke. The peak deficit in strokes occurs almost immediately, but in a small percentage of patients, the deficit progresses gradually—over 24 to 48 hours in the carotid system and over 96 hours in the vertebrobasilar system. Progressive carotid system lesions may be secondary to a severe hemispheric deficit producing cerebral edema, which causes gradual obtundation, leading to coma and signs of cerebral herniation. An overall mortality of 10% to 12% within the first few weeks of onset is seen in carotid system

infarction. In patients with a course typical of cerebral edema, mortality is 40%. In most of these patients, a dense hemiplegia, often with homonymous defect, and aphasia associated with a compromised consciousness level are seen within the first 36 hours of illness.

A progressive or remitting, relapsing course, although uncommon, may be twice as frequent in vertebrobasilar system infarction than in carotid artery system infarction. Edema in vertebrobasilar infarction becomes clinically important mainly with cerebellar lesions (Plate 11). The 27% overall mortality in vertebrobasilar system infarction increases to 80% to 90% in patients who become comatose. □

Stenosis or Occlusion of Carotid Artery

The most common location for atherosclerosis within the anterior circulation is at the bifurcation of the common carotid artery. The lesion usually begins just below the bifurcation and extends 1.5 to 3.0 cm into the internal carotid artery or external carotid artery, or both.

The earliest lesion is a fatty intimal streak that stains positively for fat with Sudan dyes. With further atheromatous buildup, a raised, flat *plaque* develops and encroaches on the arterial lumen. Fatty cholesterol material, hypertrophied medial and subintimal smooth muscle, and fibrous connective tissue contribute to luminal stenosis. Fresh hemorrhages are sometimes visible within plaques removed at surgery, and small nidi of agglutinated platelets or small red thrombi can be seen (Plate 2).

Severe atherosclerosis at the origin of the internal carotid artery is usually proportional to disease in the coronary and iliac arteries and aorta. Atherosclerotic lesions at the origin of the internal carotid artery produce neurologic symptoms when blood flow to the ipsilateral cerebral hemisphere is decreased or when embolism occurs in the distal intracranial branches. Most often, *clot formation* decreases blood flow in the compromised lumen. Similar but less severe atherosclerotic changes sometimes affect the origin of the common carotid artery. Atherosclerotic occlusion at this site is rare, but *aortic arch arteritis* (Takayasu's disease) can obliterate the proximal common carotid artery and other aortic branches.

Atheroma usually does not affect the internal carotid artery in the neck above the carotid bifurcation, but does affect the siphon portion after the vessel has begun its intracranial course. The carotid siphon rarely ulcerates, but its inner surface may contain bony, hard pits and shiny, smooth, heavily calcified zones. A lesion of the siphon can begin before the ophthalmic artery branch or within the cavernous sinus. Atherosclerotic stenosis or occlusion can also occur at the bifurcation of the internal carotid artery into its middle and anterior cerebral artery branches.

Fibromuscular dysplasia also affects the cerebral vasculature and is most often found in the pharyngeal portion of the internal carotid artery. Varying degrees of intimal fibroplasia, medial fibroelastosis, fibromuscular hyperplasia and subadventitial fibrosis are seen. The lesions are usually mixed and are probably caused by a fibroblastlike transformation of smooth muscle cells. Angiography shows long regions of smooth, concentric, tubular arterial narrowing; aneurysmal bulges; and alternating bands of medial contraction, which give the vessel a beaded appearance. Fibromuscular dysplasia can also affect the nuchal vertebral artery, as well as the intracranial internal carotid artery and its middle, anterior and posterior cerebral artery branches.

Dissection of the internal carotid artery is also most common in the pharyngeal segment just below the skull base. Blood dissects within the arterial wall, compressing the lumen. If the intima is torn, the clot reenters the lumen and can

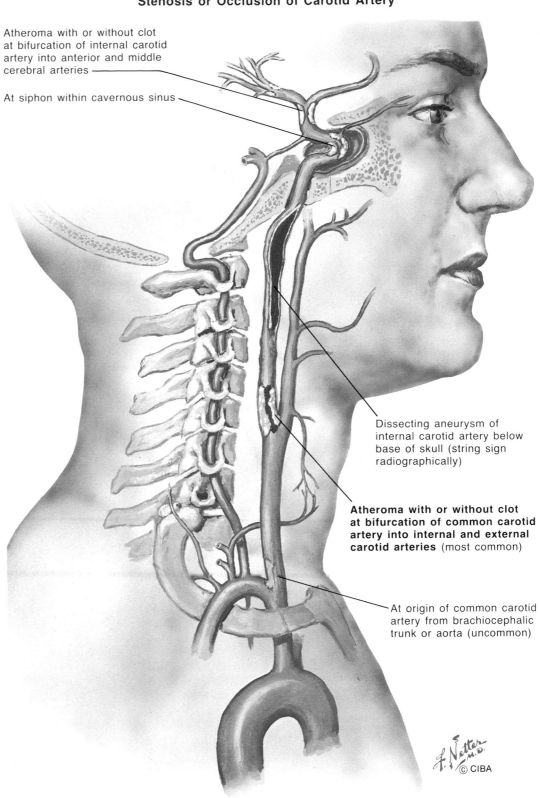

Atheroma with or without clot at bifurcation of internal carotid artery into anterior and middle cerebral arteries

At siphon within cavernous sinus

Dissecting aneurysm of internal carotid artery below base of skull (string sign radiographically)

Atheroma with or without clot at bifurcation of common carotid artery into internal and external carotid arteries (most common)

At origin of common carotid artery from brachiocephalic trunk or aorta (uncommon)

cause neurologic signs when it embolizes to the intracranial branches. Pain in the ipsilateral side of the neck, face or head; ipsilateral dysfunction of the sympathetic nervous system fibers along the wall of the internal carotid artery; and transient ischemic attacks (TIAs) are the most common symptoms of dissection. Angiography shows a long tapered narrowing of the vessel lumen (string sign), and aneurysmal outpouchings are common. Intracranial arteries dissect less frequently.

Cerebral emboli can block any vessel, but the most common sites are within the distal superficial pial branches and at the bifurcation of arteries, especially at the intracranial bifurcation of the internal carotid artery and at the origin and

trifurcation of the middle cerebral artery. Angiography often shows that the recipient artery is terminated abruptly, without atherosclerotic narrowing proximal to the block. Later examination sometimes shows that the clot has moved or disappeared. Clots at the origin of the internal carotid artery or in situ occlusions of the multiple intracranial small-branch vessels may occur in patients with coagulopathies.

Inflammatory and drug-induced *arteritis* causes irregular beading of intracranial branches. Tuberculous arteritis often narrows the internal carotid artery as it pierces the dura, and temporal arteritis affects this artery within the siphon, sometimes producing bilateral stenosis. ☐

Ischemia in Internal Carotid Artery Territory: Clinical Manifestations

A. Ocular

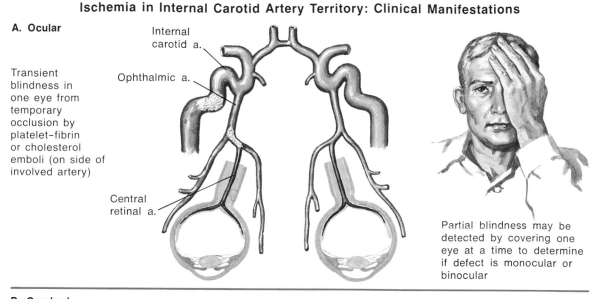

Transient blindness in one eye from temporary occlusion by platelet-fibrin or cholesterol emboli (on side of involved artery)

Internal carotid a.

Ophthalmic a.

Central retinal a.

Partial blindness may be detected by covering one eye at a time to determine if defect is monocular or binocular

Visual disturbance associated with lesions in the internal carotid artery occurs on the same side as the lesion, separate from, or coincident with, contralateral motor or sensory changes, or both. This type of monocular blindness, known as *amaurosis fugax*, is usually transitory. It has been described as a shade being pulled down over one eye and, as vision returns, the shade is raised.

Cerebral hemisphere involvement is manifested by contralateral motor or sensory changes, which may affect the upper or lower limb, or both. If the dominant cerebral hemisphere is affected, language disturbances (aphasia) may be noted. Headache, when it occurs, is supraorbital or temporal and is on the side of the arterial occlusion.

Pathogenesis. The most widely accepted hypothesis for the pathogenesis of transient ischemic attacks (TIAs) involving the internal carotid artery territory is the *embolic theory* (Plate 3). However, embolization is difficult to document, because emboli that have become lodged in small vessels usually fragment and disappear distally in the arterial system.

Occasionally, fundoscopic examination in the patient having an attack of monocular blindness reveals an embolus lodged at a bifurcation of one of the branches of the retinal arteries. Such emboli appear as bright plaques if they are cholesterol fragments, or white if they are platelet-fibrin aggregates dislodged from an ulcerated lesion.

In many patients with TIAs, angiographic examination shows that the lumen of the internal carotid artery or the common carotid artery at its bifurcation is narrowed (Plates 22–23). This narrowing is the basis of the *stenotic (hemodynamic) theory* of ischemic episodes.

Isolated stenosis of an artery is considered to impair blood flow only when the lumen is narrowed by at least 80%. However, if one carotid artery is occluded, stenosis of 50% in the other carotid artery may be significant. Stenosis alone is not sufficient evidence that the narrowed lumen is responsible for the TIAs. Some additional event probably alters cerebral hemodynamics so that a previously nonsignificant stenotic lesion becomes transiently significant and produces cerebral ischemia. Such an event might be an episode of *systemic hypotension*, as in acute myocardial infarction, acute blood loss, Adams-Stokes syndrome, use of certain medications, etc. Obviously, the hypotensive episode itself is frequently recogniz-

B. Cerebral hemisphere

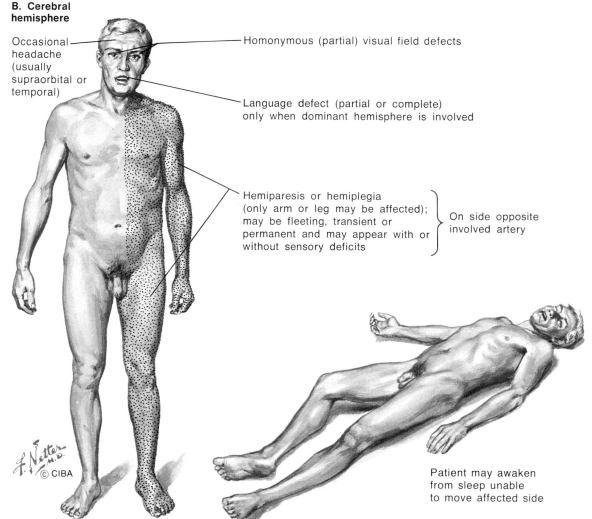

Occasional headache (usually supraorbital or temporal)

Homonymous (partial) visual field defects

Language defect (partial or complete) only when dominant hemisphere is involved

Hemiparesis or hemiplegia (only arm or leg may be affected); may be fleeting, transient or permanent and may appear with or without sensory deficits

On side opposite involved artery

Patient may awaken from sleep unable to move affected side

able as the primary clinical condition. However, only a few patients with recurrent TIAs have known attacks of hypotension. Thus, the episodic nature of the ischemia in many patients remains unexplained.

The concept of *vasospasm* in the distal arterial branches has been proposed but has now been largely discarded. Like transient episodes of hypotension without a known primary cause, vasospasm is extremely difficult to document. It may play a part, however, during episodes of sudden transient hypertension.

Nevertheless, an analysis of the results of arterial reconstructive surgery in one series of patients (Plate 25) provides indirect evidence that

the stenotic lesion plays a significant role in the recurrence of cerebral ischemia. When the appropriate carotid artery was involved, ischemic attacks were significantly reduced or ceased in patients in whom surgery was performed, compared with a similar group of nonsurgical patients.

The chief importance of the stenotic atheromatous lesion probably lies in the fact that it is the site for the development of ulceration and subsequent embolization of platelet-fibrin aggregates or atheromatous debris. However, even this explanation is not entirely satisfactory, because the events occurring at the time of the TIA cannot be documented. For the present, therefore, the pathogenesis of TIAs remains unsettled. □

Potential Collateral Circulation Following Occlusion of Internal Carotid Artery

The term "collateral circulation" is used to describe blood flow in the subsidiary vascular channels present throughout the circulatory network, which provide a secondary defense mechanism against failure of the primary vessels. However, the morphologic patterns and the capability of these channels to transport blood when the primary vessels become obstructed vary considerably, and not all anastomoses are of sufficient caliber to provide collateral circulation. Genetic factors may be important in the development of collateral vessels, and there is some indication that vascular channels are formed where needed. Thus, capillaries appear to be attracted to some regions and repelled by others.

The foundations of arterial collateral circulation are established early in embryologic development. All the vessels that play a role in collateral circulation in postnatal life develop in the prenatal period, and open in response to occlusion of a primary vessel. Thus, collateral circulation patterns for each specific vascular bed are predictable to a certain degree. However, the pattern may be influenced by embryologic variations in vascular morphologic relationships and, to a lesser extent, by physiologic factors.

When a primary artery becomes obstructed, a clot develops distal to the site of occlusion. However, the clot does not usually extend beyond the next major branch of the primary artery, provided that blood is reentering the primary channel through that branch. Collateral circulation is more likely to develop distal to the obstruction in thrombosis superimposed on a gradually increasing atherosclerotic stenosis than in acute embolic obstruction.

The principal *extracranial sources* of collateral circulation when the internal carotid artery is occluded are anastomoses between the *ophthalmic artery* and *branches of both external carotid arteries.*

The most important *intracranial anastomoses* are those of the *circle of Willis.* Ordinarily, there is little flow from one side to the other or between the posterior and anterior segments. Like all anastomoses, the circle of Willis is of potential rather than actual value, because it does not open up rapidly. Its functional value is enhanced if the primary vessel on one side becomes gradually stenotic rather than abruptly occluded. Whether cerebral ischemia and possible infarction follow major extracranial artery occlusion depends to a great extent on the adequacy of this configuration at the base of the brain.

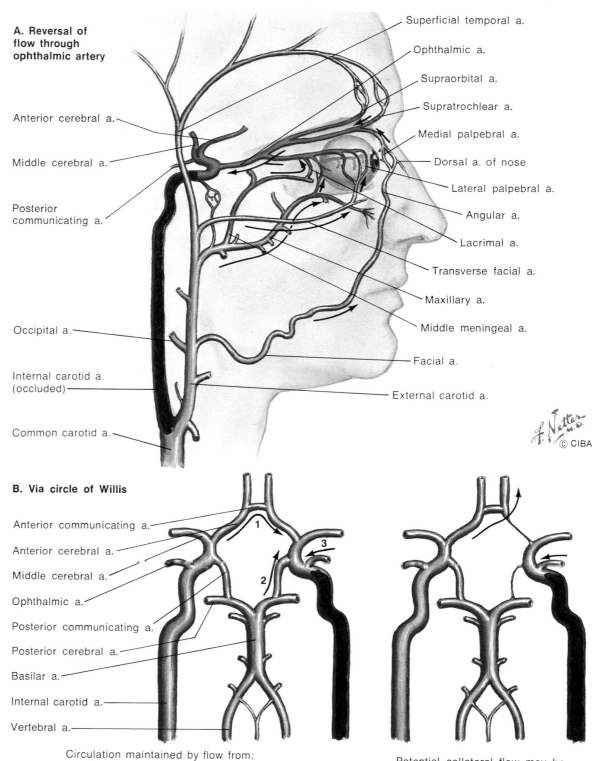

A. Reversal of flow through ophthalmic artery

Anterior cerebral a.
Middle cerebral a.
Posterior communicating a.
Occipital a.
Internal carotid a. (occluded)
Common carotid a.

Superficial temporal a.
Ophthalmic a.
Supraorbital a.
Supratrochlear a.
Medial palpebral a.
Dorsal a. of nose
Lateral palpebral a.
Angular a.
Lacrimal a.
Transverse facial a.
Maxillary a.
Middle meningeal a.
Facial a.
External carotid a.

B. Via circle of Willis

Anterior communicating a.
Anterior cerebral a.
Middle cerebral a.
Ophthalmic a.
Posterior communicating a.
Posterior cerebral a.
Basilar a.
Internal carotid a.
Vertebral a.

Circulation maintained by flow from:
1. Opposite internal carotid artery (anterior circulation)
2. Vertebrobasilar system (posterior circulation)
3. Ophthalmic artery (see **A**)

Potential collateral flow may be reduced by anomalous insufficiency of segments of circle of Willis

The pattern of collateral circulation that may be established if vertebrobasilar occlusion occurs depends largely on the side of the occlusion. If the basilar artery is occluded, the internal carotid arteries may supply the posterior circulation through the posterior communicating arteries. Alternatively, blood flow through anastomotic channels between the posterior inferior cerebellar arteries and the superior cerebellar vessels may provide a bypass route. In the latter situation, the vertebral arteries continue to supply the posterior circulation.

Occlusion of the proximal vertebral artery may promote the opening of a number of anastomotic channels, including those between the occipital

artery (from the external carotid) and the muscular branches of the vertebral artery. Both ascending cervical arteries as well as the opposite vertebral artery are also important sources of blood supply.

In obstruction of the proximal segment of the subclavian artery, the vertebral artery on the same side is one of the potential channels that may maintain distal subclavian flow. Retrograde flow in this vertebral artery is established by connections with the opposite vertebral artery. Flow into the vertebral artery on the side of the occlusion is also maintained by anastomoses between the muscular branches of this vertebral artery and the occipital artery. □

Occlusion of Middle and Anterior Cerebral Arteries

Lesion		Artery occluded	Infarct, surface	Infarct, coronal section	Clinical manifestations
Middle cerebral artery	Entire territory	Anterior cerebral, Superior division, Lenticulostriate Medial Lateral, Internal carotid, Middle cerebral, Inferior division			Contralateral gaze palsy, hemiplegia, hemisensory loss, spatial neglect, hemianopsia Global aphasia (if on left side) May lead to coma secondary to edema
	Deep				Contralateral hemiplegia, hemisensory loss Transcortical motor and/or sensory aphasia (if on left side)
	Parasylvian				Contralateral weakness and sensory loss of face and hand Conduction aphasia, apraxia and Gerstmann's syndrome (if on left side) Constructional dyspraxia (if on right side)
	Superior division				Contralateral hemiplegia, hemisensory loss, gaze palsy, spatial neglect Broca's aphasia (if on left side)
	Inferior division				Contralateral hemianopsia or upper quadrant anopsia Wernicke's aphasia (if on left side) Constructional dyspraxia (if on right side)
Anterior cerebral artery	Entire territory				Incontinence Contralateral hemiplegia Abulia Transcortical motor aphasia or motor and sensory aphasia Left limb dyspraxia
	Distal				Contralateral weakness of leg, hip, foot and shoulder Sensory loss in foot Transcortical motor aphasia or motor and sensory aphasia Left limb dyspraxia

Slide 3350

Occlusion of Middle and Anterior Cerebral Arteries

Shortly after entering the cranial cavity, the internal carotid artery gives rise to the *ophthalmic, anterior choroidal* and *posterior communicating artery branches*. It then bifurcates into the anterior cerebral artery (which supplies the anterior paramedian cerebral hemisphere) and the larger middle cerebral artery (which supplies the lateral hemisphere and most of the basal ganglia). The middle cerebral artery provides penetrating lenticulo-striate branches that arise from its horizontal main stem, and trifurcates as it nears the lateral cerebral (sylvian) fissure into major superior and inferior division trunks and a smaller anterior temporal artery. The superior trunk supplies most of the lateral surface of the brain above the lateral cerebral fissure, and the inferior trunk supplies the brain below the lateral cerebral fissure and part of the inferior parietal lobe.

Occlusion of the main stem of the middle or anterior cerebral artery or their superficial branches is most often caused by an embolus from the heart or proximal vessels, especially from the cervical segment of the internal carotid artery. Occlusion of deep penetrating branches is most often caused by lipohyalinosis resulting from hypertension. Occasionally, atherosclerosis narrows the lumina of the major intracranial arteries, leading to thrombosis and occlusion. Intracranial atherosclerosis, in the absence of severe extracranial disease, usually involves the proximal main stem of the middle cerebral artery and is more common in black and Japanese patients.

The extent of infarction following occlusion of the middle or anterior cerebral artery and their branches is extremely variable and depends on the location and rapidity of the occlusive process; the anatomic features of the circle of Willis; previous occlusive lesions; and systemic circulatory, hematologic and serologic factors. □

Lacunar Infarction

Small (100 μm) artery within brain parenchyma showing typical pathologic changes secondary to hypertension. Vessel lumen almost completely obstructed by thickened media and enlarged to about three times normal size. Pink-staining fibrinoid material within walls

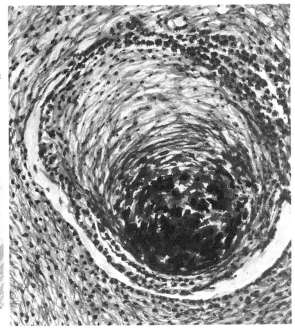

Lacunar Infarction

Lacunar infarcts in base of pons interrupting some corticospinal (pyramidal) fibers. Such lesions cause mild hemiparesis

Atherosclerosis usually affects large extracranial and intracranial arteries such as the carotid, vertebral and basilar arteries and their anterior, middle and posterior cerebral artery branches. In contrast, hypertension leads to disease of the small penetrating arteries of the brain that is qualitatively quite different from atherosclerosis of larger vessels.

The smaller vessels become occluded by a process known as *lipohyalinosis*, which disorganizes and disrupts the lumen of the vessel. Hyaline material accumulates subintimally and obliterates the lumen, leading to ischemia distal to the lesion. Because the ischemic lesions are generally small and round, the term "lacune" (hole) has traditionally been used to describe them. Penetrating arteries branch perpendicularly from the middle cerebral arteries to supply the basal ganglia and internal capsule, from the posterior and basilar communicating arteries to supply the midbrain and thalamus, and from the basilar artery to supply the pons.

Lacunes are the most common lesions found in the brain at necropsy. Patients with such lesions usually have a history of elevated blood pressure. Because the lesions are small and deep, they do not produce headache, disturb alertness, or cause slowing on an electroencephalogram (EEG). The most common lacunar syndrome is *pure motor hemiplegia*. The causative lesion, a small infarct in the base of the pons or internal capsule, produces contralateral weakness of the face, arm and leg, but no sensory, visual or intellectual dysfunction. At times, the weak limbs are also clumsy or ataxic. Dysarthria is caused by weakness and incoordination of the facial, buccal and lingual muscles.

In *pure sensory strokes*, the patient complains of contralateral paresthesias in the face, arm and leg. Often, there is little objective evidence of loss of touch, pain, temperature or position sense. Motor power, visual fields, intellectual functions and gait are well preserved. The causative lesion is in the ventral posterior medial and lateral nuclei of the thalamus.

Multiple bilateral lacunes and scars of healed lacunar infarcts in thalamus, putamen, globus pallidus, caudate nucleus and internal capsule. Such infarcts produce diverse symptoms

Several lacunar syndromes result from penetrating small lesions in the pons. *Ataxic hemiparesis* describes a syndrome of incoordination of an arm or leg, or both, accompanied by weakness and pyramidal signs in the same extremities. The *dysarthria-clumsy hand syndrome* refers to slurred speech and clumsiness of the contralateral hand. Toppling to the side when erect and pure dysarthria also can be caused by brainstem lacunes.

In some patients, accumulation of many lacunes leads to a syndrome of parkinsonianlike rigidity, weakness, hyperreflexia, pseudobulbar palsy and dementia.

Diagnostic criteria include a history of hypertension, a deficit accumulation of short duration, and anatomic localization of the infarct to deep territories. Computed tomography (CT) may document a small deep infarct, but may show no abnormality if the lesion is too small for imaging. A normal or symmetrically abnormal EEG is also a helpful diagnostic finding. In occasional cases when the clinical syndrome is not typical, angiography is required to exclude significant occlusion of the parent arteries.

Treatment of the acute lesion includes bed rest and maintenance of blood pressure. Later, control of blood pressure and of blood sugar abnormalities is important. Neither surgical correction of proximal vessel disease nor anticoagulant therapy is of proved or hypothetical value in treating lacunes. □

Ischemia in Vertebrobasilar Territory: Clinical Manifestations

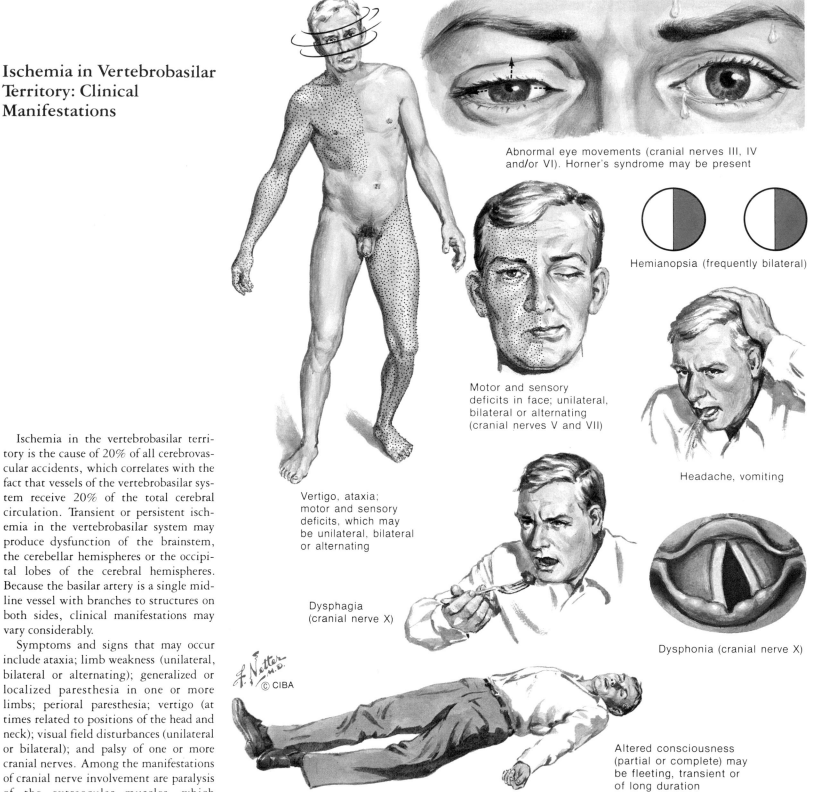

Abnormal eye movements (cranial nerves III, IV and/or VI). Horner's syndrome may be present

Hemianopsia (frequently bilateral)

Motor and sensory deficits in face; unilateral, bilateral or alternating (cranial nerves V and VII)

Headache, vomiting

Vertigo, ataxia; motor and sensory deficits, which may be unilateral, bilateral or alternating

Dysphagia (cranial nerve X)

Dysphonia (cranial nerve X)

Altered consciousness (partial or complete) may be fleeting, transient or of long duration

Ischemia in the vertebrobasilar territory is the cause of 20% of all cerebrovascular accidents, which correlates with the fact that vessels of the vertebrobasilar system receive 20% of the total cerebral circulation. Transient or persistent ischemia in the vertebrobasilar system may produce dysfunction of the brainstem, the cerebellar hemispheres or the occipital lobes of the cerebral hemispheres. Because the basilar artery is a single midline vessel with branches to structures on both sides, clinical manifestations may vary considerably.

Symptoms and signs that may occur include ataxia; limb weakness (unilateral, bilateral or alternating); generalized or localized paresthesia in one or more limbs; perioral paresthesia; vertigo (at times related to positions of the head and neck); visual field disturbances (unilateral or bilateral); and palsy of one or more cranial nerves. Among the manifestations of cranial nerve involvement are paralysis of the extraocular muscles, which produces diplopia (oculomotor [III], trochlear [IV] and abducens [VI] nerves); facial paralysis of one or both sides (facial [VII] nerve); difficulty in phonation (somatic motor portion of vagus [X] nerve); dysphagia (glossopharyngeal [IX] and vagus nerves); and dysarthria (vagus and hypoglossal [XII] nerves).

It is not uncommon to see a patient whose symptoms are confined to dysfunction of one specific cranial nerve but without associated complaints that suggest involvement of other cranial nerves or adjacent ascending or descending tracts, ie, the spinothalamic or corticospinal tracts. For example, vertigo or dizziness, with or without other symptoms and signs, is frequently seen in older patients. These patients should be observed carefully, particularly for a 6-week period following the vertiginous episode, for signs of other abnormalities in the multiple structures supplied by the vertebrobasilar system. If the symptoms continue to appear isolated, they should not be attributed to vertebrobasilar ischemia. The course in such patients should be benign.

If alteration of consciousness occurs, it may be preceded by fading vision (dimout or blackout) or a sense of giddiness, followed by loss of postural tone and falling. The presence of coma implies ischemia of the midbrain reticular activating system, which is then unable to alert the cerebral cortex. Rarely, patients may undergo a transient ischemic attack (TIA), which affects only the corticospinal tracts and is manifested by a simple drop attack or a sudden fall to the ground without impairment of consciousness. This differs from the common brief syncopal episode seen in patients with cardiac arrhythmias who suddenly fall but always experience an accompanying, although brief, loss of consciousness.

Hyperextension and concomitant rotation of the head and neck also reduce blood flow in one or both vertebral arteries. This may happen during chiropractic manipulation.

Tortuous segments, coils and kinks of the vertebral arteries are often observed on angiograms of the extracranial circulation, but have not been specifically related to vertebrobasilar ischemia. □

Ischemia in Vertebrobasilar Territory: Clinical Manifestations Related to Site

The vertebral and basilar arteries and their branches supply the brainstem and cerebellum. The posterior cerebral arteries are the terminal branches of the basilar artery, and supply the medial, temporal and occipital lobes and also the splenium of the corpus callosum. Within the vertebrobasilar circulation may be found an unusually high number of congenital anomalies, such as an atypical origin of the vertebral artery, unilateral hypoplasia of a vertebral artery, and persistent fetal vessels connecting the anterior and posterior circulations. There is also a plethora of potential collateral channels.

Symptoms of vascular insufficiency within the posterior circulation depend on (1) the rostral-caudal level of the ischemia, ie, whether the medulla oblongata, pons, midbrain, temporal lobes, etc, are involved; (2) the focus of ischemia within the brainstem, ie, whether tegmental or basal structures are involved; and (3) the adequacy of collateral circulation.

The *basal portion of the brainstem* is the major pathway for the descending corticospinal tracts and also contains crossing cerebellar fibers and extrapyramidal pathways. Dysfunction of the base at any rostral-caudal level causes loss of motor function. A unilateral lesion results in contralateral hemiparesis, occasionally with accompanying ataxia, whereas bilateral lesions cause quadriparesis.

The cranial nerve nuclei are in the *tegmentum*, and a lesion of any of these structures affects various motor or sensory functions. The hypoglossal nucleus (tongue function) is in the medial medulla. More lateral in the medulla are the nucleus ambiguus (pharyngeal and palatal muscle function) and the solitary tract nucleus (taste). The facial nucleus (facial muscle function), motor nucleus of the trigeminal nerve (jaw function), abducens nucleus (abduction of the eye), and the vestibular (equilibrium) and cochlear (hearing) nuclei are in the pontine tegmentum.

The descending spinal tract of the trigeminal (V) nerve and its nucleus (controlling ipsilateral facial pain and temperature) course through the lateral medulla and pons. The oculomotor and trochlear nuclei (eye motion except abduction) are in the midbrain tegmentum just ventral to the cerebral aqueduct (of Sylvius). Also traversing the tegmentum laterally are descending sympathetic fibers (a lesion of which leads to Horner's syndrome) and the spinothalamic tract, which carries pain and temperature fibers from the contralateral trunk and limbs. Near the base in the tegmentum is the medial lemniscus (controlling position sense from the contralateral limbs). The reticular formation courses through the medial tegmentum, and bilateral destruction of this entity leads to coma.

The relay stations for the various afferent sensory functions, as well as the most rostral level

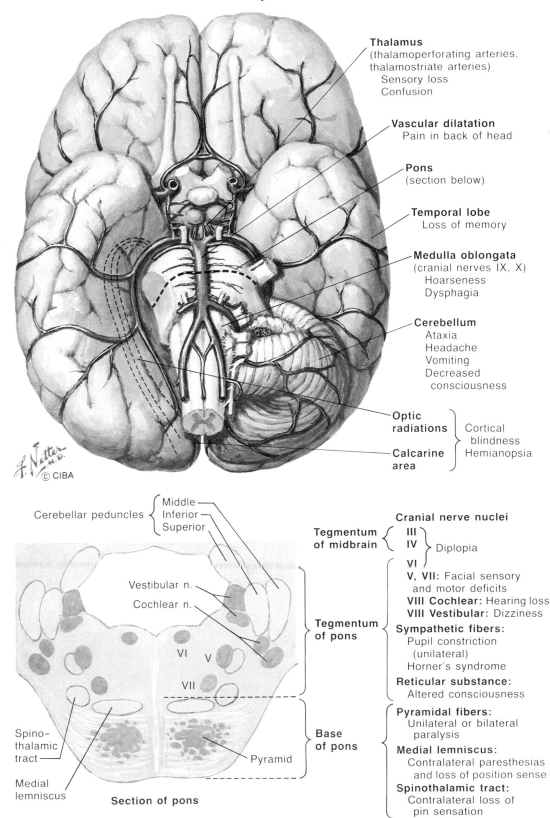

Thalamus
(thalamoperforating arteries, thalamostriate arteries)
Sensory loss
Confusion

Vascular dilatation
Pain in back of head

Pons
(section below)

Temporal lobe
Loss of memory

Medulla oblongata
(cranial nerves IX, X)
Hoarseness
Dysphagia

Cerebellum
Ataxia
Headache
Vomiting
Decreased
consciousness

Optic radiations ⎱ Cortical
Calcarine ⎰ blindness
area ⎰ Hemianopsia

Cerebellar peduncles { Middle / Inferior / Superior

Vestibular n.
Cochlear n.

VI V
VII

Spino-thalamic tract
Medial lemniscus
Pyramid

Section of pons

Cranial nerve nuclei

Tegmentum of midbrain { III / IV } Diplopia

VI
V, VII: Facial sensory and motor deficits
VIII Cochlear: Hearing loss
VIII Vestibular: Dizziness

Tegmentum of pons

Sympathetic fibers:
Pupil constriction (unilateral)
Horner's syndrome

Reticular substance:
Altered consciousness

Base of pons

Pyramidal fibers:
Unilateral or bilateral paralysis

Medial lemniscus:
Contralateral paresthesias and loss of position sense

Spinothalamic tract:
Contralateral loss of pin sensation

of the reticular activating system, are located in the thalamic nuclei. The occipital lobe, which is supplied by the posterior cerebral arteries, contains the primary visual cortex. The hippocampi and medial temporal lobes are important in the function of memory. A lesion in the posterior cerebral artery territory usually causes hemianopsia, hemisensory loss and, occasionally, amnesia and dyslexia.

Symptoms of several systemic and nonvascular neurologic conditions may mimic vertebrobasilar territory ischemia. For example, syncope, hypotension and hypoglycemia cause lightheadedness, dizziness and dimming of vision and hearing.

Diseases of the labyrinth and peripheral vestibular system cause episodic attacks of vertigo, sometimes with nausea and disequilibrium. Temporal lobe epilepsy can cause visual, memory or behavioral alterations similar to ischemic attacks in the posterior cerebral artery territory. Classic migraine, for uncertain reasons, particularly affects the posterior circulation vasculature and may cause vertigo, diplopia, visual disturbances and facial and limb paresthesias. Differentiating migraine from atherosclerotic ischemia is sometimes difficult, because some patients with ischemia have prominent headache in addition to neurologic symptoms. ☐

Extracranial Occlusive Disease of Vertebral and Subclavian Arteries

Stenosis or occlusion of the proximal subclavian artery before the origin of its vertebral artery branch may cause intermittent ischemic attacks referable to the vertebrobasilar system. Atherosclerosis, temporal arteritis, Takayasu's "pulseless" disease, and use of the subclavian artery in surgical repairs in congenital heart disease are the most common causes of ischemia at this site.

The most frequent signs and symptoms relate to the ischemic arm, which is often cool, has a decreased pulse and blood pressure, and is painful during arm exercise. Neurologic manifestations are uncommon. When present, dizziness, diplopia and altered vision are the predominant neurologic symptoms, and are occasionally precipitated by exercising the ischemic arm. Diminished blood flow into the vertebral system is caused by plaque extending into and blocking the orifice of the vertebral artery. If the subclavian or innominate artery is occluded and the major cranial vessels are patent, blood flow may be reversed in the ipsilateral vertebral artery, the so-called subclavian steal syndrome.

Noninvasive tests such as venous occlusive plethysmography and Doppler ultrasonography (Plates 20–21) accurately detect diminished flow in the arm. When right-sided aortic arch involvement affects the brachiocephalic trunk, embolic fragments of clot or plaque may interrupt flow in the carotid artery in addition to causing vertebral territory attacks. Neurologic symptoms of subclavian artery disease are usually transient; serious infarction is rare because of the rich collateral circulation available. However, subclavian artery atherosclerosis is a good indication of the presence of severe atherosclerosis, and other extracranial vessels such as the carotid arteries should be carefully screened for more serious lesions.

The most common site of atherosclerotic disease in the posterior circulation is the origin and first few millimeters (*first*, or *prevertebral*, *segment*) of the vertebral artery. Plaque either originates at this site or extends into the vessel from the subclavian artery. Congenital variations, eg, direct origin from the aortic arch, unilateral hypoplastic artery, and residual primitive connections with the carotid system, are common. Rich collateral networks of vessels originate from the thyrocervical trunk and external carotid arteries and are available should the proximal vertebral artery become occluded. These networks probably account for the fact that, in most cases, occlusion of the proximal vertebral artery causes dizziness and diplopia but usually does not cause permanent neurologic deficits. Occlusion of the proximal vertebral artery can be a source of embolization to the intracranial vertebrobasilar system, especially when the clot is newly formed and is loosely adherent to the vessel.

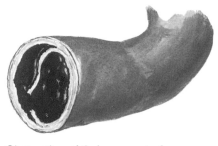

Obstruction of 3rd segment of vertebral artery is most often result of trauma or manipulation causing dissecting aneurysm

Obstruction of 1st or 2nd segment of vertebral artery may produce no or only mild functional impairment because of extensive collaterals, chiefly via ascending cervical, deep cervical and occipital arteries and muscular branches, or by reversal of flow from circle of Willis

Second segment of artery (opened) is only slightly ridged as it passes through transverse foramina. Severe obstruction by osteophytes is rare

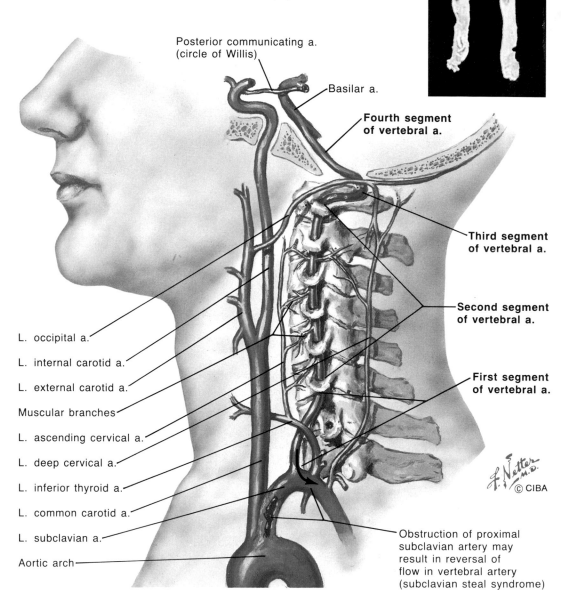

Posterior communicating a. (circle of Willis)

Basilar a.

Fourth segment of vertebral a.

Third segment of vertebral a.

Second segment of vertebral a.

First segment of vertebral a.

L. occipital a.

L. internal carotid a.

L. external carotid a.

Muscular branches

L. ascending cervical a.

L. deep cervical a.

L. inferior thyroid a.

L. common carotid a.

L. subclavian a.

Aortic arch

Obstruction of proximal subclavian artery may result in reversal of flow in vertebral artery (subclavian steal syndrome)

The *second (cervical) segment* of the vertebral artery courses through the intervertebral foramina and is seldom the site of serious atherosclerosis. Minor ridges and plaques may develop at sites of indentation by the osteophytic spurs of cervical arthritis, but occlusion of this portion of the vertebral artery is rare. The artery, in which blood flows at systemic blood pressure, is more likely to indent bone than is the bony arthritic disorder to obstruct the artery.

The *third (atlantic) segment* of the vertebral artery pursues a tortuous course after exiting from the intervertebral foramina. After circling around the posterior arch of the atlas, it pierces the dura mater and enters the posterior fossa. Although short, this segment of the artery is fixed at each end and is particularly vulnerable to trauma, especially during sudden neck movement as in chiropractic manipulation. The artery is easily dissected or torn, which may cause clot formation within one or both vertebral arteries. Ischemia most often occurs at the time of injury and is limited to the ipsilateral cerebellum and lateral brainstem. Less frequently, symptoms are delayed and are bilateral and often fatal. Atherosclerosis of the third segment is unusual. When angiography shows obstruction of the third segment of the vertebral artery, it is usually the result of occlusion of the *fourth (intracranial) segment*, with retrograde extension of the clot into the neck. □

Intracranial Occlusion of Vertebral Artery

Occlusion or stenosis of the fourth (intracranial) segment of the vertebral artery is quite common. If the *proximal* portion is occluded before the posterior inferior cerebellar artery branch, ischemia usually affects the lateral medulla oblongata or the ipsilateral side of the cerebellum. The medial medulla and more rostral brainstem are spared because of collateral blood flow through the contralateral vertebral artery.

The *lateral medullary syndrome*, or *Wallenberg syndrome*, resulting from occlusion in this area is common. The most consistent symptoms include sharp jabs of pain in the face, nose or eye and ipsilateral facial numbness; dizziness, often with a sense of turning; clumsiness of the ipsilateral arm and leg; staggering gait, with falling toward the side of the lesion; hoarseness; and dysphagia. Examination reveals ipsilateral loss of pain and temperature sensation in the face; horizontal nystagmus, often with coarse, large-amplitude jerks toward the side of the lesion; slight ipsilateral facial weakness; ipsilateral weakness of the pharynx and palate; hypotonia and ataxia of the ipsilateral limbs; ptosis and miosis of the ipsilateral eye; and decreased pain and temperature sensation in the contralateral limbs and side of the body.

The patient generally does not complain of loss of feeling in the body or limbs; this defect is determined only by sensory testing. Sometimes, because of the distribution of fibers within the spinothalamic tract, there is a sensory level on the contralateral side of the trunk. At times, involvement of the contralateral quintothalamic tract (ventral trigeminal lemniscus), which is adjacent to the spinothalamic tract, produces contralateral facial insensitivity to pin. Occlusion of the vertebral artery can produce pain behind the mastoid or in the upper neck or occiput. Vomiting, tachycardia and hiccups are also commonly associated symptoms.

The lateral medullary syndrome is usually benign unless a large portion of the cerebellum is also infarcted, causing severe pressure on the posterior fossa.

Infarction of the *cerebellum* is most frequently caused by occlusion of the intracranial segment of the vertebral artery. Dizziness, disequilibrium, vomiting, headache and diplopia are the most common symptoms. The symptoms and signs of cerebellar infarction are often difficult to distinguish from those of labyrinthitis or other disorders of the peripheral vestibular system. On examination, ocular findings may point toward an intracranial lesion. Nystagmus, sixth cranial nerve palsy, or conjugate gaze paralysis when looking toward the side of the lesion are helpful

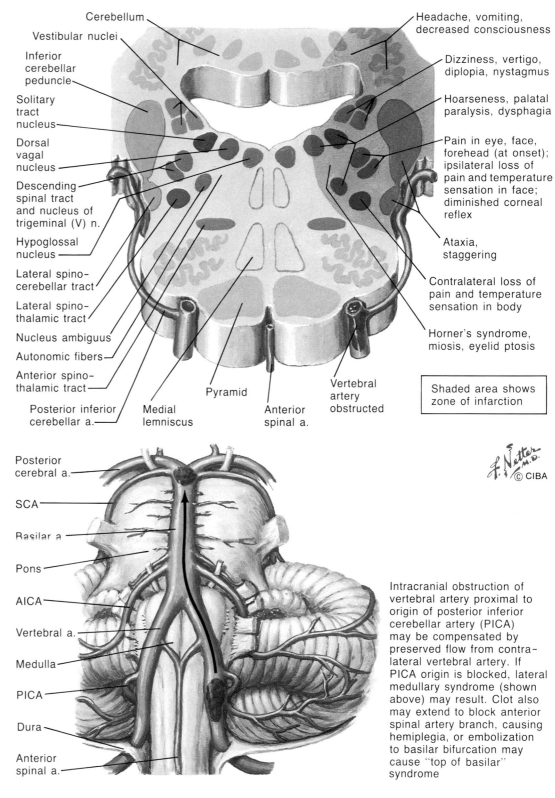

Shaded area shows zone of infarction

f. Netter © CIBA

Intracranial obstruction of vertebral artery proximal to origin of posterior inferior cerebellar artery (PICA) may be compensated by preserved flow from contralateral vertebral artery. If PICA origin is blocked, lateral medullary syndrome (shown above) may result. Clot also may extend to block anterior spinal artery branch, causing hemiplegia, or embolization to basilar bifurcation may cause "top of basilar" syndrome

clues. Gait ataxia is especially prominent on turning. When the patient is asked to quickly elevate both arms and then stop suddenly, continued motion and clumsiness of the ipsilateral arm are evident. Computed tomography (CT) confirms the diagnosis of cerebellar infarction and also provides useful information about hydrocephalus and crowding of posterior fossa structures. When hydrocephalus and brainstem compression occur, treatment includes corticosteroids, osmotic diuretic agents, drainage of the ventricles, and removal of the necrotic cerebellar hemisphere during posterior fossa decompressive surgery. Small cerebellar infarcts usually cause only slight symptoms, with good return to normal function.

If the intracranial segment of the vertebral artery is occluded *distally*, near the junction with the contralateral vertebral artery, the anterior spinal artery branch may be compromised. The resulting ischemia of the *medial medulla* causes contralateral hemiplegia. At times, the vertebral artery clot extends into the *basilar artery*, leading to the syndrome of lower basilar artery occlusion. Embolization of the clot to the more distal basilar artery can also occur. Bilateral intracranial occlusion of the vertebral artery or unilateral occlusion and a congenitally hypoplastic contralateral vertebral artery is usually very serious and leads to bilateral, often fatal, ischemia of the medulla and cerebellum. □

Occlusion of Basilar Artery and Branches

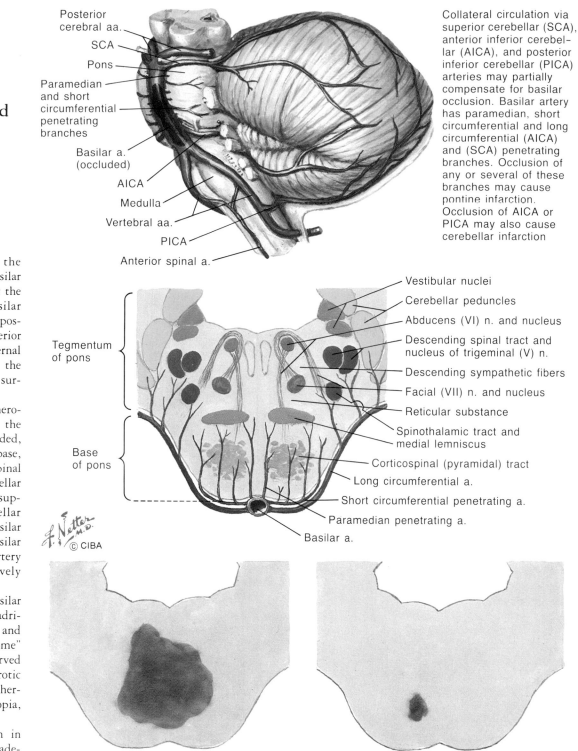

Posterior cerebral aa.

SCA

Pons

Paramedian and short circumferential penetrating branches

Basilar a. (occluded)

AICA

Medulla

Vertebral aa.

PICA

Anterior spinal a.

Collateral circulation via superior cerebellar (SCA), anterior inferior cerebellar (AICA), and posterior inferior cerebellar (PICA) arteries may partially compensate for basilar occlusion. Basilar artery has paramedian, short circumferential and long circumferential (AICA) and (SCA) penetrating branches. Occlusion of any or several of these branches may cause pontine infarction. Occlusion of AICA or PICA may also cause cerebellar infarction

Vestibular nuclei

Cerebellar peduncles

Abducens (VI) n. and nucleus

Descending spinal tract and nucleus of trigeminal (V) n.

Descending sympathetic fibers

Facial (VII) n. and nucleus

Reticular substance

Spinothalamic tract and medial lemniscus

Corticospinal (pyramidal) tract

Long circumferential a.

Short circumferential penetrating a.

Paramedian penetrating a.

Basilar a.

Tegmentum of pons

Base of pons

Large pontine infarction resulting in pupillary and other ocular abnormalities, facial weakness, quadriplegia and coma

Small infarction in base of pons, evidenced chiefly by hemiparesis

The two vertebral arteries unite at the medullary-pontine junction to form the basilar artery. The basilar artery in turn bifurcates at the pontomesencephalic junction into the basilar communicating arteries, which become the posterior cerebral arteries after receiving the posterior communicating artery branches of the internal carotid arteries. The basilar artery supplies the pons and the anterior inferior and superior surfaces of the cerebellar hemispheres.

The basilar artery is a common site of atherosclerosis, especially near its origin. When the proximal portion of the artery becomes occluded, the most vulnerable region is the pontine base, through which travel the descending corticospinal and corticobulbar motor pathways and cerebellar connections. The tegmentum of the pons is supplied principally by the superior cerebellar arteries, the most distal branches of the basilar artery, which originate just proximal to the basilar artery bifurcation. When the distal basilar artery remains patent, the tegmentum is relatively spared.

The clinical deficit in patients with basilar artery occlusion is primarily motor, with quadriplegia and weakness of the facial, tongue and pharyngeal muscles. The "locked-in syndrome" can result, with eye movement the only preserved means of communication. As in atherosclerotic lesions elsewhere, the final occlusion is often heralded by transient spells of dizziness, diplopia, weakness, ataxia and occipital headache.

Occlusion precipitates a critical situation in which survival hinges on the development of adequate collateral circulation, chiefly through the long circumferential cerebellar vessels and the carotid arterial system via the posterior communicating artery branches. If adequate collateral vessels develop, the patient may survive with little or no deficit. The critical period for development of deficits is at the time of the basilar artery occlusion. The collateral circulation is sometimes so tenuous that even the simple act of sitting up or a drop in blood pressure may extend the ischemia.

Atherosclerosis of the basilar artery can block the orifice of branches emanating from the artery, and atheroma may originate in the orifice of these branches. Occlusion of branches of the basilar artery is more common in patients with hypertension and diabetes. The branches most commonly affected are the *large paramedian pontine arteries*, which supply the median pontine base. Contralateral hemiplegia results occasionally, and is

accompanied by tingling of the contralateral limbs and an ipsilateral internuclear ophthalmoplegia.

The *thalamogeniculate artery branches* of the basilar communicating artery are also frequently affected, leading to a syndrome of contralateral face and limb paresthesias and clumsiness and ataxia of the contralateral limbs resulting from infarction in the ventrolateral thalamus.

Less often, atherosclerosis leads to blockage of an *anterior inferior cerebellar artery*. The resultant infarct in the lateral pontine tegmentum causes a deficit quite similar to the lateral medullary syndrome. Signs and symptoms include ipsilateral facial numbness and paralysis, with diminished pin and temperature sensation; ipsilateral Horner's

syndrome; horizontal nystagmus; contralateral loss of pain and temperature sensation in the limbs; ipsilateral limb ataxia; staggering gait; and deafness in the ipsilateral ear. When these findings are not accompanied by other signs of more widespread brainstem ischemia, the prognosis is quite good.

Localization of obstruction to the basilar artery or to a branch is determined by the patient's history, analysis of the anatomy of the neurologic deficit, and in some cases, angiographic visualization of the vascular occlusion. Precise localization of the obstruction is important, because treatment of basilar artery occlusion is quite different from treatment of occlusive disease of the branches. □

Occlusion of "Top of Basilar" and Posterior Cerebral Arteries

Internal carotid a.
Middle cerebral a.
Posterior communicating a.
Thalamoperforating aa. to medial thalamus
Thalamogeniculate aa. to lateral thalamus
Posterior cerebral a.
Superior cerebellar a.
Basilar a. and obstruction
Anterior inferior cerebellar a.
Vertebral a.

Areas supplied by posterior cerebral arteries (blue) and clinical manifestations of infarction

Medial thalamus and midbrain
Hypersomnolence
Small, nonreactive pupils
Bilateral third cranial
 nerve palsy
Behavioral alterations
Hallucinosis

Lateral thalamus and posterior limb of internal capsule
Hemisensory loss

Hippocampus and medial temporal lobes
Memory loss

Splenium of corpus callosum
Alexia without agraphia

Calcarine area
Hemianopsia (or bilateral blindness if both posterior cerebral arteries occluded)

Occlusion of "Top of Basilar" and Posterior Cerebral Arteries

The basilar artery is widest at its origin and gently tapers as it nears its bifurcation into the posterior cerebral artery tributaries. Emboli that originate in the heart or in the proximal vertebral system and are large enough to pass through the intracranial segments of the vertebral arteries usually do not block the larger proximal basilar artery but may obstruct the apex of the basilar artery, thus leading to ischemia in the midbrain, thalami and occipital and temporal lobes.

Numerous small penetrating arteries originate at or near the basilar apex and course through the posterior perforated substance to supply the median and paramedian midbrain tegmentum and the thalami. Interruption of this vascular supply usually causes *dysfunction of the rostral reticular activating system*, resulting in coma or excessive sleepiness. When awake, some patients report vivid visual, auditory and tactile hallucinations and describe dream or thought experiences as if they actually occurred or were happening. The pupillary reflex arc is also disrupted, leading to large, midposition or tiny pupils that react poorly to light. Eyelid ptosis, retraction of the eyelid (Collier's sign), vertical gaze paralysis, and bilateral complete or partial third cranial nerve palsies are the result of dysfunction of oculomotor pathways. Signs of unilateral or bilateral infarction of the posterior cerebral artery territory hemisphere frequently accompany brainstem dysfunction.

The posterior cerebral arteries supply the occipital lobes, thalami, splenium of the corpus callosum, and medial and inferior temporal lobes. The most common finding in occlusions of these arteries is hemianopsia contralateral to the infarction, resulting from ischemia of the visual cortex, which is located along the banks of the calcarine fissure. Patients complain of limited vision in the hemianopic field, but nevertheless are often able to read or copy objects without omitting or neglecting material in the hemianopic field of vision.

Bilateral calcarine infarction leads to cortical blindness. The sensory fibers passing from the somatosensory nuclei in the ventrolateral thalamus and headed for the sensory cortex in the parietal lobe are also disturbed. This leads to numbness, paresthesias and loss of sensation in the opposite limbs. When the hippocampi and other medial temporal structures are bilaterally infarcted, the patient exhibits a Korsakoff-like amnestic syndrome. Although able to understand and repeat language and to perform complex intellectual tasks, the patient cannot form new memories or give an account of recent events. Dysfunction of the left temporal lobe can produce a temporary amnestic syndrome lasting as long as 6 months.

The patient who has an infarction of the *left posterior cerebral artery territory* may lose the ability to read words despite a preserved ability to write, spell and name letters and numbers. Although able to write a letter to a relative, the patient cannot read back the same letter minutes later. Accompanying the syndrome of alexia without agraphia is an inability to name colors and difficulty in naming objects and people. Alexia without agraphia is caused by disconnection of visual information perceived in the right visual cortex from the left temporal speech regions, which is used to apply language to visual perceptions. Writing and spelling functions are preserved in the left speech cortex, but reading and color naming depend on visual input.

A patient who has an infarction of the *right posterior cerebral artery territory* may lose the ability to revisualize people or objects, and dreams are sometimes devoid of visual imagery. Spatial disorientation and neglect of left-sided visual stimuli accompany a large right posterior cerebral artery territory infarct. Bilateral infarction of the lower calcarine regions may cause color agnosia and inability to recognize faces. Agitated delirium, usually with memory loss, and cortical blindness are caused by bilateral temporooccipital ischemia. □

Cardiac Sources of Cerebral Emboli

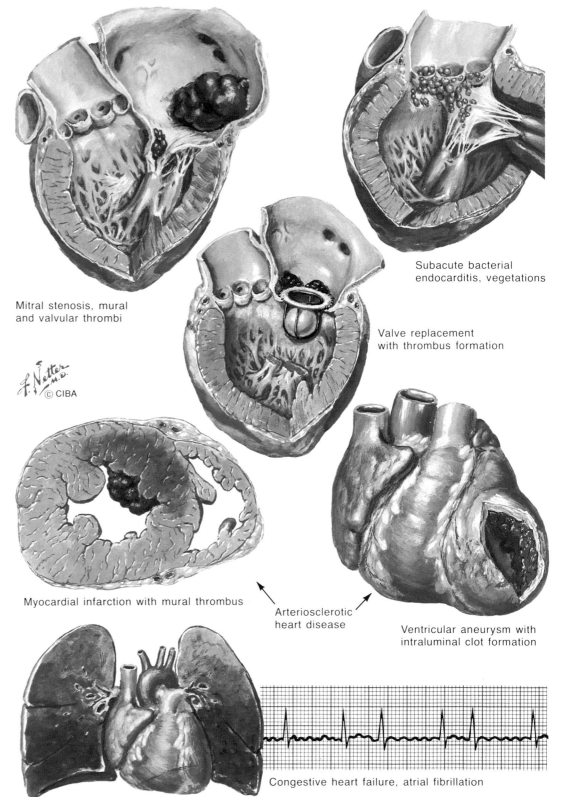

Mitral stenosis, mural and valvular thrombi

Subacute bacterial endocarditis, vegetations

Valve replacement with thrombus formation

Myocardial infarction with mural thrombus

Arteriosclerotic heart disease

Ventricular aneurysm with intraluminal clot formation

Congestive heart failure, atrial fibrillation

The classic clinical hallmark suggestive of an embolic cause of stroke is the precipitous loss of neurologic function confined to the distribution of a major cerebral vessel or one of its primary branches. In one study, cerebral angiographic examination within the first 48 hours following an acute stroke demonstrated findings suggesting an embolic mechanism in 65% of patients. However, in most large series of patients, identifiable sources of cerebral emboli were found in only 25% to 30% of patients. Often in these patients, cerebral angiography either was not done at all or was not done within the 48 hours preceding the period during which the emboli normally dissolve. The two major sources for cerebral emboli are carotid artery lesions (Plate 5) and a variety of cardiac lesions, shown in this illustration.

Atrial fibrillation is the most common cardiac pathophysiologic mechanism predisposing to cerebral emboli. The noncontracting left atrium provides a potential for the formation of intracardiac thrombi, with subsequent embolization. Rheumatic heart disease, particularly mitral stenosis with a dilated left atrium, was formerly a major cause of cerebral embolization associated with atrial fibrillation. However, as the incidence of rheumatic heart disease has declined, atrial fibrillation associated with atherosclerotic heart disease has become somewhat more important as a cause of embolic stroke. In one postmortem study, 33 of 100 consecutive patients with idiopathic atrial fibrillation had sustained a cerebral embolus and infarct.

Systemic emboli develop in about 2% of patients with *acute myocardial infarction*. Most commonly, this occurs 1 to 3 weeks after the infarction. As the infarct heals, the endocardial surface adjacent to the myocardial lesion forms a thrombus. Because myocardial infarcts may be clinically silent, any patient hospitalized with signs of a cerebral embolus should immediately have an electrocardiogram (ECG) and studies of cardiac enzymes to exclude a recent painless myocardial infarction. Rarely, chronic residua of a myocardial infarction, namely, a hypokinetic segment or a ventricular aneurysm, may provide a source of cerebral emboli.

Valve replacements, usually done for rheumatic heart disease, have the potential to develop thrombi, with a further potential for cerebral embolization.

Patients with *bacterial endocarditis* are at risk of septic emboli. Neurologic complications occur in

about 30% of all patients with this disorder, stroke being the most common. A transient ischemic attack or stroke may be the initial sign of endocarditis. Septic emboli usually affect the smaller distal branches, producing occlusion and septic infarction. Rarely, the bacteria may cause arteritis, which destroys the vessel wall and leads to the formation of a mycotic aneurysm with a potential for rupture and subarachnoid hemorrhage. Endocarditis or, rarely, atrial myxoma (Plate 17) should always be considered when angiography demonstrates a distal branch (mycotic) aneurysm, in contrast to the much more common berry aneurysm located near the circle of Willis (Plate 30).

Some clinical clues that indicate the presence of bacterial endocarditis include a heart murmur; click suggestive of mitral valve prolapse; low-grade fever; and subconjunctival, subungual or retinal petechial hemorrhages associated with an elevated erythrocyte sedimentation rate, often in the range of 60 to 100 mm/hr. A history of events predisposing to sepsis may also provide a clue, eg, recent dental work; other surgical procedures, particularly genitourinary; and use of infected syringes for narcotic abuse.

It is important to search carefully for possible signs of bacterial endocarditis in any patient with a stroke. When there is the slightest suspicion, blood cultures should be obtained. □

Uncommon Etiologic Mechanisms in Stroke

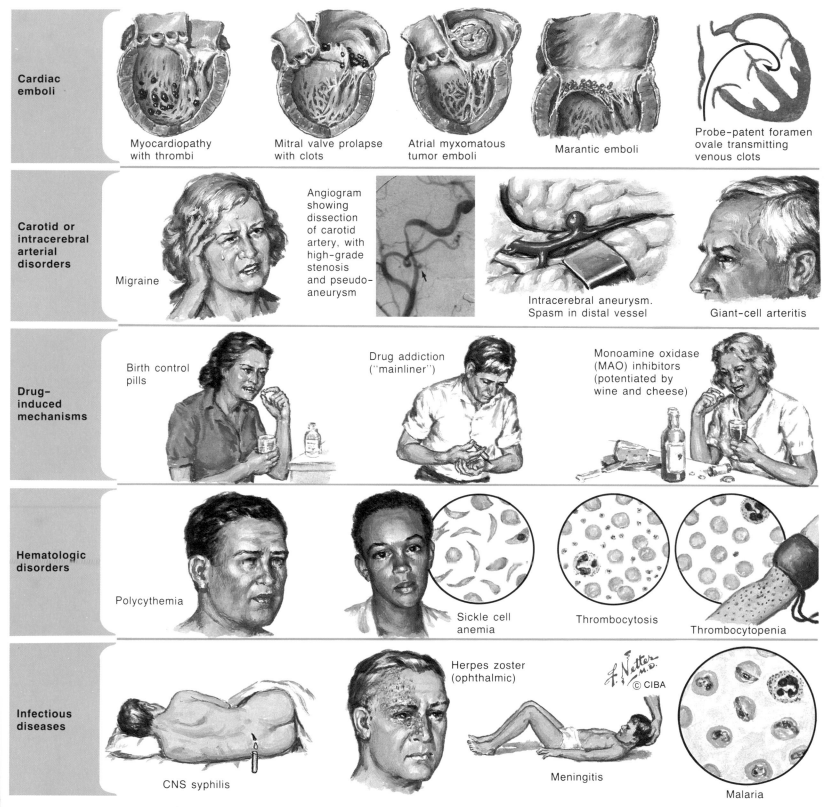

Cardiac emboli

Myocardiopathy with thrombi

Mitral valve prolapse with clots

Atrial myxomatous tumor emboli

Marantic emboli

Probe–patent foramen ovale transmitting venous clots

Carotid or intracerebral arterial disorders

Migraine

Angiogram showing dissection of carotid artery, with high-grade stenosis and pseudo-aneurysm

Intracerebral aneurysm. Spasm in distal vessel

Giant-cell arteritis

Drug-induced mechanisms

Birth control pills

Drug addiction ("mainliner")

Monoamine oxidase (MAO) inhibitors (potentiated by wine and cheese)

Hematologic disorders

Polycythemia

Sickle cell anemia

Thrombocytosis

Thrombocytopenia

Infectious diseases

CNS syphilis

Herpes zoster (ophthalmic)

Meningitis

Malaria

SECTION III   PLATE 17   *Slide 3359*

Uncommon Etiologic Mechanisms in Stroke

Although the cause of stroke in many patients can be easily identified (ie, cardiac or carotid emboli, hypertensive lacunes or intracerebral hemorrhage), in a number of other patients, the cause is not obvious. Before assuming that such strokes are idiopathic, the physician should consider less common but treatable mechanisms.

Echocardiography may define a few types of *heart disease* with embolic potential that are not immediately apparent on clinical examination.

These include *mitral valve prolapse; idiopathic myocardiopathy; intraventricular clots* in patients with painless myocardial infarction or residual aneurysm, or both; and, rarely, *atrial myxoma.* Marantic *endocarditis* in patients with mucin-secreting carcinoma is another possible source of emboli, but cannot be identified by echocardiography.

Paradoxical emboli are secondary to *venous thrombosis* in the pelvis or leg, which have entered the systemic circulation through a probe-patent foramen ovale or occult atrial septal defect. This occurs in disorders that predispose to venous stasis, ie, prolonged bed rest for neurologic or orthopedic conditions, use of birth control pills, marked obesity or underlying carcinoma.

Angiography may define *unusual arterial lesions* predisposing to stroke, including carotid and/or vertebral artery dissection; nonruptured berry aneurysms, providing sources of emboli; and critical stenosis of the carotid siphon or the proximal middle cerebral artery.

An elevated *erythrocyte sedimentation rate* may suggest mechanisms such as intracranial temporal arteritis, other vasculitides, bacterial endocarditis or atrial myxoma. The presence of *cerebrospinal fluid (CSF) pleocytosis* should lead to evaluation for tertiary syphilis; fungal, bacterial or viral infections (particularly ophthalmic herpes zoster); and meningitis. Abnormalities affecting platelets or red blood cells may also contribute to stroke. □

CT Diagnosis in Cerebrovascular Disease

Right middle cerebral artery territory: evolution of stroke

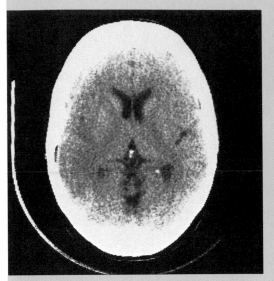

12 hours after onset of symptoms: barely perceptible loss of gray matter–white matter differentiation in right postero-temporal area

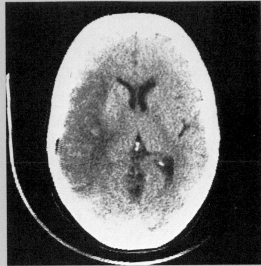

7 days after onset: generalized loss of attenuation, with resultant clearer demarcation between infarct and brain tissue

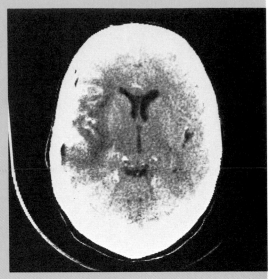

8 days after onset: CT with contrast medium showing confluent gyral pattern of enhancement

Old infarction

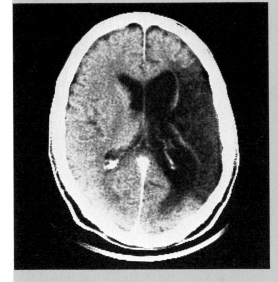

Involved area of brain shows loss of attenuation and bulk, with sharp delineation between infarct and brain tissue

Left middle cerebral artery infarct with mass effect and hemorrhage

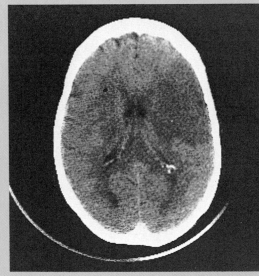

16 hours after onset of symptoms: low attenuation well demarcated. Expansion of lesion indicated by effacement of sulci

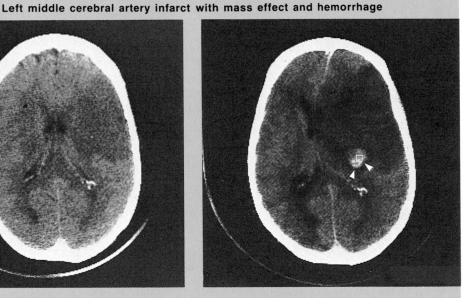

3 days after onset: left lateral ventricle compressed, with shift to midline. Hemorrhage seen in region of posterior limb of internal capsule (arrowheads)

© CIBA

SECTION III PLATE 18 *Slide 3360*

Computed Tomography Diagnosis in Cerebrovascular Disease

Many of the brain parenchymal changes that occur in the clinical setting of stroke may be detected and monitored by computed tomography (CT). Such information is important to the neuro-logic understanding and eventual treatment of stroke. However, the major value of this revolutionary, nearly risk-free technique is to document or exclude intracranial hemorrhage and to exclude tumor or other diseases that may mimic ischemic stroke.

Because the density of subarachnoid or intra-parenchymal blood differs sufficiently to be contrasted with normal brain mass, intracranial hemorrhage is readily recognized on CT. Even relatively small hemorrhages are easily seen.

The parenchymal changes that occur with nonhemorrhagic ischemic brain disease or stroke are less strikingly monitored by CT. This is especially true if the event was a transient ischemic attack (TIA). Ischemic brain infarction, though, may be diagnosed by CT done several hours or days following the acute event. The ease of and temporal course of detection vary depending upon site and extent of damage, the reestablishment of blood flow and the development of edema.

The earliest change is often a subtle decrease in x-ray attenuation, as shown in Plate 18, upper left scan, in which loss of the normal gray matter-white matter delineation is barely perceptible. Intracellular and/or extracellular edema is thought to be responsible for this loss in attenuation. If an infarct is large, such changes may be detected in the first 12 to 24 hours. Delineation between normal brain and infarct usually is more clear-cut in 3 to 4 days. By 7 to 10 days, nearly 75% of infarcts can be detected by CT. Many infarctions progress with further loss of attenuation, sharper delineation between diseased and normal brain, and enlargement of adjacent subarachnoid or ventricular spaces (Plate 18).

68

THE CIBA COLLECTION, VOLUME 1

Computed Tomography Diagnosis in Cerebrovascular Disease
(Continued)

CT Diagnosis in Cerebrovascular Disease (continued)

Embolic infarction with *Staphylococcus epidermidis* endocarditis

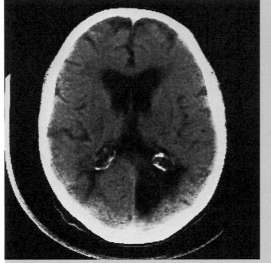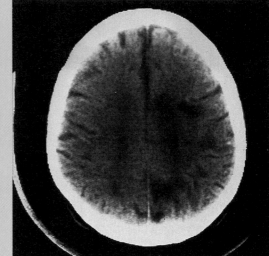

Multiple areas of low but varying attenuation in both hemispheres. Lowest attenuation infarct (left occipital, arrows) is older than 4 weeks; other infarcts, less well defined, are of more recent onset

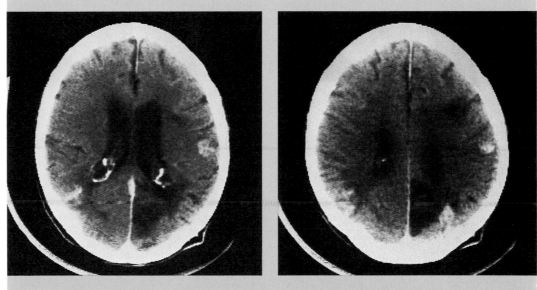

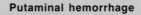

8 days after onset of ictus: CT scan with contrast medium shows several enhancing lesions in both hemispheres, indicating several areas of recent infarction

Putaminal hemorrhage

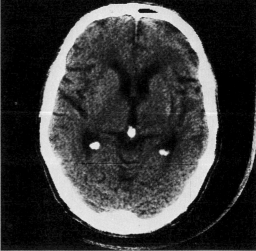

Early stage: well-circumscribed putaminal hemorrhage, with narrow lucent halo

Late stage: smaller zone of low attenuation is residuum of hemorrhage

© CIBA

This loss of attenuation may be somewhat modified in the presence of petechial hemorrhage. However, with hemorrhage, a focal accumulation of blood (hematoma) often becomes apparent and the hemorrhagic condition is recognized. Hemorrhage with infarction, if it occurs, usually does so in the first 4 to 5 days post infarction. Following ischemic infarction, hemorrhage occurs about 6% of the time.

Edema or hemorrhage may produce significant mass effect in nearly 25% to 50% of infarcts. Rarely, edema or bleeding is massive for reasons not well understood (Plate 18). Expansion is usually maximal by the end of the first week and gradually subsides over the next 2 to 3 weeks.

Following a nonenhanced CT study, a contrast-enhanced scan may yield a higher detection rate or provide additional information. Enhancement is rare before 3 days and is maximal 7 to 10 days post infarction. The most typical pattern of enhancement is a confluent or patchy enhancement of gray matter in a gyral configuration (Plate 19). Unfortunately, almost any pattern of enhancement may occur, and certain patterns are indistinguishable from neoplasm. As such, the contrast-enhanced examination infrequently yields information useful in patient management.

Intracerebral hemorrhage with resultant stroke can occur in the setting of hypertension or with a variety of vascular lesions, such as aneurysms, arteriovenous malformations, tumors, trauma or bleeding disorders. The majority of the so-called hypertensive hemorrhages involve the basal ganglia, thalamus, brainstem or, more rarely, the brain cortex (Plate 19). Identification is simple on a nonenhanced CT scan. The major diagnostic consideration is to exclude other lesions that may also bleed. □

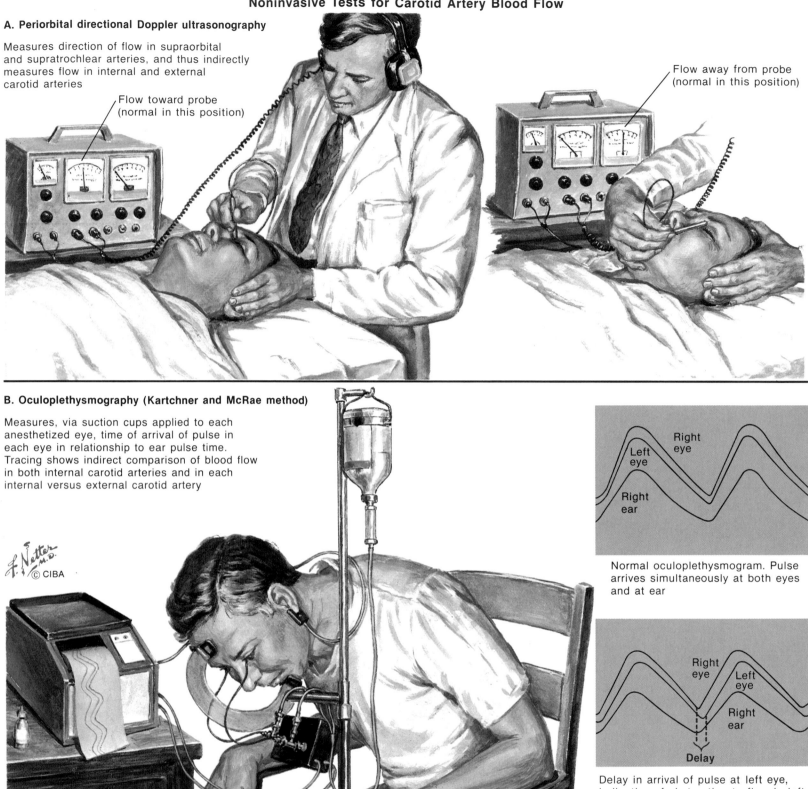

A. Periorbital directional Doppler ultrasonography

Measures direction of flow in supraorbital and supratrochlear arteries, and thus indirectly measures flow in internal and external carotid arteries

Flow toward probe (normal in this position)

Flow away from probe (normal in this position)

B. Oculoplethysmography (Kartchner and McRae method)

Measures, via suction cups applied to each anesthetized eye, time of arrival of pulse in each eye in relationship to ear pulse time. Tracing shows indirect comparison of blood flow in both internal carotid arteries and in each internal versus external carotid artery

Right eye

Left eye

Right ear

Normal oculoplethysmogram. Pulse arrives simultaneously at both eyes and at ear

Right eye

Left eye

Right ear

Delay

Delay in arrival of pulse at left eye, indicative of obstruction to flow in left internal carotid artery

SECTION III   PLATE 20   *Slide 3362*

Noninvasive Tests for Carotid Artery Blood Flow

Various arteriographic procedures are available for diagnosing lesions of the common and internal carotid arteries (Plates 22–23). However, because of the risks involved in these procedures, a search continues for safe, accurate noninvasive diagnostic methods. A large number of such tests have been developed, but some clinicians remain skeptical about noninvasive diagnosis because hemodynamic tests cannot provide anatomic information about atheromatous plaques, and tests designed to provide anatomic information cannot delineate many ulcerated lesions. Noninvasive testing may never replace conventional arteriography, but it can be extremely useful as a preliminary measure in selecting patients for whom arteriography is imperative.

The techniques for noninvasive diagnosis are readily classified as *indirect* and *direct* procedures. Indirect techniques are used to determine hemodynamic changes in distal arterial beds, such as those in the orbital and cerebral circulations. Direct tests provide either anatomic or physiologic information about the carotid artery itself.

Indirect Tests. The most commonly used indirect tests measure changes in the orbital bed. These procedures are *periorbital directional Doppler ultrasonography* and two types of *oculoplethysmography* (Plate 20). One method of oculoplethysmography (Gee method) combines a pulse volume recording with determination of the absolute systolic ophthalmic artery pressure. The other method (Kartchner and McRae method) monitors the relative arrival times of the ocular pulse waves in relationship to ear pulse time and is thus concerned with flow rather than pressure. Attempts have been made to incorporate both techniques

Noninvasive Tests for Carotid Artery Blood Flow
(Continued)

into a single instrument, but these efforts have been unsuccessful.

Indirect tests depend on a hemodynamic change, and for this reason yield negative results in the presence of nonobstructing atheromatous lesions, particularly those that are ulcerated. Moreover, both types of indirect tests are non-specific for the carotid artery because they monitor two major circulatory beds and cannot distinguish between an abnormality in the ophthalmic artery and one in the carotid artery itself.

Direct Tests. The direct physiologic tests include bruit analysis and transcutaneous imaging techniques. The two most common methods of bruit analysis, which are quite distinct, are both referred to as *phonoangiography.* One presents a display of the intensity of the bruit as a function of time, *direct bruit analysis* (Plate 21); the other, *spectral bruit analysis,* uses spectral analysis to describe the relationship of the intensity to the frequency of the bruit, assisting in the derivation of accurate numerical estimates of the residual diameter of the vascular lumen.

For either method to be useful, a bruit must be present. In approximately 30% of patients with carotid lesions, no bruit is audible when the residual lumen is 2 mm or less. Another 10% of patients who have bruits are unable to hold their breath long enough for satisfactory analysis.

Direct pathoanatomic tests produce an image of the cervical carotid bifurcation and may demonstrate atheromatous lesions, including those that may not yet have produced a hemodynamic change detectable by indirect testing. Furthermore, these tests may provide information as to whether or not an abnormality detected in an indirect test is the result of extracranial carotid artery disease. There are two distinct groups of imaging techniques suitable for the carotid artery. One includes the high-frequency *B-scan;* the other, the continuous or pulse-wave *Doppler* devices. Both systems use ultrasonic waves.

B-scanners record echoes that are related to variations in acoustic impedance of the tissues under investigation and provide instantaneous imaging of the vessel wall in real time so that it is seen while pulsating. Their principal diagnostic value is in delineating extensive lesions that distort sound waves. Thus, accurate determination of the width of the residual lumen is not feasible with phonoangiography.

The Doppler systems register frequency shifts that are related to flow velocity. Some clinicians consider that the audio information obtained with Doppler systems is more useful diagnostically than the video information, and methods have been developed to enhance the audio value.

Virtually the same limitations are inherent in the B-scan and Doppler imaging systems as in the indirect hemodynamic measuring devices. Neither can consistently demonstrate ulceration on atheromatous plaques, information that may be extremely important in determining the pathogenesis of transient ischemic attacks (TIAs).

C. Phonoangiography: direct bruit analysis

Operator applies microphone over three levels of carotid artery (angle of jaw, bifurcation and just above clavicle). Arterial sounds are detected by electronic stethoscope; resultant oscilloscopic waves are photographed by attached Polaroid camera

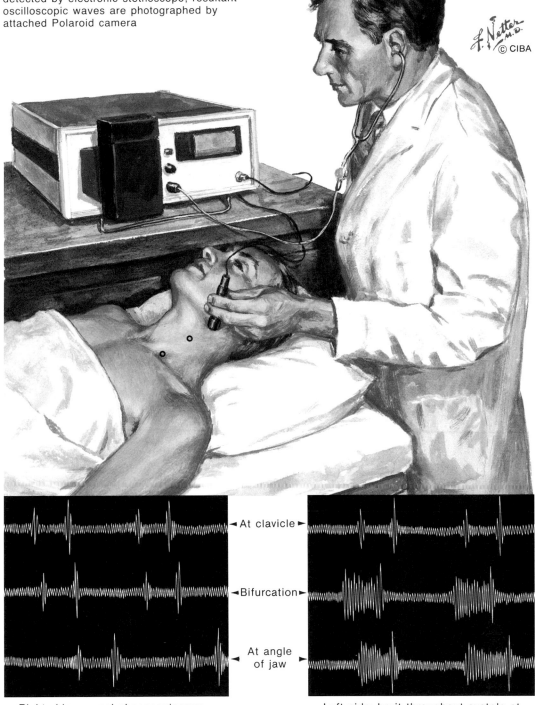

‹At clavicle›

‹Bifurcation›

At angle of jaw›

Right side: normal phonoangiogram. No bruit in carotid artery at any of three levels

Left side: bruit throughout systole at carotid bifurcation transmitted upward to angle of jaw

With the B-scan system, some lesions that have the same acoustic impedance as moving blood cannot be imaged because they are sonically translucent. An image of a vessel with such a lesion may suggest that the lumen is normal. The Doppler system, however, can provide some indication of this type of lesion.

Unfortunately, neither system can consistently differentiate a "subocclusive" lesion from a complete occlusion of the carotid artery. Nevertheless, it is potentially possible to obtain high-resolution images and important hemodynamic information by developing a real-time B-scan imager with a Doppler interface. Thus far, attempts to build such an instrument applicable to clinical use have not been successful.

Test Criteria. An ideal noninvasive test for carotid artery disease should be (1) practicable, (2) safe, (3) productive of highly specific, reproducible hemodynamic and pathoanatomic data, and (4) cost-effective.

Direct and indirect noninvasive tests can complement each other physiologically, and in an effective diagnostic workup, a battery of both types of tests is used. In general, noninvasive diagnosis should be used to determine which patients should have an arteriogram rather than to determine which should not. □

Angiography of Cervical and Cerebral Vessels

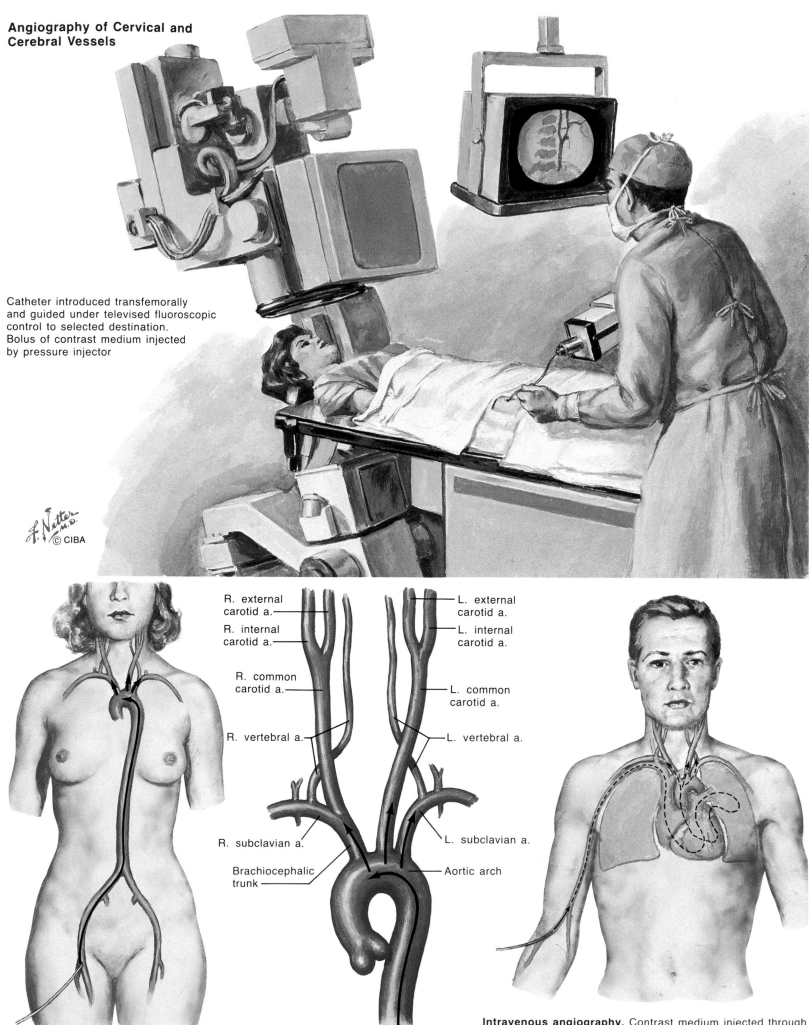

Catheter introduced transfemorally and guided under televised fluoroscopic control to selected destination. Bolus of contrast medium injected by pressure injector

R. external carotid a.

R. internal carotid a.

R. common carotid a.

R. vertebral a.

R. subclavian a.

Brachiocephalic trunk

L. external carotid a.

L. internal carotid a.

L. common carotid a.

L. vertebral a.

L. subclavian a.

Aortic arch

Retrograde transfemoral arterial angiography. Catheter passed up aorta to arch, then selectively into carotid or vertebral artery for injection of contrast medium and visualization by conventional or digital subtraction radiography

Intravenous angiography. Contrast medium injected through catheter in antecubital or subclavian vein, passes via superior vena cava to right side of heart, then through lungs, back to left side of heart, to aorta and its brachiocephalic branches for visualization by digital subtraction imaging

Angiographic Techniques

Angiography, the radiographic monitoring of an intravascular injection of a radiopaque contrast medium, is the most accurate diagnostic procedure for evaluating vascular anatomy and abnormalities. Angiography accurately defines and localizes arterial luminal abnormalities, assesses collateral vessel potential, and excludes coexisting pathologic processes. However, any type of angiographic technique used entails some degree of risk or morbidity; thus, angiography is usually the final diagnostic test before definitive treatment.

Selection of Patients. Information provided by angiography is used to determine the most effective treatment of cerebrovascular obstructive or ulcerative disease. Patients who have transient cerebral or retinal ischemic attacks (TIAs) that clear within 24 hours should be strongly considered for angiography. About 10% to 50% of strokes are preceded by TIAs, and in most patients, a surgically accessible lesion is responsible for these episodes. Patients with a minor stroke, or residual ischemic neurologic deficit (RIND), are also candidates for angiography after they have stabilized. In these patients, as well as in those in whom the diagnosis of stroke is in question, computed tomography (CT) should always precede any decision about angiography.

More controversial is the role of angiography in patients with asymptomatic bruits or in whom noninvasive diagnostic tests show that stenosis is worsening as monitored. The procedure is also questionable when such patients must undergo major surgery, in which the risk of prolonged hypotension is possible.

Intravenous Digital Subtraction Angiography (IDSA). For this procedure, a moderately large amount of contrast medium is injected rapidly into an antecubital vein (Plate 22) or more centrally into either the vena cava or the right atrium. After traversing the pulmonary vascular system, the contrast medium is visualized in the systemic vascular circulation. For subtraction, a digitalized fluoroscopic image is made just before the arrival of the dye bolus. This is subtracted from an image with contrast medium, leaving only the contrast-filled vessels. The image may be enhanced by computer techniques that greatly improve detail and sensitivity. For diagnosing cerebrovascular disease, the aortic arch, the brachiocephalic vessels and, to a lesser degree, the intracranial vessels may be visualized.

Although IDSA avoids many of the risks and discomforts of conventional angiography, detail is poor and vessels often appear to overlap. Poor patient cooperation (movement) and poor cardiac output also severely affect these images, and renal toxicity is a potential hazard.

Arterial Digital Subtraction Angiography (ADSA). ADSA and conventional film angiography are commonly performed using the trans-

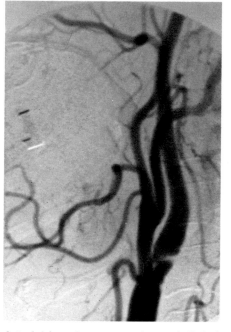

Arterial imaging: comparison of digital subtraction versus 2 ×-magnification film angiography

Above: digital subtraction image provides diagnostically clear visualization of marked stenosis and ulceration at origin of left internal carotid artery

Right: 2 ×-magnification film technique provides larger field of view and better image quality in same patient

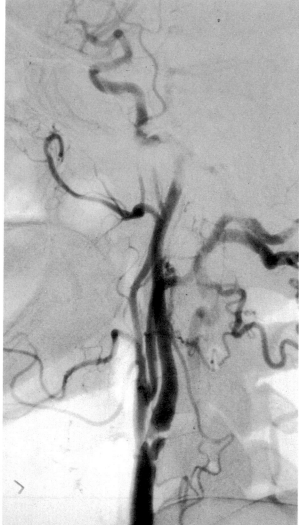

© CIBA

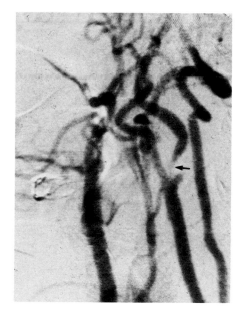

Intravenous digital subtraction angiography
High-grade stenosis (arrow) and possible proximal ulceration of left internal carotid artery are clearly delineated. Total occlusion of right internal carotid artery is less well demonstrated on this film because of swallowing artifact and projection. Note that intravenous angiography of necessity opacifies all arteries on both left and right sides

femoral approach, with the transaxillary approach used rarely (Plate 22). The implementation of smaller, more flexible catheters has greatly reduced the risks of this procedure. Nonetheless, iatrogenic embolization of clot about the catheter system or of friable material from the diseased vessel may occur.

The trade-off between ADSA and conventional angiographic film techniques is the use of smaller amounts of contrast medium and the increased speed in ADSA versus the finer detail of film angiography (Plate 23). Since angiographic risks are especially high in patients with arteriosclerotic vascular disease and since exquisite small-vessel arterial detail is rarely important, ADSA is fast

becoming the more popular choice in this group of patients.

Risks in Angiography. Before any vascular imaging procedure is recommended, the risks must be carefully weighed against the benefits. Allergy to contrast medium is a relative contraindication to all these techniques, but is about twice as common in intravenous as in intraarterial techniques. Because of the large amounts of contrast medium used, IDSA techniques may adversely affect renal function or, rarely, precipitate cardiac failure. On the other hand, risks of intraarterial catheterization include local injury to the vessel at the puncture site or distally, and the possibility of embolism and stroke. □

Clinical Evaluation and Therapeutic Options in Stroke

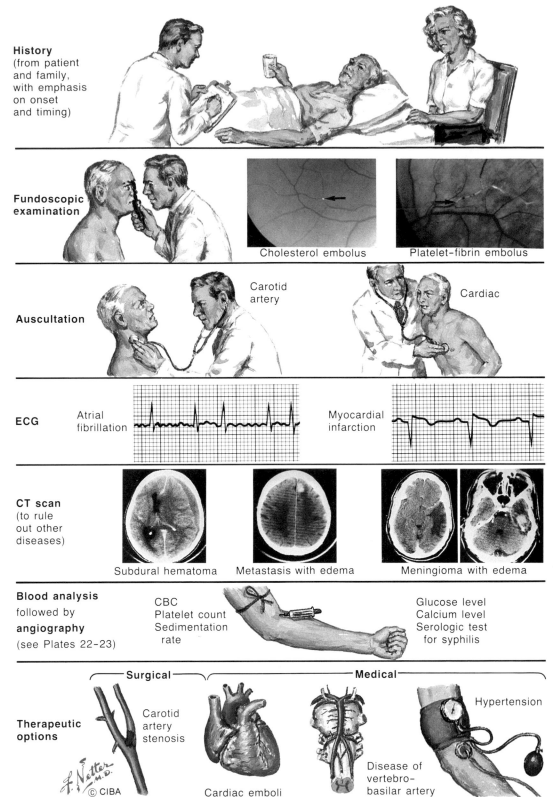

History (from patient and family, with emphasis on onset and timing)

Fundoscopic examination

Cholesterol embolus   Platelet-fibrin embolus

Auscultation   Carotid artery   Cardiac

ECG   Atrial fibrillation   Myocardial infarction

CT scan (to rule out other diseases)

Subdural hematoma   Metastasis with edema   Meningioma with edema

Blood analysis followed by angiography (see Plates 22-23)   CBC Platelet count Sedimentation rate   Glucose level Calcium level Serologic test for syphilis

Therapeutic options

Surgical   Medical

Carotid artery stenosis   Cardiac emboli   Disease of vertebro-basilar artery   Hypertension

In the differential diagnosis of a focal neurologic deficit, the physician must consider not only primary cardiovascular and cerebrovascular causes of stroke but also other pathophysiologic mechanisms that cause symptoms mimicking a stroke.

A carefully elicited history, including interviews of the patient's relatives and friends, and a thorough examination help to differentiate a cerebrovascular event from less common neurologic lesions. Cardiac auscultation, an electrocardiogram (ECG) and, sometimes, echocardiography help identify possible cardiac sources of cerebral emboli. Auscultation of the various arteries in the neck, in conjunction with noninvasive studies, yields important information about potential carotid emboli. Fundoscopic examination may demonstrate cholesterol or platelet-fibrin emboli, which usually originate from the carotid bifurcation.

Diagnostic Studies. Laboratory evaluation should include a complete blood count, including platelet count; determination of the erythrocyte sedimentation rate and levels of serum glucose, creatinine and calcium; and a serologic test for syphilis.

Computed tomography (CT), which should be done on admission and before a spinal tap, is of particular value in differentiating hemorrhagic and nonhemorrhagic stroke and in excluding the uncommon causes of acute focal neurologic deficit, ie, subdural hematoma and primary or metastatic brain tumors. Cerebrospinal fluid (CSF) analysis is of value chiefly in confirming a subarachnoid hemorrhage not seen on CT or infection in a febrile patient in whom CT does not show a mass lesion.

If a mass lesion or intracerebral/subarachnoid hemorrhage is not demonstrated and the patient does not have a dense hemiplegia or aphasia, intravenous administration of heparin may be considered during the evaluation in the hope of preventing progression or recurrence of the cerebral ischemic event.

Angiography is of help in (1) defining the carotid bifurcation; (2) demonstrating an embolus within a cerebral artery branch, providing the study is performed within the first 48 hours after onset of symptoms; (3) delineating other possible intracranial lesions such as at the carotid siphon or a stenotic atherosclerotic lesion of the middle cerebral artery; and (4) demonstrating cerebral aneurysms.

Treatment. The underlying mechanism and the severity of the deficit dictate the treatment. Patients with a transient ischemic attack (TIA) or residual ischemic neurologic deficit (RIND) who have an operable carotid lesion on the side appropriate to the symptoms and findings are generally considered candidates for endarterectomy (Plate 25). If no operable carotid lesion is found, if the TIA or RIND is in the vertebrobasilar system, or if a cardiac source of emboli is demonstrated, a course of anticoagulants or antiplatelet therapy is usually considered.

The treatment of choice is controversial because of the inherent risk of intracerebral hemorrhage, particularly when anticoagulants are used for more than 10 months. Some neurologists prefer to first try the more benign antiplatelet therapy, such as *acetylsalicylic acid* or *dipyridamole*, and to use anticoagulants only if the patient has recurrent focal ischemic events during antiplatelet therapy. If nonseptic cardiac emboli have been documented, early anticoagulation is generally advocated, providing there is no large infarct demonstrated by CT. Duration of therapy depends on the mechanism; it is usually 6 to 12 weeks in the patient with a recent myocardial infarction versus long-term in the patient with chronic atrial fibrillation. Blood pressure should be carefully controlled in the patient sustaining lacunar infarctions. ☐

Endarterectomy for Extracranial Carotid Artery Atherosclerosis

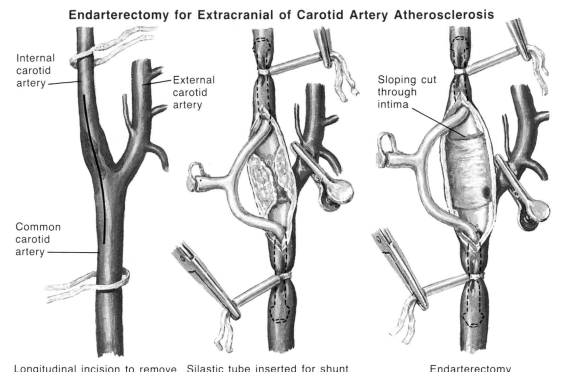

Longitudinal incision to remove atherosclerotic obstruction at carotid bifurcation

Silastic tube inserted for shunt during endarterectomy. T permits clearance of air from tube

Endarterectomy performed

Transient cerebral ischemic attacks (TIAs) indicate a significant risk of subsequent stroke. When these episodes involve the brain and eye territory served by the carotid arteries, they may be caused by a correctable obstruction of the origin of the ipsilateral internal carotid artery. Timely recognition of transient cerebral hemispheric ischemia, or amaurosis fugax (transient dimming or loss of vision in the ipsilateral eye), is important, because effective measures can be taken to prevent stroke. Cerebral angiography, a safe procedure when done by an experienced person, can demonstrate whether the obstructing lesion is significantly impairing carotid blood flow, whether an ulcerated plaque may be the source of obstruction, and whether the obstructing lesion is amenable to surgery.

Occasionally in asymptomatic patients, a carotid bruit is detected as part of a routine examination. In these patients, noninvasive testing by Doppler ultrasonography and oculoplethysmography can help to determine whether an obstruction is hemodynamically significant (Plate 20). To impair flow, the lesion must obstruct 70% or more of the vessel lumen.

A safe surgical technique, carotid endarterectomy, has been devised to remove the obstructing lesion. To provide optimal controlled conditions for adequate cerebral perfusion during this procedure, the patient should be placed under general anesthesia. Many surgeons elect to monitor the electroencephalogram (EEG) while the common, internal and external carotid arteries are clamped, a procedure that should require about 7 to 15 minutes. Ordinarily, collateral blood flow under general anesthesia is sufficient to maintain the cerebral circulation if adequate blood pressure levels are maintained. If the EEG slows over the ipsilateral hemisphere, signifying ischemia, a shunt can be done as shown in the illustration. When this criterion is used, a shunt is needed in only about 10% of patients. A shunt can be used in any patient, if EEG monitoring is not available.

Surgical Technique. An incision is made parallel to the anterior border of the sternocleidomastoid muscle, and the common, external and internal carotid arteries are identified. Tapes are passed around the common and internal carotid arteries in case a shunt is needed. The nerves of the carotid bifurcation (nerves of Hering), which arise from the carotid sinus receptors, are locally

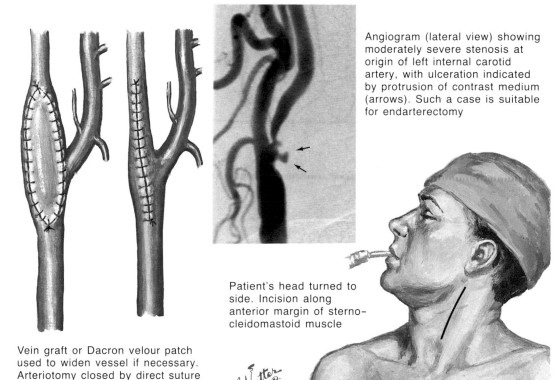

Vein graft or Dacron velour patch used to widen vessel if necessary. Arteriotomy closed by direct suture

Angiogram (lateral view) showing moderately severe stenosis at origin of left internal carotid artery, with ulceration indicated by protrusion of contrast medium (arrows). Such a case is suitable for endarterectomy

Patient's head turned to side. Incision along anterior margin of sterno-cleidomastoid muscle

infiltrated with lidocaine to prevent fluctuations of blood pressure as the carotid bifurcation is manipulated. A longitudinal arteriotomy of the internal carotid artery is extended above the level at which atherosclerotic plaque is palpated, ordinarily within 1 cm of the origin of the internal carotid artery. If necessary, a shunt can be placed at this point.

The atherosclerotic plaque is dissected from within the lumen. A clear cleavage plane is dissected between the intima involved with plaque and the media, and the inner wall of the vessel is then picked clean. Plaque is dissected from the origin of the external carotid artery, with care to avoid an intimal flap that could later obstruct the

carotid artery. If the vessel is unusually narrow, a Dacron velour patch or a vein graft can be used to widen the artery. Continuous suture is used for tight closure.

Maintenance of adequate blood pressure is critical in the early postoperative period, because patients with carotid artery obstruction may well have coronary or other vascular disease that could decrease perfusion if hypotension develops.

When done by an experienced surgeon, the surgical risks of this procedure are low. In properly selected patients, endarterectomy reduces the likelihood of stroke, but the main determinant of life expectancy is the presence and severity of other vascular disease. □

Intracerebral Hemorrhage (Hypertensive): Pathogenesis

Intracerebral Hemorrhage

Hypertension is the most common etiologic factor in intracerebral hemorrhage. Blood pressure may be only moderately elevated and need not be in the "malignant hypertension" range. During the initial stages of arterial hypertension, blood pressure rises, causing rupture of intracerebral arterioles and capillaries. When an arteriole ruptures, blood is extravasated into local tissues and creates pressure on adjacent tiny vessels, which in turn also rupture. An avalanchelike effect follows, with local bleeding increased by high arterial pressure causing a gradually enlarging hemorrhage. Tissue turgor and pressure work to tamponade and stop the bleeding. Later in the course, small arteries and arterioles become hypertrophied, which protects the capillaries from high systemic pressure but increases vascular resistance, leading to a higher cardiac workload.

As hypertension becomes chronic, degenerative lesions develop in the vessels. Small outpouchings, or microaneurysms, create weak points in the small penetrating cerebral arteries, and breaks in these diseased vessels cause intracerebral hemorrhage (Plate 26).

Hemorrhages often dissect along white matter tracts, undercutting and disconnecting the cerebral cortex. The enlarging hematoma may discharge itself through the cerebral surface or into the ventricles, providing internal decompression and leaking blood into the cerebrospinal fluid (CSF). Old healed hypertensive hemorrhages appear as healed slits consisting of hemosiderin-lined cavities.

Hypertensive intracerebral hemorrhage most commonly occurs in regions with a predilection for lacunes: putamen (lateral ganglionic) 50%, cerebral lobar white matter 16%, thalamus 12%, pons 8%, cerebellum 8% and caudate nucleus 6%. The first symptoms relate to the region involved (Plate 27). For example, hemorrhage into the right putamen is initially manifested by weakness or tingling in the left limbs. Hemorrhages usually, but not always, begin while the patient is awake and active, when the circulation is presumably more vigorous. As the hematoma enlarges, the focal neurologic deficit gradually increases over a period of minutes or a few hours. Headache, vomiting and diminished alertness ensue if the hemorrhage is large. In small hematomas, signs of pressure are absent, often leading to the mistaken diagnosis of cerebral infarction.

Other Causes of Intracerebral Hemorrhage. *Arteriovenous malformations (AVMs)* and capillary angiomas can also rupture into brain tissue and cause intracerebral hemorrhage. The diagnosis should be considered especially in young normotensive individuals who have brain hemorrhage in a location atypical for hypertensive intracerebral hemorrhage. A history of headaches and seizures also favors the diagnosis of AVM (Plates 28–29).

Bleeding diatheses, especially treatment with warfarin compounds, can also cause intracerebral hemorrhage. Intracranial bleeding in patients with hypoprothrombinemia (resulting from cirrhosis or anticoagulant therapy) develops insidi-

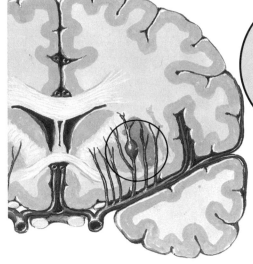

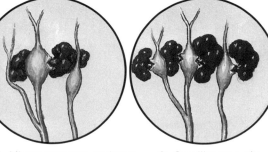

B. Microaneurysm ruptures, causing pressure on adjacent (satellite) vessels

C. Satellite vessels rupture

A. Microaneurysm formed in parenchymal artery of brain as result of hypertension. Lenticulostriate vessels (shown) most commonly involved, but similar process may occur in other parts of brain, especially lobar white matter, thalamus, pons and cerebellum

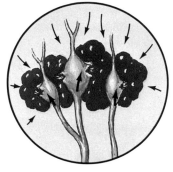

D. Amount of blood extravasated into brain tissue depends on tissue turgor opposed to intravascular blood pressure

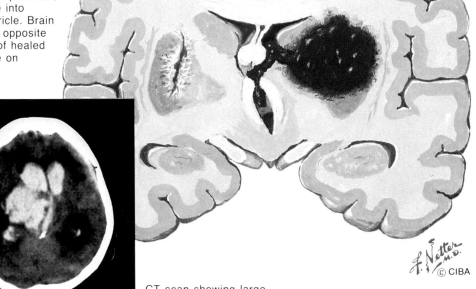

Moderate-sized intracerebral hemorrhage involving left putamen, with rupture into lateral ventricle. Brain distorted to opposite side. Scar of healed hemorrhage on right side

CT scan showing large putaminal hemorrhage with blood in ventricles

ously but can be fatal. Furthermore, a history of transient ischemic attacks (TIAs) that precipitated the use of warfarin, or confusion, amnesia, aphasia or stupor in a patient who has received anticoagulant therapy but has failed to report it, can make the correct diagnosis difficult. In this situation, anticoagulation should be immediately reversed with use of vitamin K. An intracranial episode in any patient who has been taking anticoagulants should be considered an intracerebral hemorrhage or subdural hematoma until proved otherwise. Other causes are leukemia, thrombocytopenia and hemophilia.

Trauma, sometimes not reported by the patient or denied by others, can result in intracerebral

hemorrhage. *Amyloid angiopathy*, a degenerative vasculopathy seen in elderly persons, is an increasingly recognized cause. In this disorder, hemorrhages develop, usually within cerebral lobes, and ischemic infarcts coexist. In younger patients, *drug abuse*, especially of amphetamines or cocaine, can cause hemorrhages. Amphetamines may also be etiologic in older patients who use these drugs for energy or weight control.

Diagnostic Studies. Clinical recognition of intracerebral hemorrhage has been greatly aided by computed tomography (CT). Hemorrhages appear as round, well-circumscribed lesions of uniform high density. With time, the circumference of the lesions becomes more irregular, and

Intracerebral Hemorrhage: Clinical Manifestations Related to Site

	Pathology	CT scan	Pupils	Eye movements	Motor and sensory deficits	Other
Caudate nucleus (blood in ventricle)			Sometimes ipsilaterally constricted	Conjugate deviation to side of lesion. Slight ptosis	Contralateral hemiparesis, often transient	Headache, confusion
Putamen (small hemorrhage)			Normal	Conjugate deviation to side of lesion	Contralateral hemiparesis and hemisensory loss	Aphasia (if lesion on left side)
Putamen (large hemorrhage)			In presence of herniation, pupil dilated on side of lesion	Conjugate deviation to side of lesion	Contralateral hemiparesis and hemisensory loss	Decreased consciousness
Thalamus			Constricted, poorly reactive to light bilaterally	Both lids retracted. Eyes positioned downward and medially. Cannot look upward	Slight contralateral hemiparesis, but greater hemisensory loss	Aphasia (if lesion on left side)
Occipital lobar white matter			Normal	Normal	Mild, transient hemiparesis	Contralateral hemianopsia
Pons			Constricted, reactive to light	No horizontal movements. Vertical movements preserved	Quadriplegia	Coma
Cerebellum			Slight constriction on side of lesion	Slight deviation to opposite side. Movements toward side of lesion impaired, or sixth cranial nerve palsy	Ipsilateral limb ataxia. No hemiparesis	Gait ataxia, vomiting

CIBA

SECTION III PLATE 27   *Slide 3369*

Intracerebral Hemorrhage
(Continued)

gradually the hematoma becomes a low-density lesion. CT scans also yield information of prognostic value about the location of the hemorrhage, its size, presence of surrounding edema, displacement of nearby and distant structures, and spread of blood into the ventricular system. When the hemorrhage is in an atypical location and there is no definite history of hypertension, angiography is necessary to exclude an arterial aneurysm or

AVM. Studies of bleeding function and inquiry into drug abuse should also be routine in patients with intracerebral hemorrhage.

Treatment. Large hemorrhages are often rapidly fatal. Small hemorrhages need no treatment other than control of arterial blood pressure. Surgical drainage of medium-sized hemorrhages can occasionally be lifesaving. Cerebellar, lobar and right putaminal hemorrhages are particularly amenable to surgical drainage, but decompression usually leaves a large hole, and the resulting residual neurologic deficit must be considered before it is used. "Medical" decompression using forced hyperventilation, corticosteroids and osmotic diuretics is sometimes helpful.

Most important is careful patient observation. It the hematoma exceeds 3 cm and the patient's condition worsens, developing signs of herniation, the outcome is usually fatal if no treatment is rendered. Blood pressure should be lowered, but the physician should remember that the elevated intracranial pressure causes increased venous pressure. Arterial pressure increases to help provide an arteriovenous difference capable of perfusing the remainder of the brain. If blood pressure falls too low or if it falls too precipitously, the patient's condition may worsen. The best indication of the patient's progress is a careful neurologic examination, not a blood pressure chart. □

NERVOUS SYSTEM, PART II

77

Vascular Malformations

Vascular malformations are congenital anomalies that can cause intracerebral or subarachnoid hemorrhage. These lesions can be divided into four categories.

Arteriovenous malformations (AVMs) are vascular malformations in which there are direct communications between arteries and veins without an intervening capillary network. The venous blood is arteriolized and is under higher than normal pressure.

Capillary angiomas, or telangiectases, are malformations of arterioles and capillaries within brain substance, usually without obviously dilated feeding arteries.

Cavernous angiomas are dilated abnormal vessels of various sizes, with no intervening neural tissue. Focal calcification, thrombosis and reactive gliosis are common.

Venous angiomas are profuse collections of veins, frequently short and straight but sometimes dilated and undulated, that appear to converge abruptly onto a main dilated venous trunk. The term "caput medusae" has been applied to this configuration. Classically, no arterial or capillary abnormality is present, and the blood flow sequence is normal. Although the basic vascular defect of these lesions is congenital, they may enlarge with time.

Dilatation of vessels and augmented blood flow in AVMs involving the brain can cause *headache* indistinguishable from migraine. Unilateral pounding or pulsatile headaches occur consistently on the side of the AVM, in contrast to migraine, in which headache usually changes sides. The abnormal vascular channels in AVMs also irritate the cortical regions, causing *epileptic seizures*. Since the malformations are focal, the seizures are often focal (temporal lobe epilepsy). Bruits may be heard over the cranium or neck vessels.

Clearly, the most serious problem related to AVMs is *bleeding*. Symptoms of hemorrhage from AVMs depend on the location of the hemorrhage. If the lesion is superficial and adjacent to the brain surface, bleeding is primarily into the cerebrospinal fluid (CSF) or ventricular system. The bleeding is usually slow (more like an ooze) compared with the instantaneous high-pressure leak associated with arterial aneurysmal rupture. When an AVM bleeds into the brain, it causes a *parenchymal deficit*, depending on the location of the lesion.

At times, an AVM or telangiectasis destroys itself when it bleeds. Smaller lesions such as telangiectasis usually produce smaller hemorrhages; however, strategically located telangiectasis, eg, in the pontine tegmentum, can produce fatal hemorrhage. Repeated leakage of blood into the CSF can cause *hydrocephalus*. Very large AVMs, especially in young children, can have sufficient arteriovenous shunting to create high-output *heart failure*.

Diagnostic Studies. Hemorrhage from a ruptured AVM is visible on computed tomography (CT) as a high-density area of 60 to 100 Hounsfield units. Large unruptured AVMs may be seen on CT as areas slightly denser than brain tissue, but visualization is greatly enhanced

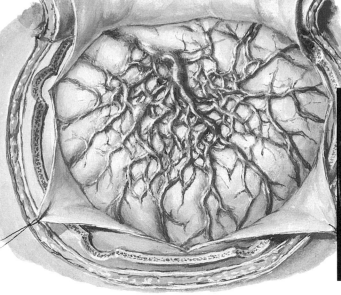

Arteriovenous malformations on surface of brain, covered by arachnoid

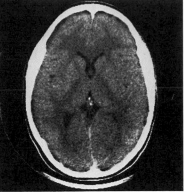

CT scan without contrast medium does not clearly demonstrate arteriovenous malformation

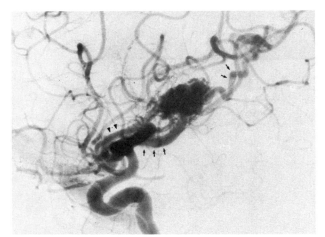

Right internal carotid angiogram: dense cluster of vessels in sylvian fissure. Main feeding artery (arrowheads), large draining veins (arrows)

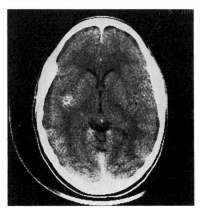

CT scan with contrast medium clearly demonstrates arteriovenous malformation

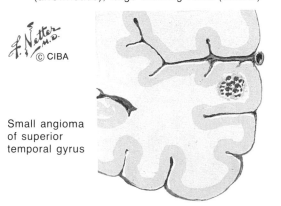

Small angioma of superior temporal gyrus

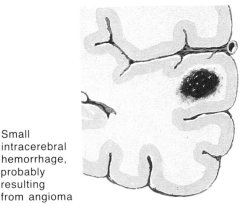

Small intracerebral hemorrhage, probably resulting from angioma

by the injection of contrast medium. Cerebral angiography identifies most AVMs but often fails to delineate telangiectasis or cavernous hemangiomas. To aid in subsequent treatment, it is important to define the feeding arterial vessels and draining veins.

Treatment. There are many ingenious new methods of treating AVMs. Surgical removal is the treatment of choice. The operating microscope now allows easier and more complete surgical extirpation of these lesions. Embolization with foreign materials may aid surgical removal. Injection of glues and plastics can obliterate the lesion. Radiation therapy, especially with a proton beam, can be effective in destroying the lesion.

The decision of whether or not to treat an AVM is frequently difficult. AVMs that have not ruptured and are causing symptomatic headache or seizures should probably be managed medically. Intraventricular shunts are indicated in patients with hydrocephalus. Because surgery, embolization and radiation therapy can damage brain tissue and cause a neurologic deficit, it is usually best not to operate on patients who have no neurologic deficit unless they have had multiple serious hemorrhages.

The decision as to which specific treatment to use depends on the location, size and angiographic features of the AVM and the surgeon's experience and capability. □

Embolization Techniques

Embolization of cerebral arteriovenous malformation (AVM) with polyvinyl alcohol sponge

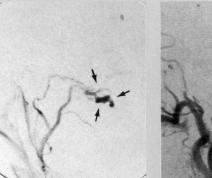

Before embolization (left): small AVM at base of skull fills only from external carotid artery. After embolization of occipital artery with very small particles of polyvinyl sponge (right): AVM no longer fills

Presurgical embolization of cerebral AVM with Silastic balls

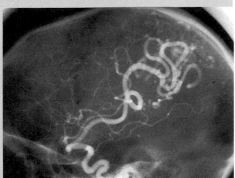

Before embolization: large AVM of parietal lobe fills primarily from large branches of middle cerebral artery

After embolization: considerable reduction in size of AVM

Balloon occlusion of carotid–cavernous fistula

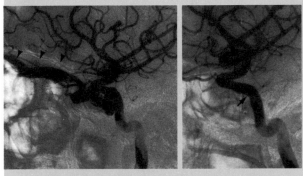

Before occlusion (left): shunt occurs between cavernous portion of internal carotid artery and cavernous sinus, with major outflow via superior ophthalmic vein (arrowheads). After occlusion (right): fistula closed by detachable balloon. Only minor irregularity of internal carotid artery seen at site of fistula (arrow)

Partial embolization of cerebral AVM with bucrylate

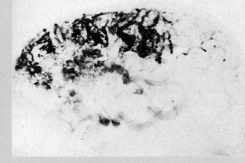

Before embolization: extensive AVM involves most of anterior portion of hemisphere

After embolization with bucrylate by use of variable-leak balloon catheter: portion of AVM no longer fills

Embolization of spinal cord AVM with polyvinyl alcohol sponge

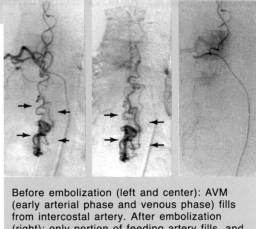

Before embolization (left and center): AVM (early arterial phase and venous phase) fills from intercostal artery. After embolization (right): only portion of feeding artery fills, and no AVM is seen

© CIBA

Slide 3371

Embolization Techniques

Some vascular processes may prove difficult to manage with surgery alone; thus, transarterial embolization methods have been developed and have gained importance as either an adjunct to surgery or a primary treatment modality. The spectrum of vascular abnormalities treated varies from high-flow arteriovenous fistulas and arteriovenous malformations to slow-flow but highly vascular, sometimes inaccessible, tumors. Because no single technique is suitable for all lesions, a number of embolic agents and delivery techniques are needed.

Nearly all these techniques are designed to deliver an agent that will block blood vessels within the lesion. It is important to confine, as much as possible, the blockage to the lesion; thus, it may be necessary to advance the delivery system as close to the abnormality as possible. Often,

highly selective catheterization techniques are used. In high-flow processes with no capillary beds, prevention of distal migration of emboli to the venous system or lungs poses an additional problem. Thus, the choice of delivery system and agent must be tailored to the anatomic and hemodynamic characteristics of the lesion, as well as to the final goal, ie, a preoperative adjunct versus sole treatment or palliation.

Absorbable particulate embolic agents are frequently selected for preoperative occlusion of vascular tumors or for treatment of nosebleed. Conventional or coaxial catheter systems are advanced to the proximity of the abnormality, and the embolic material is injected under close radiographic monitoring. In facial lesions or those at the base of the skull, some normal vessels may be temporarily blocked, but because collateral supply is rich in these areas and the occlusion is temporary, the risk of damage to normal tissue and blood vessels is low. It is imperative that emboli are not allowed to enter the vascular pathways leading to the brain or spinal cord.

If embolization is the primary treatment, nonabsorbable particulate material such as polyvinyl alcohol (PVA) sponge is used for permanent occlusion. The delivery system in this case is the same as for the absorbable particulate emboli. Temporary occlusion of the large vessel may be accom-

plished by use of a deflatable balloon catheter system, while detachable balloons or coils may occlude large vessels permanently.

High-flow arteriovenous malformations of the brain pose special problems. Flow-guided embolization with Silastic spheres has been successfully used as a prelude to surgical removal or, more rarely, as a primary treatment. The other method used requires advancement of a calibrated leak balloon far into the intracerebral circulation. Fluid embolic agents that quickly solidify, such as bucrylate or silicon, are injected from the balloon into the malformation. More direct injection may be performed with surgical assistance. □

Congenital Intracranial Aneurysms

Aneurysms are localized dilatations of the blood vessels of congenital, traumatic, arteriosclerotic or septic (infectious) origin. Congenital and traumatic aneurysms are most commonly found in cerebral blood vessels and are a major cause of stroke-related morbidity and mortality.

Over 90% of intracranial aneurysms are congenital. They are found in 4% of adults at autopsy, and are multiple in 20% of cases. Although congenital aneurysms affect males and females equally, in some sites they are more common in one sex than in the other.

Etiology

Although saccular, or berry, aneurysms are commonly referred to as congenital aneurysms, they are actually caused by a combination of congenital and acquired factors. An important congenital factor is a maldevelopment of the media that allows the intima to bulge, particularly at arterial bifurcations, where the muscular coat is incomplete. The site of these medial defects correlates with the location of aneurysms.

The number of aneurysms associated with anomalies of the circle of Willis has led some researchers to conclude that congenital aneurysms are remnants of the embryonic vessels that normally would have disappeared when the vessels fused to become larger intracranial arteries. This particularly applies to anterior communicating artery aneurysms, which are commonly associated with hypoplasia of one anterior cerebral artery.

The low incidence of aneurysms in infants and children emphasizes the importance of acquired factors and age. The most important acquired change is fragmentation of the elastica, the strongest layer of the vessel wall. Early intimal proliferative changes associated with atherosclerosis may cause degeneration of the elastica, and hypertension may speed its fragmentation.

Anatomic Sites

Three basic anatomic principles apply to all the common sites of congenital intracranial aneurysms. First, aneurysms arise at a branching site in the parent artery. Second, aneurysms arise at a turn or curve in the artery, which creates unusual stresses on the arterial wall. Third, saccular aneurysms point in the direction the blood would have gone had there not been a curve in the artery. Plate 30 details the relative distribution of aneurysms in the cerebral circulation.

Ruptured aneurysms of the anterior communicating artery occur more frequently in males, while those of the internal carotid and middle cerebral arteries are seen more often in females.

Clinically, it is important to remember that 95% of aneurysms are found at one of the following five sites: (1) the internal carotid between the posterior communicating and anterior choroidal arteries, (2) the anterior communicating area, (3) the first or second bifurcation of the middle cerebral artery, (4) the internal carotid bifurcation, and (5) the basilar bifurcation. It is also important to recognize that aneurysms are multiple in 15% to 20% of patients.

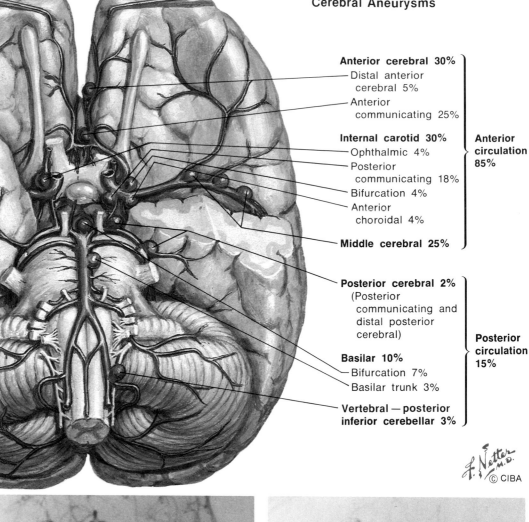

Distribution of Congenital Cerebral Aneurysms

Anterior cerebral 30%		
— Distal anterior cerebral 5%		
— Anterior communicating 25%		**Anterior circulation 85%**
Internal carotid 30%		
— Ophthalmic 4%		
— Posterior communicating 18%		
— Bifurcation 4%		
— Anterior choroidal 4%		
Middle cerebral 25%		
Posterior cerebral 2% (Posterior communicating and distal posterior cerebral)		**Posterior circulation 15%**
Basilar 10%		
— Bifurcation 7%		
— Basilar trunk 3%		
Vertebral — posterior inferior cerebellar 3%		

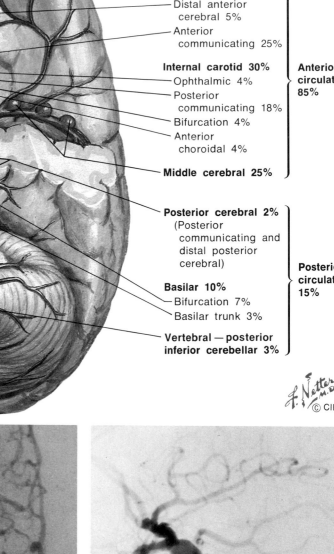

Frontal carotid arteriogram disclosing bilobate aneurysm of anterior communicating artery

Different patient: lateral view showing large aneurysm of internal carotid artery at origin of posterior communicating artery

Unruptured Congenital Aneurysms

Unruptured aneurysms detected clinically or at autopsy are usually less than 6 to 7 mm in diameter. Giant aneurysms expand to 2.5 cm in diameter or more without rupturing. Aneurysms of this size are less likely to rupture than smaller ones.

Atherosclerosis may develop in the walls of large aneurysms in any location and may lead to calcification. Laminated thrombi may also develop in the walls of a giant aneurysm, causing blood to circulate in only a small portion of the mass of the aneurysm.

Clinical Manifestations. Giant unruptured aneurysms, like tumors, produce symptoms by compressing different parts of the brain, brainstem or cranial nerves (Plate 31).

Oculomotor nerve palsy, the most frequent symptom of an unruptured aneurysm (Plate 32), occurs in 20% of patients. It is usually secondary to an aneurysm of the internal carotid artery at or near its junction with the posterior communicating artery. Less frequently, an unruptured aneurysm may cause visual disturbances by compressing the optic (II) nerve, the optic chiasm or the optic tract. Such compression is usually secondary to internal carotid or anterior communicating aneurysms and may cause optic atrophy, together with unilateral visual field defects or bitemporal hemianopsia.

Congenital Intracranial Aneurysms
(Continued)

Rupture of Aneurysms

Congenital aneurysms may be microscopic or the size of an orange, and they expand with time. Although rupture may occur in any size aneurysm, it is rare in those less than 5 mm in diameter. Usually, only an internal carotid aneurysm compressing the oculomotor (III) nerve produces pressure symptoms when it is less than 3 cm in diameter.

Subarachnoid hemorrhage usually follows rupture of a congenital aneurysm because most aneurysms lie free in the subarachnoid cisterns under the brain. Although subarachnoid hemorrhage can cause sudden death in an otherwise healthy person, it rarely causes death after rupture if there are no other complications.

Intracerebral hemorrhage occurring with subarachnoid hemorrhage is more likely to cause death than subarachnoid hemorrhage alone. The brain area affected depends on the site of the rupture. Anterior communicating and basilar aneurysms are more likely to rupture into the ventricle than are other aneurysms, causing sudden death or acute hematocephalus.

Subdural hematomas may follow aneurysm rupture, especially if the aneurysm is adherent to and breaks through the arachnoid (in up to 20% of cases), but the resulting hematoma is clinically significant in only 2% to 3% of cases.

Infarction and vasospasm are also secondary results of aneurysm rupture. Infarction, found in 75% of patients dying after rupture, is ascribed to vasospasm because thrombi are rarely found.

Vasospasm is thought to result from combined mechanical and chemical changes. Significant mechanical factors include pressure of the hematoma against the arteries and periarterial nerve stimulation by blood clot; chemical factors include the liberation of serotonin, prostaglandins and catecholamines into the subarachnoid blood. Vasospasm leads to damage to the blood-brain barrier, causing vasogenic edema, which in turn causes local increases in tissue pressure, increased intracranial pressure, further alteration of the blood-brain barrier, local tissue acidosis, focal vasodilatation, and a loss of autoregulation.

Hydrocephalus occurs when subarachnoid or ventricular blood or scarring following bleeding blocks the pathways for absorption of cerebrospinal fluid (CSF). The resulting condition may be acute or delayed. Slowly developing hydrocephalus may not cause symptoms for months after rupture. But in 15% of patients, symptomatic hydrocephalus appears soon after rupture and may require a shunt (see Section IV, Plate 10).

Clinical Manifestations. Because most ruptured congenital aneurysms cause subarachnoid

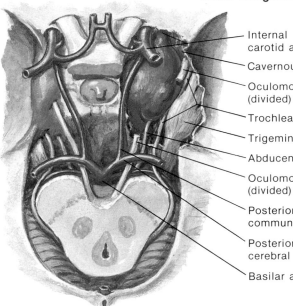

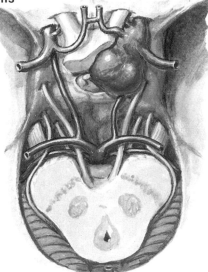

Internal carotid a.
Cavernous sinus
Oculomotor (III) n. (divided)
Trochlear (IV) n.
Trigeminal (V) n.
Abducens (VI) n.
Oculomotor (III) n. (divided)
Posterior communicating a.
Posterior cerebral a.
Basilar a.

A. Intracavernous (infraclinoid) internal carotid aneurysm compressing abducens (VI) nerve. Oculomotor (III), trochlear (IV) and trigeminal (V) nerves may also be affected. Trigeminal involvement may cause facial pain

B. Aneurysm of supraclinoid segment of internal carotid artery elevating optic chiasm, distorting infundibulum and compressing oculomotor (III) nerve

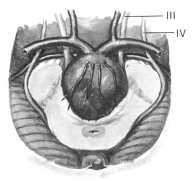

III
IV

C. Aneurysm of basilar bifurcation projecting posteriorly, invading peduncles and compressing cerebral aqueduct. Corticospinal tracts may be affected, resulting in paralysis or paresis

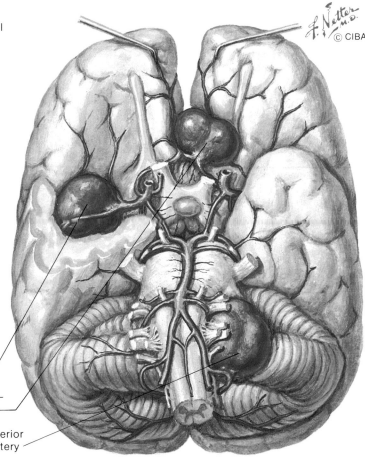

D. Aneurysm of middle cerebral artery

E. Aneurysm of anterior cerebral-anterior communicating arteries

F. Aneurysm of posterior inferior cerebellar artery

hemorrhage, a syndrome typical of this type of hemorrhage is the most common manifestation. Over 90% of patients with an aneurysm will have no symptoms preceding rupture. But in a few patients, vague prodromal manifestations may be attributed to enlarging of the aneurysm or to a small leak. These include a generalized, mild headache; alterations in preexisting migrainous headaches; or localized pain in the distribution of the ophthalmic nerve in and above the eye.

The onset of symptoms after aneurysm rupture is abrupt and rapid (Plate 33). *Headache* is dramatic, sudden and severe; the patient describes it as violent, bursting or explosive and of an intensity never before experienced. Some patients

hear a burst or snap inside the head. The pain rapidly spreads to the neck and may also extend into the back and lower extremities. A careful history defining the side and site of headache may help localize the leak. However, the headache may begin or be worse on the opposite side.

In approximately 50% of patients, *altered consciousness* follows rupture, although many patients recall the onset of symptoms. Approximately one third of those with altered consciousness exhibit mild disturbances, with confusion and confabulation, and are poorly cooperative; another third are responsive only to painful stimuli; and the remaining third exhibit only reflex responses or no response to painful stimuli.

Congenital Intracranial Aneurysms
(Continued)

Mental disturbances short of loss of consciousness may range from mild disorientation to a sleepy, semicomatose state. Manifestations may include irritability, delirium, incoherence, disorientation, confusion, apathy, depression, restlessness, disturbances of mood, or involuntary picking at the bedclothes or sexual organs. A specific mental disturbance related to a clot within or around the hypothalamus and third ventricle or to spasm of diencephalic arteries is Korsakoff's syndrome (loss of recent memory with confabulation). The classification of these mental states is discussed in connection with patient grading (page 83).

Meningeal irritation, caused by the presence of subarachnoid blood, often follows rupture. The clinical manifestations are secondary to the displacement, distention, irritation or hypersensitivity of the arteries, nerves, and meninges in the cranial or spinal subarachnoid space. The severity depends on the intensity of the hemorrhage.

Hematogenic meningeal irritation often causes irritability and subjective sensory aberrations such as photophobia, hyperacusia and hyperesthesia. Postural manifestations are also quite common. Following a subarachnoid hemorrhage, the patient often rests quietly in bed, resisting neck and extremity movement, with his eyes closed because of photophobia and his back and legs flexed to reduce tension on the irritated nerves and meninges.

Nuchal rigidity, the most frequent sign of meningeal irritation, may vary from slight resistance to flexion to complete resistance to all movement. Passive flexion (inability to place the chin on the chest) is affected more than extension. Because of rigidity of the extensor muscles, the neck may be drawn into a hyperextended position of opisthotonus, and in the characteristic supine position, passive extension of the legs may be resisted. Kernig's and Brudzinski's signs are usually present.

Autonomic disturbances, especially fever, frequently follow aneurysm rupture. Fever often develops after 24 hours, indicating meningeal irritation when mild, and hypothalamic disturbance when high.

Other autonomic disturbances related to alterations of hypothalamic regulatory mechanisms include vomiting, sweating, chills and alterations in heart rate. (Vomiting occurs in 25% of patients and is the most common symptom after headache and alteration of consciousness.) The disturbances may be severe enough to lead to gastric ulceration with hematemesis and melena, high fever and urinary retention. Increased blood glucose levels,

A. Neuromuscular disorders

Abducens nerve palsy: affected eye turns medially. May be first manifestation of intracavernous carotid aneurysm. Pain above eye or on side of face may be secondary to trigeminal (V) nerve involvement

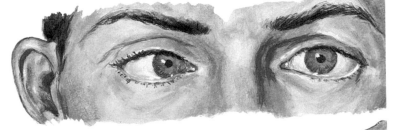

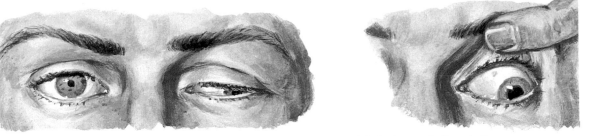

Oculomotor nerve palsy: ptosis, eye turns laterally and inferiorly, pupil dilated. Common finding with cerebral aneurysms, especially carotid–posterior communicating aneurysms

B. Visual field disturbances

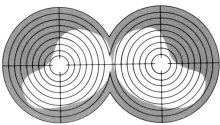

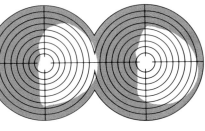

Superior bitemporal quadrantanopia caused by supraclinoid carotid aneurysm compressing optic chiasm from below

Inferior bitemporal quadrantanopia caused by compression of optic chiasm from above

Right (or left) homonymous hemianopsia caused by compression of optic tract. Unilateral amaurosis may occur if optic (II) nerve is compressed

C. Retinal changes

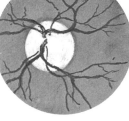

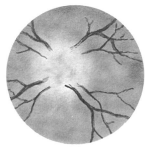

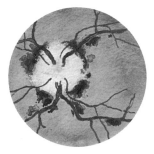

Optic atrophy may develop as result of pressure on optic (II) nerve from a supraclinoid carotid, ophthalmic or anterior cerebral aneurysm

Papilledema may be caused by increased intracranial pressure secondary to rupture of cerebral aneurysm

Hemorrhage into optic (II) nerve sheath after rupture of aneurysm may result in subhyaloid hemorrhage, with blood around disc

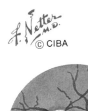

glycosuria, albuminuria and electrocardiographic abnormalities often accompany the symptoms. Although slowing of the pulse would be expected because of increased pressure, pain and hypothalamic dysfunction often cause paradoxical tachycardia.

Focal neural damage occurs in approximately 50% of patients after aneurysm rupture, and is caused by direct compression of neural tissue by hematoma, infarction as a result of vasospasm, or hydrocephalus. The nature of the symptoms is determined by whether the damage is in the cerebrum, brainstem or cerebellum or to the cranial nerves. Symptoms related to focal neural damage

include weakness or paralysis, speech and sensory disorders, seizures and visual alterations.

The pattern of focal weakness may give a clue to the site of the offending lesion. Weakness in one leg, and especially in both legs, suggests hemorrhage from the anterior communicating area, while arm and facial weakness suggests a middle cerebral aneurysm. A rare, dense hemiplegia suggests bleeding into the internal capsule from either an upward-extending internal carotid or middle cerebral aneurysm. Speech and receptive disturbances such as aphasia, dysphasia, apraxia and agnosia suggest rupture of an aneurysm into the dominant hemisphere.

Congenital Intracranial Aneurysms
(Continued)

Convulsions occur in 5% to 10% of patients at the time of rupture. Most of these seizures are generalized, although they may be focal, causing twitching in one extremity or the face.

Visual disturbances are often the result of focal neural damage (Plate 32). Diplopia is common, and is caused by extraocular nerve palsy, especially of the oculomotor and abducens (VI) nerves. Blurring or loss of vision may also occur as a result of bleeding into the visual pathways, sudden increases in intracranial pressure, or spasm of the arteries supplying the visual pathway.

The most common visual defect is homonymous hemianopsia, which may be caused by spasm of the posterior cerebral artery or by an intracerebral hematoma. Another frequent sign of rupture into the frontal lobe is forced deviation of the head and the eyes toward the side of the hematoma. Pupillary changes, either miosis or mydriasis, usually follow injury to the oculomotor centers in the upper brainstem. These centers may be damaged by a clot distending the third ventricle and hypothalamus or by vasospasm.

A clinical syndrome resulting from *hydrocephalic enlargement* of the ventricles may be superimposed on other symptoms following aneurysm rupture. Common findings include dementia, flat affect, gait disturbances and urinary incontinence. These symptoms may appear soon after rupture or develop months after what appeared to be a satisfactory recovery.

Course. The clinical state immediately after aneurysm rupture is extremely unstable. Rebleeding, cerebral swelling, infarction with vasospasm, or hydrocephalus may lead to fast or slow deterioration. Rebleeding may cause sudden death at any point, although the incidence is greatest the first week after the rupture.

Without treatment, the mortality within the first 2 months after the hemorrhage is approximately 50% in patients surviving long enough to reach a hospital. Nearly one third of the deaths occur within 2 days after rupture, half within 7 days, and three fourths within 6 weeks. After the first 2 weeks, the risk of recurrent hemorrhage and death decreases.

Grading. The patient's condition following rupture or discovery of the aneurysm has important predictive value in determining the outcome, and recognition of this relationship has led to various systems of patient grading. The following is a common classification: *grade 1*, alert patients without neurologic deficit and with minimal signs of meningeal irritation; *grade 2*, alert patients with minimal deficit or increased signs of

meningeal irritation; *grade 3*, drowsy or confused patients with or without deficit; *grade 4*, stuporous or semicomatose patients with or without deficit; *grade 5*, deep coma, moribund appearance or decerebrate rigidity.

Diagnostic Studies. A *lumbar puncture* is helpful in the diagnosis of ruptured aneurysm (Plate 33). After subarachnoid hemorrhage, the CSF is blood-stained, does not clot on standing, and does not clear as fluid is removed. Bilirubin appears as a breakdown product on the third or fourth day and gives the fluid a characteristic yellow color. Xanthochromia can be present within 2 hours of hemorrhage. Even if no further bleeding occurs,

the fluid may not completely clear for several weeks or even a month.

After subarachnoid hemorrhage, the *CSF pressure* is elevated above 150 mm in approximately 75% of patients and above 250 mm in approximately 50%. The elevation is usually proportionate to the severity of bleeding.

The *protein content* of the CSF is elevated immediately after hemorrhage as a result of the serum liberated into the fluid. Later, as the blood products break down, protein content increases further because of the released hemoglobin and the irritating effect of the subarachnoid blood. In measurement of red blood cells,

Clinical Manifestations of Congenital Aneurysm Rupture

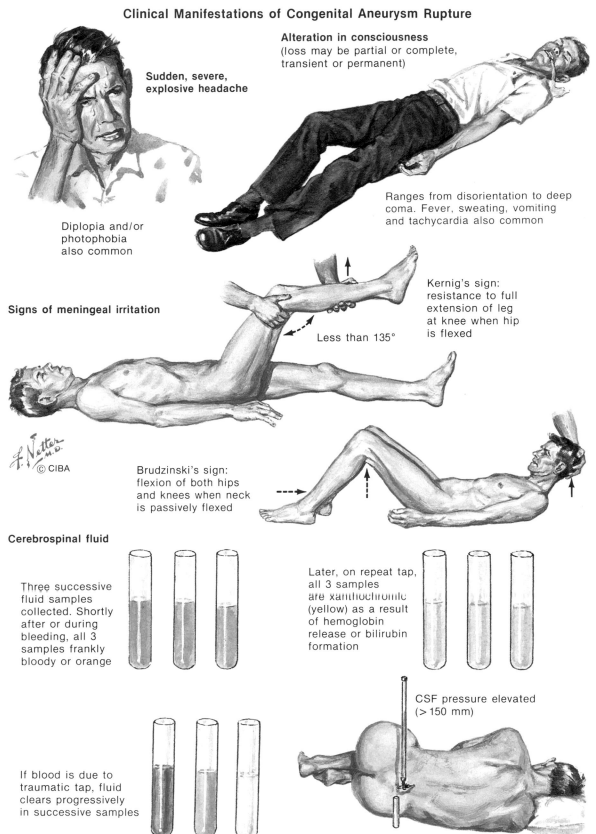

Sudden, severe, explosive headache

Diplopia and/or photophobia also common

Alteration in consciousness
(loss may be partial or complete, transient or permanent)

Ranges from disorientation to deep coma. Fever, sweating, vomiting and tachycardia also common

Signs of meningeal irritation

Kernig's sign: resistance to full extension of leg at knee when hip is flexed

Less than 135°

Brudzinski's sign: flexion of both hips and knees when neck is passively flexed

Cerebrospinal fluid

Three successive fluid samples collected. Shortly after or during bleeding, all 3 samples frankly bloody or orange

Later, on repeat tap, all 3 samples are xanthochromic (yellow) as a result of hemoglobin release or bilirubin formation

If blood is due to traumatic tap, fluid clears progressively in successive samples

CSF pressure elevated (>150 mm)

Frontotemporal Approach for Internal Carotid, Ophthalmic, Anterior Communicating, and Middle Cerebral Aneurysms

Congenital Intracranial Aneurysms
(Continued)

10,000 RBC/mm³ would give a protein count of 15 mg/100 ml. Protein elevation after hemorrhage is usually 80 to 130 mg/100 ml, but may be above 300 mg/100 ml.

White blood cells in the CSF after hemorrhage are initially proportionate in number to the red cells, but increase later as a result of meningeal irritation. These elevated levels may persist until the xanthochromia clears.

CSF glucose levels are depressed in about 25% of patients, especially in those with severe hemorrhage.

Ruptured aneurysms usually produce no signs on a plain *skull x-ray film* except for evidence of a pineal shift caused by hematoma. Giant unruptured aneurysms may be seen as shell-like curvilinear calcifications that are often incomplete. Less commonly, multiple mottled calcifications suggestive of a craniopharyngioma are seen in the aneurysm wall.

Large aneurysms arising from the anterior part of the circle of Willis, especially from the internal carotid artery, may erode the clinoid processes, sellar floor and sellar dorsum, and x-ray films suggest a sellar tumor. Others may erode the optic foramen and widen the superior orbital fissure.

Dynamic radioisotope brain scanning may demonstrate slowed circulation as a result of vasospasm, and conventional scans may demonstrate areas of abnormal uptake caused by clot and infarction. However, only giant aneurysms may be seen on the scan.

Computed tomography (CT) does not define aneurysms smaller than 5 mm in diameter but does demonstrate larger ones and those with calcium in the wall. The value of the CT scan includes demonstration of subarachnoid blood, aneurysm, outlining areas of clot, infarction and edema. The CT scan can differentiate parenchymatous, subdural or intraventricular hemorrhage from edema and infarction. It also clearly outlines the ventricles and aids in determining the degree to which hydrocephalus is a contributing factor.

In 80% of patients with subarachnoid hemorrhage, a congenital aneurysm is detected on *cerebral angiography*. Consequently, early angiography is indicated even if surgery is delayed, so that in the event of deterioration in the patient's condition, angiograms are still available.

Patients with subarachnoid hemorrhage or suspected aneurysm are best studied by transfemoral catheterization, which allows visualization of both carotids and the vertebrobasilar system through one puncture site.

Oblique and submental vertical views, in addition to conventional biplane anteroposterior (AP)

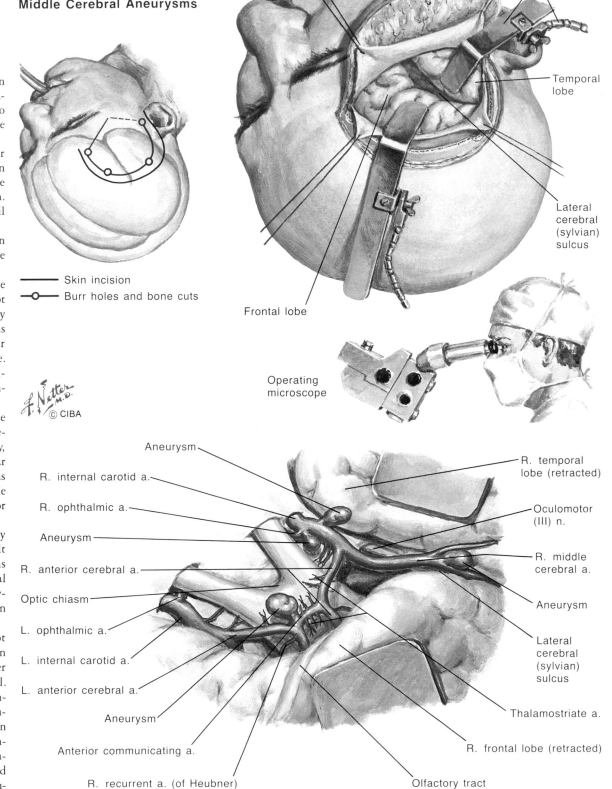

Skin incision

Burr holes and bone cuts

Self-retaining retractor

Temporal lobe

Lateral cerebral (sylvian) sulcus

Frontal lobe

Operating microscope

Aneurysm

R. internal carotid a.

R. ophthalmic a.

Aneurysm

R. anterior cerebral a.

Optic chiasm

L. ophthalmic a.

L. internal carotid a.

L. anterior cerebral a.

Aneurysm

Anterior communicating a.

R. recurrent a. (of Heubner)

R. temporal lobe (retracted)

Oculomotor (III) n.

R. middle cerebral a.

Aneurysm

Lateral cerebral (sylvian) sulcus

Thalamostriate a.

R. frontal lobe (retracted)

Olfactory tract

and lateral views, are necessary to identify aneurysms at bifurcations or in the presence of tortuous or overlapping blood vessels. Oblique views are especially useful in defining anterior communicating aneurysms that are difficult to see on conventional AP or lateral views. Use of digital subtraction angiography may also be helpful in delineating an aneurysm (Plates 22–23).

During injection of one carotid artery, it may be necessary to compress the opposite carotid to obtain filling of aneurysms of the anterior communicating artery. Knowledge of the extent of cross-filling may also help in planning the surgical approach.

In the presence of multiple congenital aneurysms, it is important that x-ray films of the kidneys be taken because of the association of congenital intracranial aneurysms with polycystic kidney disease.

Medical Therapy Following Rupture

The high mortality rate resulting from aneurysm rupture makes surgery the treatment of choice whenever feasible. However, a dilemma exists. On the one hand, mortality is higher in early surgery than in surgery 7 to 14 days after hemorrhage; on the other hand, the delay of 7 to 14 days allows rebleeding, with death in some

Temporal Approach for Basilar Trunk or Posteriorly Directed Basilar Apex Aneurysm

Congenital Intracranial Aneurysms
(Continued)

———— Skin incision

—o— Burr holes and bone cuts

▓▓▓ Additional bone removed

cases. Because of this dilemma, medical therapy has been developed so that surgery can be postponed until the risks are reduced.

Medical therapy is designed to prevent recurrent hemorrhage, to reduce or prevent cerebral edema and increased intracranial pressure, and to prevent and control vasospasm. Medical therapy alone is used after subarachnoid hemorrhage when angiography reveals no bleeding abnormality; when the bleeding lesion is inaccessible; in patients classified as grade 3, 4 or 5 (see page 83) who are not improving; in the presence of multiple aneurysms when it is impossible to determine which one has bled (multiple surgical approaches are possible and preferred in most of these cases); and when surgery is refused.

The cornerstones of medical treatment for cerebral hemorrhage are absolute bed rest for at least 4 weeks if surgery is not performed, excellent nursing care to prevent complications, institution of antifibrinolytic therapy, and maintaining a reduced blood pressure (approximately 100 mm Hg systolic in normotensive patients). Other factors are control of intracranial pressure with steroid therapy and institution of anticonvulsant therapy.

Antifibrinolytic drugs, designed to prevent perianeurysmal clot lysis, are being increasingly used to prevent rebleeding. With their use, it may be possible to delay surgery until cerebral circulation has stabilized. The drug used most frequently is ∈-aminocaproic acid (EACA), which reduces the incidence of rebleeding to below 10%.

Surgical Therapy Following Rupture

The prognosis after aneurysm rupture is so bleak that surgical treatment must be considered in almost every case. The two most important factors determining surgical mortality are the time that has elapsed since subarachnoid hemorrhage occurred and the patient's condition at the time of surgery. The earlier the operation is undertaken, the more dangerous it is, and the sicker the patient when operation is advised, the higher is the risk.

Some surgeons operate on patients in the grade 1 or 2 category within the first few days after hemorrhage, hoping that eliminating the chance for the often fatal rebleeding will compensate for the somewhat higher mortality associated with earlier operation. The chief problem is that in many patients, early operation is followed by arterial spasm and infarction. Therefore, most surgeons prefer to wait 5 to 7 days after hemorrhage, to reduce the chance that vasospasm will complicate the patient's response to surgery. The

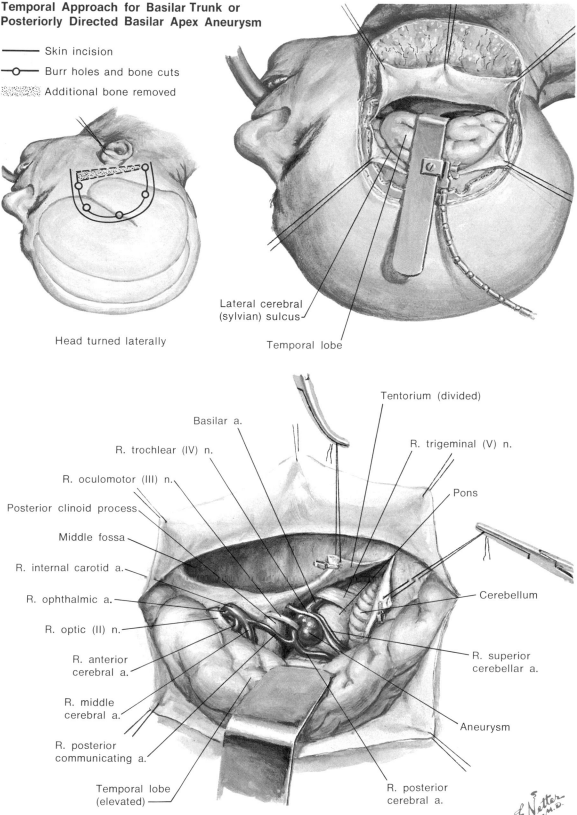

Head turned laterally

Lateral cerebral (sylvian) sulcus

Temporal lobe

Tentorium (divided)

Basilar a.

R. trochlear (IV) n.

R. oculomotor (III) n.

Posterior clinoid process

Middle fossa

R. internal carotid a.

R. ophthalmic a.

R. optic (II) n.

R. anterior cerebral a.

R. middle cerebral a.

R. posterior communicating a.

Temporal lobe (elevated)

R. trigeminal (V) n.

Pons

Cerebellum

R. superior cerebellar a.

Aneurysm

R. posterior cerebral a.

©CIBA

recent use of antifibrinolytic and hypotensive agents has reduced the risk of waiting until the patient is in the best condition for surgery. If angiography shows vasospasm, surgery should be delayed until the spasm starts to subside.

Patients graded 3, 4 or 5 (confused, semicomatose or comatose) should not be operated on until they have improved, unless they have an intracranial clot that causes a significant intracranial shift or appears to be life-threatening.

Basic principles of congenital aneurysm surgery, which involve clipping and other means of forestalling further bleeding from an aneurysm, include the following 10 procedures.

1. The patient should be anesthetized without inducing stress, coughing or rise in blood pressure, to avoid rebleeding.

2. The parent artery should be exposed proximal to the aneurysm to allow control of flow to the aneurysm if it ruptures during dissection.

3. If possible, the side of the parent vessel opposite that of the aneurysm should be exposed prior to dissection of the aneurysm neck, so that the dissection can be carried around the side of the parent vessel to the origin of the aneurysm.

4. The aneurysm neck should be dissected before the fundus, because the neck can tolerate the greatest manipulation, has the least tendency

Congenital Intracranial Aneurysms
(Continued)

to rupture, and is the area to be clipped. Unfortunately, it is also the portion of the aneurysm that is most likely to incorporate the origin of a vessel. Therefore, the neck and proximal part of the fundus should be dissected carefully and with full visualization to prevent passage of a clip around an arterial branch arising from the base near the neck. The dissection should not start at the dome, because this is the area most likely to rupture before or during surgery.

5. All perforating arterial branches should be separated from the aneurysm neck before the clip is passed around the aneurysm.

6. Bleeding during microdissection should be controlled by reducing mean arterial pressure and by local measures, if possible, or by interrupting the proximal supply with temporary clips for the briefest possible time.

7. The bone flap should be placed as low as possible to expose the area where most congenital aneurysms are found (the circle of Willis and surrounding area) and thus minimize the need for brain retraction.

8. A noncrushing type of clip with a spring mechanism that allows it to be removed, repositioned and reapplied should be used. Care should be taken to avoid kinking or obstruction of a major vessel or any perforating branches.

9. If the neck of an aneurysm is broad-based and use of a clip is therefore impractical, the aneurysm may be reduced by bipolar coagulation, with care to protect nearby perforating arteries.

10. If a clip or ligature cannot be applied to obliterate the neck of the aneurysm, the sac may be encased with surgical gauze or plastic. Muscle packing is probably ineffective.

The *craniotomy* used to expose most aneurysms can be (1) frontotemporal or pterional or (2) temporal.

The *frontotemporal or pterional craniotomy* along the sphenoid ridge is suitable with slight modification for 90% of aneurysms that arise from the anterior part of the circle of Willis and the carotid branches, and for some aneurysms arising from the upper part of the basilar artery (Plate 34).

The *temporal approach* is used for aneurysms arising from the posterior aspect of the upper part of the basilar artery and can also be used to expose the area under the temporal lobe (Plate 35). In contrast to the approach along the sphenoid ridge, the temporal approach provides better exposure of the perforating arteries that commonly arise from the posterior aspect of the basilar artery. These arteries are especially vital because they supply the diencephalic areas controlling consciousness.

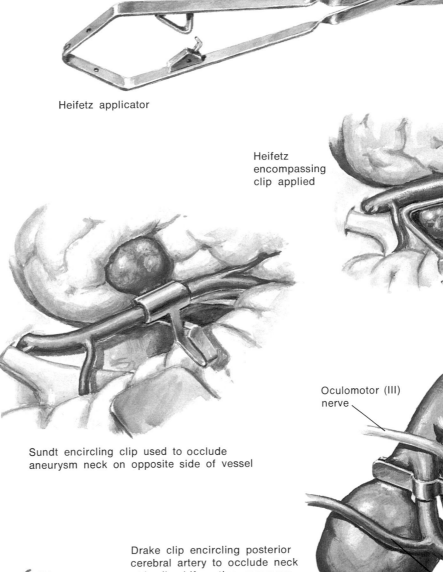

Yasargil clip positioned with Yasargil applicator on anterior communicating aneurysm. Perforating branches avoided (mandatory in all cases)

Heifetz applicator

Heifetz angled clip used for less accessible aneurysm

Heifetz encompassing clip applied

Sundt encircling clip used to occlude aneurysm neck on opposite side of vessel

Drake clip encircling posterior cerebral artery to occlude neck of basilar bifurcation aneurysm

Basilar artery

Oculomotor (III) nerve

Superior cerebellar artery

Posterior cerebral artery

Posterior communicating artery

This approach beneath the temporal lobe can also be combined with section of the tentorium cerebelli posterior to the trochlear (IV) nerve to expose and clip aneurysms as low as at the origin of the basilar artery from the vertebral arteries.

Ventricular drainage and shunting procedures also have a place in aneurysm surgery. Acutely developing ventricular enlargement in patients grades 3 to 5 may be treated temporarily by external ventricular drainage through a twist drill or burr hole. Repeated lumbar punctures may also be used for temporary relief. If hydrocephalus persists after the CSF has cleared, a permanent shunt between the ventricle or lumbar subarachnoid space and the peritoneal cavity must be established (see Section IV, Plate 10).

Postoperative Care. Following surgery, the patient should be carefully observed in an intensive care unit. The head is elevated, and steroid therapy is continued for several days. Intravascular volume should be aggressively maintained to reduce the incidence of postoperative vasospasm. Anticonvulsants are administered for at least 6 months after surgery.

The outlook for patients with congenital aneurysms has improved over the past 2 decades as a result of improvements in diagnostic and therapeutic technology. □

Hypoxic Brain Damage and Brain Death

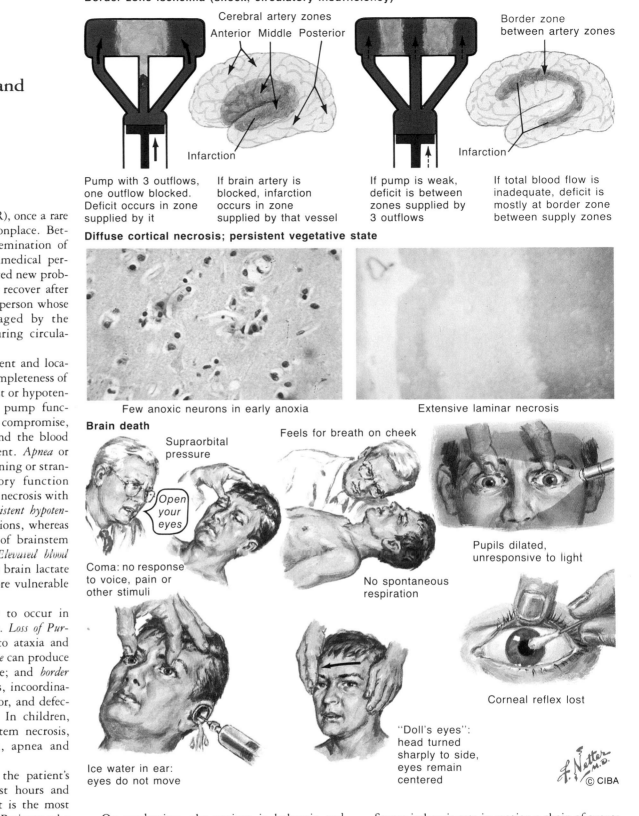

Hypoxic Brain Damage and Brain Death

Border zone ischemia (shock, circulatory insufficiency)

Cerebral artery zones
Anterior Middle Posterior

Border zone between artery zones

Infarction

Infarction

Pump with 3 outflows, one outflow blocked. Deficit occurs in zone supplied by it

If brain artery is blocked, infarction occurs in zone supplied by that vessel

If pump is weak, deficit is between zones supplied by 3 outflows

If total blood flow is inadequate, deficit is mostly at border zone between supply zones

Diffuse cortical necrosis; persistent vegetative state

Few anoxic neurons in early anoxia

Extensive laminar necrosis

Brain death

Supraorbital pressure

Feels for breath on cheek

"Open your eyes"

Coma: no response to voice, pain or other stimuli

No spontaneous respiration

Pupils dilated, unresponsive to light

Ice water in ear: eyes do not move

"Doll's eyes": head turned sharply to side, eyes remain centered

Corneal reflex lost

Cardiopulmonary resuscitation (CPR), once a rare occurrence, has now become commonplace. Better techniques and widespread dissemination of knowledge to paramedical and nonmedical personnel have saved lives but have created new problems and dilemmas. The heart may recover after cardiac arrest, only to beat within a person whose brain has been irreversibly damaged by the ischemic-anoxic insult sustained during circulatory failure.

Many variables determine the extent and location of hypoxic brain damage: the completeness of circulatory collapse (full cardiac arrest or hypotension, with some preserved cardiac pump function); the duration of circulatory compromise, accompanying respiratory failure; and the blood glucose level at the time of the event. *Apnea* or *hypoxia* (as in carbon monoxide poisoning or strangulation) with preserved circulatory function often results in pallidal and thalamic necrosis with preservation of cerebral cortex. *Persistent hypotension* leads to border zone ischemic lesions, whereas *cardiac arrest* often causes necrosis of brainstem nuclei and hippocampal damage. *Elevated blood glucose* at the time of arrest increases brain lactate production and makes the brain more vulnerable to ischemia.

Ischemic damage is more likely to occur in certain brain regions than in others. *Loss of Purkinje cells* in the cerebellum leads to ataxia and action myoclonus; *hippocampal damage* can produce a Korsakoff-like amnestic syndrome; and *border zone ischemia* results in arm weakness, incoordination during visually directed behavior, and defective visual and spatial perception. In children, *severe hypotension* can lead to brainstem necrosis, loss of brainstem reflex function, apnea and decerebrate rigidity.

Careful, repeated assessment of the patient's neurologic function within the first hours and days after a hypoxic-ischemic insult is the most reliable way of judging prognosis. Patients who have sustained severe damage usually remain deeply comatose after resuscitation and do not respond to painful stimuli. Brainstem reflex functions (corneal, pupillary, oculocephalic and oculovestibular) are absent.

Shortly after arrest and resuscitation, patients with less severe cerebral injury show some reaction to the environment. Restless limb motions and eye opening develop. When the examiner raises the patient's eyelids, the eyes rove from side to side and later temporarily fixate. Painful stimuli evoke an alerting or withdrawal response. Brainstem reflexes are preserved. As stupor decreases, periods of agitation or delirium occur.

On awakening, the patient is lethargic and unable to persevere with a task; concentration is poor. Memory deficit and visual dysfunction are common. The patient complains of inability to "see" and cannot integrate the features of large objects or scenes but may be able to identify small objects or fragments. Words and phrases are missed in reading. Hand movements are poorly coordinated, and the patient often reaches past an object or misjudges distance. An especially important prognostic clue is the patient's response to deep supraorbital ridge or interphalangeal pain. Failure to respond by opening the eyes or by verbal or motor responses within the first 24 hours indicates a poor prognosis.

Severe ischemia sets in motion a chain of events leading to irreversible *brain death*. Brain swelling becomes intense and blocks the entrance of blood into the cranium, increasing the ischemia. Brain death is a clinical diagnosis. Absent brainstem reflexes, failure to initiate respiration when off the respirator, and absent cortical function are accepted criteria of brain death. The cause and potential reversibility of the brain damage should be considered. A flat electroencephalogram (EEG) for longer than 12 hours (in the absence of hypothermia or sedative drugs) and absence of vascular filling of the cerebral vessels on radionuclide or cerebral angiography corroborate the diagnosis of brain death. □

Section IV

Central Nervous System Trauma

Frank H. Netter, M.D.

in collaboration with

William A. Friedman, M.D. *Plates 1–24*
H. Royden Jones, Jr., M.D. *Plate 25*

Compound Depressed Skull Fractures

Head Injuries

Head injury, a serious health problem in all industrialized nations, is a significant factor in approximately half of all deaths related to trauma. Trauma is the leading cause of death in persons aged 1 to 44, and accounts for more deaths than stroke in persons aged 45 to 64. In 1976, 7,560,000 head injuries were reported in the United States. Even though most of these were minor, 1,255,000 were major injuries, including concussion, contusion and hemorrhage.

The causes of head trauma include road accidents, assaults, falls, sports injuries and industrial accidents. Various factors influence the incidence of serious head injuries. For example, alcohol intoxication has been implicated in half of all fatal road accidents. On the other hand, lowering the highway speed limit, use of seat belts in cars, and use of headgear by industrial workers and motorcyclists have reduced the number of serious accidents.

If the morbidity and mortality caused by head injuries are to be reduced, it is essential that all physicians understand the pathophysiologic aspects of head trauma and the appropriate treatment of injuries of the scalp, skull and brain.

Scalp Injuries

Scalp injuries are common, and although usually minor, must be carefully investigated and properly treated. The extent of investigation and treatment depends on the depth of the injury.

The least severe scalp injury is the simple *abrasion/contusion*, which usually responds well to local measures such as cleansing of the wound and application of antibiotic ointment and cold compresses. A more forceful blow may produce bleeding in the subgaleal or the subperiosteal space, with formation of a *cephalhematoma*; this is most common in neonates. If large enough, a cephalhematoma may cause a significant decrease in the infant's hematocrit. Other than monitoring of blood volume and watching for hyperbilirubinemia, no specific treatment is required. A cephalhematoma should not be routinely aspirated. Rarely, a subperiosteal hematoma calcifies, requiring surgical removal. Occasionally after major head trauma, an epidural hematoma extrudes through an overlying skull fracture and periosteal laceration and produces a subgaleal collection of blood.

Scalp lacerations account for the majority of emergency room visits related to head trauma. Since the scalp is well vascularized, these injuries usually heal quite well.

The hair surrounding a laceration should be shaved circumferentially so that the wound can be prepared in a surgical fashion. The "prep" should include irrigation with copious quantities of sterile saline and vigorous scrubbing with a standard skin-sterilizing solution (ie, a povidone-iodine compound).

After infiltration of the area with local anesthetic, the wound should be explored under a good light. If the laceration does not penetrate the galea aponeurotica, one-layer skin closure is

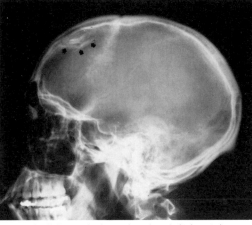
Left lateral view showing left frontal depressed fracture

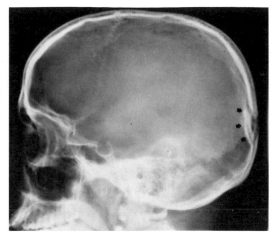
Left lateral view showing occipital depressed fracture

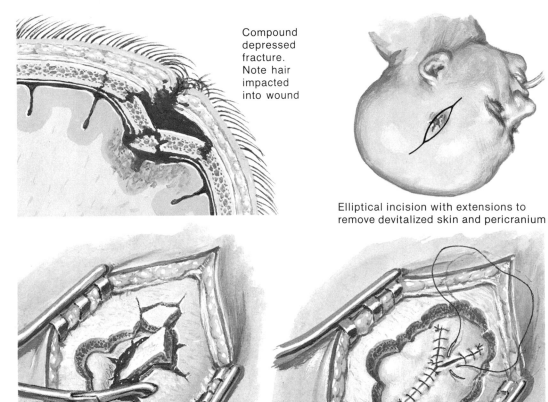
Compound depressed fracture. Note hair impacted into wound

Elliptical incision with extensions to remove devitalized skin and pericranium

Burr hole placed at margin of fracture to facilitate elevation of depressed bone fragments. Bone edges, dura and brain then debrided

Watertight dural closure. Optionally, bone fragments may be cleaned and wired in place. Skin is closed in one layer

usually done. If the galea aponeurotica is lacerated, the underlying skull must be carefully examined for evidence of a fracture. Any hint of a fracture is an indication for skull x-ray films and neurosurgical consultation before the wound is closed, since more extensive surgical debridement or extended antibiotic treatment may be necessary. If skull trauma is not detected, the wound may be closed in one or two layers. If the wound initially appeared contaminated, a one-layer closure is preferable, because buried stitches may become infected.

Tetanus toxoid should be administered according to each patient's immunization status. Although some physicians advise the routine

prophylactic use of antibiotics, no study has proved their efficacy in reducing the incidence of infection. Extensive lacerations may bleed profusely and, especially in children, may produce anemia or, rarely, hypovolemic shock.

Skull Fractures

A variety of terms are commonly used to describe skull fractures. A *linear* fracture produces radiographically distinct, straight lines with parallel margins. Unlike vascular markings, the lines do not taper or branch. Since the fracture affects both tables of the skull, an x-ray film taken at right angles shows a more sharply defined line than a vascular groove. A fracture that produces

Head Injuries
(Continued)

multiple fragments of bone is termed *comminuted*. Comminuted fracture fragments may sometimes be driven in, compressing or tearing the underlying dura and brain. Such a fracture is then termed *depressed*.

A fracture line that runs into a cranial suture may split the suture–a phenomenon called *diastasis*, which is most common in children. A fracture of the base of the skull–a *basilar* fracture–is often difficult to see on routine skull x-ray films, but characteristic clinical signs lead to the diagnosis (Plate 2). Rarely, in children, a fracture lacerates the dura mater, allowing the arachnoid to herniate into the fracture line; the cerebrospinal fluid (CSF) pulsations may subsequently enlarge the fracture (a *growing* skull fracture). Finally, any skull fracture that communicates with a scalp laceration, the paranasal sinuses or the middle ear cavity is termed a *compound* fracture.

In the International Data Bank series, a linear vault fracture was reported in 77% of all patients with intracranial hematomas, and a skull fracture was found in 91% of patients with an epidural hematoma. (These percentages were somewhat lower in children.) The cost-efficiency of obtaining skull x-ray films in patients unlikely to have a fracture (ie, those with concussion) is controversial and is currently the subject of a national study. Yet, because the presence of a linear fracture in a conscious patient increases the risk of intracranial hemorrhage about 400 times, skull x-ray films seem justified.

Treatment. A *closed linear fracture* in an otherwise normal patient requires no specific treatment besides initial observation. However, children must be reexamined later for evidence of a growing fracture, since this rare lesion requires surgical repair.

A *compound linear fracture* requires thorough debridement to prevent osteomyelitis or scalp infection. The most common infectious agent is *Staphylococcus*, which produces a lesion called "Pott's puffy tumor." If the wound is relatively clean and the patient is cooperative, the wound can usually be irrigated and scrubbed in the emergency room. When contamination is obvious or when a patient cooperates poorly (eg, a child), surgical debridement in the operating room should be considered. Most physicians recommend a subsequent course of antibiotic treatment.

Depressed fractures may also be either closed or compound. Closed depressions up to 5 mm often are only observed. However, if the fracture is in a readily visible area (eg, frontal), even a small depression may be cosmetically unacceptable. In infants, closed depressions often produce a characteristic greenstick fracture, termed a "ping-pong fracture." Fractures producing greater degrees of depression are frequently reduced surgically because dural laceration and cerebral injury are more likely in these fractures.

Compound depressed fractures are always treated surgically (Plate 1). Even a wound that appears clean often contains impacted fragments of dirt and hair. Surgical debridement in the operating room is required. Depending on the location and

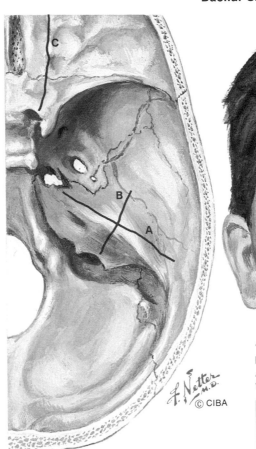

"Panda bear" or "raccoon" sign due to leakage of blood from anterior fossa into periorbital tissues. Absence of conjunctival injection differentiates fracture from direct eye trauma

Longitudinal (**A**) and transverse (**B**) fractures of petrous pyramid of temporal bone, and anterior basal skull fracture (**C**)

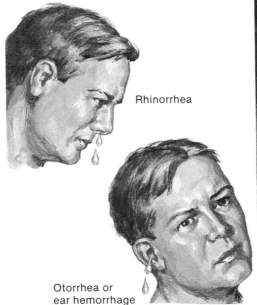

Rhinorrhea

Otorrhea or ear hemorrhage

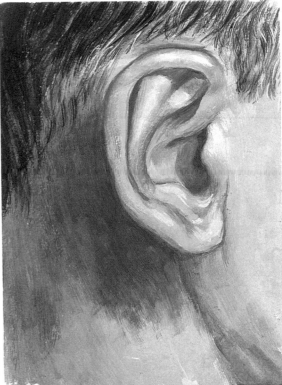

Battle's sign: postauricular hematoma

size of the fracture, a curvilinear incision, including the scalp laceration, or a more cosmetic scalp flap may be used. The scalp is debrided and a burr hole is generally placed adjacent to the depression. In a ping-pong fracture, the depression can often be easily pried up, but in most other fractures, the fragments must be elevated piecemeal to avoid further compression of the brain while one edge of a bone fragment is elevated. If the dura mater has been lacerated, the underlying brain should be thoroughly inspected and debrided.

The dura mater should then be closed in a watertight fashion. Some surgeons cleanse and replace the bone fragments; others perform an elective cranioplasty later. The wound is copiously irrigated and the skin is closed in one or two layers. Antibiotics are administered for a variable period following surgery. As the overall incidence of late posttraumatic epilepsy in such patients is 15%, many physicians routinely prescribe long-term anticonvulsant therapy; others treat only certain high-risk patients (eg, those with a dural laceration).

Basilar fractures often involve the *petrous portion of the temporal bone*. The most common type (usually from a temporal blow) begins in the squamous portion of the temporal bone and extends longitudinally along the petrous pyramid. This fracture often produces an obvious

Slide 3382

Temporal fossa hematoma

Head Injuries
(Continued)

deformity of the external ear canal or rupture of the tympanic membrane, or both. If the adjacent dura mater is torn, leakage of CSF from the ear canal (otorrhea) is characteristic. If the eardrum remains intact and the fracture extends more medially, blood may collect behind the membrane (hemotympanum) or CSF may collect in the middle ear cavity and drain, through the eustachian tube, into the nose (rhinorrhea). The ossicular chain may be disrupted, producing a conductive hearing loss. Injury to the facial (VII) nerve produces paresis or complete paralysis in 20% of patients with such fractures.

Finally, if the fracture extends more posteriorly, the sigmoid sinus may be damaged, causing bleeding into the mastoid air cells and beneath the pericranium overlying the mastoid. This postauricular swelling and hematoma, known as Battle's sign (Plate 2), becomes clinically evident 24 to 48 hours after injury.

Occipital blows may cause fractures extending down the occipital bone and transversely across the petrous pyramid. These *occipital transverse fractures* are less commonly seen, partly because they often cause immediate death. They almost always damage the inner ear, but because the middle ear, tympanic membrane and external ear canal are rarely injured, bleeding from the ear canal or otorrhea is seldom seen. The facial nerve, however, is injured in 50% of transverse fractures. Major vascular structures at the base of the skull may also be injured, resulting in high mortality.

The *anterior skull base* is a common fracture site. Dural lacerations in this area may cause drainage of CSF into the paranasal sinuses and rhinorrhea. Damage to anterior venous sinuses may cause leakage of blood into the periorbital tissues, producing the characteristic "raccoon" or "panda bear" sign (Plate 2). Absence of subconjunctival hemorrhage usually distinguishes this injury from direct ocular trauma. Although any cranial nerve crossing the anterior skull base may be affected, the olfactory (I) nerve is the most commonly injured. Indirect evidence of anterior basilar fractures includes an air-fluid level in one of the sinuses or the presence of intracranial air on skull x-ray films or on computed tomography (CT) scans.

The major complications of basilar skull fractures are, therefore, cranial nerve injury and CSF leakage (leading to meningitis). Because these complications may be delayed, every patient with a basilar fracture should be hospitalized for observation. For traumatic Bell's palsy, some physicians recommend decompression of the facial nerve; however, many treat these cranial nerve injuries

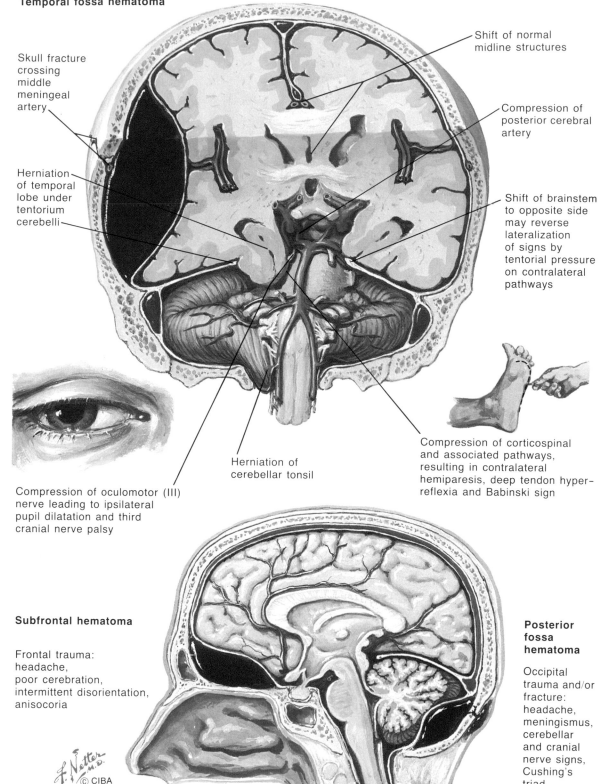

Skull fracture crossing middle meningeal artery

Herniation of temporal lobe under tentorium cerebelli

Shift of normal midline structures

Compression of posterior cerebral artery

Shift of brainstem to opposite side may reverse lateralization of signs by tentorial pressure on contralateral pathways

Compression of corticospinal and associated pathways, resulting in contralateral hemiparesis, deep tendon hyper-reflexia and Babinski sign

Herniation of cerebellar tonsil

Compression of oculomotor (III) nerve leading to ipsilateral pupil dilatation and third cranial nerve palsy

Subfrontal hematoma

Frontal trauma: headache, poor cerebration, intermittent disorientation, anisocoria

Posterior fossa hematoma

Occipital trauma and/or fracture: headache, meningismus, cerebellar and cranial nerve signs, Cushing's triad

conservatively. Steroids are often prescribed, although their use has never been proved beneficial. Most cases of rhinorrhea and otorrhea resolve after several days of bed rest with the patient's head elevated.

The treatment of prolonged CSF leakage is controversial. Generally, if the leakage persists beyond 1 week, further investigation is done to locate the site of the dural tear. Diagnostic procedures include skull tomography, radioisotope cisternography, pneumoencephalography and metrizamide cisternography. After the site has been identified, a craniotomy is done so that the leak can be patched. Prophylactic use of antibiotics after basilar fracture is also controversial.

Because the incidence of meningitis (with leakage of CSF) is approximately 10% to 15% and the most common organism implicated is *Pneumococcus*, many physicians recommend the prophylactic use of penicillin. However, several studies have failed to demonstrate any beneficial effect.

Intracranial Injuries

Concussion. The most minor brain injury is concussion. This results in loss of consciousness for a short period and some degree of amnesia, either retrograde (before the accident) or antegrade (posttraumatic amnesia). Experimental models and the scant neuropathologic data relating to concussed patients dying from other causes

Initial Management of Severe Head Injuries

Head Injuries
(Continued)

have failed to delineate any reliable evidence, on light microscopy, of pathologic lesions in the brain. Trauma that causes some rotation of the head is more likely to produce loss of consciousness.

Although early studies implicated physiologic dysfunction of brainstem centers in these injuries, no case of an isolated brainstem pathologic lesion has come to light. In fact, most head injuries appear to be centripetal; that is, superficial brain structures are damaged before deeper structures. The frequent observation of profound postconcussion amnesic deficits in patients with the most minimal alteration of consciousness confirms the centripetal nature of the injury. Although the precise cellular mechanism underlying concussion remains unknown, the aforementioned facts suggest a physiologic disconnection between the cortex and brainstem.

Concussion has been classified according to the severity of the primary injury and the resultant neurologic dysfunction. A *grade I lesion* causes transient confusion, with a rapid return to normal consciousness and no amnesia; *grade II*, increased confusion and some residual amnesia (posttraumatic only), *grade III*, more pronounced initial confusion, with a greater degree of residual amnesia (posttraumatic and retrograde); and *grade IV* (classic concussion), brief loss of consciousness, a variable period of subsequent confusion, and some degree of both posttraumatic and retrograde amnesia.

Initial evaluation of all concussed patients includes a complete history and physical examination. Many physicians obtain routine skull x-ray films, to screen for possible intracranial hematoma. Some physicians routinely order x-ray films of the cervical spine as well, but these should *always* be obtained in any patient who has neck pain or in any patient with persistent alteration of consciousness. Other laboratory investigations should be undertaken as indicated for each patient.

If the period of confusion has passed, if results of the various investigations are negative, and if someone reliable is available to observe the patient with the aid of a "head sheet" over the next 24 hours, the patient may be discharged. (The head sheet instructs the observer to return the patient to the hospital should certain complications develop [eg, somnolence, vomiting, etc].) If the patient is even mildly confused, radiographic findings are positive, a reliable observer is not available, or any additional problems occur, the patient should be admitted for observation. These

"ABC" assessment

A—airway: suction to free pharynx from blood and other material; intubate after cervical spine evaluation

B—breathing: evaluate rate, rhythm and breath sounds; ventilate to raise PaO_2 and reduce $PaCO_2$ (to lower ICP); monitor ABG levels

C—circulatory status: start intravenous infusion of lactated Ringer's or normal saline solution, followed by blood if indicated; obtain immediate laboratory work and x-rays; administer steroids and phenytoin, plus pressor agent if required (shock rarely due to head injury alone; search for cause)

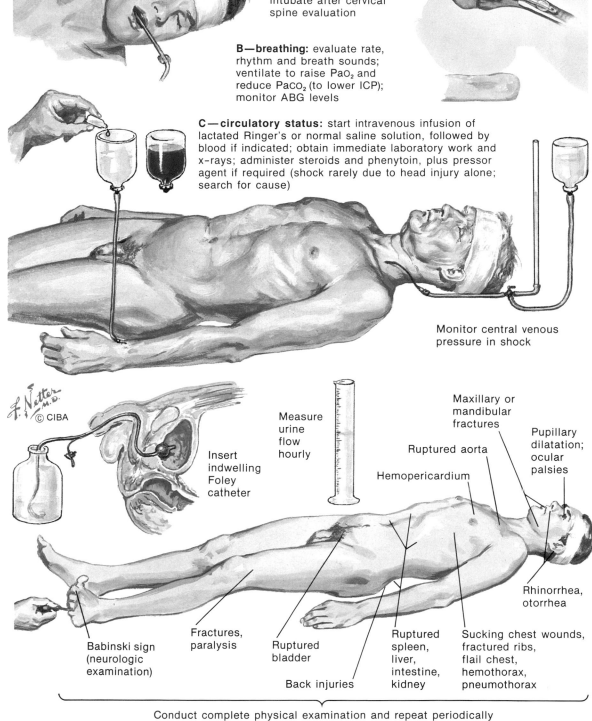

Monitor central venous pressure in shock

Insert indwelling Foley catheter

Measure urine flow hourly

Maxillary or mandibular fractures

Ruptured aorta

Hemopericardium

Pupillary dilatation; ocular palsies

Rhinorrhea, otorrhea

Babinski sign (neurologic examination)

Fractures, paralysis

Ruptured bladder

Back injuries

Ruptured spleen, liver, intestine, kidney

Sucking chest wounds, fractured ribs, flail chest, hemothorax, pneumothorax

Conduct complete physical examination and repeat periodically

precautionary measures are necessary, even after an apparently trivial head injury, because such patients may, rarely, have a life-threatening intracranial hemorrhage and deteriorate quite rapidly.

A small percentage of patients return after discharge complaining of persistent headache, nausea, difficulty in concentrating, poor memory, insomnia and depression. This constellation of symptoms constitutes the *postconcussive syndrome*. In most of these patients, results of cursory neurologic examinations and radiographic studies (such as CT scans) are normal, but recent studies indicate that detailed neuropsychologic testing reveals abnormalities in many concussed patients, even those without overt postconcussive symptoms. No

specific therapy is available for this problem, but with reassurance and symptomatic treatment, most patients do well.

Epidural Hematomas. In 1% to 3% of major head injuries, epidural hematomas develop. Although they may occur in persons of any age, they are most common in the second and third decades of life. The male-female ratio is as high as 4:1. Automobile accidents are the most common cause, but trivial causes, such as minor falls and sports injuries, are notorious as precipitating events. The source is usually arterial (85%), but epidural hematomas may follow injury to a meningeal vein or dural sinus. Common locations of epidural hematomas include the temporal fossa,

Head Injuries
(Continued)

subfrontal region and occipital-suboccipital area (Plate 3).

The *temporal fossa epidural hematoma*, which results from damage to the middle meningeal artery, is the most common epidural hematoma. Fracture of the temporal skull is the cause in at least 80% of such cases. The classic and long-recognized sequence of clinical signs of this type of hematoma is seen in only a minority of patients. Classically, the concussion causes an initial period of unconsciousness; subsequently, because the dura mater is quite adherent to the skull, accumulation of blood is delayed and a lucid interval follows, during which the patient's neurologic function is relatively normal. Finally, as the lesion enlarges, the level of consciousness deteriorates rapidly. This characterizes the so-called talk-and-die patient. The lucid interval is longer if the source of the hemorrhage is venous (under lower pressure) rather than arterial.

As the hematoma enlarges, it pushes the temporal lobe medially, causing herniation of the uncus and hippocampal gyrus over and through the tentorial notch. The *uncal herniation syndrome* is characterized by a decreasing level of consciousness, early dilatation of the ipsilateral pupil, and hemiparesis. The hemiparesis is usually contralateral, because of the decussation of the descending pyramidal tracts; however, if the opposite cerebral peduncle is compressed against the tentorial edge (Kernohan's notch), ipsilateral hemiparesis may result. Other evidence suggesting an epidural hematoma includes a scalp contusion at the site of injury, a temporal skull fracture, or a temporal subgaleal hematoma secondary to extravasation of epidural blood through the skull fracture and lacerated periosteum.

The *frontal or subfrontal epidural hematoma* is most common in the young or elderly, and is often associated with direct frontal blows. The injury may involve the anterior branch of the middle meningeal artery, the anterior meningeal artery or a venous sinus. Common symptoms and signs include headache, personality changes and anisocoria (difference in pupillary diameters). The lucid interval is characteristically longer and the evolution of the lesion slower than with temporal lesions. Recent evidence suggests that some of these lesions may be treated conservatively.

The *posterior fossa epidural hematoma* usually results from an occipital blow, and is associated with a fracture that crosses the transverse sinus. Clinical presentation may be acute or chronic. Common symptoms and signs include headache, meningismus, dysmetria, ataxia and cranial nerve deficit. Herniation of the posterior fossa contents through the foramen magnum can produce *Cushing's triad*—respiratory depression, an increase in blood pressure, and a decrease in pulse rate.

Epidural hematomas are rarely bilateral, but are sometimes associated with subdural lesions. This diagnosis can be confirmed by CT; occasionally however, there is no time for delay, and the diagnosis and treatment must be simultaneous, in the form of a temporal craniectomy. Although the

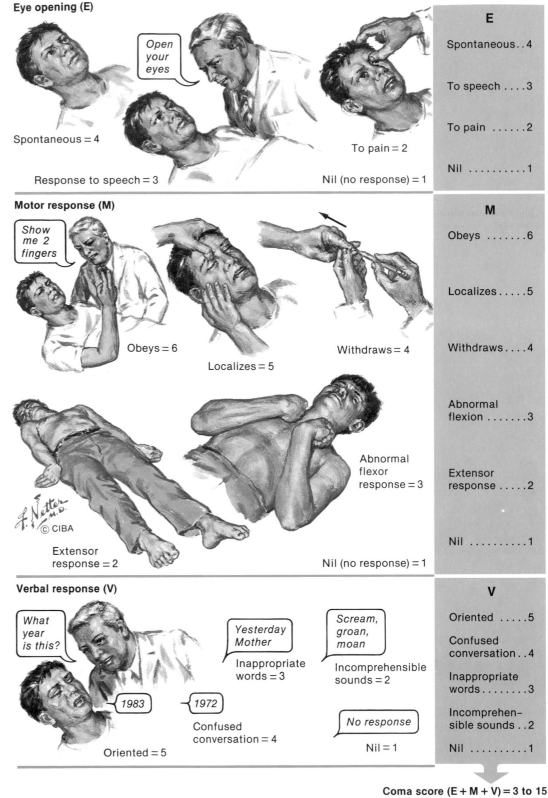

Glasgow Coma Scale

Eye opening (E)

"Open your eyes"

Spontaneous = 4

Response to speech = 3

To pain = 2

Nil (no response) = 1

E	
Spontaneous	4
To speech	3
To pain	2
Nil	1

Motor response (M)

"Show me 2 fingers"

Obeys = 6

Localizes = 5

Withdraws = 4

Extensor response = 2

Abnormal flexor response = 3

Nil (no response) = 1

M	
Obeys	6
Localizes	5
Withdraws	4
Abnormal flexion	3
Extensor response	2
Nil	1

Verbal response (V)

"What year is this?"

1983   1972

Oriented = 5

Confused conversation = 4

"Yesterday Mother"

Inappropriate words = 3

"Scream, groan, moan"

Incomprehensible sounds = 2

"No response"

Nil = 1

V	
Oriented	5
Confused conversation	4
Inappropriate words	3
Incomprehensible sounds	2
Nil	1

Coma score (E + M + V) = 3 to 15

mortality reported in most older clinical series is as high as 50%, more recent studies, describing aggressive diagnostic and therapeutic techniques, have been more encouraging, reporting a mortality of about 20%.

Subdural Hematomas. A subdural hematoma is usually the result of an acute venous hemorrhage caused by rupture of cortical bridging veins. Less common sources include cortical arteries, aneurysms, arteriovenous malformations and metastatic tumors.

Acute subdural hematomas develop within 1 week after injury (usually within hours). Fifty percent are associated with skull fractures; vehicular accidents are the most common cause. Frequently

associated massive cerebral or brainstem contusions, or both, account for the distressingly high mortality (50%). Common signs include decreasing level of consciousness, ipsilateral pupillary dilatation, and contralateral hemiparesis. As with an epidural hematoma, the hemiparesis is occasionally ipsilateral. Other so-called false localizing signs include homonymous hemianopsia from thrombosis of the posterior cerebral artery in uncal herniation, abnormalities of gaze secondary to brainstem injuries and, rarely, contralateral pupillary dilatation secondary to oculomotor nerve compression against the tentorium. Acute subdural hematomas are almost always located over the cerebral convexities and are bilateral in

Head Injuries
(Continued)

15% to 20% of patients. The definitive diagnosis can be made by CT or angiography.

Subacute subdural hematomas usually develop within 7 to 10 days after injury. The symptoms and signs are similar to those of acute subdural hematomas, but the course is slower and the mortality correspondingly lower. The definitive diagnosis can usually be made by CT, although, because of the isodensity of these hematomas, angiography is occasionally required.

Chronic subdural hematomas are most common in elderly patients and chronic alcoholics who usually have some degree of brain atrophy, with a resultant increase in the size of the subdural space. Patients who are receiving long-term anticoagulant therapy or who have a blood dyscrasia are also at risk. The precipitating trauma is often so trivial it has been forgotten. Initially, a small hemorrhage fills the preexisting subdural space and, after approximately 2 weeks, a vascular membrane forms around the lesion. It was originally theorized that the blood products within the subdural hematoma osmotically attracted CSF, increasing the size of the hematoma, stretching the membrane, and causing further hemorrhage. Subsequently, it was shown that there is no osmotic gradient across the membrane. Nevertheless, in some patients, the hematoma apparently enlarges until it produces symptoms.

The symptoms and signs of a chronic subdural hematoma are often confused with those of cerebrovascular accident, encephalitis, metabolic encephalopathy or psychosis, and tend to wax and wane remarkably. Chronic headache and percussion tenderness over the lesion occur in 80% of patients, and most patients manifest progressive dementia with generalized rigidity (paratonia). Skull x-ray films show abnormalities in 25% of patients, the electroencephalogram (EEG) characteristically shows decreased voltage over the lesion, and the concentration of protein in the CSF is often increased. The diagnosis can be confirmed by CT or angiography.

Initial Management and Evaluation. An acute intracranial injury is often associated with severe neurologic impairment. In most instances, the patient is comatose on arriving in the emergency room—that is, "unable to open the eyes, make any recognizable sound, or follow any commands." The initial management of these severe head injuries is based on the ABC approach that is central to modern emergency medicine (Plate 4).

The first step is to assess the *airway* (A) and clear it of all obstructive material (eg, dentures, vomitus). Because of the possibility of an associated cervical spine injury, lateral x-ray films of the cervical spine should be obtained before the neck is manipulated for tracheal intubation. However, if the breathing appears at all compromised, nasotracheal or endotracheal intubation with the neck in neutral position should be carefully performed without delay. Occasionally, facial trauma prevents intubation, and cricothyroidotomy or tracheostomy is necessary.

CT Scans and Angiograms of Intracranial Hematomas

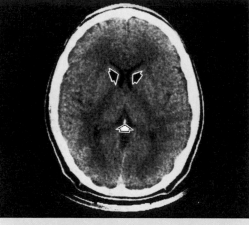

A. Normal brain. CT scan demonstrating normal anatomy at level of frontal horns of lateral ventricles (black arrows). Pineal gland (white arrow) is in normal midline location

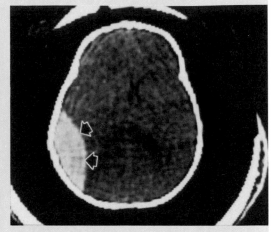

B. Epidural hematoma. CT scan demonstrating hyperdense right parietal epidural hematoma (black arrows), which has assumed classic lenticular configuration secondary to adherence of dura to inner table of skull. Other structures are compressed and shifted

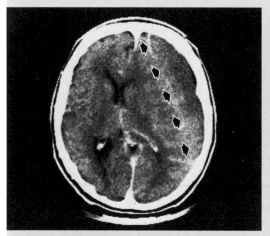

C. Subacute subdural hematoma. CT scan demonstrating large isodense mass over left cerebral convexity. Compressed cerebral cortex (black arrows) shows enhanced density delineating inner border of subacute subdural hematoma. Normal structures are shifted across midline

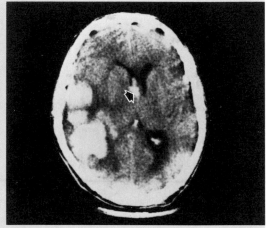

D. Acute intracerebral hematoma. CT scan demonstrating hyperdense mass in right parietotemporal area. Large acute intracerebral hematoma has shifted lateral ventricle toward midline. Blood is visualized within ventricular system (black arrow)

© CIBA

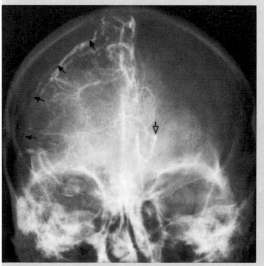

E. Acute subdural hematoma. Cerebral angiogram, venous phase, demonstrating displacement of cortical veins (solid arrows) away from skull by acute subdural hematoma. Typical shape is due to relatively free spread of blood within subdural space. Internal cerebral vein (open arrow) is shifted across midline

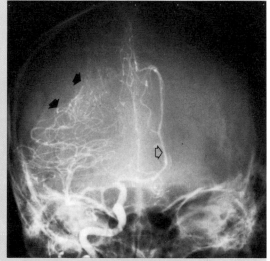

F. Chronic subdural hematoma. Cerebral angiogram, arterial phase, demonstrating displacement of cortical vessels (solid arrows) away from inner table of skull by chronic subdural hematoma. Lenticular shape is secondary to subdural membrane formation. Anterior cerebral artery (open arrow) is shifted across midline

Head Injuries
(Continued)

After a clear airway has been ensured, the patient's *breathing* (B) is assessed. The rate and rhythm of respiration, as well as the breath sounds, are evaluated. Alterations in the respiratory pattern may reflect the relative level of central nervous system (CNS) dysfunction. Bilateral deep hemispheric and basal ganglia lesions may cause Cheyne-Stokes respiration (alternating periods of hyperventilation and apnea), and central neurogenic hyperventilation may result from mesencephalic or high pontine lesions. Ataxic respiration develops terminally, when only medullary function remains. Arterial blood gases should be analyzed in every patient with a head injury, as hypoxemia is common. Sufficient oxygen should be administered to keep the PaO$_2$ within normal range; hyperventilation is recommended to keep the PaCO$_2$ between 25 and 30 mm Hg, as hypocarbia is a potent cerebral vasoconstrictor, reducing cerebral blood volume and, hence, intracranial pressure. A baseline chest x-ray film should be obtained to screen for chest injuries such as pneumothorax, pulmonary contusion or aspiration.

Attention is then directed to the patient's *circulatory status* (C), as reflected by the blood pressure. Because shock rarely results from head injury alone, a rigorous search must be made for other causes (eg, rupture of the spleen or fracture of a long bone). A central venous catheter, placed in either a subclavian or internal jugular vein, is often invaluable in evaluating and treating patients with multiple injuries. Along with a rapidly determined hematocrit, central venous pressure readings may help to distinguish hypovolemic shock from those few instances of neurogenic shock caused by an associated spinal cord injury.

In *neurogenic shock*, cervical cord dysfunction disrupts the sympathetic outflow to the tissues, causing venous pooling and hypotension. This type of shock is usually characterized by hypotension, bradycardia, relatively normal central venous pressure, and a normal hematocrit; *hypovolemic shock* causes tachycardia, low central venous pressure, and a decreased hematocrit. Neurogenic shock can usually be corrected by tilting the patient head downward and administering modest amounts of fluid; occasionally, atropine or vasopressor agents are required. In contrast, the patient in hypovolemic shock needs large amounts of intravenous fluids.

During and following institution of ABC therapy, a complete physical examination is performed. The neurologic evaluation should be directed particularly toward assessing the level of

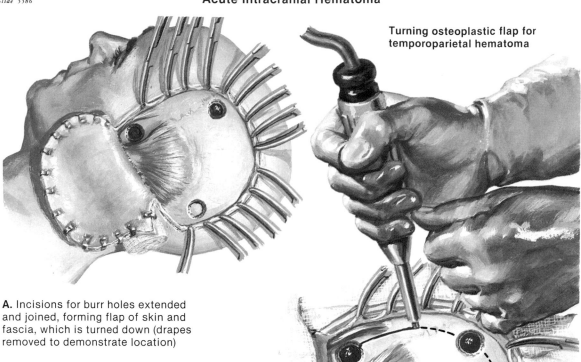

Turning osteoplastic flap for temporoparietal hematoma

A. Incisions for burr holes extended and joined, forming flap of skin and fascia, which is turned down (drapes removed to demonstrate location)

B. Skull opened by connecting burr holes with craniotome

C. Bone flap turned down by cracking uncut segment of margin, exposing epidural hematoma, which is removed by suction, spoon or Penfield dissector

consciousness, pupillary reactions, extraocular movements and motor response. These features can be reliably recorded at the scene of the trauma, in the emergency room, and subsequently in the intensive care unit. Thus, any change can be recognized early and effective therapy can be instituted more rapidly.

A variety of terms, such as coma, semicoma, stupor and obtundation, have been used to describe the *level of consciousness*, but such terms are not uniformly used among examiners or centers. Therefore, the development by Teasdale and Jennett, in 1974, of what has become known as the *Glasgow Coma Scale* was an important advance. On this scale, the patient's ability to perform three

tests of neurologic function—*eye opening, motor response* and *verbal response*—determines the total score (Plate 5). The standard definition of coma—"unable to open the eyes, make any recognizable sound, or follow any commands"—corresponds to a maximum score of 8. The Glasgow Coma Scale rating is easily and reproducibly determined, allowing for ready recognition of changes in individual patients and comparison of groups of patients within an institution or among many institutions. It has become an integral part of the modern diagnosis and treatment of head trauma.

Various *pupillary abnormalities* may develop after head trauma. The best known is unilateral third

Head Injuries
(Continued)

cranial nerve palsy from uncal herniation, which characteristically causes early dilatation of the ipsilateral pupil and a poor response to light (Hutchinson's pupil). Subsequently, the extraocular muscle function of the third cranial nerve is lost, resulting in a maximally dilated ("blown") pupil displaced to an inferolateral position. On the other hand, anisocoria may reflect Horner's syndrome. Traumatic Horner's syndrome is usually associated with injury to the cervicothoracic spinal cord, brachial plexus or carotid artery. This results in sympathetic denervation of the ipsilateral eye, leading to the classic triad: miosis, ptosis and anhidrosis (loss of sweating).

Bilateral small (miotic) pupils, although often indicative of drug intoxication, may also reflect pontine injury. Damage to the retina or optic nerve may produce the Marcus Gunn afferent pupillary defect, in which the consensual pupillary response is stronger than the response to direct light in the damaged eye. Swinging a flashlight from the normal to the damaged eye causes seemingly paradoxical pupillary dilatation. Other abnormal pupillary responses, such as tectal pupils and hippus, occasionally develop after head trauma.

When evaluating *extraocular motility*, it is helpful to remember that two major areas govern horizontal eye movements. Within the pontine reticular formation is a horizontal gaze center. It is connected, via the medial longitudinal fasciculus, to the upper cervical spinal cord and to the vestibular and extraocular cranial nuclei. Damage to this gaze center causes conjugate deviation of the eyes to the opposite side. The other center is located within the frontal lobe (the frontal eye fields, Brodmann's area 8). Damage to this center is signaled by conjugate deviation of the eyes and head toward the side of injury. If the site of injury is in the frontal lobe, the eyes deviate away from the hemiparetic side (the motor tracts cross in the medulla); in brainstem injury, the eyes deviate toward the hemiparetic side.

Whether or not ocular deviation is seen, the presence or absence of full ocular motility must be assessed. If the cervical spine is undamaged, the doll's-eyes phenomenon may be used. Moving the head from side to side stimulates the cervical nerve roots and vestibular nuclei and, when the brainstem centers are intact, causes an opposite movement of the eyes so that they maintain their relative position in space. If the brainstem centers are injured, the eyes remain fixed in relationship to the head (a poor prognostic sign).

Alternatively, the ice-water caloric test may be used. The head is raised 30 degrees from supine, so that the horizontal semicircular canal is in a vertical position. If the canal is clear and the tympanic membrane is intact, ice water is introduced. In a conscious patient, this stimulates the vestibular nuclei, inducing nystagmus with the fast phase toward the contralateral side. (Recall the mnemonic, Cold Opposite Warm Same, COWS.) But in a comatose patient, the fast phase is abolished, so that the eyes actually deviate

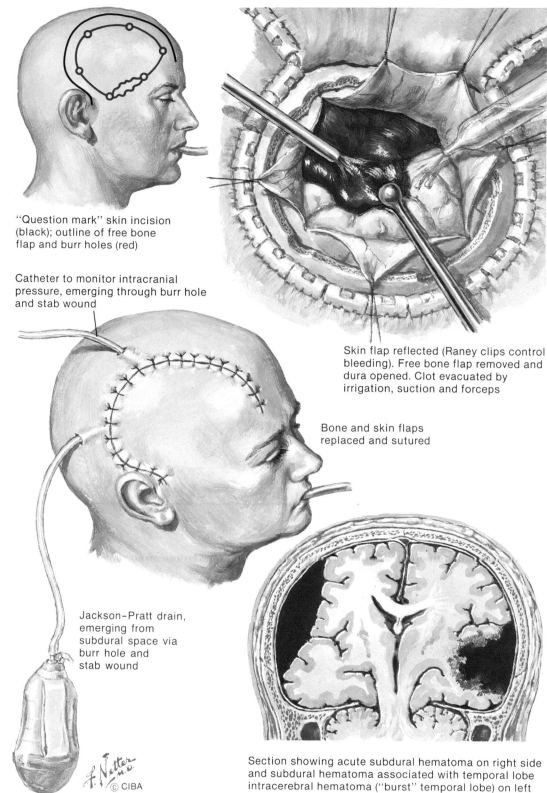

"Question mark" skin incision (black); outline of free bone flap and burr holes (red)

Catheter to monitor intracranial pressure, emerging through burr hole and stab wound

Skin flap reflected (Raney clips control bleeding). Free bone flap removed and dura opened. Clot evacuated by irrigation, suction and forceps

Bone and skin flaps replaced and sutured

Jackson–Pratt drain, emerging from subdural space via burr hole and stab wound

Section showing acute subdural hematoma on right side and subdural hematoma associated with temporal lobe intracerebral hematoma ("burst" temporal lobe) on left

conjugately toward the cold. Absence of a caloric response is also a poor prognostic sign.

Some categories of *motor response* are included in the Glasgow Coma Scale in Plate 5. Although somewhat simplistic, the following schema is helpful in understanding the relative severity of injury. If the patient obeys commands, localizes painful stimuli, or withdraws from pain, all descending motor pathways are intact. The rubrospinal pathways subserve flexion responses but innervate only the upper extremities in humans. Decortication (flexion of the arms and extension of the legs), therefore, reflects a physiologic level of injury between the cortex and the red nuclei. The vestibulospinal pathways subserve

extension in all four extremities. Decerebration (extension of all four limbs), therefore, reflects a level of injury between the red nuclei and vestibular nuclei. Absence of motor response indicates that the functional level of injury is below the vestibular nuclei. Other motor patterns (such as monoplegia, paraplegia or quadriplegia) reflect injury to various areas of the nervous system.

Depending on the severity of the injury, a more or less detailed examination may be done following initial evaluation. Simultaneously, skull x-ray films are obtained. Standard laboratory tests should be ordered routinely on every trauma patient.

Attention is then directed to definitive radiographic or therapeutic measures, or both. The

Head Injuries
(Continued)

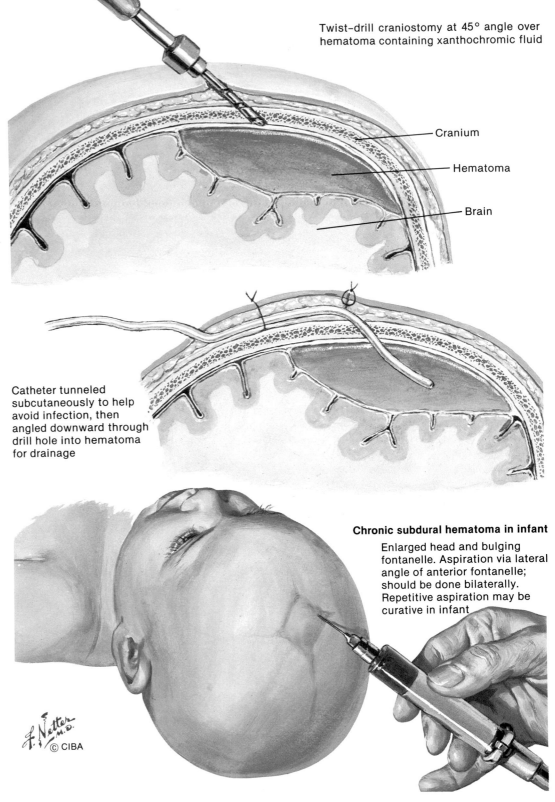

Twist-drill craniostomy at 45° angle over hematoma containing xanthochromic fluid

Cranium

Hematoma

Brain

Catheter tunneled subcutaneously to help avoid infection, then angled downward through drill hole into hematoma for drainage

Chronic subdural hematoma in infant

Enlarged head and bulging fontanelle. Aspiration via lateral angle of anterior fontanelle; should be done bilaterally. Repetitive aspiration may be curative in infant

former include CT of the brain, which in recent years has revolutionized the diagnosis of intracranial lesions (see CIBA COLLECTION, Volume 1/I, page 62). Because the head must remain motionless during the procedure, a general anesthetic is occasionally required for agitated, very young, or otherwise uncooperative patients. As the scanner rotates around the head, x-rays traverse the intracranial contents at many different angles but in one horizontal plane. By analyzing the degree to which the intracranial structures attenuate the x-ray beam, a computer produces a composite video or printed picture of the radiodensities within the section scanned. Plate 6 illustrates CT features of a normal brain and of various types of intracranial hematomas.

CT scans show the normal differences in density between intracranial structures. The cerebrum is arbitrarily designated as isodense. Hyperdense structures include the skull, pineal gland and fresh blood; hypodense structures include CSF, fat and air. Adjoining structures must have different densities in order to be easily distinguishable on a CT scan. In addition, shift of normal structures, such as the pineal gland or ventricular system, may indicate the presence of a lesion.

Epidural and subdural hematomas are both hyperdense but often differ in shape. Epidural hematomas are *lenticular* in shape because of the dura mater's adherence to the inner table of the skull at the edges of the lesion. They may displace the ventricular system and the pineal gland.

Acute subdural hematomas are generally *crescentic* (biconcave). They are usually located over the cerebral convexity, and commonly displace portions of the ventricular system. Subacute subdural hematomas, if isodense, may be difficult to distinguish on a CT scan. They can usually be detected because of the shift of normal structures, but this may not occur if the hematomas are bilateral, as in 15% to 20% of cases. In such cases, contrast-enhanced CT may delineate the cortical margin. Otherwise, carotid angiography (Plate 6), frequently performed via a transfemoral catheter, may be necessary to demonstrate the characteristic displacement of the cortical vessels away from the inner table of the skull at the site of the hematoma. Chronic subdural hematomas are usually hypodense and, therefore, easily detected on CT. Their configuration is occasionally lenticular, because of their confinement within a subdural membrane.

Intracerebral hematomas are hyperdense and usually develop within the temporal and frontal lobes after trauma. Normal structures may be displaced. Sometimes, an intracerebral hemorrhage of the temporal lobe is seen in conjunction with an overlying subdural hematoma—the so-called burst temporal lobe (Plate 8), which carries a relatively poor prognosis. Not infrequently, CT after major head trauma fails to reveal any lesion. Alternatively, areas of relative hypodensity may be seen within the white matter structures, indicating posttraumatic cerebral edema.

Surgical Management. The decisions regarding surgical removal of lesions identified on CT scans are complex and controversial. Suffice it to say that most extracerebral and many traumatic intracerebral hematomas are initially treated surgically.

Although intracranial hematomas account for a relatively small percentage (10%) of "serious" head injuries, they are found in approximately 50% of patients brought to emergency facilities in coma. Any delay in treating these critically ill patients can be fatal. Comatose patients should be evaluated and scanning done as expeditiously as possible. If a lesion requiring surgery is identified, mannitol (or another diuretic) should be

administered and the patient transported to the operating room immediately.

The technique used to evacuate an *acute intracranial hematoma* varies, but the following principles generally apply (Plates 7–8). If appropriate neurodiagnostic studies have proved that the lesion is unilateral, the patient's body is placed supine and the head positioned laterally, with the side of the lesion uppermost. To reduce venous bleeding, the head is always positioned higher than the chest; a cerebellar headrest or Mayfield head holder may be used. The lines of the prospective skin incision and the midline are marked on the shaved scalp with a needle. The area is then surgically "prepped" and draped.

Head Injuries
(Continued)

The initial incision is usually made from the zygomatic arch upward, remaining within 1 fingerbreadth of the ear to avoid cutting branches of the facial nerve. The temporalis fascia and muscle are divided with cutting cautery and retracted. A burr hole is made in the temporal fossa with a gas- or electric-powered drill, and is enlarged with bone rongeurs. If an epidural hematoma is present, it can be removed with suction and the middle meningeal artery coagulated. Occasionally, it is necessary to trace the artery back to the foramen spinosum, which is packed with bone wax or a cotton pledget. If a subdural hematoma is present, the dura mater is opened in a cruciate fashion, which allows rapid decompression of the brain.

Exposure provided by a temporal craniectomy is often inadequate for the removal of a large epidural, subdural or intracerebral hematoma. In this case, the skin flap must be extended and a formal craniotomy performed. Two flaps are commonly used. One is horseshoe-shaped and centered over the ear (Plate 7); the other is the "question mark" skin incision (Plate 8). Hematomas in unusual locations (ie, subfrontal or posterior fossa lesions) require appropriately positioned skin flaps. As the scalp is opened, skin clips or hemostats are applied to control skin bleeding. Additional burr holes are drilled in appropriate locations and the dura mater is carefully stripped from the inner table of the skull. Bone cuts are then made between the burr holes, with use of the craniotome. When the cuts are complete, the bone flap can be "cracked back" while still connected to the periosteum and temporalis muscle (osteoplastic flap) (Plate 7), or the temporalis muscle can be elevated and a free bone flap cut (Plate 8). The dural flap is usually opened with its base toward the sagittal sinus. The epidural, subdural or intracerebral clot can then be removed and all sources of bleeding meticulously controlled. In addition, severely traumatized brain (eg, a burst temporal lobe) should be removed.

Frequently, it is advisable to leave a closed drainage system within the subdural or epidural space for several days. In addition, an intracranial pressure monitor should be inserted to facilitate postoperative management. The dura mater is then reapproximated and the skull flap replaced. Finally, the temporalis muscle and skin are closed in layers.

Chronic subdural hematomas in adults have traditionally been treated either by burr-hole drainage or by craniotomy, with stripping of the subdural membranes. Many of these patients, however, are medically infirm, and surgical mortality and morbidity are high. In addition, the atrophic brain often fails to reexpand rapidly, leading to persistence of the subdural collections. More recently, treatment based on a *percutaneous drainage technique* has been successful (Plate 9).

At the bedside, the patient's head is surgically "prepped." With the patient under local anesthetic, a small hole is made with a twist drill over

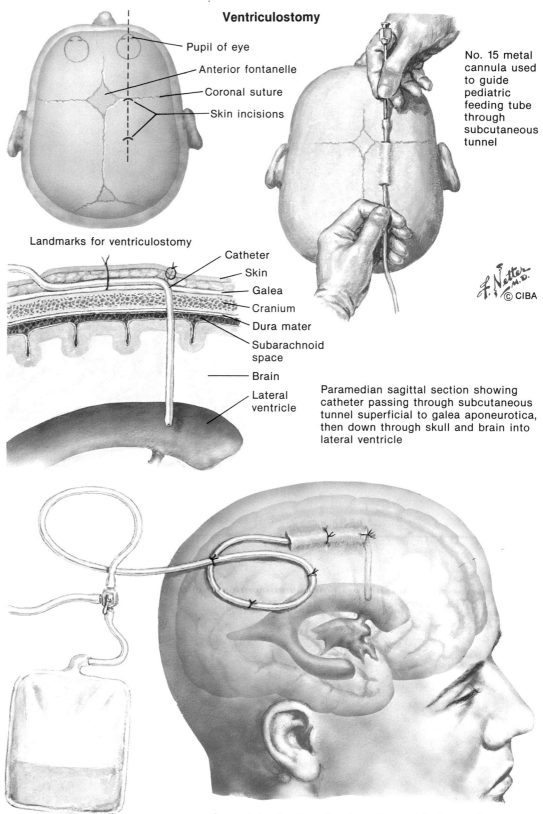

Ventriculostomy

Landmarks for ventriculostomy

- Pupil of eye
- Anterior fontanelle
- Coronal suture
- Skin incisions

No. 15 metal cannula used to guide pediatric feeding tube through subcutaneous tunnel

- Catheter
- Skin
- Galea
- Cranium
- Dura mater
- Subarachnoid space
- Brain
- Lateral ventricle

Paramedian sagittal section showing catheter passing through subcutaneous tunnel superficial to galea aponeurotica, then down through skull and brain into lateral ventricle

Superolateral schematic view of completed procedure

the area of maximal subdural collection. The bit is angled at 45 degrees to the skull surface, so that it travels through the dura mater and into the subdural space. A No. 5 French catheter is threaded through a subcutaneous tunnel and into the subdural space. A sample of fluid is sent for analysis and culture, and the fluid then is drained continuously into a closed system positioned below the head. Another technique used occasionally in the treatment of refractory chronic subdural hematoma is the *subdural-peritoneal shunt*.

Chronic subdural hematomas in children constitute a special category. These lesions are usually traumatic, and occur more often in boys than in girls. The symptoms and signs are those of increased intracranial pressure (tight fontanelle, increased head size, irritability and vomiting) and cortical irritation (seizures). The diagnosis can be confirmed by CT or ultrasonography. Although older studies recommend craniotomy and stripping of the membranes, recent series favor repeated subdural taps, with subdural-peritoneal shunting for refractory cases. Neurologic development is normal in 75% of all children with chronic subdural hematomas if they are properly treated.

Nonsurgical Management. The mortality from intracranial injuries has remained distressingly high. Early diagnosis and surgery for intracranial hemorrhage are, of course, crucial, but

Head Injuries
(Continued)

recent studies have demonstrated the additional importance of intensive medical therapy during the postoperative course as well as in comatose head trauma patients without surgical lesions.

Intracranial pressure monitoring is the cornerstone of medical therapy. It is hoped that this procedure, with aggressive measures to control the pressure, will improve the outcome of patients with severe head injury. Monitoring clearly constitutes an effective early warning system for these patients. For example, intracranial hypertension may be an early reflection of inadequate ventilation, hyponatremia or delayed intracranial hemorrhage.

A variety of monitoring devices are available, including ventriculostomy catheters, subarachnoid screws, subdural catheters and epidural sensors. Percutaneous ventriculostomy offers several advantages, including therapeutic CSF drainage, diagnostic CSF sampling (eg, daily cultures), an intrathecal route for drug administration, and the possibility of testing the compliance of the CSF system by injecting small quantities of fluid and measuring the pressure response.

Many methods of draining the ventricles have been devised. In 1927, Adson first used a metal cannula, secured in an occipital burr hole by means of a bolt threaded into the skull. Other devices used have included woven-silk ureteral catheters, silver cannulas and rubber catheters. Polyethylene catheters have also been used, with increasing success. Infection, however, has remained a problem, despite use of a meticulous technique and prophylactic administration of antibiotics. The addition of a percutaneous tunnel has largely obviated this difficulty.

Plate 10 shows the landmarks for *ventriculostomy*. The ventricular catheter is inserted at the junction of the coronal suture and a parasagittal plane passing through the pupil of the ipsilateral eye. From this site, the needle used for the ventricular tap is directed toward the nasion on a trajectory leading toward the interventricular foramen (of Monro). After the ventricle has been tapped, a pediatric feeding tube is tunneled subcutaneously from a second incision over the parietal bone, superficial to the galea aponeurotica and beneath the skin, until it emerges at the first incision. The tip of the tube is then directed into the lateral ventricle down the tract of the prior ventricular tap. The tube is sutured in place and connected to a drainage or pressure-monitoring device. This procedure is easily done at the bedside, with the use of local anesthetic. The catheter may be left in place for up to 1 week with minimal risk of infection.

Use of the *subarachnoid screw* (Plate 11) is a technically easier alternative if the lateral ventricles are small (as with diffuse cerebral edema). With a special drill bit, a hole is made in the skull and the dura mater is opened. A precisely machined bolt is then screwed into the hole, until the tip rests against the brain. After the system has been filled with fluid, the intracranial pressure can be easily determined.

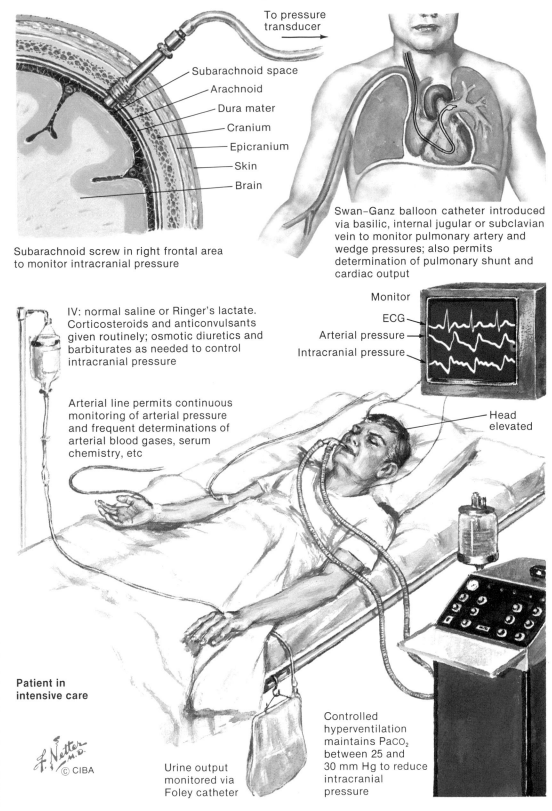

Subarachnoid screw in right frontal area to monitor intracranial pressure

Swan–Ganz balloon catheter introduced via basilic, internal jugular or subclavian vein to monitor pulmonary artery and wedge pressures; also permits determination of pulmonary shunt and cardiac output

IV: normal saline or Ringer's lactate. Corticosteroids and anticonvulsants given routinely; osmotic diuretics and barbiturates as needed to control intracranial pressure

Arterial line permits continuous monitoring of arterial pressure and frequent determinations of arterial blood gases, serum chemistry, etc

Patient in intensive care

Urine output monitored via Foley catheter

Head elevated

Controlled hyperventilation maintains PaCO₂ between 25 and 30 mm Hg to reduce intracranial pressure

Another alternative device is the *subdural intracranial pressure monitor catheter* (Plate 8). This plastic catheter is placed on the brain at the time of surgery and tunneled out through a burr hole and separate skin incision. Epidural sensors can also be placed through a burr hole, but they are more expensive and calibration is more difficult.

If the intracranial pressure remains normal, intensive supportive care is provided (Plate 11). If the pressure is elevated, vigorous medical measures are needed to reduce it. Controlled ventilation is routinely used to maintain the PaCO₂ between 25 and 30 mm Hg. This relative hypocarbia constricts the cerebral vessels, decreases the cerebral blood volume, and hence lowers the

intracranial pressure. Steroid therapy may prevent intracerebral edema, although the beneficial effects of such therapy remain to be proved. Since hyperthermia increases the cerebral metabolic rate and hypothermia leads to additional medical complications, most physicians maintain their patients in a normothermic state. Osmotic diuretics, such as mannitol, may be given by bolus or continuous infusion to reduce the intracranial pressure. Close monitoring of serum electrolyte concentrations and osmolality is required if osmotic agents are used repeatedly.

If the measures previously described do not control intracranial pressure, the prognosis is uniformly poor. Under these circumstances, other

Head Injuries
(Continued)

agents and techniques to further reduce the intracranial pressure have been used, with varying success. *Barbiturate coma* is now the most commonly used of these adjuncts. Barbiturates decrease the cerebral metabolic rate, suppress catecholamine synthesis, and increase free-radical scavenging. Probably more important is the potent constrictive effect these drugs have on cerebral vessels. Whatever the mechanism, barbiturates often reduce, at least temporarily, otherwise intractable intracranial hypertension.

The medical management of severe head trauma is the subject of intensive research, and it remains to be proved whether controlling intracranial pressure alone will improve the outcome in large numbers of trauma patients. One area of investigation concerns the use of *cortical evoked potentials*. These electrical signals are much smaller than the background electroencephalographic activity, but can be readily extracted using special computer averaging techniques. A variety of stimuli (auditory, visual and somatosensory) are used to elicit these responses, and early data indicate that abnormalities in multimodality evoked potentials may reflect the actual site of injury. For example, if the injury is primarily hemispheric, visual evoked potentials may be more abnormal than brainstem auditory evoked potentials. Evoked potentials may also be useful in monitoring patients under barbiturate coma and in predicting the ultimate outcome after head injury.

Respiratory Exchange in Head Injuries

Crucial to the medical management of head trauma victims is an understanding of the frequent derangements of respiratory exchange (Plate 12). The brain is completely dependent on aerobic metabolism in physiologic and most pathologic situations. The normal cerebral metabolic rate for oxygen is 3.5 ml/100 g·min, which represents 20% of the body's total oxygen requirement. In addition, cerebral blood flow and hence intracranial pressure are dependent on the $PaCO_2$ and blood pH. For instance, the inhalation of 5% carbon dioxide increases the cerebral blood flow by 50%, whereas the hypocapnia that results from hyperventilation may reduce cerebral blood flow by 60%. After cerebral injury, therefore, the hypoxemia, hypercarbia and acidosis associated with abnormalities of respiration may lead to both deterioration in neuronal metabolism and intracranial hypertension. This further impairs respiration, which leads to a vicious cycle of deterioration.

Respiration is under both voluntary and automatic control (see CIBA COLLECTION, Volume 7, pages 76–77). The higher voluntary centers have not been well localized, although three automatic centers have been identified within the brainstem: the pneumotaxic center, which is located in the rostral pons and fine-tunes the other centers; the apneustic center, which is in the midpontine reticular formation and is probably the terminal for the stimuli that end inspiration; and the medullary center, which maintains the intrinsic rhythmicity of respiration. Afferent stimuli from peripheral receptors (carotid and aortic bodies and lungs) and central receptors provide the input to these centers. The output of the voluntary system

lies within the corticospinal tract, while the output of the automatic system lies within the ventrolateral quadrant. A lesion placed in the cervical spinothalamic tract to eliminate intractable pain (cordotomy) may affect these pathways. Rarely, this results in "Ondine's curse," a condition that causes the patient to stop breathing during sleep.

Specific abnormalities in the respiratory rate and pattern may reflect the physiologic or anatomic level of dysfunction of the CNS. Bilateral deep hemispheric or basal ganglia lesions, or both, may lead to *Cheyne-Stokes respiration*, which is also associated with metabolic encephalopathy or impending uncal herniation. Mesencephalic or

Respiratory Exchange in Head Injury

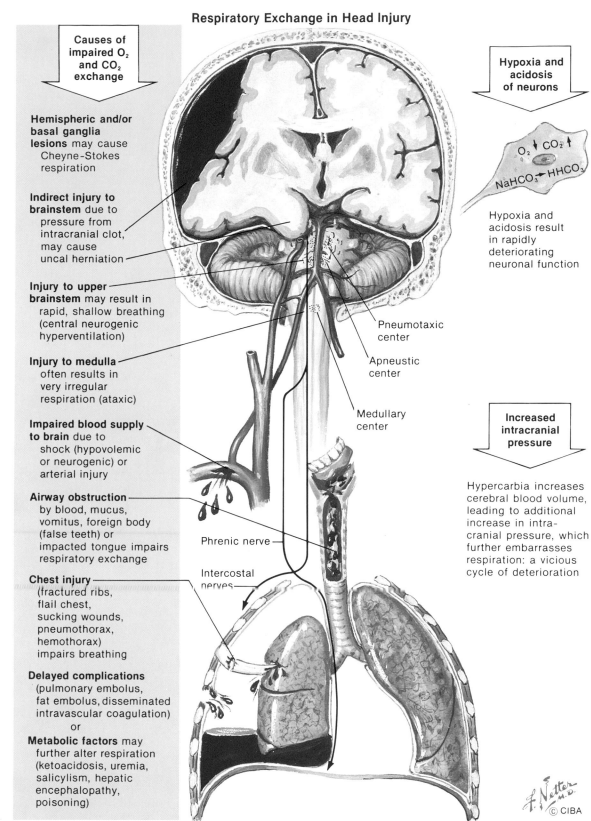

Causes of impaired O_2 and CO_2 exchange

Hemispheric and/or basal ganglia lesions may cause Cheyne-Stokes respiration

Indirect injury to brainstem due to pressure from intracranial clot, may cause uncal herniation

Injury to upper brainstem may result in rapid, shallow breathing (central neurogenic hyperventilation)

Injury to medulla often results in very irregular respiration (ataxic)

Impaired blood supply to brain due to shock (hypovolemic or neurogenic) or arterial injury

Airway obstruction by blood, mucus, vomitus, foreign body (false teeth) or impacted tongue impairs respiratory exchange

Chest injury (fractured ribs, flail chest, sucking wounds, pneumothorax, hemothorax) impairs breathing

Delayed complications (pulmonary embolus, fat embolus, disseminated intravascular coagulation) or **Metabolic factors** may further alter respiration (ketoacidosis, uremia, salicylism, hepatic encephalopathy, poisoning)

Pneumotaxic center

Apneustic center

Medullary center

Phrenic nerve

Intercostal nerves

Hypoxia and acidosis of neurons

$O_2 \downarrow CO_2 \uparrow$

$NaHCO_3 \rightleftharpoons HHCO_3$

Hypoxia and acidosis result in rapidly deteriorating neuronal function

Increased intracranial pressure

Hypercarbia increases cerebral blood volume, leading to additional increase in intracranial pressure, which further embarrasses respiration: a vicious cycle of deterioration

Head Injuries
(Continued)

high pontine lesions may result in central *neurogenic hyperventilation*, which may also be caused by hypoxia and acidosis. *Apneustic respiration*, characterized by prolonged inspiration, is related to lesions of the apneustic respiratory center; it develops in patients with pontine infarcts, hypoglycemia or anoxia. An *ataxic respiratory pattern* may result from mass lesions affecting the medullary respiratory center.

Monitoring of arterial blood gases is essential to the diagnosis and treatment of respiratory abnormalities in comatose patients. Hypoxemia develops in many such patients, and changes in arterial blood gas concentrations often precede radiographic changes by 12 hours or more. Monitoring arterial blood gases can also be extremely valuable in determining the cause of coma. *Metabolic acidosis* may signal uremia, diabetic ketoacidosis, lactic acidosis or poisoning. *Metabolic alkalosis* may point to ingestion of alkali, prolonged emesis or hypokalemia. *Respiratory acidosis* may be secondary to severe depression of the CNS (as with trauma or drugs) or pulmonary failure. *Respiratory alkalosis* complicates salicylism, hepatic encephalopathy and sepsis. *Acute pulmonary edema* sometimes occurs with head injuries, probably because hypothalamic damage causes massive sympathetic discharge, with consequent vasoconstriction and shunting of large quantities of blood into vascular areas of relatively low resistance, including the lungs.

Many other factors cause respiratory difficulty in patients who have sustained multiple trauma (Plate 12). Vigorous medical and pulmonary care may alleviate all such abnormalities, improving the outcome in patients with injuries of the CNS.

Salt and Water Metabolism in Head Injuries

The brain, via the hypothalamus and neurohypophysis, is crucial in regulating the body's salt and water metabolism. Any derangement of this delicate system can produce severe hypertonicity or hypotonicity of the blood, which in turn can exacerbate the original neurologic insult (Plate 13).

Normal sodium metabolism depends on three factors. First, man and other mammals prefer salty foods in quantities that greatly exceed their homeostatic needs. Second, aldosterone, a mineralocorticoid secreted by the adrenal cortex—primarily in response to the renin-angiotensin system but also in response to adrenocorticotropic hormone (ACTH)—conserves sodium by enhancing its renal absorption. Finally, some have postulated the existence of a central natriuretic factor,

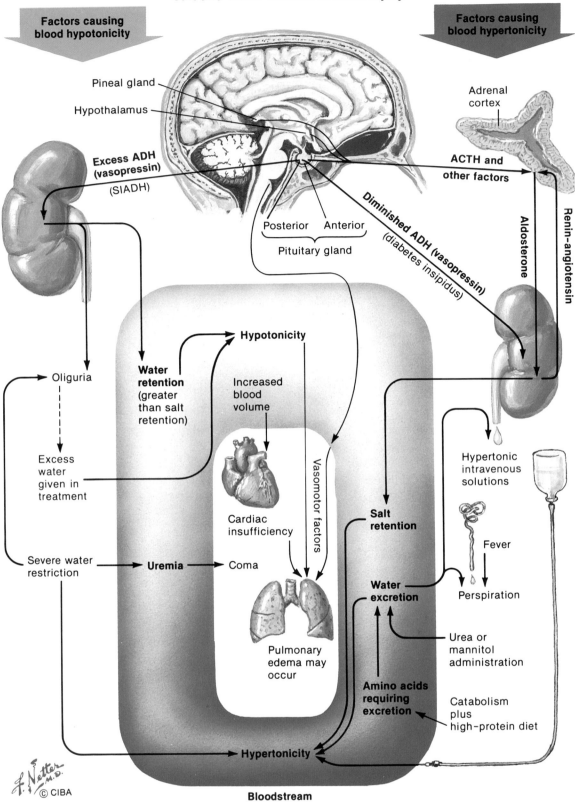

Salt and Water Balance in Head Injury

possibly antidiuretic hormone (ADH, vasopressin), oxytocin, melanocyte-stimulating hormone or neurophysine.

Many factors can affect sodium and water turnover in CNS disease. The administration of hypertonic solutions (eg, mannitol) or excessive fluid restriction to reduce cerebral edema may cause severe dehydration. Conversely, the intravenous administration of excessive quantities of hypotonic fluids may result in hyposmolality and increased cerebral edema. Fever, pulmonary problems and shock can greatly alter fluid requirements, and these conditions must be dealt with appropriately. The frequent *monitoring of serum electrolyte levels and urine output* is invaluable.

The most common derangements of salt and water metabolism in a CNS disorder (head trauma, encephalitis or tumor) are related to disturbances in the elaboration of ADH. In the absence of ADH, the patient will excrete large quantities (8 to 10 L/day) of dilute urine (specific gravity, <1.005), a condition known as diabetes insipidus. If conscious, the patient experiences extreme thirst and drinks sufficient fluid to replace the urinary losses. However, if consciousness is altered or the thirst mechanism is impaired, or both, as is often the case in head injuries, the patient will become severely dehydrated. Mild cases can be treated with drugs that enhance the action of circulating ADH; these

Head Injuries
(Continued)

include chlorpropamide, carbamazepine and clofibrate.

Treatment of severe acute dehydration is appropriate *fluid replacement*. If this is inadequate or if the condition continues beyond 24 to 48 hours, *hormone replacement* therapy can be started with aqueous vasopressin or vasopressin tannate in oil, the latter having a longer effect. Chronic severe diabetes insipidus is now best treated by the nasal insufflation of a synthetic analogue of vasopressin, desmopressin acetate (DDAVP).

Excessive secretion of ADH is a sequela of head trauma, brain tumors, infections of the CNS and hydrocephalus, among many other conditions. It has been estimated that this condition, called the *syndrome of inappropriate ADH secretion* (SIADH or the Schwartz-Bartter syndrome), occurs sometime during the hospital course of 30% of neurosurgical patients. If severe, it can lead to water intoxication, as indicated by nausea, weakness, lethargy, confusion, coma and seizures. Laboratory criteria for the diagnosis of SIADH include a serum sodium concentration lower than 135 mEq/L, a urinary sodium concentration exceeding 25 mEq/L, serum hyposmolality, and inappropriately concentrated urine. These criteria exclude other causes of serum hyponatremia, which include dehydration, congestive heart failure, cirrhosis, adrenal or renal disease and administration of diuretics.

In asymptomatic patients, fluid restriction (600 to 800 ml/day) decreases glomerular filtration and increases sodium absorption in the kidney. If the patient is symptomatic, careful intravenous administration of *hypertonic saline solution* rapidly corrects the serum sodium level. Alternatively, *furosemide* can be administered, with replacement of subsequent urinary electrolyte losses. Chronic SIADH can be successfully treated with *demeclocycline*, a tetracycline drug that acts on the distal renal tubule, creating a "nephrogenic" form of diabetes insipidus.

Traumatic Cerebrovascular Lesions

Although CT provides a rapid and precise approach to the diagnosis of traumatic intracranial hemorrhage, in a few patients, either the neurologic deficit is out of proportion to the lesions detected on a CT scan, or symptoms and signs obviously referable to cerebrovascular disease develop later. A high degree of suspicion about such patients and the use of improved angiographic techniques have led to the identification of an increasing number of traumatic cerebrovascular lesions, the most common of which are dissecting aneurysms of the cervical segment of

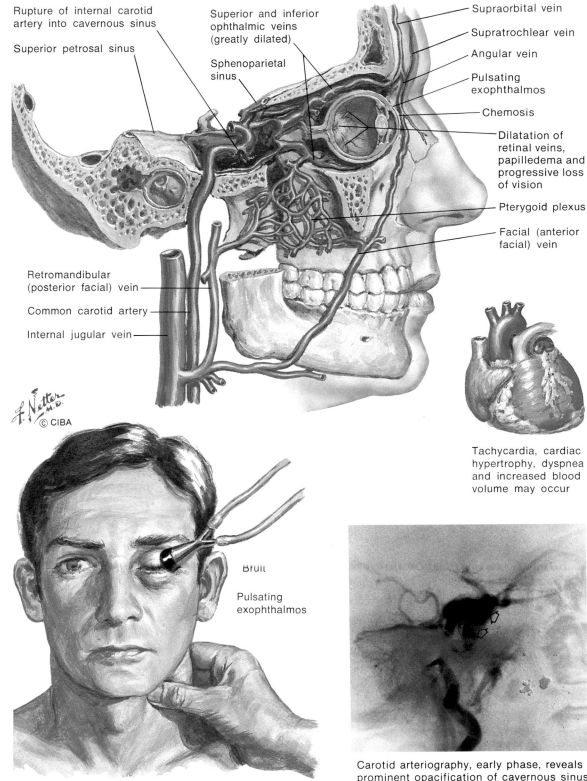

Bruit obliterated by carotid compression

Tachycardia, cardiac hypertrophy, dyspnea and increased blood volume may occur

Carotid arteriography, early phase, reveals prominent opacification of cavernous sinus (arrows) via carotid-cavernous fistula

the internal carotid artery, aneurysms of the cavernous segment of the internal carotid, and carotid-cavernous fistulas.

Aneurysms. Although degenerative medial disease has been implicated in the pathogenesis of dissecting aneurysms, which occur most commonly in the aorta, the precise cause of this degeneration remains unknown. In any case, the primary event is an intramedial hemorrhage. Enlargement of the hemorrhage reduces the caliber of the lumen of the artery. Rupture of the hemorrhage through the intima into the true lumen may create a false lumen, and dissection of the hemorrhage into the plane between the media and the adventitia may create a pseudoaneurysm.

Dissecting aneurysms of the cervical carotid artery occur most commonly following percutaneous angiography and trauma; other associated conditions include Marfan's syndrome, fibromuscular dysplasia and pediatric stroke. An increasing number of "spontaneous" dissections also have been identified, probably resulting from occult trauma or from erosion of an isolated atheromatous plaque.

A sufficiently large aneurysm may present as a pulsatile mass, causing compressive symptoms such as dysphagia. The neurologic signs and symptoms of cervical carotid dissections reflect three factors. First, the disruption of sympathetic fibers in the carotid artery wall may produce

Balloon Embolization of Carotid-Cavernous Fistula

Head Injuries
(*Continued*)

ipsilateral *Horner's syndrome* and hemicranial *headache*. Second, the intimal disruption at the site of the dissection provides a potent stimulus for platelet aggregation, which may lead to embolic *transient ischemic attacks* (TIAs) or *stroke*. Third, the decrease in the caliber of the true lumen reduces cerebral blood flow; depending on the collateral blood supply available, the result may be a TIA, stroke or no symptoms at all.

Because of the paucity of such cases in the literature, the natural history of dissections has remained obscure. As a result, many different therapeutic procedures have been tried. A patient who has an acute neurologic deficit secondary to reduction in blood flow may be a candidate for emergency revascularization. It has become increasingly apparent, however, that these lesions often behave in a benign manner. Many of them resolve spontaneously and cannot be seen on repeat angiograms.

Head trauma may also damage the *intrapetrous, intracavernous* or *supraclinoid segment of the carotid artery*. A traumatic aneurysm forms most commonly in the cavernous segment. Typically, the patient has sustained a severe closed head injury, usually associated with an anterior basilar skull fracture; unilateral blindness and anosmia are often present. The aneurysm, although not initially symptomatic, enlarges until it ruptures into the sphenoid sinus, causing massive epistaxis. Because further hemorrhage may be fatal, angiography and early surgical treatment should be undertaken. Likewise, a traumatic aneurysm of the meningeal vessels can rupture, with catastrophic consequences, and should be treated as soon as the lesion is suspected.

The least common traumatic cerebrovascular lesions are *traumatic aneurysms and arteriovenous malformations of scalp vessels*. These present as pulsatile scalp masses that produce easily heard bruits. They can be visualized by external carotid angiography and are amenable to surgical excision.

Carotid-Cavernous Fistulas. First described by William Hunter in 1757, carotid-cavernous fistulas (Plate 14) are more common than symptomatic intracavernous aneurysms, but considerably less common than subarachnoid saccular aneurysms. Traumatic carotid-cavernous fistulas are 3 times more common than the spontaneous type, occur most often in men, are most common in the third and fourth decades of life, and frequently follow severe head trauma. These are high-pressure, high-flow lesions, and their effects are secondary to the resultant increased pressure on neighboring neural and venous structures.

The most common symptom of a carotid-cavernous fistula is an *orbital bruit*, which is often particularly bothersome. *Exophthalmos and ocular pulsations* may result from venous engorgement. *Chemosis* is a consequence of conjunctival engorgement and exposure ophthalmitis. *Extraocular muscle palsies* may occur secondary to pressure on the third, fourth and sixth cranial nerves within the cavernous sinuses. *Visual failure* may follow initial trauma to the optic nerve, corneal ulceration,

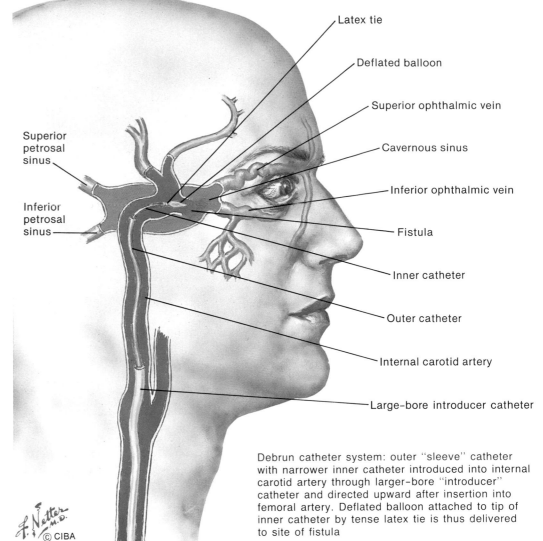

Latex tie

Deflated balloon

Superior ophthalmic vein

Cavernous sinus

Inferior ophthalmic vein

Fistula

Inner catheter

Outer catheter

Internal carotid artery

Large-bore introducer catheter

Superior petrosal sinus

Inferior petrosal sinus

Debrun catheter system: outer "sleeve" catheter with narrower inner catheter introduced into internal carotid artery through larger-bore "introducer" catheter and directed upward after insertion into femoral artery. Deflated balloon attached to tip of inner catheter by tense latex tie is thus delivered to site of fistula

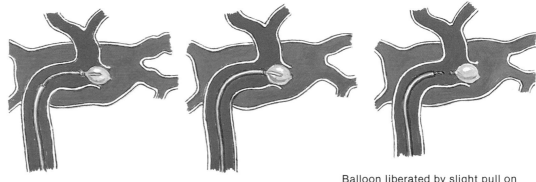

Balloon inflated with radiopaque fluid occluding fistula

Outer catheter advanced over inner catheter to engage balloon cuff

Balloon liberated by slight pull on inner catheter. Balloon neck spontaneously constricted by tense latex tie. All catheters then withdrawn

increased intraocular pressure, or hypoxemia from decreased ophthalmic arterial flow. Rarely, these features affect the eye contralateral to the fistula, because of transmission of pressure across the midline through the intercavernous sinuses. Occasionally, hemispheric symptoms result from reduced cerebral blood flow.

The definitive diagnosis requires angiography. Because of the high-flow nature of the lesion, injection of the vertebral artery with simultaneous compression of the ipsilateral carotid artery may be necessary to delineate the exact site of the fistula. Complete cerebral angiography should be done to rule out any anomalous vasculature and to assess the state of the collateral circulation in

case subsequent carotid artery ligation becomes necessary.

Catastrophic complications of carotid-cavernous fistulas are rare. Intracranial hemorrhage occurs in less than 3% of patients. Surgery is indicated only for an intolerable bruit, progressive visual loss or frank hemorrhage, since occlusive procedures can cause acute or long-term ischemic complications. In addition, ablative treatment occasionally increases ocular hypoxia, leading to further deterioration in visual function. The ideal therapy, therefore, obliterates the fistula while maintaining patency of the carotid artery.

Traditional surgical approaches, involving sacrifice of the ipsilateral carotid artery, include

Head Injuries
(Continued)

ligation of the cervical part of the artery, "trapping" of the artery (cervical and intracranial ligation), embolization of the fistula with ligation of the cervical part of the artery, and embolization with trapping. More recently, Prolo has introduced a balloon catheter technique in which the catheter is inserted into the exposed cervical carotid artery and directed to the site of the fistula. The balloon is then inflated and the carotid artery ligated with the catheter in situ. Thus trapping is done without intracranial surgery.

Newer operative procedures permit preservation of the carotid artery. Parkinson has had some success in approaching the fistula directly while the patient is in induced cardiac arrest. Mullan has used a number of approaches to thrombose portions of the cavernous sinus. Most recently, Debrun and others have devised catheters with detachable balloons. In this technique, the balloon is introduced into the circulation percutaneously, floated into the fistula, inflated and detached (Plate 15). Often the fistula can be obliterated without sacrificing the carotid artery. Initial reports of results of this technique have been promising.

Prognosis in Head Injuries

The Glasgow Outcome Scale is commonly used to rate the results of treatment after severe head trauma. The outcome categories include death, a persistent vegetative state, severe disability (dependent on others for activities of daily living), moderate disability (independent in activities of daily living), and good recovery (able to resume previous employment). In Becker's series, which is representative of aggressive surgical and medical management, the results were as follows: mortality, 32%; severe disability/vegetative state, 11%; and moderate disability/good recovery, 57%. All these patients were comatose on admission.

A variety of pretrauma factors affect the prognosis of severe head injury (Plate 16). *Age* is the most important factor, as mortality after head injury increases with advancing age. The higher incidence of medical complications in severely injured older patients accounts for most of this; in addition, intracranial mass lesions develop more frequently in the older patients. The presence of *previous or coexistent brain disease* or injury also worsens the prognosis (eg, the "punch-drunk" syndrome in boxers, in whom repeated "minor" head injuries produce a cumulatively poor outcome).

Various aspects of coma are strongly correlated with outcome. The Glasgow Coma Scale rating correlates with the prognosis. Death or a vegetative state is the outcome in 80% of patients with a score of 3 to 4, in 54% with a score of 5 to 7, in 27% with a score of 8 to 10, and in 6% with a score of 11 to 15. In addition, signs of *brainstem dysfunction* are poor prognostic factors. If the pupillary responses to light are bilaterally absent, mortality is 65% in patients with mass lesions and 82% in those with diffuse brain injuries. If oculovestibular responses are absent, mortality

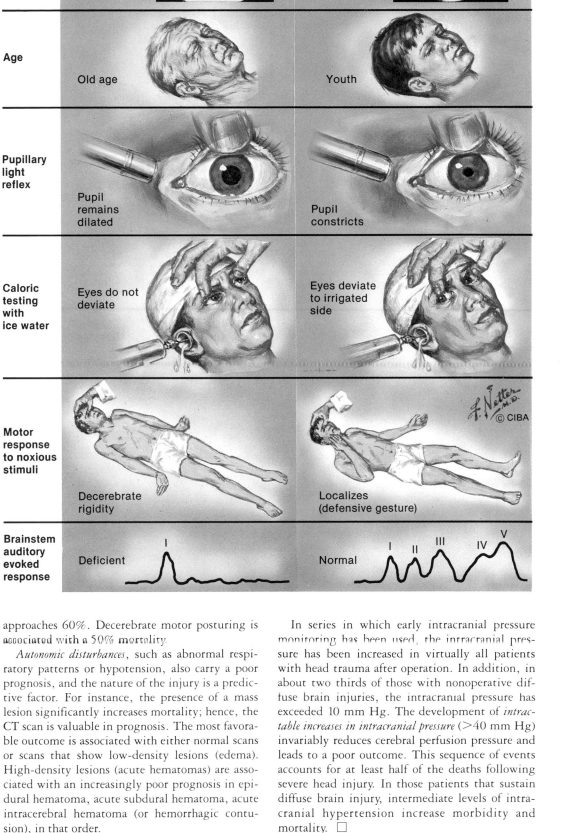

Prognosis in Severe Head Injuries

	Poorer	**Better**
Glasgow Coma Scale	<7	>7
CT scan	Subdural hematoma	Normal
Age	Old age	Youth
Pupillary light reflex	Pupil remains dilated	Pupil constricts
Caloric testing with ice water	Eyes do not deviate	Eyes deviate to irrigated side
Motor response to noxious stimuli	Decerebrate rigidity	Localizes (defensive gesture)
Brainstem auditory evoked response	Deficient	Normal

approaches 60%. Decerebrate motor posturing is associated with a 50% mortality.

Autonomic disturbances, such as abnormal respiratory patterns or hypotension, also carry a poor prognosis, and the nature of the injury is a predictive factor. For instance, the presence of a mass lesion significantly increases mortality; hence, the CT scan is valuable in prognosis. The most favorable outcome is associated with either normal scans or scans that show low-density lesions (edema). High-density lesions (acute hematomas) are associated with an increasingly poor prognosis in epidural hematoma, acute subdural hematoma, acute intracerebral hematoma (or hemorrhagic contusion), in that order.

In series in which early intracranial pressure monitoring has been used, the intracranial pressure has been increased in virtually all patients with head trauma after operation. In addition, in about two thirds of those with nonoperative diffuse brain injuries, the intracranial pressure has exceeded 10 mm Hg. The development of *intractable increases in intracranial pressure* (>40 mm Hg) invariably reduces cerebral perfusion pressure and leads to a poor outcome. This sequence of events accounts for at least half of the deaths following severe head injury. In those patients that sustain diffuse brain injury, intermediate levels of intracranial hypertension increase morbidity and mortality. □

Cervical Spine Injury: Incomplete Spinal Cord Syndromes

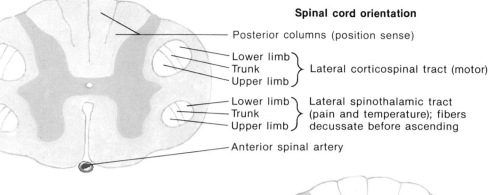

Spinal cord orientation

Posterior columns (position sense)

Lower limb ⎫
Trunk   ⎬ Lateral corticospinal tract (motor)
Upper limb ⎭

Lower limb ⎫ Lateral spinothalamic tract
Trunk   ⎬ (pain and temperature); fibers
Upper limb ⎭ decussate before ascending

Anterior spinal artery

Cervical Spine Injury

Spinal cord injuries are a major health problem in the United States and other developed countries. In 1974, the National Head and Spinal Cord Injury Survey recorded approximately 10,000 spinal cord injuries in the United States. The incidence in other industrialized nations ranges between 13 and 50 persons per million. In most series, the majority of victims are male.

The cost of treating these injuries in the United States is approximately $380 million annually, with an expense of $70,000 per patient for the first year of therapy. In addition, the victim of spinal cord injury pays an enormous price in terms of suffering, emotional trauma and loss of years of productivity.

History

Spinal cord injury and its treatment have been mentioned throughout recorded medical history. The Edwin Smith papyrus describes spinal injury as "a disease not to be treated," and Guy de Chauliac and other medieval physicians also regarded this problem as incurable. Galen was among the first to demonstrate that disruption of the spinal cord did, in fact, produce paralysis, and paraplegia is even briefly discussed in the Talmud.

Paré and his contemporaries advocated closed reduction via traction, and reported variable results. Cline performed the first laminectomy for spinal trauma in 1814, and in 1933, Crutchfield invented a practical device for skeletal traction. The historical controversy regarding conservative versus surgical treatment continues to this day, although the need for a comprehensive and multidisciplinary approach to management, as pioneered by Munro, Guttmann and Bors, is receiving increasing recognition.

Research regarding the pathophysiology of spinal cord injury and its possible treatment began in 1911, when Allen developed the falling weight model most commonly used today. In addition, he postulated that the spinal cord suffered not only direct but delayed injury. Unfortunately, his ideas lay fallow for many years.

Osterholm et al ignited interest in this field with their biogenic amine theory. They reported increased norepinephrine levels at the site of experimental injury and purported to reproduce the histologic findings in the lesion by injecting norepinephrine into the normal spinal cord. Although subsequent investigators failed to confirm these observations, other biogenic amines may indeed be crucial to the pathophysiology of this process.

Etiologic and Pathologic Mechanisms

Motor vehicle accidents account for up to 50% of spinal cord injuries. Other accidental causes

Central cord syndrome

Central cord hemorrhage and edema. Parts of 3 main tracts involved on both sides. Upper limbs more affected than lower limbs ▷

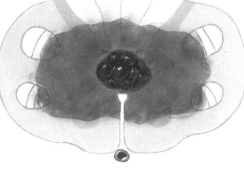

Anterior spinal artery syndrome

Artery damaged by bone or cartilage spicules (shaded area affected). Bilateral loss of motor function and pain sensation below ◁ injured segment; position sense preserved

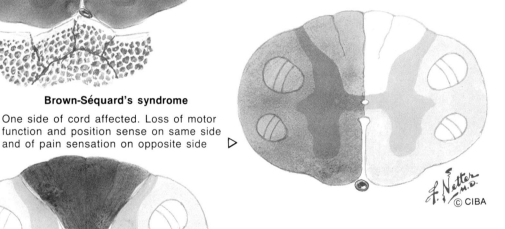

Brown-Séquard's syndrome

One side of cord affected. Loss of motor function and position sense on same side and of pain sensation on opposite side ▷

Posterior column syndrome (uncommon)

Position sense lost below lesion; motor ◁ function and pain sensation preserved

include diving, missile or knife wounds, athletic injuries, birth injury, the "clay-shoveler's" fracture, electrical trauma, seat belt injury and the "bends."

Conditions predisposing to spinal cord symptoms include spinal stenosis, rheumatoid arthritis, ankylosing spondylitis, achondroplasia, Paget's disease, arachnoiditis and spondylosis.

The exact mechanism remains unknown; however, considerable evidence implicates a vascular pathologic process in the mediation of spinal injury. A wide variety of techniques, including microangiography, xenon clearance blood flow studies, hydrogen ion clearance and autoradiography, have consistently demonstrated dramatic

decreases in spinal cord blood flow after trauma, even at sites distant from the direct injury. In addition, studies of spinal cord metabolism confirm the presence of a severe metabolic injury after spinal cord trauma.

Thus, pathologic, blood flow and metabolic studies indicate that spinal cord injury involves not only direct neuronal trauma but also both direct and delayed injury to the vasculature. The basis of theoretical treatment methods for spinal cord injury involves the prevention of the delayed component of injury.

Spinal cord injury can result in a number of neurologic deficits. The most frequent levels of injury involve the lower cervical vertebrae and the

Cervical Spine Injury: Flexion and Flexion-Rotation

Mechanism

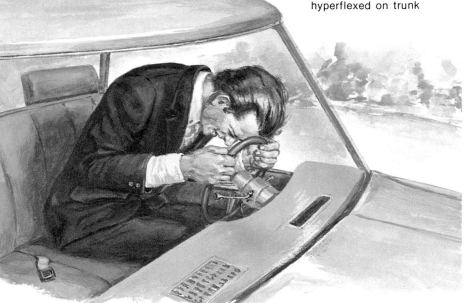

Head-on collision with stationary or moving object. Occupant not restrained by seat belt: head strikes steering wheel, windshield or roof. Head hyperflexed on trunk

Cervical Spine Injury
(Continued)

thoracolumbar junction, reflecting the vulnerability of the most mobile segments of the spine to injury. The neurologic deficits sustained have been reported as follows: 43% complete functional interruption, 18% partial functional interruption, 12% nerve root deficit, 3% Brown-Séquard's syndrome, 3% central cord damage, and 21% other deficits.

Incomplete Spinal Cord Syndromes

Because of the unique anatomy and vascular supply of the spinal cord, a variety of incomplete syndromes are encountered in cervical spinal cord injuries. In these syndromes, certain sensory and motor functions are impaired or eliminated while others are spared.

The *central cord syndrome* is most commonly seen after a cervical hyperextension injury (Plates 17, 19). For a variety of reasons, including the mechanical properties and vascular supply of the cord, the central portion can be contused even though the lateral components receive little injury.

Characteristically, the patient complains of severe burning dysesthesia in the arms, which is thought to result from damage to spinothalamic fibers, perhaps as they cross in the anterior commissure. Physical examination reveals arm weakness, with preservation of lower extremity strength. In addition, pain and temperature sensation is lost in a capelike distribution. Any lesion causing primary injury to the central spinal cord can produce this constellation of deficits. Such lesions include syringomyelia, intrinsic spinal cord tumors and hydromyelia. In addition, the syndrome can, rarely, affect the lower spinal cord (conus medullaris). (See also Section X.)

The *anterior spinal artery* supplies the gray matter as well as the white matter in the ventrolateral and posterolateral portions of the spinal cord. Damage to the anterior spinal artery produces the distinct clinical syndrome of bilateral paralysis and loss of pain and temperature sensation below the level of injury, but position sense and vibration sense (posterior column function) are spared. Lesions affecting the anterior spinal artery include vertebral trauma, anteriorly located neoplasms (usually metastases) and aortic injuries.

The *Brown-Séquard syndrome*, in its pure form, represents the consequence of spinal cord hemisection. Neurologic deficits include ipsilateral loss of motor function, as well as of vibration sense and position sense. In addition, contralateral pain and temperature sensation is lost. Stab and missile wounds can produce a "complete" Brown-Séquard syndrome, but the incomplete manifestations of the syndrome are seen with a variety of other lesions, including trauma and neoplasms.

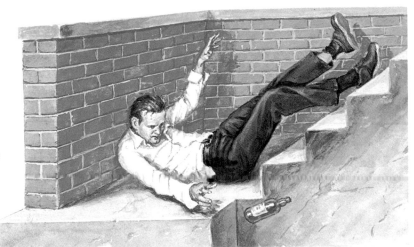

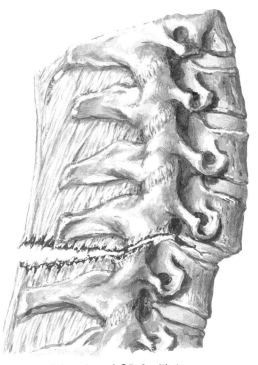

Blow to back of head from falling against hard surface when balance is compromised

Anterior dislocation of C5-6 with tear of interspinal ligament, facet capsules and posterior fibers of intervertebral disc

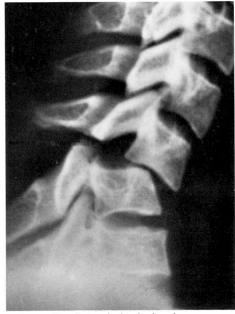

X-ray film (lateral view) showing bilateral interfacet dislocation at C5-6

Cervical Spine Injury: Hyperextension

Individual (usually elderly) falls forward, striking chin or face, causing forceful hyperextension and backward thrust of neck

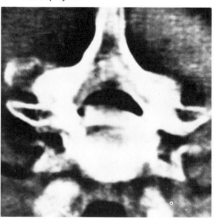

Cervical Spine Injury
(Continued)

The *posterior column syndrome* occurs when the posterior columns are selectively damaged, producing bilateral loss of vibration sense and proprioception below the lesion (Plate 17). These findings are most commonly encountered secondary to certain systemic diseases (eg, neurosyphilis), but have been infrequently described after spinal cord trauma alone.

Classification of Injuries

Most spinal cord injuries are a consequence of spinal fractures or dislocations, or both. Of the variety of classifications proposed for these injuries, the most useful is divided according to the mechanisms that produce the fracture, including flexion, flexion-rotation, hyperextension, extension-rotation and vertical compression.

Flexion Injuries. Anterior subluxation, bilateral interfacet dislocation, wedge fracture, "teardrop" fractures and clay-shoveler's fractures are classified as flexion injuries. These injuries usually result from blows to the back of the head or the forceful deceleration experienced in motor vehicle accidents (Plate 18).

Anterior subluxation results from the least amount of flexion force that causes a radiographically recognizable injury. The lesion disrupts the posterior longitudinal ligament, the interspinal ligament and the interfacet joint capsules. Because the anterior longitudinal ligament and the disc space are relatively intact, the injury is not acutely unstable. Patients with this injury often have severe neck pain and spasm at the time of injury. Recovery is usually uneventful, but if the lesion is not discovered on initial evaluation, progressive anterior subluxation of the involved vertebrae may develop. If subluxation develops despite adequate conservative therapy, stabilization of the spine, usually via posterior fusion, is recommended.

Bilateral *interfacet dislocation* results from complete disruption of the posterior ligamentous complex. The disc space and, usually, the anterior longitudinal ligament are also disrupted. The superior facets pass upward and over the inferior facets of the joint, which always causes anterior dislocation of the upper vertebral body by at least the distance of one half the anteroposterior (AP) diameter of the body. Because of the extensive ligamentous disruption, these injuries are unstable and are associated with a high incidence of cord damage.

Flexion trauma often results in *wedge fractures* of vertebral bodies, without ligamentous disruption. X-ray films reveal loss of vertebral height anteriorly and widening of the paraspinous soft-tissue shadow. Such injuries are stable, rarely associated with neurologic injury, and often treated conservatively with halo bracing.

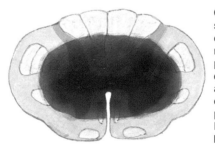

Section of cervical spinal cord showing orientation of fibers in lateral corticospinal tracts

Osteophytes compressing spinal cord. Hyperextension injury results in cord contusion, self-destructive edema and intramedullary hemorrhage with rapidly developing quadriplegia

Lower limb
Trunk
Upper limb

Central cord syndrome: central hemorrhage may damage medial part of lateral corticospinal tract and anterior horn cells resulting in paralysis of upper limbs, leaving lower limbs intact

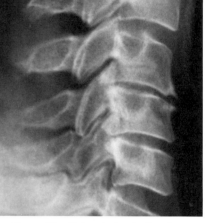

X-ray film (lateral view) showing osteophytes

CT scan showing fragments of disc in spinal canal causing cord compression

Another relatively minor injury resulting from flexion trauma is the *clay-shoveler's fracture*. This injury involves the spinous processes of C6, C7 or T1, and results from flexion of the head and neck against tensed posterior cervical muscles.

The most severe of the flexion injuries is the so-called *teardrop fracture*. The involved vertebral body is fractured, with the anteroinferior corner constituting the teardrop. The anterior and posterior longitudinal ligaments, as well as the disc space and posterior ligamentous complex, are totally disrupted. In addition, the interfacet joints are bilaterally subluxed. The injury is totally unstable and is associated with severe neurologic dysfunction. Treatment consists of stabilization with a halo brace, and fusion and decompression, if appropriate.

Flexion-Rotation Injuries. Injuries causing flexion combined with rotation produce unilateral interfacet dislocation. In these injuries, the posterior ligamentous complex is disrupted. On one side, the superior facet is dislocated anterior to the tip of the inferior facet of the joint. The subluxated facet lies within the intervertebral foramen and may be fractured. Subluxation of the involved vertebral body is never greater than one half of its AP diameter. Although cervical nerve root deficits are commonly seen, they are stable and rarely associated with spinal cord injury. Closed reduction and posterior fusion are often utilized.

Cervical Spine Injury
(Continued)

Hyperextension Injuries. Cervical spine injuries with normal radiographic appearance, fracture-dislocations, posterior atlantal arch fractures, extension teardrop fractures and the "hangman's" fracture are all examples of hyperextension injuries.

Forceful hyperextension of the cervical spine usually results from a forward fall with a blow to the anterior part of the head (Plate 19). If the spinal canal was previously narrowed as a result of chronic degenerative arthritis (cervical spondylosis), the hyperextension may be sufficient to compress the spinal cord, even in the absence of actual fracture or dislocation. This type of injury frequently causes selective injury to the central gray matter of the spinal cord.

Initial treatment of this injury includes immobilization of the spine, with absolute avoidance of further hyperextension. If subsequent investigation reveals spinal cord compression, surgical treatment via either the anterior or posterior route may be indicated.

Hyperextension combined with compressive forces may cause a *fracture-dislocation*. This injury frequently fractures the lateral vertebral masses, pedicles and laminae. In addition, the posterior ligamentous complex and disc space are disrupted, so that this injury is unstable. Even though the mechanism of injury involves hyperextension, characteristically the vertebra is subluxed anteriorly. The degree of spinal cord injury varies.

Severe hyperextension may fracture the *posterior arch* of the atlas (C1) between the occiput and the arch of the axis (C2). This injury is stable and does not cause neurologic injury. Similarly, hyperextension may lead to avulsion of the anteroinferior corner of C2, resulting in an extension teardrop fracture. This injury is stable in flexion but unstable in extension because of disruption of the anterior longitudinal ligament.

Violent hyperextension may result in bilateral fracture of the pedicles of C2, with anterior dislocation of C2 on C3. As the injury is often produced by hanging, it is known as the *hangman's fracture*. The degree of subluxation, as well as the presence of pedicular fractures, may be subtle or striking. Widening of the prevertebral shadow is frequently seen on an x-ray film. The injury is unstable, but the degree of neurologic compromise is highly variable, probably because even though significant vertebral dislocation may be present, the bilateral pedicular fractures perform an "autolaminectomy," decompressing the spinal cord at the point of injury. The hangman's fracture can often be successfully treated by immobilizing the patient in a halo body jacket.

Extension-Rotation Injuries. The combination of extension and rotational forces may

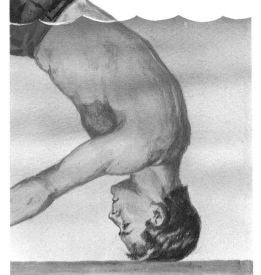
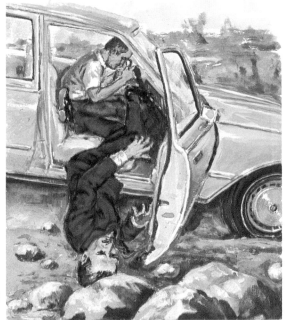

Mechanism. Vertical blow on head as in diving or surfing accident, being thrown from car, or football injury

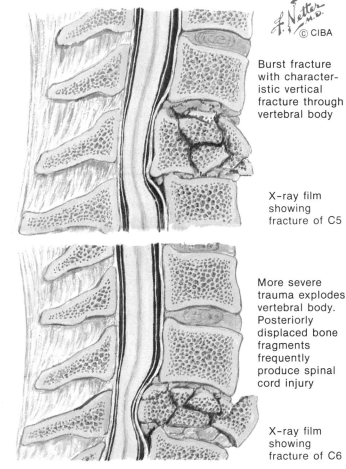

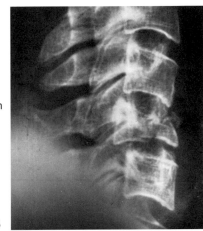

Burst fracture with characteristic vertical fracture through vertebral body

X-ray film showing fracture of C5

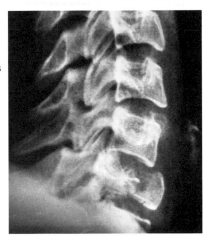

More severe trauma explodes vertebral body. Posteriorly displaced bone fragments frequently produce spinal cord injury

X-ray film showing fracture of C6

produce a fracture of the lateral masses known as the *pillar fracture*. This is a stable injury, amenable to conservative treatment with halo bracing.

Compression Injuries. The *Jefferson fracture* of C1 and the *burst fracture of the lower cervical vertebrae* are compression fractures. Such injuries are uncommon because vertical compression must be applied at a time when the spine is perfectly straight. They usually result from vertical blows to the head during motor vehicle accidents, diving or sports injuries (Plate 20). Falling objects also can cause compression trauma.

The *burst fracture of C1* was first described by Jefferson in 1920. The compressive force causes bilateral fractures of the anterior and posterior arches of C1 and disruption of the transverse atlantal ligament, with resultant subluxation of C1 on C2. Special "odontoid" radiographic views are necessary to exclude this fracture, which is unstable and variably associated with neurologic injury. External immobilization with halo bracing is often therapeutically successful.

The *burst fracture of the lower cervical vertebrae* results from explosion of compressed disc material into the vertebral body. The resultant comminution of the vertebral body may impinge on the ventral aspect of the spinal cord, leading to neurologic deficit. Because the posterior ligamentous complex remains intact, the injury is usually stable.

Cervical Spine Injury: Management at Accident Site

Cervical Spine Injury
(Continued)

Treatment

Emergency Treatment. The emergency treatment of cervical spine injuries is predicated on the fact that currently there is no cure for spinal cord damage. The extent of recovery from spinal cord injury depends on the extent of the initial trauma, the prevention of further trauma during rescue, the prevention of complications that would extend the injury (such as hypoxia or hypotension), and the thoroughness of rehabilitation.

At the scene of injury, immobilization of the spine is of paramount importance, particularly in dealing with an unconscious patient, who may well have a spinal injury. After a cervical collar has been applied, the victim should be carefully placed on a spine board by a three- or four-man lift (Plate 21). During this movement, great care is taken to avoid manipulation of any portion of the spine. After being placed on the board, the victim is further immobilized by the placement of sandbags or use of halter traction. These precepts should be violated only for life-threatening reasons.

Evaluation and Early Management. After transportation to a hospital facility, the patient undergoes a detailed evaluation, including careful neurologic and spinal examinations. X-ray films of the cervical spine should be taken as early as possible. Occasionally, forceful downward traction on the arms may be required to depress the shoulders for adequate visualization to T1. If necessary, x-ray films of the thoracic and lumbar spine are obtained. If intubation is required before the radiographic examination, great care should be taken to avoid undue manipulation of the spine. If a neurologically normal patient, with apparently normal x-ray films of the spine, complains of spinal pain, a spinal injury should be suspected and the patient treated accordingly. Appropriate treatment includes continued immobilization with a cervical collar and bed rest and more detailed radiography, such as flexion-extension views or computed tomography (CT).

If trauma to the cervical spine and spinal cord trauma are excluded, residual pain may be safely attributed to a cervical *soft-tissue injury*, known as a cervical strain. Because this injury is often caused by violent hyperextension followed by flexion, the popular term "whiplash" is used to describe it. This injury may produce stretching or tearing of the scalene muscles, esophagus, larynx, temporomandibular joints, disc space or sympathetic fibers. Symptoms may include cervical pain and stiffness, dysphonia, dysphagia and vertigo. If a cervical disc fragment is extruded, upper extremity radiculopathy may result. The vast majority of patients with such injuries can be successfully treated at home with rest, mild analgesia, use of a soft cervical collar, and cervical

Three-man lift: useful if limited help available for placing patient on board or carrying patient short distances. Head, trunk and legs must be aligned in straight line, and head must be supported from underneath and laterally

Prolo cervical stabilization traction board applied in sitting position before patient is removed from car

Patient's head held securely between attendant's elbows; shoulders supported by attendant's hands during lift. Cervical collar applied before lift

traction. The traction (usually 7 to 10 lb) can be applied for 20 minutes 3 or 4 times per day with the patient in either the supine or the sitting position. If symptoms and signs persist, further investigation, including myelography and electromyography, may be indicated.

When a cervical fracture-dislocation or spinal cord injury, or both, is identified, the spinal column should be promptly realigned. This is usually done with skeletal traction. A variety of devices have been developed since Crutchfield first described his skull tongs in 1933. Those currently available (including the Gardner-Wells and Heifetz tongs) can be quickly applied in the emergency room, with a minimum of discomfort

to the patient (Plate 22). Varying amounts of weight, up to 5 lb per level in the vertebral column counting downward (ie, 20 lb for a C4-5 dislocation) are applied until realignment is satisfactory. The weight is then reduced until a definitive course of therapy is determined.

Even after direct trauma to other body systems has been excluded, appropriate measures must be taken in anticipation of the *multisystem effects* of cervical spinal cord injury.

Such an injury disrupts sympathetic outflow to the body, which may result in pooling of blood and hypotension. This syndrome, known as *spinal shock*, must be distinguished from hypovolemic shock, because the administration of large

Cervical Spine Injury
(Continued)

amounts of fluid helps only the latter. Characteristically, spinal shock victims manifest bradycardia, as a result of sympathetic blockade, whereas those in hypovolemic shock have tachycardia. In addition, the central venous pressure in hypovolemia is very low, whereas it may be normal or only mildly depressed in spinal shock.

Spinal shock can be effectively treated by placing the patient in a Trendelenburg position. Fluid should be cautiously replaced only after placement of a central venous pressure monitor. The accompanying bradycardia can be reversed with the administration of atropine or low-dose adrenergic agents. If the pulse rate remains below 45, placement of a temporary transvenous pacemaker should be considered. Vagal stimulation, such as by vigorous nasotracheal suctioning, should be avoided at this stage, as it may precipitate cardiac arrest.

Pulmonary function is often compromised after cervical spinal injury because of loss of intercostal muscle function. In addition, an upper spinal cord lesion (C3-5) may damage the phrenic nerve output and further compromise respiration. A patient with this injury requires intensive pulmonary toilet and very careful observation. If the vital capacity drops below 1 L, mechanical ventilation may be required.

Following spinal cord injury, the *gastrointestinal system* is usually paralyzed for several days, or longer if an associated retroperitoneal hemorrhage is present. A nasogastric tube should be placed until the ileus resolves; this prevents emesis and possible aspiration, which would further compromise the already tenuous pulmonary reserve. The patient should be given intravenous hyperalimentation of at least 3,000 calories per day. The administration of high-dose steroids in the hope of reducing spinal cord edema is a generally accepted, although questionably effective, mode of therapy in spinal cord injuries. Even so, the incidence of gastrointestinal hemorrhage is very low. Subsequent therapy involves the development of a bowel regimen with stool softeners, laxatives and intermittent rectal stimulation.

The *genitourinary system* is also nonfunctional after spinal injury. An indwelling Foley catheter should be used initially in all patients, with great care to maintain sterile technique. This is helpful in monitoring fluid status as well as in preventing urinary retention. The patient must be watched closely for urinary tract infection and treated vigorously if one occurs. Subsequent management of the urinary system depends on the patient's functional ability and the degree of automatic bladder function that returns. If the patient is able to tolerate it, intermittent catheterization is

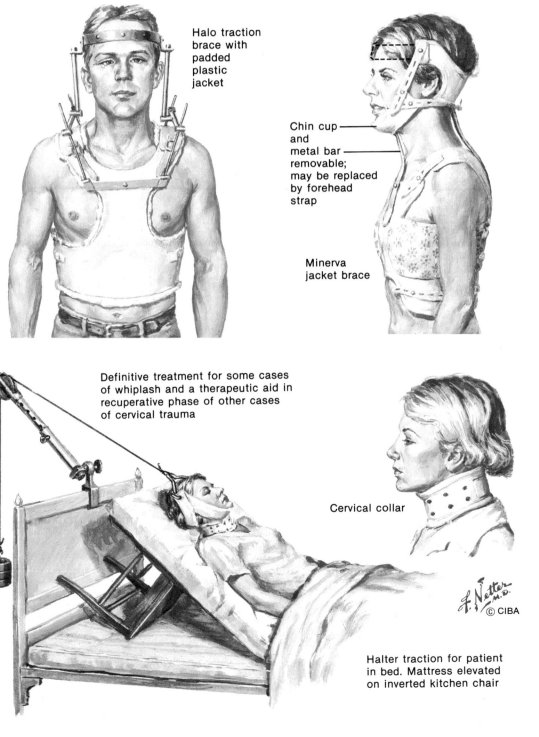

Cervical Spine Injury: Traction and Bracing

Gardner-Wells tongs applied in emergency room. Cervical traction pulley with adjustable arm clamped to examining table

Gardner-Wells tongs: preferred because they can be rapidly and easily applied through intact skin

Spring-loaded pin

Crutchfield tongs: require skin incision and drill holes in skull for application

Halo traction brace with padded plastic jacket

Chin cup and metal bar removable; may be replaced by forehead strap

Minerva jacket brace

Definitive treatment for some cases of whiplash and a therapeutic aid in recuperative phase of other cases of cervical trauma

Cervical collar

Halter traction for patient in bed. Mattress elevated on inverted kitchen chair

Cervical Spine Injury
(Continued)

preferred. If a permanent indwelling catheter is required, efforts should be made to ensure a high urine output, an unobstructed catheter and a clean perineum.

Great care should be taken to prevent *skin breakdown*, a frequent complication after the loss of protective sensation. The bony prominences (sacrum, iliac crests, trochanters, etc) should be padded. Most important, the bed must be clean and the patient must be turned every 2 hours. A variety of beds that can be mechanically turned have been developed to minimize this problem; however, there is no substitute for meticulous nursing care.

Conservative Versus Surgical Management. Almost all physicians are in agreement regarding the general methods for the early management of spinal cord injury. However, there is serious dissent concerning the merits of subsequent conservative versus surgical management of such lesions. Those who urge early operative intervention cite as its benefits the following factors: reduction of the distorted spine, decompression of the spinal canal, and internal stabilization of the fracture-dislocation with consequent earlier mobilization of the patient. Cloward, a prominent proponent of this approach, operates on all quadriplegics, stating: "There is nothing to lose and everything to gain."

Those who favor conservative therapy counter that closed reduction is almost always possible. If skeletal traction alone is not sufficient, the spine may be manipulated under general anesthesia. Closed reduction of a bilateral interfacet dislocation involves manual traction with the neck flexed, gradual extension of the neck until the facets reengage, and then further extension and decreased traction.

A unilateral locked facet is reduced by neck flexion and rotation to the side opposite the dislocation, followed by rotation and flexion of the head toward the side of dislocation and extension with relaxation of traction. The conservative school of thought further argues that decompression of the spinal canal rarely helps because the spinal cord injury cannot be reversed. Further, proponents of this view feel that many spinal injuries are inherently stable, rendering operative stabilization unnecessary.

In recent years, an increasing number of physicians have used external stabilization devices, including the halo and Minerva braces, to immobilize cervical spine injuries and thus allow early mobilization (Plate 22). The more common indications include odontoid fracture, Jefferson's fracture, hangman's fracture, wedge fracture and burst fracture. The greater the degree of bony

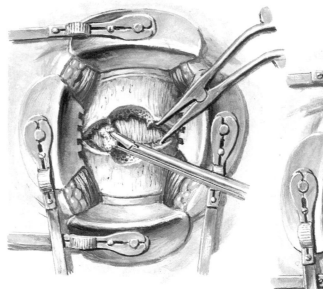

Spine exposed by progressive dissection and self-retaining retractors inserted. Disc, osteophytes and bone fragments removed under direct vision

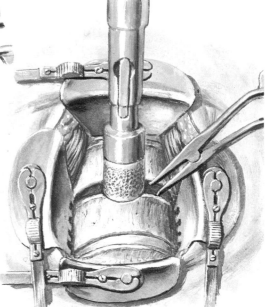

Dowel bone graft obtained from ilium or bone bank is cut 2 mm wider and 2 mm shorter than drill hole. It is impacted after hole is widened with vertebra spreader

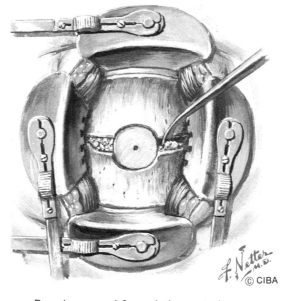

Dowel recessed 2 mm below anterior margin of drill hole. When spreader is removed, graft is locked securely in place. Cortical end plates lateral to dowel are perforated and interspace packed with bone dust removed from drill

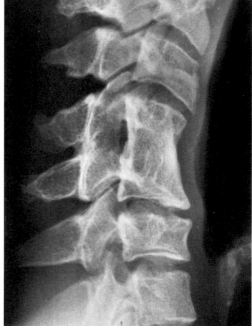

Follow-up x-ray film. Dowel graft fusion of C5–6 with good union

injury, the smaller is the degree of ligamentous injury, and the younger the patient, the greater is the chance of nonoperative fusion with this technique.

All physicians agree that surgery is indicated in the following situations: unsuccessful reduction, penetrating wounds, treatment of uncooperative patients and progressive neurologic deficit. Adequately controlled studies of operative versus conservative therapy for other indications have not been done.

Surgical Techniques. The surgical treatment of cervical spine injury involves a number of techniques. Foremost among these are the approaches to the vertebrae via the anterior and posterior

routes. The *anterior cervical discectomy and fusion* (Plate 23) was developed by Cloward and associates in the mid-1950s, and has subsequently proved to be a versatile and safe procedure. Ideally, it is applied in circumstances in which the posterior ligamentous complex is still intact and the lesion is anterior in the spinal canal, ie, disc or disrupted vertebral body. Otherwise, a simultaneous posterior stabilization procedure may also be necessary. It has been used in the treatment of almost every type of cervical spine injury.

The patient is placed in the supine position and given general anesthesia. A transverse skin incision is made at the level of the disc space concerned, and dissection is continued along the

Cervical Spine Injury: Posterior Fusion

Posterior fusion of C1 and C2 (Brooks)

Midline incision from lower occiput to spine of C4. Laminae of C1 and C2 exposed by gentle subperiosteal dissection. Twisted double strands of wire passed around laminae of C1 and C2 and fastened over prism-shaped corticocancellous bone grafts taken from iliac crest. Wedge-shaped graft fits between laminae without compressing dura or spinal cord

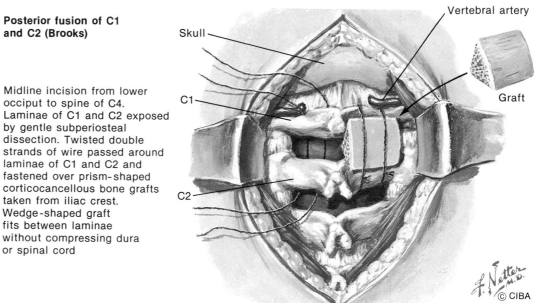

Cervical Spine Injury
(Continued)

anterior border of the sternocleidomastoid muscle. The fascial plane between the carotid sheath and the esophagus is bluntly dissected and the anterior surface of the cervical spine exposed. Self-retaining retractors are inserted after mobilization of the longus colli muscles. The appropriate disc space is entered and the injured disc material removed. A drill hole is placed in the space, a disc-space spreader is inserted, and further fragments of bone or disc are removed from the spinal canal. A specially cut bone dowel is obtained from the iliac crest or a bone bank, and placed in the previously made drill hole. The wound is then closed in layers, and a drain is left in place. The spine is immobilized with either a hard collar or halo bracing.

The other widely employed access route for operating on cervical spine injuries is the posterior approach (Plate 24). The two most commonly performed procedures are the posterior C1-2 fusion (Brooks) and the posterior interspinous fusion of the lower cervical spine (Rogers).

The *Brooks fusion* is by far the most popular technique used to treat odontoid fractures and ligamentous subluxations of C1 and C2. The patient undergoes nasotracheal intubation while awake, and is given local anesthesia while a three-pin head holder is applied. The patient is then turned to the prone position on the operating table and placed in a "military" posture. General anesthesia is administered only after it has been verified that the patient can move his extremities normally and after an intraoperative x-ray film has been obtained. Alternatively, the patient is initially placed under general anesthesia and spinal cord function is monitored by somatosensory evoked responses. A midline skin incision is made from the lower occiput to the level of C4. The incision is then extended deeply to the spinous processes, and gentle subperiosteal dissection is used to fully expose the laminae of C1 and C2. Twisted strands of 24-gauge wire are passed under the laminae. Appropriate bone grafts are taken from the posterior iliac crest and are wired in place (Plate 24). The wound is then closed in layers. The rate of fusion with this technique is exceedingly good.

The *Rogers posterior interspinous technique* is used for unstable injuries in the lower cervical spine, and is much more widely employed than the technique involving cervical laminectomy and fusion of the lateral masses (posterolateral facet fusion). Again, the patient is carefully positioned

Posterior interspinous fusion of lower cervical vertebrae (Rogers)

A. Holes drilled in spinous processes of vertebrae to be fused

B. Wires passed through holes in each pair of adjacent vertebrae and secured by twisting

C. Another wire passed, encompassing all spinous processes of vertebrae to be fused

D. Corticocancellous bone graft strips from iliac crest laid down over area of intended fusion

for surgery. A generous midline incision is made and extended to the spinous processes. The involved spinous processes and laminae are exposed by gentle subperiosteal dissection, and holes are drilled in the appropriate spinous processes. Wires are passed and tightened as shown in Plate 24. Corticocancellous bone graft material from the posterior iliac crest is laid down around the area of intended fusion. There is no need to denude the cortical surfaces to obtain a good fusion in the cervical spine. The posterior approach is particularly useful when disruption is more extensive in the posterior ligamentous structures than in the anterior structures (ie, unilateral locked facet).

Comment

Spinal cord injury not only affects the spine but also causes dysfunction of other body systems, which must constantly be considered during all phases of treatment. The physician who can care most effectively for a patient is the "generalist for the spinal cord-injured," who understands all the systems likely to be affected by the injury and who can consult with medical specialists and coordinate the activities of allied health professionals. Evaluation of the long-term effects of the medical or surgical programs allows comprehensive care and gives the patient the best possible chance for successful adjustment.

Cervical Spine Injury
(Continued)

Rehabilitation of Patient

Because of the multiple support systems available today, the person who sustains a spinal cord injury that results in paraplegia or quadriplegia can now have a more meaningful life than was possible a few decades ago. The many spinal cord injuries that occurred during World War II and subsequent wars, and the large number of persons with spinal cord injury caused by motor vehicle accidents have increased public awareness of these persons' needs.

Establishment of spinal cord injury centers has provided a team approach to the medical management of these patients that permits a relatively independent existence for a significant percentage. The vigorous lobby generated by these handicapped persons has resulted in the widespread availability of accessible public transportation, housing and restrooms, and of automobiles fitted with hand controls. Higher education for handicapped persons is now readily available at many universities; competitive athletic events have been developed for them; and above all, many have achieved a successful family life.

These accomplishments have been made possible by use of a combination of orthopedic appliances, as shown in the illustration, and by careful medical management by a team of neurologists, neurosurgeons, orthopedic surgeons, plastic surgeons, urologists, physiatrists and psychiatrists. Paramedical personnel, including physical and occupational therapists, social workers and nurses, greatly aid in the rehabilitation program.

Bladder training should be started early after injury. Philosophies of appropriate techniques may vary from one spinal cord injury center to another. Reflex function may return and aid elimination even though skeletal function is absent. Early mobilization and prevention of infection have significantly reduced the incidence of urinary calculi. Previously, the effects of genitourinary complications led to renal failure, which contributed to significant mortality in paraplegic patients.

Bowel paralysis also follows spinal cord trauma. The use of bulk-forming substances may prevent impaction. Small enemas early after injury and later use of suppositories may be effective. Eventually, control of defecation is possible in most patients.

A good level of nutrition is also important, and prevention of decubitus ulcers is vital. Frequent turning of the patient prevents pressure necrosis. Meticulous care is indicated at the first sign of any skin breakdown.

With time, the spinal cord below the level of the transection develops the potential for reflex spasms. Most common are those of paraplegia in flexion, resulting from afferent sensory signals generated by urologic infections or decubiti. Early mobilization in combination with compulsive

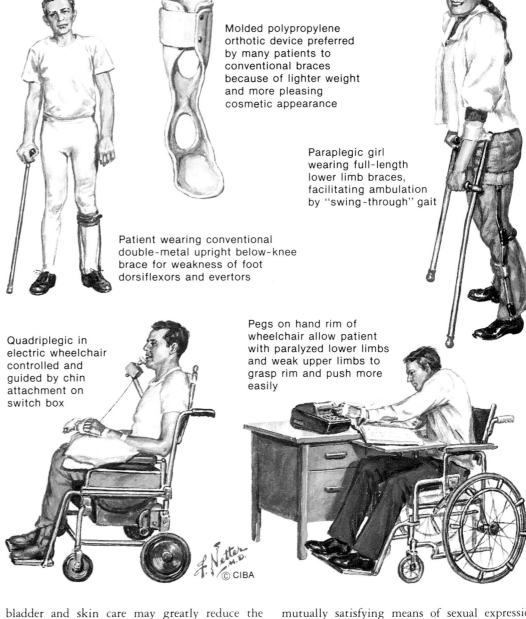

Functional wrist orthotic device aids in prehension and in maintaining metacarpophalangeal alignment. Extension of wrist opposes fingers to thumb, providing grasping action

Molded polypropylene orthotic device preferred by many patients to conventional braces because of lighter weight and more pleasing cosmetic appearance

Patient wearing conventional double-metal upright below-knee brace for weakness of foot dorsiflexors and evertors

Paraplegic girl wearing full-length lower limb braces, facilitating ambulation by "swing-through" gait

Quadriplegic in electric wheelchair controlled and guided by chin attachment on switch box

Pegs on hand rim of wheelchair allow patient with paralyzed lower limbs and weak upper limbs to grasp rim and push more easily

bladder and skin care may greatly reduce the severity of these spasms.

Successful management of these problems has allowed more vigorous rehabilitation programs. A number of patients have married, and the question of sexual function is important. Females are still capable of becoming pregnant, although many may not experience a true sensory orgasm. Erection representing a spinal reflex and allowing possible intromission may occur in more than half of the male patients. However, as in females, normal sensory appreciation is absent in most males. Counseling has allowed these patients to overcome their feelings of sexual inadequacy, directing a significant number of them to a

mutually satisfying means of sexual expression with their partners.

Depression is a recurrent problem for any patient with spinal cord injury. The spinal cord injury centers provide significant group support for these patients. Battery-powered wheelchairs and personal computers connecting home and office have added to their independence, self-esteem and potential for economic and social independence. Although it may be many years before major advances are made to allow significant medical therapy directed at the spinal cord injury per se, continued development of sophisticated electronic devices undoubtedly will expand the horizons of the patient with spinal cord injury. □

Section V

Brain Tumors

Frank H. Netter, M.D.

in collaboration with

J. Paul Badami, M.D. and Michael Brant-Zawadzki, M.D. *Plate 17*

Richard A. Baker, M.D. *Plate 16*

Louis R. Caplan, M.D. *Plate 2*

Marc A. Flitter, M.D. *Plate 1*

Stephen R. Freidberg, M.D. *Plates 3–7, 9–10, 14–15*

Stephen R. Freidberg, M.D. and Roger L. Hybels, M.D. *Plate 8*

Edward Tarlov, M.D. *Plates 11–13*

Common Manifestations of Brain Tumors

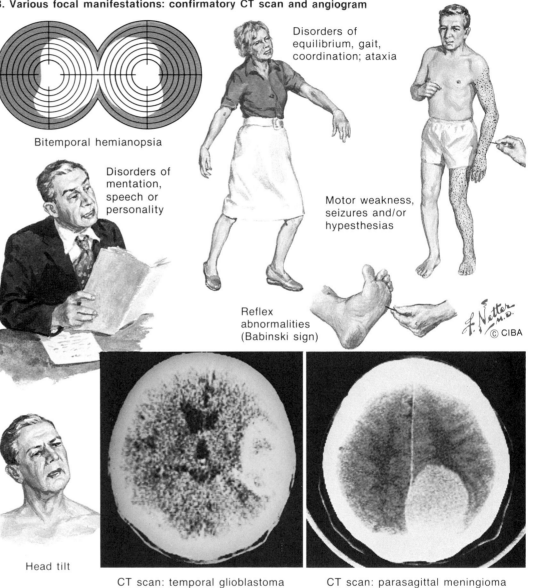

Some Common Manifestations of Brain Tumors

A. Intracranial pressure triad

Headache (may be frontal, parietal or occipital)

Nausea and/or vomiting

Papilledema

B. Various focal manifestations: confirmatory CT scan and angiogram

Bitemporal hemianopsia

Disorders of equilibrium, gait, coordination; ataxia

Disorders of mentation, speech or personality

Motor weakness, seizures and/or hypesthesias

Reflex abnormalities (Babinski sign)

Head tilt

CT scan: temporal glioblastoma

CT scan: parasagittal meningioma

The symptoms of a brain tumor result from either elevated intracranial pressure or focal brain dysfunction. The former is caused directly by the enlarging tumor mass or can be secondary to the hydrocephalus that results from obstruction of the cerebrospinal fluid (CSF) pathways in the ventricular system by tumor.

Clinical Manifestations. *Headaches, nausea and vomiting,* and *papilledema* comprise the cardinal clinical triad seen with elevated intracranial pressure. Clearly, not every patient complaining of headache has a brain tumor. However, by the time a patient has become somnolent and papilledema and focal signs and symptoms have developed, the correct diagnosis is only too obvious.

The headache caused by elevated intracranial pressure is usually generalized and tends to awaken the patient from sleep. Pressure in the region of the fourth ventricle causes vomiting; however, the frequently described "projectile" vomiting is rarely seen. Any vomiting associated with a headache should alert the attending physician to the possibility of increased intracranial pressure. Blurring of the optic disc margin or papilledema (swelling of the optic [II] nerve head caused by partial obstruction of venous outflow from the optic nerve secondary to elevated intracranial pressure) can be detected by ophthalmoscopic examination.

Local effects of a brain tumor on adjacent meningeal, vascular or neural tissues commonly produce focal symptoms and signs before the tumor enlarges to the degree necessary to increase intracranial pressure. The location and character of these symptoms and signs depend on the particular intracranial tissue being compressed or displaced and on the character and growth rate of the tumor. Knowledge of the course and clinical behavior of various intracranial tumors permits accurate anatomic or even histologic diagnosis.

Disturbances of mentation in the absence of elevated intracranial pressure usually imply the presence of bilateral frontal lobe tumors; unilateral frontal lobe tumors seldom produce such symptoms. *Disorders of equilibrium* can occur with either posterior fossa tumors or frontal lobe tumors. Well-defined *motor or sensory symptoms*, as well as *focal seizures*, clearly relate to the particular cortical areas involved by the tumor. A diagnostic impression of unilateral cerebral tumor may be confirmed during the neurologic examination by the observation of contralateral mild drift of an upper extremity and a positive Babinski sign. When a pituitary tumor has extended superiorly to compress the optic chiasm, the visual field

examination may demonstrate a *bitemporal hemianopsia*. In children, as well as adults, *head tilt* may be the first symptom. This is caused by a torticollislike syndrome of pain and neck spasm provoked by a tumor of the posterior fossa or foramen magnum.

Diagnostic Studies. Once the suspicion of a brain tumor has been raised, computed tomography (CT) should provide the definitive diagnosis; this procedure detects all but the smallest lesions. If the CT scan is positive, an angiogram may then be done to help refine the differential diagnosis, as well as to provide the critical information required for planning an appropriate therapeutic approach. □

Pseudotumor Cerebri

Pseudotumor Cerebri

Pseudotumor cerebri, also called benign intracranial hypertension, is a nonneoplastic disorder that causes signs and symptoms of increased intracranial pressure closely mimicking those in brain tumor. Pseudotumor is a diagnosis of exclusion made in patients with headache and papilledema when appropriate investigations have ruled out tumor; central nervous system (CNS) inflammatory disease; and space-occupying lesions of vascular, traumatic or infectious origin.

Etiology. Pseudotumor cerebri is probably caused by a chronic imbalance between cerebrospinal fluid (CSF) production and absorption. It most commonly affects young, obese women with menstrual irregularities. The female:male ratio is between 2:1 and 3:1. Pregnancy, amenorrhea or use of birth control pills, endocrinopathies such as hypoparathyroidism or Addison's or Cushing's disease, exogenous administration of corticosteroids, use of tetracycline or nalidixic acid, systemic lupus erythematosus, hypocomplementemia and hypervitaminosis A are known to be associated with pseudotumor cerebri. It can also develop secondary to occlusion of the dural sinuses in children with otitis media. Increased venous pressure following radical neck dissection is another mechanism of pseudotumor, and the empty sella syndrome has been radiographically documented in some patients with this disorder.

Clinical Manifestations. The most important and constant symptom of pseudotumor is *headache*. Although the headache may be slight or intermittent in some patients, most patients feel steady, pressurelike discomfort in the forehead or top or back of the head. The headache is often worse at night or when arising, and may be increased by bending or performing the Valsalva maneuver. In many patients with pseudotumor, vision becomes transiently obscured. These episodes usually affect both eyes, last 10 to 15 seconds, and are sometimes precipitated by bending, coughing or straining. Momentary sparkles or visual flashes also occur, especially with changes in position. Constant blurring of vision, diplopia, tinnitus and syncopal spells may occur, but less frequently.

On examination, the cardinal sign is *papilledema*. Rarely, pseudotumor is correctly diagnosed at an early stage, when diminished venous pulsation or early blurring of the nasal disc margins precedes frank papilledema. Decreased visual acuity in one or both eyes, enlarged blind spots, concentric decrease in the visual fields, and sixth cranial nerve palsy can also be present. Visual loss from increased intracranial pressure can be permanent, sometimes to the point of blindness. Tests show no evidence of mental deficit, motor or sensory symptoms, gait disturbance or reflex abnormalities.

Diagnostic Studies. The diagnosis of pseudotumor depends on the documentation of increased

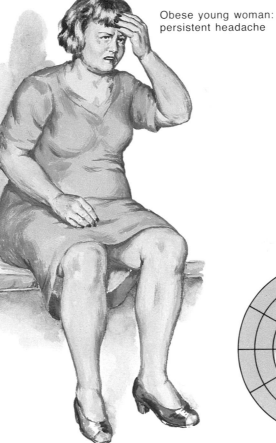

Obese young woman: persistent headache

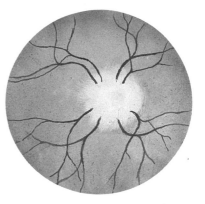

Papilledema: nasal blurring of optic disc vessels

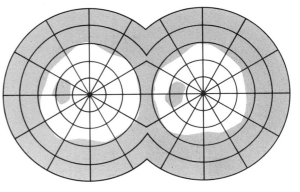

Concentrically contracted visual fields, large blind spots

Often related to pregnancy; menstrual disturbances; hypervitaminosis A; use of steroids, tetracycline or nalidixic acid; chronic otitis media with dural sinus occlusion; endocrinopathy (Addison's or Cushing's disease, hypoparathyroidism)

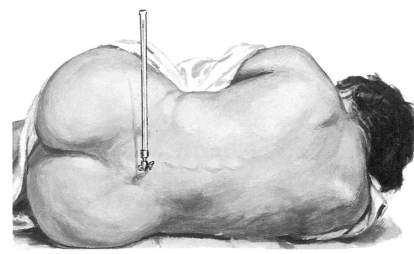

Cerebrospinal fluid pressure elevated

CSF pressure measured during lumbar puncture. In some patients, abnormalities of the optic disc (pseudopapilledema) are sometimes difficult to distinguish from papilledema, and direct ophthalmoscopy by an ophthalmologist or fluorescein angiography may be necessary to make this distinction. The CSF should be under elevated pressure (200 to 500 mm H_2O), with few or no cells and normal protein and glucose content. Brain imaging (computed tomography [CT], radionuclide scan, magnetic resonance imaging [MRI]) should exclude tumor. The ventricles are usually normal or small in size, and angiography shows no abnormalities other than occasional occlusive disease of the dural sinus.

Treatment. Single or multiple lumbar punctures significantly reduce intracranial pressure and provide symptomatic relief. Acetazolamide can be used to decrease CSF production, and use of glycerol and corticosteroids possibly increases CSF absorption. In patients who do not respond to these conservative measures, lumboperitoneal shunts, ventriculoperitoneal or ventriculoatrial shunts, subtemporal decompression, or optic nerve sheath decompression is necessary to reduce CSF pressure. In some patients with pseudotumor, CSF pressure remains chronically high for years and does not always return to normal after apparently successful treatment of the acute symptoms. □

Gliomas

Gliomas are the most common tumors of the brain, accounting for approximately 40% of all primary brain tumors in combined series. They arise from the supporting tissue in the brain rather than from neurons. Although the classification of these tumors is somewhat controversial, current concepts suggest that they originate from a common stem cell that differentiates into a more mature glial cell or neuron. Any of these cells can form tumors: astrocytoma, ependymoma, oligodendroglioma, and even ganglioneuroma.

Tumors in any cell group range from fairly well-differentiated, slow-growing neoplasms to histologically pleomorphic, rapidly growing tumors, the most common of which is glioblastoma multiforme. Examination of an entire biopsy specimen of glioblastoma may show a mixed cell pattern, with areas of undifferentiated tumor near areas of well-differentiated astrocytoma and oligodendroglioma.

Clinical Manifestations. The clinical picture depends on the location, size and growth rate of the tumor. Small tumors superficial to the motor area of the cerebrum may initially cause seizures, while a deeper tumor may reach enormous size before producing focal neurologic symptoms. Headache and dementia are early symptoms of these deep tumors, especially if the corpus callosum is involved. Tumors affecting the brainstem or optic chiasm produce symptoms related to local involvement of the brainstem nuclei or optic apparatus.

Diagnostic Studies. Computed tomography (CT) has revolutionized the diagnosis of gliomas. Treatment can usually be planned without other testing, although angiographic demonstration of the blood supply is occasionally useful. However, although CT, with angiography if necessary, can frequently predict the histologic type of the tumor, histologic examination is necessary for accurate diagnosis and treatment.

Treatment. The prognosis in gliomas located in the cerebral hemispheres varies with the location and type of tumor. A well-differentiated, slow-growing tumor located in a neurologically silent pole may occasionally be cured by surgical excision. On the other hand, a glioblastoma involving nonresectable structures is usually fatal in approximately a year, regardless of treatment. In general, wide surgical resection, if possible, is the appropriate treatment, followed by radiation therapy (5,500 R) to the tumor.

In deep, nonresectable tumors, the histologic diagnosis should be established by examination of a specimen obtained by CT-guided stereotactic biopsy before radiation therapy is initiated. The ability to interface accurate stereotactic frames with the information from CT has provided an extremely safe method of obtaining a sample.

While the ultimate outlook for deep anaplastic gliomas is still dismal, recent developments are encouraging. Chemotherapy combined with irradiation has improved survival. In fact, there appears to be a small but definite long-term survival. Work with tissue culture of the glioma cell and immunotherapy is exciting and promising. □

Gliomas

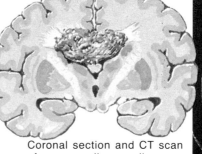

Large, hemispheric glioblastoma multiforme with central areas of necrosis. Brain distorted to opposite side

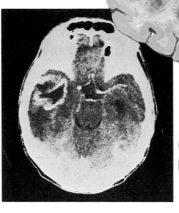

CT scan showing tumor similar to that shown above right

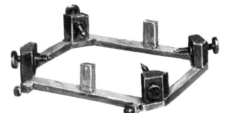

Coronal section and CT scan of corpus callosum glioma

Stereotactic brain biopsy using modified Gouda frame

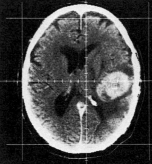

Basic frame for interfacing with CT scanner fastens to patient's head by steel pins

CT scan taken with basic frame on patient's head. Side arms, vertical and horizontal bars and arc then applied and biopsy needle directed at target according to X, Y, Z coordinates dialed directly on Gouda frame

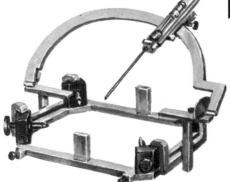

Side arms (for Y axis), vertical bars (for Z axis, which relates to level of CT cut) and horizontal bars (for X axis), plus arc with biopsy needle affixed to frame

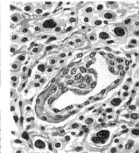

Patient, head draped, on operating table. Biopsy specimen taken via burr hole under local anesthesia

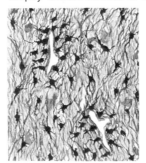

Astrocytoma

Oligodendroglioma

Ependymoma

Glioblastoma multiforme

Tumors Metastatic to Brain

Metastasis to the brain is a devastating stage in the course of disseminated cancer. In some centers, metastatic disease is the most often seen tumor of the brain. Although primary tumors of the lung and breast frequently spread to the brain, less common tumors, such as melanoma and carcinoma of the kidney also often metastasize to the brain. Most cancers are diagnosed before the onset of symptoms of central nervous system (CNS) disease, but because the period between diagnosis and metastatic spread is shorter with the more aggressive tumors, brain metastasis may occasionally be the first manifestation of an aggressive tumor such as lung cancer.

Most tumors metastatic to the brain spread through the bloodstream and lodge in the border between the white and gray matter. This implies that the tumor has either originated in the lung or has already spread there. Tumors lodge in a random pattern, their location depending on brain mass. Occasionally, a tumor may spread directly to the brain by local extension from a head and neck cancer or via Batson's venous plexus. Metastatic tumors are usually well demarcated from the brain. They are most often solid but may be cystic, or a hemorrhage into the lesion may be the first sign. The latter is more common with melanoma.

Clinical Manifestations. The focal neurologic symptoms depend on the location of the tumor in the brain. *Headache* is present in about one half of patients with metastatic brain tumor, and *seizures* are seen in one fourth. *Hemiparesis* and *mental changes* are common. *Hydrocephalus* may be present with tumors in the posterior fossa.

Diagnostic Studies. High-resolution computed tomography (CT) with injection of intravenous contrast medium demonstrates most metastatic deposits as small as 1 cm in diameter or larger. Edema with brain shift and hydrocephalus are seen. If the CT scan does not show a tumor, the cerebrospinal fluid (CSF) should be carefully examined for evidence of carcinomatous meningitis. This may be manifested by focal cerebral signs, confusion and hydrocephalus but also by

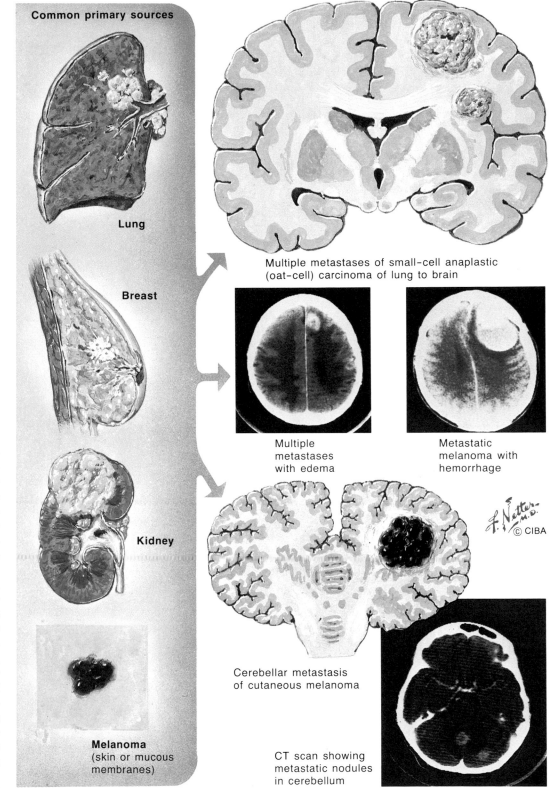

Common primary sources

Lung

Breast

Kidney

Melanoma (skin or mucous membranes)

Multiple metastases of small–cell anaplastic (oat–cell) carcinoma of lung to brain

Multiple metastases with edema

Metastatic melanoma with hemorrhage

Cerebellar metastasis of cutaneous melanoma

CT scan showing metastatic nodules in cerebellum

peripheral nerve, cranial nerve and radicular disease.

Treatment. Administration of corticosteroids and anticonvulsants is the first step in the treatment of parenchymal metastasis. If the primary tumor is known and is radiosensitive, such as breast cancer, radiation therapy is the treatment of choice. However, if the primary tumor is unknown or is known not to be radiosensitive, surgery must be considered. This, of course, depends on the demonstration of a solitary tumor and its location. Removal of lesions in noneloquent locations in the cerebrum or in the cerebellar hemisphere should be technically easy. Excision of other lesions depends on the judgment

of the neurosurgeon. In any event, if there is any doubt about the histologic type of the tumor, the lesion should be excised, or at least a biopsy, by means of a CT-guided stereotactic technique, should be carried out.

Radiation therapy is usually given postoperatively, since microscopic residual tumor is common despite an apparently total removal. While systemic chemotherapy has no place in the treatment of brain metastasis, local chemotherapy instilled through an Ommaya reservoir has been useful in patients with meningeal carcinoma.

Metastasis to the brain is a serious problem, but with judicious treatment, good palliation and even long-term survival are possible. □

Meningiomas

Meningiomas are the most common of the benign brain tumors, comprising 13% to 20% of all intracranial tumors reported in various series. Their incidence increases with age, with a female: male ratio of 2:1. Meningioma of the spine is almost unknown in men. Meningiomas arise from arachnoid cells in the meninges and are virtually always benign. Malignancy with distant metastasis is exceedingly rare, and the tumor can be surgically cured if total excision is possible. Classification can be based on histologic findings or on the tumor's location. The simplest histologic grouping divides the benign tumors into *meningotheliomatous, fibromatous* and *angioblastic* types. *Psammomatous* tumors, with the characteristic whorl pattern of the stroma (which may be calcified), are thought to belong to the meningotheliomatous group.

Clinical Manifestations

Like most brain tumors, the symptoms produced by a meningioma depend on its location, growth rate and adherence to adjacent structures rather than on its histologic type. Since most meningiomas are relatively slow-growing and produce little reaction in the brain, the early symptoms are usually related to dysfunction in that part of the brain being compressed.

Tumors over the cerebral convexity produce *focal seizures* or *hemiparesis*, while those arising in the parasagittal area cause *hemiparesis beginning in the leg* and can be diagnostically confused with spinal tumors. Many tumors arising in this location invade the sagittal sinus (Plate 5). For tumors anterior to the rolandic vein, the sinus may be ligated and excised. For more posterior tumors, however, ligation of the sinus is not possible because venous obstruction will cause brain infarction. Much of the tumor can usually be removed from the sinus.

Tumors overlying the cerebellar hemisphere may cause *ataxia* or symptoms of *obstructive hydrocephalus*. A meningioma at the base of the skull causes symptoms related to compression of adjacent neural structures. Olfactory groove, medial sphenoid wing and other parasellar tumors compress the optic (II) nerve, causing *blindness* and *optic atrophy*. These tumors may extend into the cavernous sinus, producing *extraocular palsies* and *facial numbness*. Tumors arising from the tentorium may involve structures either in the posterior fossa or in the incisure of the tentorium and cause *ataxia* or *hemiparesis* secondary to brainstem compression. Meningiomas that arise along the petrous ridge may be very adherent to the cranial nerves in the cerebellopontine angle, as well as to the branches of the basilar artery. Tumors may also extend to the clivus or arise there, producing lesions that are exceptionally difficult to remove.

Because of the brain's ability to adapt to slowly enlarging masses, tumors arising in the frontal or occipital areas may grow to enormous size before the pressure relationships suddenly decompensate. The patient who has had a tumor for many years may first experience a *personality change, hemiparesis* or even *stupor* of recent onset. Rarely, the initial clinical picture in meningioma is more characteristic of a glioma or metastasis, with a

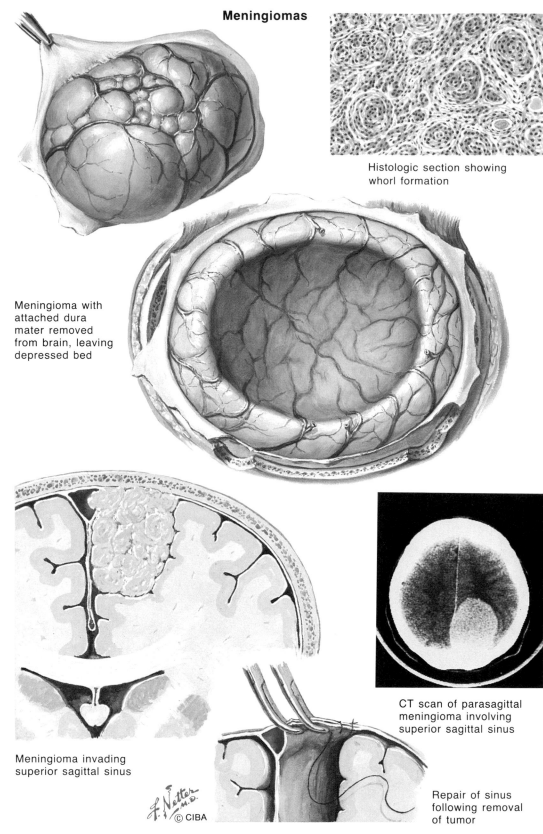

Meningiomas

Histologic section showing whorl formation

Meningioma with attached dura mater removed from brain, leaving depressed bed

Meningioma invading superior sagittal sinus

Repair of sinus following removal of tumor

CT scan of parasagittal meningioma involving superior sagittal sinus

great deal of edema surrounding a relatively small tumor. The danger in this situation lies in a decision that the tumor is malignant and therefore cannot be effectively treated. All tumors, unless there are specific contraindications, should be studied histologically. The therapeutic approach for large or edema-producing tumors is preoperative administration of corticosteroids and anticonvulsants and surgical removal.

Meningiomas arising from the sheath of the optic nerve in the optic canal can produce a slowly progressive loss of vision. These tumors may be difficult to diagnose and require meticulous examination by computed tomography (CT). In the absence of clear-cut radiographic studies,

surgical exploration of the optic canal may be indicated.

Meningiomas arising in the foramen magnum are first manifested by a unique syndrome of *neck pain, hemiparesis* and, occasionally, *atrophy of the hand*. The reason for the atrophy is unknown.

Diagnostic Studies

CT of the brain has become the primary diagnostic test. Modern equipment can demonstrate tumors as small as 1 cm in diameter. CT should be carried out with the intravenous administration of contrast medium. Unless a small tumor is adjacent to bone and is not visualized because of artifact, CT should be accurate.

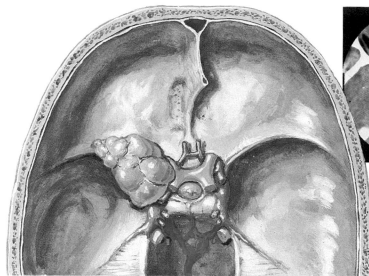

Meningioma of left medial sphenoid wing compressing optic (II) nerve and internal carotid artery

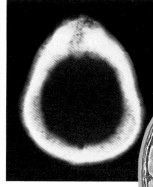

CT scan showing meningioma expanding cavernous sinus

CT scan showing meningioma eroding through hyperostotic frontal bone

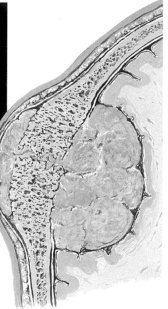

Convexity meningioma eroding through skull and producing distinct prominence

Removal of meningioma of right tentorium via temporoparietal skull flap by means of CO_2 laser interfaced with operating microscope

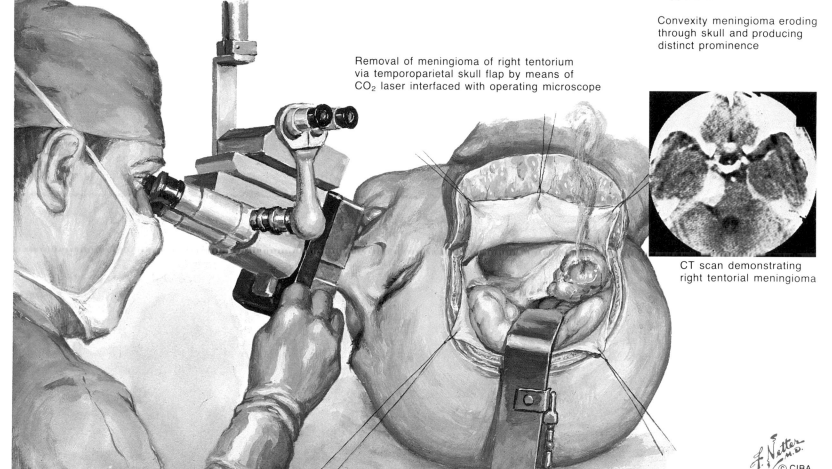

CT scan demonstrating right tentorial meningioma

Meningiomas
(Continued)

Before CT was available, angiography was the standard procedure for the diagnosis of meningiomas, but currently it is used as an adjunct. Angiography demonstrates the characteristic vascular pattern of a meningioma, a sunburst appearance with fine vessels and no arteriovenous shunting. The primary vascular supply is usually through the external rather than the internal carotid arteries, and selective angiography is therefore useful. With exceedingly vascular tumors, preoperative embolization with small particles or detachable balloons has been used.

Plain x-ray films of the skull still have a place in the diagnosis of meningioma. Because of the site of origin, the skull is invaded by the tumor in a high percentage of patients, and the radiographic changes are characteristic, showing hyperostosis. This information is helpful in planning the surgical approach.

Treatment

The treatment for meningioma is the total surgical excision of the tumor whenever possible. For tumors arising from the base of the skull or the sagittal sinus, the operating microscope and the recent development of the CO_2 laser as a surgical tool have improved the surgeon's range of operation (Plate 6). The use of spinal drainage, osmotic diuretics and hyperventilation anesthesia has been of great benefit in shrinking the brain to allow for nontraumatic retraction to expose these deep lesions.

Whether or not radiation therapy is useful for tumors that cannot be totally excised has not been resolved. Since the probability of recurrence of an incompletely excised tumor is extremely high, local radiation therapy is indicated to retard growth. □

Pituitary Tumors

The evaluation and treatment of pituitary tumors have undergone a dramatic change in recent years, brought about by better understanding of the chemistry of the nervous and endocrine systems and by improvements in radiographic techniques and surgical and medical treatment. (For a detailed discussion of the diagnosis of endocrinologic problems, see CIBA COLLECTION, Volume 4.)

Diagnostic Studies

Computed tomography (CT) has become the primary radiographic procedure used in diagnosing pituitary tumors. High-resolution CT can demonstrate even the tiny microadenoma. Three-dimensional imaging demonstrates the intimate relationships of the larger macroadenomas to the surrounding structures. Usually, a CT scan with contrast medium is adequate. However, if the suprasellar portion of the tumor is not well visualized or if there is concern about an empty sella, a subarachnoid injection of metrizamide preceding the CT scan demonstrates the anatomy. When a nonfunctioning adenoma with suprasellar extension cannot be differentiated from a giant aneurysm protruding into the sella, angiography is necessary.

Classification

Pituitary tumors are classified on both a functional and an anatomic basis (Plate 7). The classification based on the histologic staining of the tumor is flawed. The *eosinophilic adenoma* is seen with acromegaly and the *basophilic adenoma* in Cushing's syndrome. However, the most common type of tumor, the *chromophobe adenoma*, might be nonfunctioning or might represent a stage in the activity of an endocrine-active tumor.

A more rational classification divides pituitary adenomas into *functioning* and *nonfunctioning* tumors. The nonfunctioning adenomas produce symptoms caused by pressure on adjacent structures. The functioning tumors cause hyperprolactinemia, acromegaly and Cushing's syndrome. Tumors producing less common hormones, such as thyroid-stimulating hormone, and mixtures of hormones have also been described.

Prolactin-Secreting Tumor. Hyperprolactinemia suppresses the gonadotropins, causing amenorrhea, infertility and galactorrhea in women and impotence in men. Transsphenoidal removal of the prolactin-secreting tumor, with preservation of normal pituitary function, is the treatment of choice. The cure rate is high in intrasellar tumors, but decreases with larger tumors. Bromocriptine reverses the endocrinopathy and may shrink the tumor, but when the drug is stopped, prolactin rises and the tumor, if shrunken, rapidly enlarges.

Growth Hormone-Secreting Tumor. Manifestations of increased growth hormone depend on the patient's age. Gigantism develops in the child. In the adult, acromegaly develops, causing diabetes and cardiovascular and respiratory diseases, which reduce longevity. Because of the early obvious clinical manifestations, these tumors rarely attain the size of the nonfunctioning or prolactin-secreting tumor. Transsphenoidal removal of the

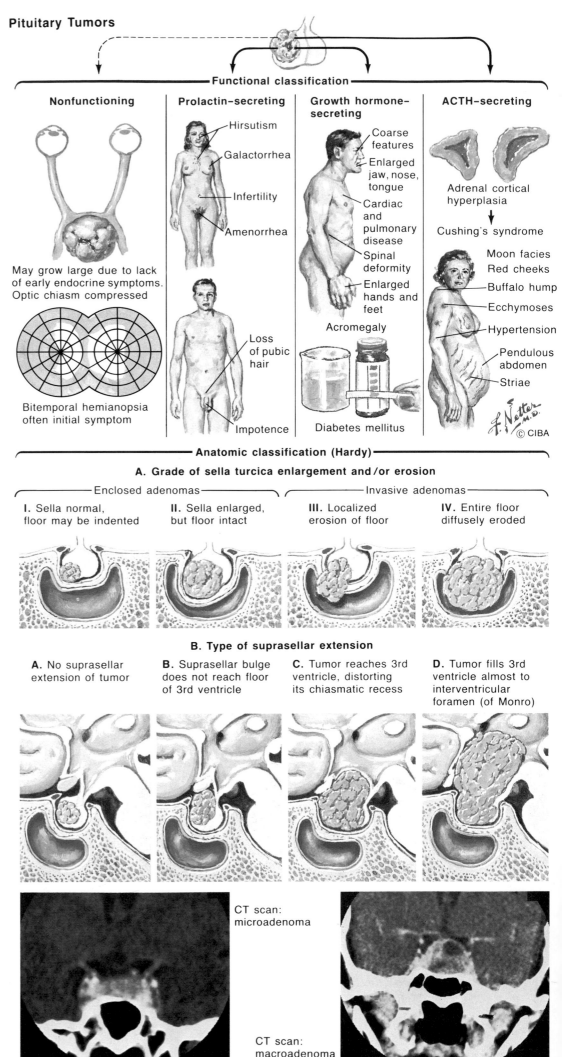

Functional classification

Nonfunctioning

May grow large due to lack of early endocrine symptoms. Optic chiasm compressed

Bitemporal hemianopsia often initial symptom

Prolactin-secreting

Hirsutism
Galactorrhea
Infertility
Amenorrhea
Loss of pubic hair
Impotence

Growth hormone-secreting

Coarse features
Enlarged jaw, nose, tongue
Cardiac and pulmonary disease
Spinal deformity
Enlarged hands and feet

Acromegaly

Diabetes mellitus

ACTH-secreting

Adrenal cortical hyperplasia

Cushing's syndrome

Moon facies
Red cheeks
Buffalo hump
Ecchymoses
Hypertension
Pendulous abdomen
Striae

Anatomic classification (Hardy)

A. Grade of sella turcica enlargement and/or erosion

Enclosed adenomas

I. Sella normal, floor may be indented

II. Sella enlarged, but floor intact

Invasive adenomas

III. Localized erosion of floor

IV. Entire floor diffusely eroded

B. Type of suprasellar extension

A. No suprasellar extension of tumor

B. Suprasellar bulge does not reach floor of 3rd ventricle

C. Tumor reaches 3rd ventricle, distorting its chiasmatic recess

D. Tumor fills 3rd ventricle almost to interventricular foramen (of Monro)

CT scan: microadenoma

CT scan: macroadenoma

Pituitary Tumors
(Continued)

tumor, with preservation of the normal gland, is usually successful unless the cavernous sinus has been invaded. Radiation therapy provides some benefit but rarely reduces growth hormone levels to normal.

ACTH-Secreting Tumor. Cushing's syndrome, resulting from an ACTH-secreting tumor, is the most serious condition produced by any pituitary tumor. This disease causes typical body deformity, myopathy, hypertension and potassium loss, and must be vigorously treated. A microadenoma can be removed and the normal gland preserved. Because the patients are often so desperately ill, this is the one hyperfunctioning pituitary tumor in which total hypophysectomy along with tumor removal may be indicated. In patients who have had bilateral adrenalectomy, a rapidly enlarging, aggressive pituitary tumor may develop, producing Nelson's syndrome with hyperpigmentation.

Surgical Techniques

The major recent therapeutic development for pituitary tumors is the transsphenoidal approach to the sella turcica (Plate 8). This technique was used by Harvey Cushing in the early years of this century and then abandoned in favor of a transcranial approach. Since the late 1960s, largely through the efforts of Jules Hardy, MD, of Montreal, the transsphenoidal approach has been widely accepted. The development of the operating microscope has permitted meticulous dissection of the pituitary tumor, with preservation of the normal gland.

Hardy has developed an anatomic classification of pituitary tumors according to their size, the presence of suprasellar extension, and invasive properties. The best results are obtained in small intrasellar tumors that have not invaded the surrounding dural structures. However, with the aid of intraoperative fluoroscopy, tumors with significant suprasellar extension can be surgically removed if the tumor remains in the midline. The transcranial approach is reserved for tumors that extend laterally out of the sella turcica and cannot be approached from below.

Most surgeons enter the sphenoid sinus through a variant of the transseptal approach. An incision is made in the nasal mucosa along the caudal edge of the septum on the right side and the entire mucoperichondrium is elevated. An incision is made through the cartilage parallel to the caudal edge of the septum, leaving a strut of cartilage about 2 cm wide, which supports the tip of the nose postoperatively. The entire septal cartilage may be left undisturbed. The mucoperichondrium is then elevated from the left side.

The cartilage and bone posterior to the strut are removed to expose the anterior wall of the sphenoid bone. Following the maxillary crest and the junction of the perpendicular plate with the vomer, the surgeon exposes the sphenoid sinus. The anterior wall is removed to enter the sinus. The operating microscope is then used for the remainder of the operation.

The position of the sella turcica is confirmed with fluoroscopy, although with large tumors it is

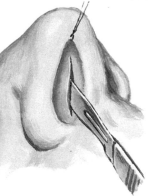

1. Incision in mucosa of nasal septum. Alternate transgingival approach indicated by arrow in figure 2

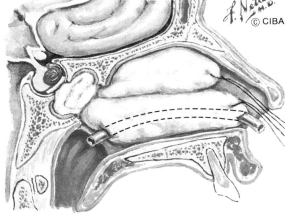

2. Septal mucosa elevated and speculum introduced. Anterior wall of sphenoid sinus removed, exposing its posterior superior wall (roof), which constitutes floor of sella turcica

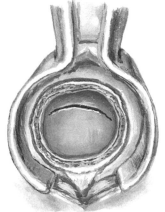

3. View through speculum into sphenoid sinus with incision in roof for opening into sella turcica

4. Bony floor of sella removed, exposing lining dura. Cruciate incision indicated (view through microscope)

5. Sellar dura opened. Tumor enucleated from remainder of pituitary gland

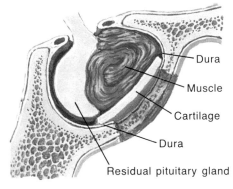

Dura
Muscle
Cartilage
Dura
Residual pituitary gland

6. After removal of tumor, muscle pack placed in cavity. Piece of cartilage from septum closes opening (enlarged sagittal view)

7. Sphenoid sinus packed with Gelfoam; Merocel packs containing airway placed in nose

often obvious, and free tumor may be present in the sphenoid sinus. If the floor of the sella is intact, it is fractured with a chisel. The bone is removed with a small punch, with care to protect the surrounding venous sinuses. The dura mater overlying the tumor is cut and coagulated.

The technique of tumor removal varies with the consistency of the tumor. Some tumors can be easily removed with suction and caught in a trap. Firmer tumors must be removed piecemeal. When it is difficult to grossly differentiate the tumor from the normal gland, multiple frozen sections are examined to insure that the entire tumor is removed and the gland preserved. With larger tumors, air injected into the cisterns before

surgery allows fluoroscopic visualization of the suprasellar extension, and angled mirrors help to visualize blind recesses. The most important aspect of the surgery is the preservation of the arachnoid membrane. Low postoperative morbidity depends on preventing blood from entering the cerebrospinal fluid (CSF) during the operation and leakage of CSF postoperatively.

For closure, muscle is placed in the tumor cavity and, if necessary, held in place with a piece of nasal cartilage. The mucosal flaps are reapproximated and the nose is packed. The single incision is closed with absorbable sutures. The packs are removed in 3 days, and the patient is discharged in 4 days. □

Craniopharyngiomas

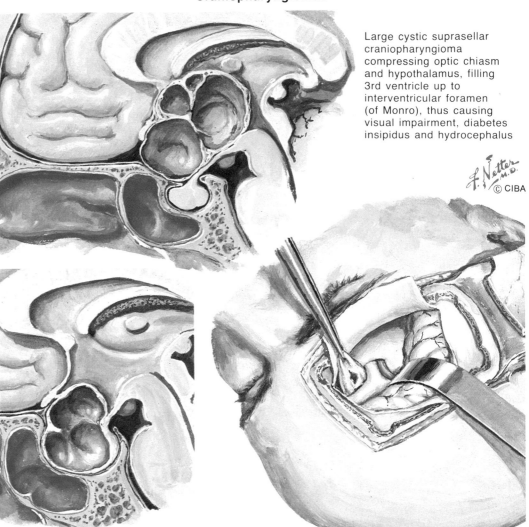

Large cystic suprasellar craniopharyngioma compressing optic chiasm and hypothalamus, filling 3rd ventricle up to interventricular foramen (of Monro), thus causing visual impairment, diabetes insipidus and hydrocephalus

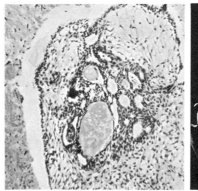

Intrasellar cystic craniopharyngioma compressing pituitary gland to cause hypopituitarism

Tumor gently teased forward from under optic chiasm after evacuation of cystic contents via frontotemporal flap

Craniopharyngiomas arise from remnants of the craniobuccal pouch, a structure originating in the embryonic pharynx. They are the most common parasellar tumors in children, accounting for 7% of pediatric brain tumors, but also occur in adults.

The tumor may be solid or cystic, containing an oily fluid that may contain cholesterol crystals. The tumor invariably extends to the optic chiasm. It may be small or enormous and extend under a frontal or a temporal lobe into the interpeduncular fossa, or it may extend to the interventricular foramen and produce obstructive hydrocephalus. Although the tumor is usually suprasellar, it may extend into the sella turcica and, rarely, may be entirely intrasellar. It can spread down the clivus or even through the incisure of the tentorium to the cerebellopontine angle.

A craniopharyngioma is comprised of masses of columnar and cuboidal epithelial cells. Degenerative areas in the tumor may contain oily fluid, calcium and keratin. Cyst walls may be easily separated from the surrounding brain, but frequently there are dense gliotic adhesions between the tumor and the undersurface of the chiasm and the hypothalamus. The gliosis may provide a plane in which the tumor can be surgically separated from the neural tissue.

Clinical Manifestations. A craniopharyngioma invariably causes *visual symptoms* secondary to compression of the optic apparatus. *Endocrine dysfunction* is seen in one half of the patients, manifested by diabetes insipidus, panhypopituitarism and gonadal deficiency in adults and by growth retardation and obesity in children. *Hydrocephalus*, often with *papilledema*, develops in 15% of children with a craniopharyngioma. *Mental deficiency, lethargy* and *motor symptoms* also occur.

Diagnostic Studies. Radiographic examination shows calcification in almost all tumors in children and in half of those in adults. Computed tomography (CT) is the primary diagnostic tool. It should be done in both the horizontal and the coronal plane, which will demonstrate the tumor's relationships to the brain, the base of the skull, the pituitary fossa and the circle of Willis. This information is essential for surgical planning. Endocrine studies are necessary to establish function of the pituitary gland and hypothalamus. Any deficiencies of cortisone, antidiuretic

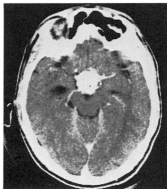

Histologic section: craniopharyngioma (H and E stain, × 125)

CT scan showing craniopharyngioma

Tomogram: flocculent calcification in craniopharyngioma

hormone, gonadotropins and thyroid must ultimately be corrected.

Treatment. In recent years, the treatment of choice, especially in children, has become complete surgical removal of the lesion if possible. The cure rate with microsurgical techniques in experienced hands has been as high as 80%. With partial resection, even followed by radiation therapy, recurrence is the rule. However, even if surgery is successful, endocrine dysfunction is common, and some surgeons have advocated postponing definitive surgery in children until after puberty if possible. Percutaneous needle drainage of cysts, with later surgery, may allow more normal growth and development. Repeated needle

drainage may also be useful in treatment of a recurrent tumor.

Radiation therapy retards the growth of the tumor and reduces the production of the cyst fluid, although irradiation of this area runs the risk of damage to the chiasm, hypothalamus and pituitary gland. In the older adult with a more solid tumor densely adherent to the optic chiasm and hypothalamus, partial removal of the lesion followed by radiation therapy is justified. This may prevent surgical damage to the chiasm, hypothalamus and pituitary gland and provide a better functional result. The rare intrasellar tumor can be approached with the transsphenoidal technique. □

Tumors of Pineal Region

Pineal tumors have long taxed clinicians because of the difficulties in classifying them pathologically, in deciding on the optimal therapy, and in determining the appropriate surgical approach.

The pineal gland is located centrally in the brain and is surrounded by vital structures, the posterior third ventricle, the mesencephalon and cerebral aqueduct (of Sylvius), and the great cerebral vein (of Galen).

Clinical Manifestations. Symptoms of a tumor in the pineal region result from increased intracranial pressure secondary to hydrocephalus, dysfunction of the mesencephalic tectum and endocrinopathy. Most patients initially have headache and ataxia, and many have papilledema. The delicate cerebral aqueduct is easily obstructed, causing hydrocephalus. Pressure on the mesencephalic tectum produces the characteristic Parinaud syndrome: paralysis of upward gaze, paresis of convergence and unequal pupils. Diabetes insipidus, caused by spread of the tumor to the anterior third ventricle and hypothalamus, develops occasionally, and precocious puberty is seen in 10% of patients, usually boys, reflecting the sex predilection of these tumors.

Classification. A rational pathologic classification divides pineal tumors into those of germ cell origin, tumors of the pineal parenchyma, and a miscellaneous group.

Tumors of germ cell origin are germinomas and teratomas. *Germinomas*, comprising 50% of all pineal region tumors, are most common in adolescence and have a marked predilection for males. Endocrinologic abnormalities may be the first indication of a germinoma. These tumors tend to spread in the cerebrospinal fluid (CSF) and seed the hypothalamic region of the third ventricle. A germinoma is extremely radiosensitive and, in this respect, resembles testicular teratoma. *Teratoma* also strikes young males and may be initially manifested by diabetes insipidus and precocious puberty. These tumors may contain elements of bone, cartilage and hair. They are not invasive.

Pinealcytoma, a tumor of the pineal parenchyma, is well circumscribed and not invasive. It occurs at any age and has no sex predilection, and it may remain localized or spread within the CSF. On the other hand, the malignant *pinealblastoma* contains primitive cells resembling medulloblastoma and spreads within the CSF.

Also seen in the pineal region are *benign meningiomas* and *cysts*. The importance of these lesions is obvious. They respond only to surgical treatment.

Diagnostic Studies. The diagnosis of tumors in the pineal region depends on radiographic examination and cytologic study of CSF obtained by ventricular puncture. Plain x-ray films of the skull may show abnormal amounts of calcium in the pineal region. Angiography is necessary if malformation of the great cerebral vein is considered a possibility. Computed tomography (CT) is the diagnostic study of choice, because it demonstrates the degree of hydrocephalus, as well as the tumor, and indicates whether the tumor is infiltrating or circumscribed.

Tumors of Pineal Region

Tumor compressing mesencephalic tectum and corpora quadrigemina, occluding cerebral aqueduct (of Sylvius) and invading 3rd ventricle

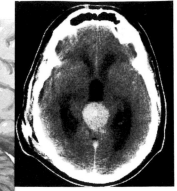

CT scan showing tumor of pineal region, with hydrocephalus

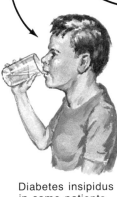

Parinaud's syndrome: paresis of upward gaze, unequal pupils, loss of convergence

Diabetes insipidus in some patients

Sexual precocity in boys may occur

Position of patient (undraped to show detail), surgeon and microscope for resection of pineal region tumors

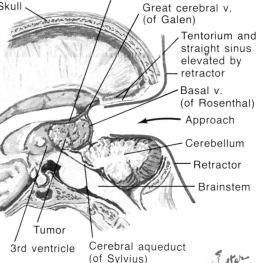

Internal cerebral v.

Skull

Great cerebral v. (of Galen)

Tentorium and straight sinus elevated by retractor

Basal v. (of Rosenthal)

Approach

Cerebellum

Retractor

Brainstem

Tumor

3rd ventricle   Cerebral aqueduct (of Sylvius)

Anatomic aspects of exposure

Treatment. The treatment of pineal tumors is controversial. Some surgeons operate directly on all lesions, and some perform a ventriculosystemic shunt and irradiate all lesions. However, these tumors are complicated, and each case must be carefully evaluated by the surgeon.

The ventricular CSF should be examined at the time of shunting. If the CSF contains malignant cells, shunting and radiation therapy are appropriate. The surgeon must take care to avoid seeding malignant cells from the CSF. The initial drainage can be external; if an internal shunt is used, a Millipore filter should be placed in the shunt line. If the CSF is clear and the tumor appears circumscribed, a direct operative approach is indicated. It is impossible to make a histologic diagnosis without study of a tissue specimen. A benign mass must not be treated incorrectly.

The operating microscope has allowed neurosurgeons to approach this lesion with more confidence and safety than was possible in the past. Most surgeons use the infratentorial-supracerebellar approach. After the cerebellar hemispheres are allowed to fall, the view of the tumor is not obstructed by the great cerebral vein. Circumscribed tumors can be totally removed, and it is usually possible to remove enough tissue from infiltrating tumors to allow for CSF drainage from the posterior third ventricle. □

Acoustic Neurinomas

The syndrome of the cerebellopontine angle, caused by a large acoustic neurinoma (Plate 11), is a paradigm of neurologic clinical diagnosis. The tumor typically arises from the Schwann cells of the vestibular nerve and slowly, often without apparently significant symptoms, impairs the vestibular and cochlear nerves. If the tumor is not recognized, it continues to expand and may cause death from brainstem compression and hydrocephalus.

Clinical Manifestations

The rate of growth of acoustic tumors varies widely. Some smaller intracanalicular tumors may be associated with symptoms of long duration, while the large lesions often have a rapid course.

In addition to hearing loss and tinnitus, early symptoms of acoustic neurinoma may include tic douloureux, ataxia, facial sensory loss or, occasionally, even dementia. However, a patient with early acoustic neurinoma is rarely totally deaf, and often is not aware of any progressive hearing loss. A vague sensation of imbalance or nonspecific dizziness, with difficulty in walking in the dark, may be present. Early symptoms can thus be minimal.

Compression of the vascular supply of the auditory nerve can occasionally result in a precipitous loss of hearing. Although the facial (VII) nerve is severely compressed and hemifacial spasm may occasionally occur, significant preoperative symptoms of facial nerve dysfunction are unusual. As the tumor expands further, the adjacent trigeminal (V) nerve superiorly becomes involved, and tic douloureux or facial sensory loss is a sign of a larger tumor. If the lower cranial nerves become involved, disturbances of swallowing and hoarseness may develop. Later, with increasing pressure on the brainstem, intracranial pressure rises; lethargy and subsequent coma develop; and death may occur due to aspiration, respiratory failure or complications of hydrocephalus. Early diagnosis is an important goal.

Diagnostic Studies

No audiometric pattern of hearing loss is absolutely characteristic of acoustic neurinoma, although a hearing loss for high tones, with impaired speech discrimination, frequently occurs. Testing by impedance audiometry has often shown an absence of acoustic reflexes on the affected side. Early audiometric diagnosis of acoustic neurinomas has been greatly aided by use of brainstem auditory evoked response (BAER) testing. Caloric testing shows reduced vestibular responses on the side of an acoustic neurinoma.

The entire clinical and radiographic workup is usually an outpatient procedure. Plain x-ray films of the skull are ordinarily not helpful. As the tumor slowly expands, it may erode the bony walls of the internal auditory meatus and commonly cause a trumpet-shaped widening. Tomograms of the internal auditory meatus are considered abnormal if there is a difference of greater than 2 mm in canal diameter on the two sides.

Computed tomography (CT) should be done with enhancement by intravenous contrast

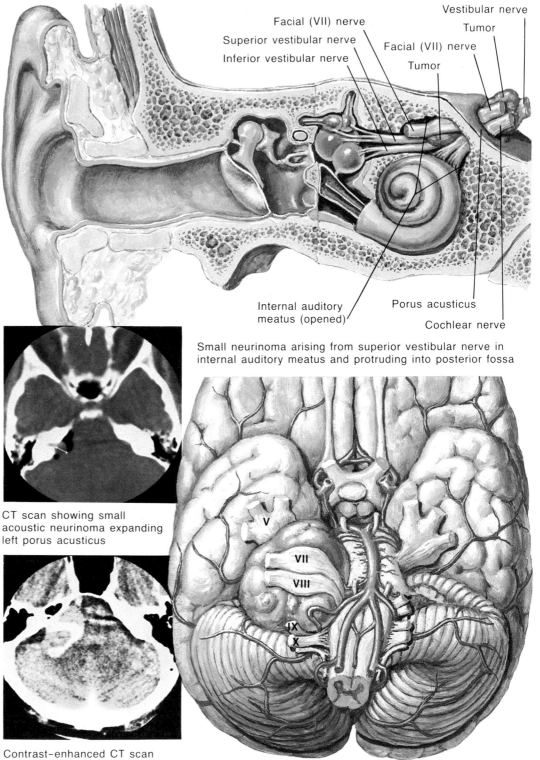

Acoustic Neurinomas

Small neurinoma arising from superior vestibular nerve in internal auditory meatus and protruding into posterior fossa

CT scan showing small acoustic neurinoma expanding left porus acusticus

Contrast-enhanced CT scan showing moderate-sized left neurinoma, with some distortion of 4th ventricle

Large acoustic neurinoma filling cerebellopontine angle, distorting brainstem and cranial nerves V, VII, VIII, IX, X

Brainstem auditory evoked response (BAER) in patient with acoustic neurinoma on right side. There is delay in action potentials of cochlear nerve (wave I) and cochlear nuclei (wave II) on affected side

Acoustic Neurinomas
(Continued)

medium, which demonstrates most medium-sized and large tumors (Plate 11). Without contrast enhancement, the scan may be negative. Tumors less than 1 cm in diameter may not be obvious even on contrast-enhanced CT scans.

Patients in whom clinical suspicion is high and contrast-enhanced CT scanning is negative should have CT pneumography. A small bubble of gas introduced into the lumbar region, with the affected ear uppermost, outlines and enters the internal auditory meatus in normal patients. Even a small acoustic neurinoma is likely to obstruct the internal auditory meatus, preventing gas from entering this region and demonstrating the presence of a tumor, as shown in the illustration.

Surgical Treatment

The advisability of surgery for large symptomatic tumors is usually not questioned. For small, minimally symptomatic tumors, the need for surgery should be carefully considered.

Microsurgery has made a tremendous difference in the treatment of acoustic neurinomas. The major problem during total removal of an acoustic tumor is preservation of the adjacent vasculature, especially the anterior inferior cerebellar artery, and the markedly thinned and displaced facial nerve. It is now possible to remove safely and completely even the largest tumors via the *posterior fossa approach* (Plate 12).

The posterior fossa approach minimizes the chance of a disabling postoperative deficit. With this technique, the tumor and the important structures medial and lateral to it are all in full view in the surgical field. In patients with a small tumor, whose hearing loss is not severe, preservation of hearing is an occasional consideration.

Plate 12 shows the posterior fossa approach to the left cerebellopontine angle. The patient is in a horizontal position, with the head turned away from the surgeon. An incision is made to the tip of the mastoid eminence; the underlying muscles are separated; and a bony opening is made, extending laterally to the sigmoid sinus. After aspiration of cerebrospinal fluid (CSF) from the cisterna magna, gravity aids cerebellar retraction. A self-retaining retractor is placed, and the microscope is brought into the field.

The surgeon carefully tries to preserve the planes of the arachnoid over the tumor, in order to protect the delicate cranial nerves and brainstem. To the right, the fifth cranial nerve and petrosal vein are seen, an area commonly involved by the larger tumors. Toward the lower portion of the field, the glossopharyngeal (IX), vagus (X) and accessory (XI) nerves are visible. They are extremely delicate, and any but the most careful manipulation in this area may produce difficulty in swallowing, hoarseness or more serious deficits.

At the level of the tumor, the facial nerve is usually displaced anteriorly, as shown in the lower part of the illustration. The facial nerve lies anteriorly in the canal, and as the tumor grows in the posterior portion of the canal on the vestibular nerve, the facial nerve tends to be pushed forward. This relationship is important in preserving

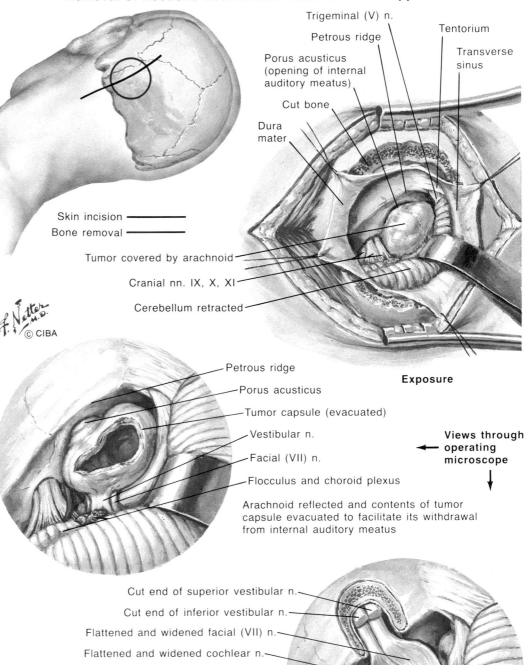

Removal of Acoustic Neurinoma: Posterior Fossa Approach

Trigeminal (V) n.
Petrous ridge
Tentorium
Transverse sinus
Porus acusticus (opening of internal auditory meatus)
Cut bone
Dura mater
Skin incision
Bone removal
Tumor covered by arachnoid
Cranial nn. IX, X, XI
Cerebellum retracted

Exposure

Petrous ridge
Porus acusticus
Tumor capsule (evacuated)
Vestibular n.
Facial (VII) n.
Flocculus and choroid plexus

Views through operating microscope

Arachnoid reflected and contents of tumor capsule evacuated to facilitate its withdrawal from internal auditory meatus

Cut end of superior vestibular n.
Cut end of inferior vestibular n.
Flattened and widened facial (VII) n.
Flattened and widened cochlear n.
Loop of anterior inferior cerebellar a.
Depressed tumor bed in brainstem
Cut end of vestibular n.

Segment of roof of internal auditory meatus removed with its superior and intrameatal dura. Superior and inferior vestibular nerves divided and tumor shelled out. Flattened and widened facial (VII) and cochlear nerves are visible

the facial nerve, which is markedly flattened and often quite adherent just medial to the internal auditory meatus.

The vestibular nerves, from which the tumor is arising, must be sectioned, and if hearing has not already been irreversibly damaged, preservation of hearing might be a consideration. In this case, the cochlear nerve should be manipulated as little as possible. The anterior inferior cerebellar artery supplies the lateral portion of the brainstem and cerebellar peduncles and must be carefully preserved. Large tumors obtain some blood supply from the labyrinthine artery, which also must be preserved if preservation of hearing is a consideration.

With a larger tumor, the capsule is gutted at an early stage to facilitate its atraumatic manipulation. In the lower part of the exposure illustrated, the ninth, tenth and eleventh cranial nerve complex is visible, passing through the jugular foramen with the accompanying sigmoid sinus. In the lower right corner of the illustration is a view after the tumor has been excised. The labyrinthine artery has been preserved and the relationship of the four main nerves in the canal is seen. Because a CSF leak through the lateral portion of the canal can develop, the lateral canal is plugged with fat and bone wax.

With improvement of surgical techniques, the treatment may soon be no worse than the disease. □

Neurofibromatosis (von Recklinghausen's Disease)

Neurofibromatosis

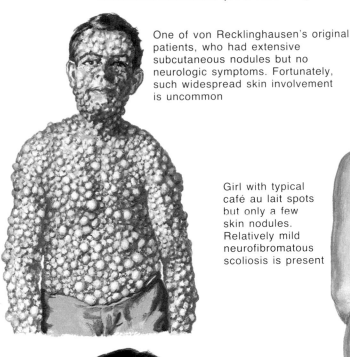

One of von Recklinghausen's original patients, who had extensive subcutaneous nodules but no neurologic symptoms. Fortunately, such widespread skin involvement is uncommon

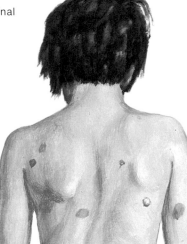

Girl with typical café au lait spots but only a few skin nodules. Relatively mild neurofibromatous scoliosis is present

Neurofibromatosis, or von Recklinghausen's disease, is the most common of the phacomatoses, a group of inherited disorders that affect the nervous system and involve tissues that arise embryologically from the neural crest. These disorders affect both skin and brain and include the Sturge-Weber syndrome, with port-wine stains on the upper face and calcifications of the cerebral cortex with seizures (see Section I, Plate 23); Hippel-Lindau disease, with cerebellar and retinal hemangioblastomas; and tuberous sclerosis, with shagreen spots on the skin and intracranial periventricular glial hematomas.

Neurofibromatosis in itself is a varied group of disorders, with differing manifestations in the nervous system. The melanin-containing cells, which form the cutaneous patches known as café au lait spots, arise from the neural crest, as do the Schwann cells, which form neurofibromas involving the cranial and peripheral nerves. Gliomas and meningiomas are frequently associated with this disorder.

Peripheral Neurofibromatosis. Von Recklinghausen's original patients, one of whom is shown in the illustration, had the peripheral form of neurofibromatosis, with multiple subcutaneous nodules arising from subcutaneous nerves, but no neurologic symptoms. Peripheral neurofibromatosis is of autosomal dominant inheritance and is perhaps the most common human genetic mutation, occurring in one of 100,000 persons. Patients with this form of the disease rarely harbor acoustic neurinomas or other tumors involving the intracranial or intraspinal nerve roots.

Central Neurofibromatosis. In the less common central form of the disease, the inheritance is also autosomal dominant. Unlike the peripheral disease, central neurofibromatosis can be extremely debilitating and even fatal. It may be manifested by bilateral acoustic neurinomas. The growth pattern of these tumors may be slow and quite unpredictable. They do not always cause severe hearing loss, but when they are bilateral, the resulting acquired deafness, as well as the brainstem compression and other signs that may develop, can be extremely debilitating. These tumors often invade the mechanism of the middle ear, and complete surgical removal is usually not

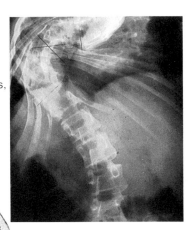

X-ray film showing severe scoliosis, with typical sharp angulation unresponsive to corrective measures, often seen in neurofibromatosis

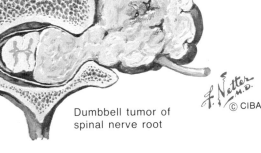

Dumbbell tumor of spinal nerve root

Young woman with bilateral facial palsy (note drooping of cheeks) due to compression of both facial (VII) nerves by acoustic neurinomas, which also caused hearing loss. Proptosis resulted from bilateral optic (II) nerve tumors. Subcutaneous nodules developed on her forehead, and masses in her neck compressed the trachea. Disease was fatal in this patient

feasible. Surgical objectives are limited to palliative measures.

Other intracranial manifestations of central neurofibromatosis may include neurofibromas on other cranial nerves, occasionally aqueductal stenosis, and optic (II) nerve glioma. Neurofibromas may also arise within the spinal canal, typically on the posterior nerve roots just central to the ganglion, and may extend into both the paraspinal region and the spinal canal, with a waistlike constriction at the level of the neural foramen. Because of their configuration, these are known as dumbbell tumors in this location. They occasionally are the only manifestation of the disorder and can be totally excised.

Surgery is indicated for relief of pain and of spinal cord compression, which may develop in the severest form of the disease. The neurofibromas may be multiple, and the entire spinal contents can be a mass of grapelike clusters.

The illustration shows the facies of a young woman with severe central neurofibromatosis. Large bilateral acoustic neurinomas have produced total deafness and have compressed the facial (VII) nerve, causing bilateral facial palsy. In addition, subcutaneous tumors are obvious over the forehead, and a large neck mass caused tracheal compression. Proptosis due to an optic nerve glioma is also evident. The disease was fatal in this patient. □

Intraventricular Tumors

Intraventricular tumors are histologically heterogeneous lesions but are grouped together because of their unique position within the ventricular system. While they may produce symptoms by local pressure and invasion, hydrocephalus is the common finding. The hydrocephalus usually develops slowly, with headache, personality change and unsteadiness, but acute deterioration, with increased intracranial pressure and brainstem herniation, may occur. When it is not possible to treat the tumor adequately, the hydrocephalus must be treated with a ventriculosystemic shunt.

Computed tomography (CT) is necessary for diagnosis of intraventricular tumor. The procedure accurately demonstrates the size of the tumor and the ventricles. Postoperative CT scans are important in following regression of the hydrocephalus and aid in the decision for shunting.

Tumors of the Lateral Ventricle. These tumors may arise from the choroid plexus (meningioma and choroid plexus papilloma) or from the substance of the brain itself (ependymoma, astrocytoma, subependymoma and the giant-cell tumor of tuberous sclerosis).

The *meningioma* and *choroid plexus papilloma* do not invade the brain and can be totally excised through a temporoparietal cortical incision into the hydrocephalic lateral ventricle. While this approach may result in a homonymous hemianopsia, it is preferred because it avoids the motor and speech areas and allows access to the vascular pedicle of the tumor before the tumor itself is encountered. The hydrocephalus caused by the papilloma is usually marked, since the tumor secretes cerebrospinal fluid (CSF).

The *subependymoma* and the *tumor of tuberous sclerosis* are slow-growing, arising from the floor of the lateral ventricle. They can be approached with a corticectomy through the hydrocephalic ventricle. Total removal is not possible, because the tumor blends into the normal thalamus and basal ganglia. Shaving the tumor to the ventricular floor produces excellent long-term results. Radiation therapy is not necessary for subependymoma.

Ependymoma and *astrocytoma* are more aggressive tumors. The surgical problems are identical to those encountered in the subependymoma, but regrowth is common. Radiation therapy is essential in treatment of both tumors and may cure the ependymoma, but the prognosis in the more malignant astrocytoma remains dismal.

Tumors of the Third Ventricle. Anterior third ventricle tumors are the *colloid cyst, giant craniopharyngioma* (Plate 9) and *pituitary adenoma* (Plate 7). The colloid cyst is a benign, nonneoplastic remnant of the embryonic paraphysis. Because of its location in the interventricular foramen (of Monro), a small mass produces massive hydrocephalus. Some neurosurgeons approach the cyst through a cortical incision into the hydrocephalic right lateral ventricle or through the corpus

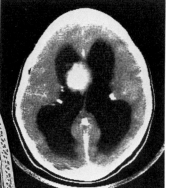

CT scan showing tumor similar to that at left

Subependymoma of anterior horn of left lateral ventricle obstructing interventricular foramen (of Monro), thus producing marked hydrocephalus

Colloid cyst of 3rd ventricle and surgical approach via right prefrontal (silent) cerebral cortex. May also be approached through corpus callosum (arrow). Note enlarged lateral ventricles (posterior view)

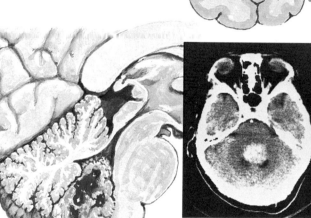

Ependymoma of 4th ventricle protruding into cisterna magna. CT scan shows similar tumor

CT scan showing colloid cyst of 3rd ventricle

callosum. Both approaches are satisfactory, although the risk of neurologic damage is significant. Thus, a reasonable approach is bilateral ventriculosystemic shunting. Unilateral shunting may cause a disastrous brain shift.

The tumor of the *posterior* third ventricle is the *pineal region tumor* (Plate 10).

Tumors of the Posterior Cranial Fossa. These tumors can be subdivided into three groups: *extraaxial, cerebellar hemispheric* and *intraaxial.* While the extraaxial and cerebellar tumors are not intraventricular in origin, they compress the fourth ventricle and may cause hydrocephalus. The extraaxial tumors are the *acoustic neurinoma* (Plate 11), the *meningioma* (Plates 5–6) and the

cholesteatoma. The type of cerebellar hemispheric tumor varies with age. The *cystic astrocytoma* and *medulloblastoma* (see Section I, Plates 21–22) occur in children, while *metastasis* (Plate 4) and the more malignant *astrocytoma* occur predominantly in adults.

The ependymoma and subependymoma arise from the roof of the medulla and fungate into the fourth ventricle. Total removal should not be attempted because of the certainty of damage to the nuclei in the roof of the medulla. Residual ependymoma and papilloma should receive radiation therapy. Should follow-up CT show that symptomatic hydrocephalus persists with any of the tumors, a shunt should be placed. ☐

Chordomas

Chordomas

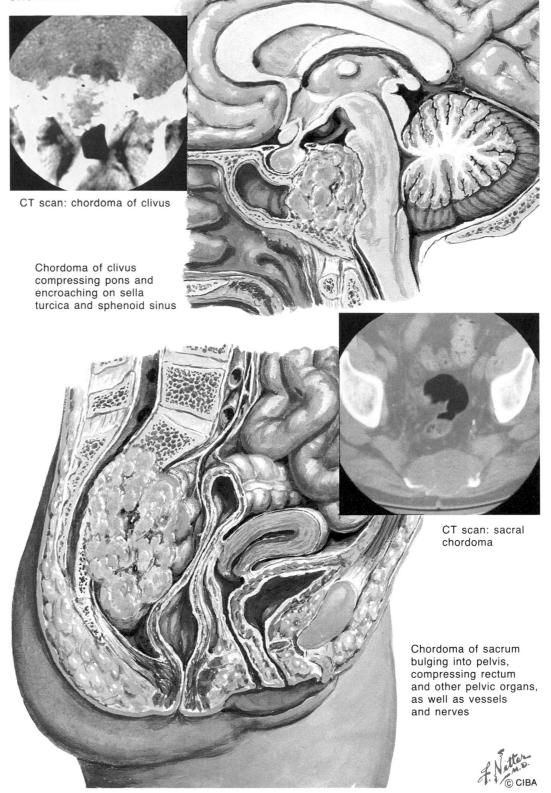

CT scan: chordoma of clivus

Chordoma of clivus
compressing pons and
encroaching on sella
turcica and sphenoid sinus

CT scan: sacral
chordoma

Chordoma of sacrum
bulging into pelvis,
compressing rectum
and other pelvic organs,
as well as vessels
and nerves

Chordomas arise from unresorbed remnants of the embryonic notochord, a mesodermal structure running through the center of the vertebrae and into the clivus. Phylogenetically, the notochord is last identified as a distinct entity in the shark, but is seen in mammalian embryos. Tumors involving this structure may arise anywhere in the spinal cord, but most often develop at the upper and lower tips: 35% on the clivus or the body of the first or the second cervical vertebra and 50% on the sacrum/coccyx. Tumors on the clivus occur most commonly in the third and fourth decades, while the sacral tumors are more common later in life. Most series demonstrate strong male predominance.

Even though these tumors are usually slow-growing, recurrence is the rule and metastases occur frequently. On occasion, however, they may contain many mitoses and recur and disseminate rapidly. The histologic appearance of the chordoma is unique. It is composed of sheets of foamy-appearing cells with clear cytoplasmic vacuoles, *physaliphorous cells*.

Clinical Manifestations. Symptoms depend on the effect the tumor has on the neural and adjacent structures. Minor symptoms may be ignored as long as 2 years. Local *pain* is the most common symptom of tumors of the clivus, sacrum and spinal column. In tumors of the clivus, *visual loss* and *paralysis* of the *extraocular* and *pharyngeal muscles* precede the effects of pressure on the brainstem. If the growth is anterior, a pharyngeal mass may be the first sign of the tumor.

The tumor of the sacrum or coccyx, which may reach enormous size, causes *constipation* by direct pressure on the rectum and involves the sciatic nerve roots and nerve branches to the anus, bladder and skin of the perineum. Spinal column tumors cause *spinal cord compression*, like any other malignant extradural tumor.

Diagnostic Studies. Plain x-ray films and tomograms of the clivus or sacrum outline the extent the tumor has encroached on the bone. Computed tomography (CT) not only accurately defines the degree of bone destruction but also demonstrates the tumor's extension outside the bone. Angiography may be useful in demonstrating the vascularity of the tumors and major vascular displacement. Myelography shows impingement or block in the spinal canal. Barium enema examination shows the relationship of the sacral tumor to the rectum, which is essential information before surgery.

Surgical Treatment. The surgical approach to the lesions of the clivus depends on the location of the tumor. A tumor in the sella turcica or in the region of the dorsum sellae can be reached by the standard *transsphenoidal approach* to the sella turcica. When the tumor arises in the cavernous sinus or extends into the floor of the middle fossa, the *subtemporal approach*, either extradural or intradural, is best. The *paramedian posterior fossa exposure* of the cerebellopontine angle may be necessary for tumors growing into this region. For the tumor involving a large portion of the clivus and growing posteriorly into the prepontine cistern and brainstem, a *transoral approach* provides the most direct access.

Tumors of the sacrum or coccyx are approached through a *sagittal midline incision* over the tumor. It is best to expose the distal dural sac and follow the nerve roots in an attempt to preserve them. All involved bone should be removed and the tumor traced laterally into the gluteal muscles if necessary. It is usually possible to peel the tumor off the posterior wall of the rectum without entering the rectum. Colostomy is usually unnecessary. Surgical cure is rarely obtained. The tumors tend to recur slowly, and repeat surgery is often indicated. Radiation therapy has been administered to the residual tumor but is rarely beneficial. In cases in which the tumor is aggressive and metastatic, the prognosis is extremely poor. □

Differential Diagnosis in Central Nervous System Tumors
Ring enhancement

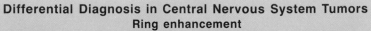

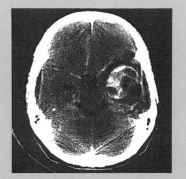 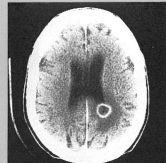 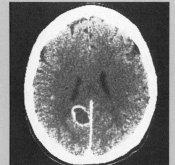 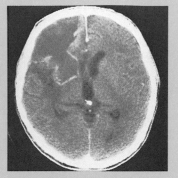

Glioma. Ring enhancement with lucent portions (cyst or necrosis). Thick regions of enhancement are characteristic. Large tumor causes small mass effect

Abscess. Spherical lesion with thin rim enhancement. Only modest edema seen. Central lucency represents pus

Remote hemorrhage. Density of original clot lost. Neovascularity and phagocytosis at periphery (enhancement) and no edema

Infarction. Thin rim enhancement associated with subacute infarction. Anatomic pattern suggests infarction

Patterns of edema

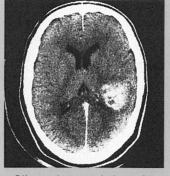 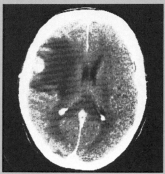 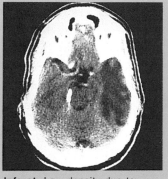 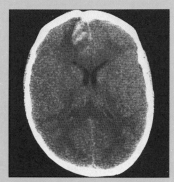

Glioma. Increased absorption (enhancement and/or hemorrhage) with small cystic or necrotic areas. Large lesion causes little edema or mass effect

Metastases. Small enhancing lesion with much edema. Gyral gray matter contrasted against edema along convexity is characteristic

Infarct. Low density due to edema and/or necrosis. Small or moderate mass effect is characteristic of infarction

Contusion associated with skull fracture. Patchy or linear streaks of blood with edema (suggest trauma). Skull fracture and subgaleal hematoma seen

Multiple lesions

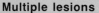

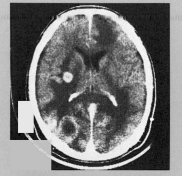 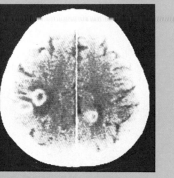 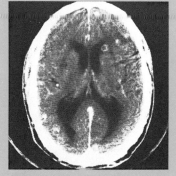 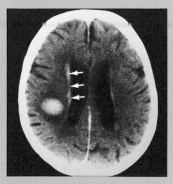

Metastases. Variably sized ring-enhancing lesions with central necrosis and striking edema

Emboli with subacute bacterial endocarditis. Multiple ring-enhancing lesions with septic emboli (either infarction and/or small abscesses)

Parasitic (cysticercosis). Many differing lesions — calcification, lucency, variable enhancement (either homogeneous or ring), variable edema

Lymphoma. Discrete, dense, and homogeneously enhancing lesions in white matter. Mass effect is minimal. Subependymal involvement may occur (arrows)

Lucent lesions

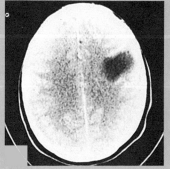 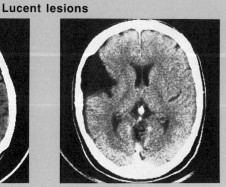 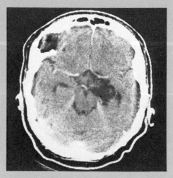

Glioma. Discrete lucent lesion with adjacent enhancing areas. Small mass effect suggests tumor

Infarct. Remote infarct has discrete borders. Vascular territorial pattern seen, with atrophy

Arachnoid cyst with agenesis. Discrete lucent lesion with thinning of skull and no displacement of normal brain

Epidermoid tumor. Lucent lesions at skull base. Frontal lesion shows remodeling of skull and calcification. Fat density is characteristic but often absent

© CIBA

Magnetic Resonance Imaging in Diagnosis of Central Nervous System Tumors

Nuclear magnetic resonance (NMR) spectroscopy was first described in 1946 by Bloch and Purcell, who received the Nobel Prize in 1952 for their work. This foundation led to the first imaging application of NMR by Lauterbur in 1973. The term "magnetic resonance imaging" (MRI) has subsequently been coined for the medical application of this technology.

Atomic nuclei containing an odd number of protons or neutrons have the potential to be imaged. However, in current clinical practice, the hydrogen nucleus, by virtue of its relatively high concentration in biologic systems and its sensitivity to the MRI process, is the preferred nuclear species for imaging.

The hydrogen nucleus, or proton, as a spinning charged particle, generates a small magnetic field. Much like small bar magnets, protons align either parallel or antiparallel to an externally applied magnetic field. The slightly greater number of nuclei aligning parallel to the applied field compared with those aligned antiparallel provides the basis for imaging.

This alignment can be perturbed via bombardment by radio frequency (RF) signal. The subsequent realignment of these magnetic dipoles results in the emission of an RF signal of the same frequency as that absorbed. This so-called Larmor frequency is specific for a given nuclear species in a specific magnetic field. In practice, an object in the magnetic field is surrounded by a wire coil that acts as both a transmitter and a receiver of these RF signals.

The addition of magnetic gradient coils creates a predictable spatial gradient in the static magnetic field. Because the Larmor frequency is proportional to the field strength, knowledge of the exact variation of the magnetic field allows the determination of the origin of a given RF signal in space. Thus a "hydrogen map" (or spin map) is created.

One determinant of the amplitude of the emitted RF signal is the *hydrogen density*, ie, the number of protons sampled at any given point. Variation in the number of protons returning the RF signal within biologic molecules (fat, brain tissue, bone, blood) contribute to MRI contrast. Molecular relationships of some protons diminish their contribution to such a signal.

The other major determinants of signal amplitude are the *magnetic relaxation times*, T1 and T2. *T1* (spin lattice, longitudinal, or thermal relaxation time) describes the time interval necessary for a nucleus to become magnetized when placed in a magnetic field. Similarly, it is the time for return of the sample to its original equilibrium magnetization following perturbation by an RF pulse. T1 varies with temperature, physical state (solid versus liquid) and magnetic field strength.

Groups of protons can change their magnetic orientation, and application of an RF pulse can make them spin coherently (in phase) in a plane perpendicular (or transverse) to the applied static magnetic field. Following RF perturbation, the loss of this "spin coherence" results in a rapid decay of RF signal intensity described by *T2* (spin-spin or transverse relaxation time). T2 varies most with local magnetic field heterogeneity; however, the physical state of the molecules and temperature also contribute to its variability.

The images shown in Plate 17 were obtained via the *spin echo technique*, which elicits both T1 and T2 information. Images are obtained by a sequence of RF pulses of varying duration repeated at a precise time interval termed *TR* (pulse repetition time). Subsequent RF signal "echoes" are sampled at discrete intervals termed *TE* (echo delay time). Short TR images (frequent RF perturbations, eg, 0.5 second) accentuate tissue differences based on T1 and may be termed "T1-weighted." Longer TR values (less frequent perturbation, eg, 2.0 seconds) accentuate T2 differences and are termed "T2-weighted." Longer values of TE (later echo sampling) also emphasize differences in T2 among species.

Simply stated, on T1-weighted images, protons with short T1 values emit a relatively higher signal intensity (appearing white) than those with long T1 values (appearing dark). On T2-weighted images, species with relatively long T2 values retain their signal strength, thus emitting a higher-intensity (brighter) signal at delayed echo times.

Clinical MRI of the central nervous system (CNS) has proved to be very sensitive to tissue alteration, whether it is secondary to demyelination, hemorrhage, ischemia or neoplasm. Local changes in molecular composition and free water content at sites of demyelination in multiple sclerosis are manifested as foci of a high-intensity signal, usually in the periventricular area of the deep white matter.

Differences in T1 and T2 values between brain tumor and associated surrounding edema have been demonstrated, allowing more precise localization of tumor foci. Often, the tumor focus itself may appear of relatively low intensity on T1-weighted images, while surrounding edema is of relatively high intensity. On T2-weighted images, differentiation between tumor and edema usually is poor. However, as longer and longer echo delays are performed, some differentiation may be noted. Calcification within tumor foci appears as an area of absent signal or "signal dropout." Because protons in a calcium crystalline lattice are relatively immobile, their signal is not available.

Differentiation between cerebrospinal fluid (CSF) or cyst fluid and CNS parenchyma has allowed good visualization of fluid spaces within both the brain and the spinal cord, including syringomyelia and those cysts associated with tumors.

Current MRI research includes chemical shift imaging, in which those protons associated with various compounds (eg, water versus fat) can be selectively imaged secondary to local magnetic field variation within these molecules. There is ongoing investigation of in vivo NMR spectroscopy and the possibility of imaging various other nuclear species (eg, sodium, phosphorus, fluorine and carbon). Further evaluation of paramagnetic contrast agents (eg, gadolinium) may also lead to increased sensitivity and specificity of MRI in the study of CNS pathology. □

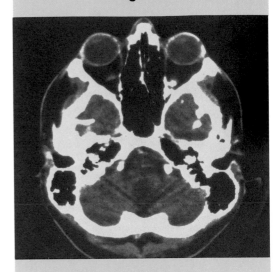

Magnetic Resonance

1a. Cystic astrocytoma. Transaxial CT scan reveals "water density" structure, which may possibly be enlarged cisterna magna

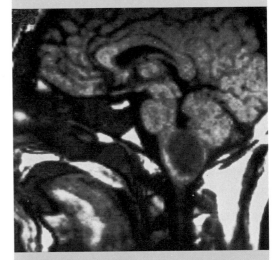

1b. Cystic astrocytoma. T1-weighted (TR 0.5 sec, TE 28 msec) direct sagittal MR image shows circumscribed low-intensity lesion emanating from medulla, with elevation of obex of 4th ventricle and compression of inferior vermis

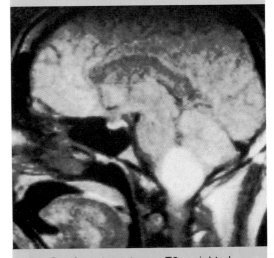

1c. Cystic astrocytoma. T2-weighted (TR 2 sec, TE 28 msec) MR image shows intense signal from lesion. This indicates prolonged T2 relaxation time, ruling out benign fluid collection and indicating presence of tumor in medulla

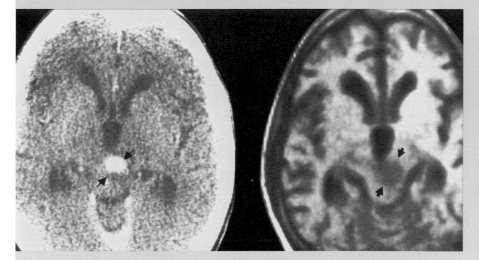

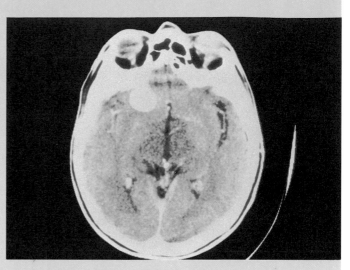

2a, b. Midbrain glioma. Left: transaxial CT scan shows focus of contrast enhancement (arrows) corresponding to tumor. Right: T1-weighted (TR 0.5 sec, TE 28 msec) MR image reveals focus of tumor as low-intensity area (arrows) corresponding to lesion seen on CT scan. Low intensity suggests T1 prolongation

4a. Meningioma. Transaxial CT scan shows well-circumscribed densely enhancing lesion originating from medial sphenoid wing

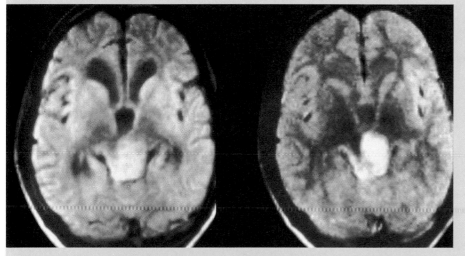

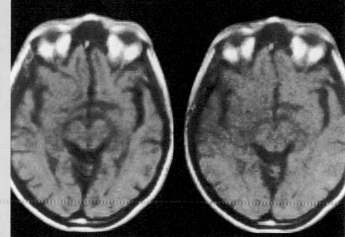

2c, d. Midbrain glioma. T2-weighted (TR 2.0 sec; TE 28 [left], 56 msec [right]) MR images show diffuse area of increased intensity involving midbrain, indicating greater tissue alteration than that seen in **2a, b.** (T1-weighted image shows good definition of CSF space vs brain tissue but poor gray matter–white matter definition. T2-weighted images show good gray matter–white matter definition but poorer CSF definition)

4b. Meningioma. T1-weighted (TR 0.5 sec; TE 28 msec [left], 56 msec [right]) MR images show that lesion is "isointense" to brain parenchyma, probably because of similar T1 characteristics. There is minimal mass effect. Note high-intensity signal from orbital fat

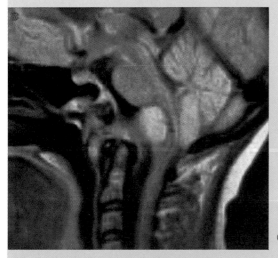

© CIBA

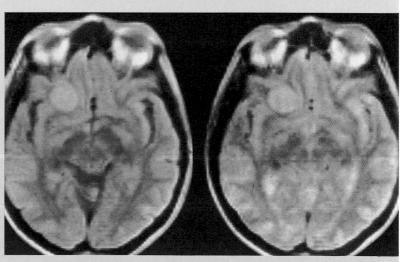

3. Chordoma of clivus. T2-weighted (TR 1.4 sec, TE 35 msec) MR image shows rounded high-intensity lesion occupying premedullary cistern. Posterior distortion of cervicomedullary junction, with elevation of floor of 4th ventricle

4c. Meningioma. T2-weighted (TR 2 sec; TE 28 msec [left], 56 msec [right]) MR images show that lesion now contrasts with normal brain parenchyma due to its relatively prolonged T2 relaxation time

Section VI

Common Problems in Psychiatry

Frank H. Netter, M.D.

in collaboration with

John R. Hayes, M.D. *Plates 1–6*

Major Depression

"I've lost interest in everything. It's even an effort to get out of bed in the morning. I don't want to go anywhere, see anybody or do anything. It's all closing in on me"

Major Depression

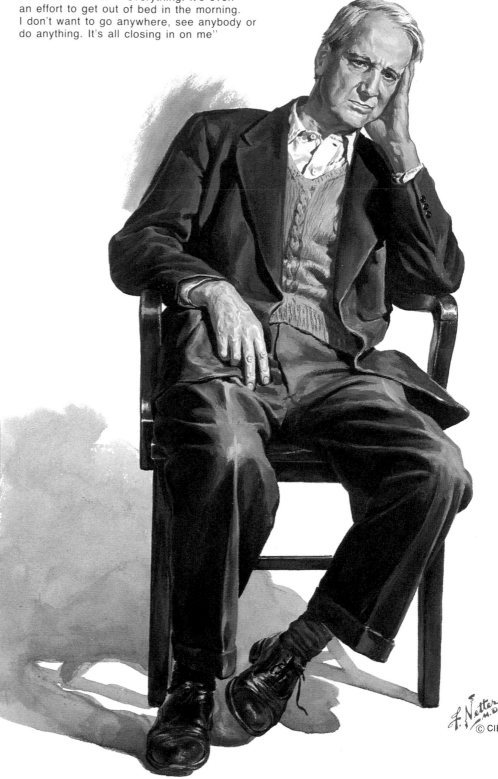

Depression is probably the most common cause of physical complaints that are really a manifestation of underlying psychiatric illness. The depressed patient's somatic complaints are exhibited in depressive concomitant symptoms, depressive equivalent symptoms or somatic delusions.

Depressive concomitant symptoms are somatic symptoms that are part of a depressive illness, such as appetite and weight changes, sleep disturbance (especially early morning awakening), loss of interest, loss of energy, fatigue and gastrointestinal complaints (especially constipation). These symptoms are not a symbolic representation of psychologic depression, but are examples of disturbed physiologic function that occur in depression.

Symptoms that are symbolic, or somatic metaphors for depression, are called *depressive equivalent* symptoms. They often occur in people for whom the idea of being "depressed" is unacceptable, and who therefore express their illness in the language of physical symptoms. For example, a patient might complain of headaches, and when asked to describe the pain, might say, "It's all closing in on me. It feels like I'm trapped and I can't get out." Asked how this pain affects him, the patient might say, "It wakes me up at 3 o'clock in the morning and I can't go back to sleep, I don't feel like eating, don't want to go anywhere, and I've even lost interest in sex. It hurts so bad I feel like crying, and I've even thought of killing myself." Clearly, the patient sounds and looks depressed, but he rejects a diagnosis of depression, claiming that "it's just this headache." Such "masked" depression is often treatable despite the patient's disavowal of the diagnosis.

Finally, major depression can affect the patient's perceptions of reality, and seriously depressed people may become psychotic. *Somatic delusions* are common in such cases, and the physical complaints usually have a ring of bizarre self-deprecation. Patients may believe irrationally, despite negative evaluations, that they are dying of cancer or have venereal disease or parasitic infestation. Frequently, patients feel that the disease is deserved punishment for some real or imagined misdeed.

Depressed patients very often have *memory complaints*, and may believe that their brain is degenerating. Differentiating genuine dementia from "depressive pseudodementia" is difficult and important in such patients. Interestingly, it has been shown that the complaint of memory loss correlates with the degree of identifiable depression, not with objective evidence of memory loss. Truly demented patients are more likely to try to hide their deficits, while those who complain of memory loss are likely to be depressed instead. Competent psychologic testing is often the reliable means of solving this common diagnostic dilemma.

The previously described symptoms of depression include appetite disturbance with weight change, sleep disturbance, loss of interest in sexual intercourse or decreased libido, fatigue, feelings of worthlessness or self-reproach and guilt, memory or thinking complaints, and thoughts of suicide or wishing to be dead. Another symptom is *psychomotor disturbance*. It may be retardation, as in the patient shown in the illustration, or agitation with restlessness, hand wringing and pacing.

The newest official psychiatric diagnostic nomenclature calls for a diagnosis of major depressive episode when four of these symptoms have been present nearly every day for at least 2 weeks, coupled with dysphoria or loss of interest or pleasure in usual activities. Major depression implies that other serious psychiatric disorders have been excluded and that the symptoms are not associated with some catastrophic event.

When all these criteria are met, such major depression should virtually always be treated with *antidepressant medications* or, in selected cases, with *electroconvulsive therapy*. *Psychotherapy* is often useful, but the somatic therapies are always indicated in this serious disease. □

Dysthymic Disorder

When patients have chronic feelings of depression or have lost interest or pleasure in usual activities but do not have symptoms of a major depressive episode, they may have a dysthymic disorder. This term has replaced the older term "neurotic depression," and implies a duration of 2 years or more. In essence, these patients are nearly always sad. They may have occasional good days or even 1 or 2 good weeks, often with only mild impairment of social and occupational functioning, but they never seem to feel happy or comfortable for long periods of time.

For several reasons, it is important to differentiate dysthymic disorder from a major depressive episode. First, although dysthymic disorder is a separate diagnosis, it is often associated with other problems that need attention. The complaint "I haven't felt happy in years" may indicate a chronic physical disorder coexisting with psychosomatic complaints. Considering both possibilities and doing an adequate but not exhaustive medical examination are part of the art of evaluating such complaints. For example, it is important to ask women with chronic mild depressive complaints to keep careful records of their menstrual cycle and to document whether mood problems are consistently noted in the second half of the cycle. Although the exact nature of the premenstrual syndrome is still undefined, most experts agree that when dysthymic complaints are clearly premenstrual, explanation of the problem and interventions aimed specifically at treating it are very useful.

Regardless of other physical problems, *chronic psychosocial* and *economic stresses* or *relational problems* are frequently associated with dysthymic disorder. Personality disorders also often coexist with dysthymic disorder. Patients whose depressive complaints have persisted for years usually need psychotherapeutic and social interventions. Developmental history, coping style, personality characteristics, current life stresses and capacity for change are important variables and must all be considered. For these reasons, consultation with mental health professionals is often indicated when dysthymic disorder is the diagnosis.

Second, treatment with antidepressant medications is not always indicated in dysthymic patients. Failure to recognize and treat major depression with appropriate antidepressants is a significant omission. Judicious use of psychopharmacologic agents is also often helpful in dysthymic disorder. However, medications are usually useful only when combined with other

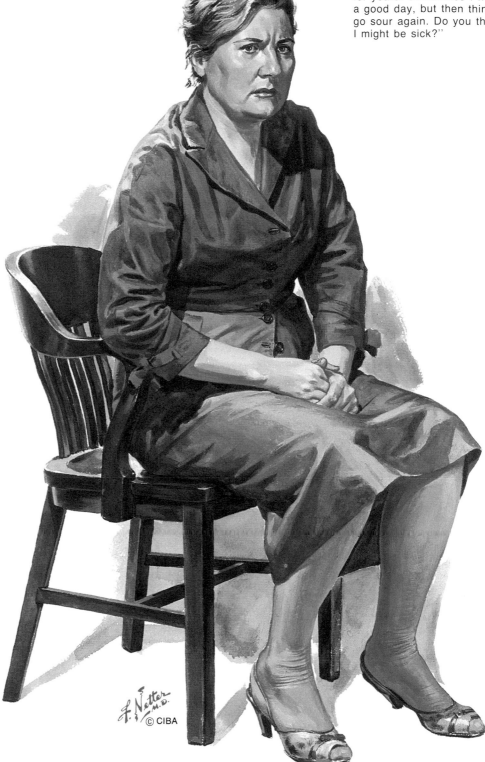

Dysthymic Disorder

"I really haven't felt happy for years. Sometimes I have a good day, but then things go sour again. Do you think I might be sick?"

medical and mental health interventions and only when the target symptoms are other than chronic sadness itself.

Finally, associated *alcoholism* or *substance abuse* is an important and often overlooked problem associated with dysthymic disorder. It is possible that persons with chronic life problems and chronic sadness begin to self-medicate with alcohol or drugs. However, it is more likely that chemically dependent persons begin to have increasing trouble with their life as their chemical dependence escalates. Job, marital, legal, economic and health problems, along with chronic depression, should always raise the index of suspicion about substance abuse. Since patients are likely to minimize the importance of chemicals in the genesis of their problems, it is useful to take some history from a family member when evaluating dysthymic patients.

All too often, failure to attend to associated physical factors, psychosocial stressors or substance abuse leads to a therapeutic failure when dysthymic patients are treated with antidepressant medications. The chronicity and complexity of associated problems make dysthymic disorder a therapeutic challenge for doctor and patient alike, but chronic depression should not be considered untreatable. The correct diagnosis and appropriate interventions can often significantly improve the life of dysthymic patients. □

Bipolar Affective Disorder: Manic Episode

The obverse of depression is mania. The depressed patient feels low, "slowed down," self-deprecating and uninterested in life. The manic patient feels high, "speeded up" and irrationally self-confident, and becomes involved in activities that often have potentially painful consequences. The patient's grandiosity and expansiveness lead to uncharacteristic sexual behavior, buying, or investment sprees, unwise political alliances or overzealous religious involvements. Manic patients exhibit loquaciousness, racing thoughts and an infectious energetic air. They are often condescending and irritable, and may become belligerent if they are thwarted in acting out their grandiose intentions.

The term "hypomania" is used to describe less severe episodes, but at the other end of the spectrum, patients with full-blown mania can become psychotic. When actual psychosis is part of the picture, an essential feature of the diagnosis is that the patient has not evidenced bizarre behavior or preoccupation with delusions or hallucinations when the other signs of inflated mood and associated behavior have not been present. Such a historical determination allows differentiation of bipolar affective disorder (as manic-depressive illness is now called) from schizophrenia. This differentiation is sometimes difficult, but is extremely important in treatment planning. Manic episodes generally respond to lithium carbonate, while schizophrenic decompensations do not. The prognosis is better in a bipolar disorder than in schizophrenia.

Manic behavior is dramatic and disruptive; occurs in persons who commonly function well between episodes; and typically begins suddenly, escalating rapidly over a few days. Because of this, many patients having a first episode are likely to be referred for neurologic evaluation before psychiatric intervention is attempted. Some toxic states, especially amphetamine ingestion, can cause hyperactive behavior, but there are medical/neurologic situations that produce not just hyperactivity, but a mental and behavioral picture virtually indistinguishable from primary mania.

Manic-type illness, often with full-blown psychosis, develops in 10% to 14% of patients treated with high-dose steroids, thus complicating the treatment of the underlying problem, often a serious rheumatologic disease. Such episodes, even though directly related to steroid administration, tend to respond to treatment with lithium carbonate and antipsychotic medications. These medications may be stopped when steroids are reduced, but may need to be used again

Bipolar Affective Disorder: Manic Episode

"I bought eleven cars last week. I'll sell them all and make a fortune. I'm going to set up my own hospital and make us both famous"

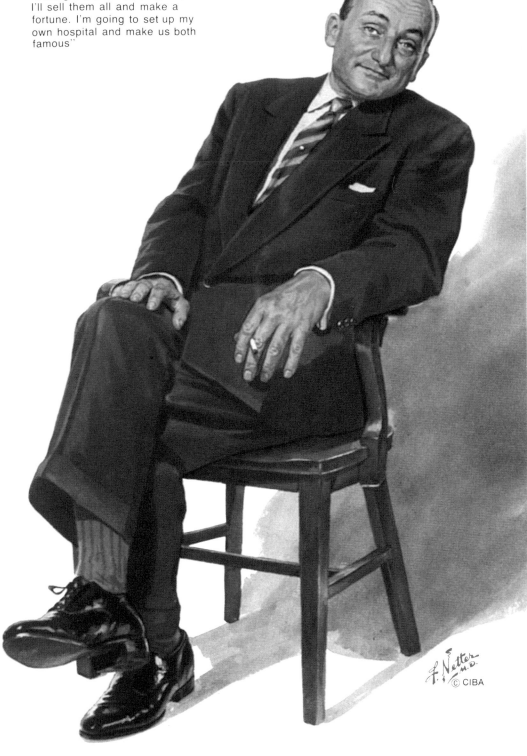

whenever a course of high-dose steroids is contemplated in susceptible patients.

An organic affective disorder indistinguishable from a manic episode also occasionally develops in patients who have a structural brain lesion. Such episodes have been reported in patients with tumor, trauma or a cerebrovascular accident in either hemisphere. Response to lithium has also been noted in patients with these lesions, but experience has suggested that when a structural brain lesion is associated with mania, even without obvious seizure activity, carbamazepine may be useful. A first manic episode in a patient who is over 50 years of age should suggest an underlying organic neurologic disease or toxic factors.

Antipsychotic medications and lithium carbonate are used to treat acute manic episodes, with a maintenance dosage of lithium alone continued as prophylaxis against repeat episodes. Although about 25% of patients with a first manic episode have no further episodes even if not treated pharmacologically, the great majority of patients with bipolar affective disorder require chronic treatment with lithium. The medication can be maintained in a therapeutic range and toxic levels avoided by monitoring blood levels. At therapeutic blood levels, long-term renal or thyroid toxic effects develop in only a few patients, and the risk of these effects is acceptably low versus the benefits of controlling a disabling mental illness. □

Anxiety State

Anxiety State

"Doctor, I'm worried, but I don't know why. I'm just worried. I have no reason to be, but I am"

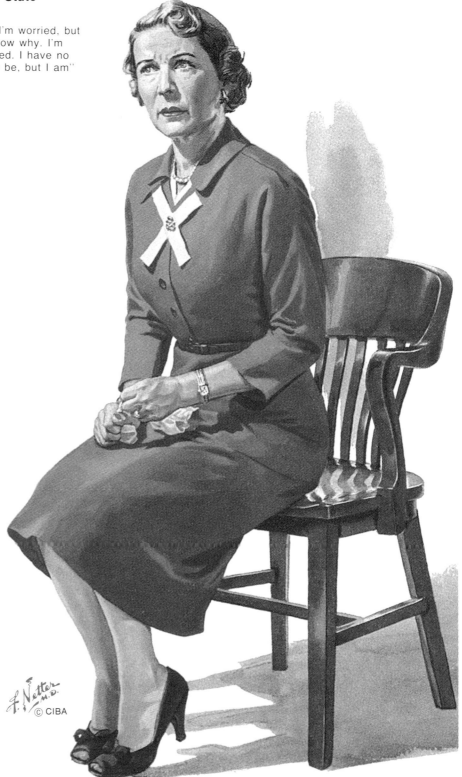

One of the major contributions of newer psychiatric nomenclature has been the separation of the concepts of panic disorder and generalized anxiety disorder (in which anxiety is the primary problem) from other anxiety states such as phobic, obsessive-compulsive and posttraumatic disorders. In the latter conditions, anxiety develops when a person tries to master other symptoms.

Such diagnostic distinctions allow more consistent communication about anxiety problems. However, given the fact that anxiety also occurs in adjustment disorders and other primary psychiatric illnesses, some clinician/researchers have begun to use a diagnostic concept previously popular in conceptualizing depression: endogenous symptoms versus exogenous symptoms. This concept allows a logical and simplified approach to patients who exhibit primary symptoms of anxiety.

The concept of *endogenous anxiety* parallels that of panic disorder. Panic attacks, with their dramatic, spontaneous and unprovoked symptoms of dyspnea, palpitations, chest pain, choking, dizziness, paresthesias, sweating, tremulousness and feelings of impending doom, are thought to be endogenous, biochemical phenomena. A history showing that such attacks are unrelated to environmental stimuli is very important and must be carefully elicited from the patient. A patient with spontaneous attacks may explain them as a response to some specific event or place. However, careful questioning may show that the symptoms have occurred at other times and in other places and situations.

Conversely, a patient may perceive symptoms of anxiety as spontaneous and inexplicable, but careful questioning may reveal a pattern of anxiety symptoms associated with specific events, situations, relationships or conflicts. This is considered *exogenous, or reactive, anxiety*. Under this rubric can also be included causes of anxiety symptoms such as abuse of caffeine, over-the-counter sympathomimetics or other substances or withdrawal syndromes. A few physical conditions such as hyperthyroidism or hypoglycemia may cause anxiety symptoms, but are usually revealed by a thorough history and physical examination and the indicated laboratory studies.

When a carefully elicited history indicates a diagnosis of endogenous anxiety, treatment is also endogenous. Biochemical/pharmacologic treatment is considered most useful. Imipramine, monoamine oxidase (MAO) inhibitors, and one

specific benzodiazepine (alprazolam) have been equally effective in reducing the frequency and severity of panic attacks. Since other benzodiazepines are not specific for panic and since the tricyclic antidepressants and MAO inhibitors are of little use in reactive anxiety, the historical differentiation of endogenous and exogenous anxiety is important.

Exogenous anxiety implies a need either to deal with the anxiety-provoking stimuli or to improve mechanisms for coping with environmental problems. Changes in stressful situations, confrontation of smoldering conflicts, relaxation training, and cognitive restructuring of the patient's views of the situation are helpful. Avoiding caffeine,

getting regular exercise, having good nutrition, and generally gaining control of those things that are amenable to control are also often useful. Any medication used to treat exogenous anxiety should be a benzodiazepine that meets the patient's requirements for rapidity of onset, duration of action, amount of sedation and method of administration. Drugs should be used with specific goals and time limitations in mind and as adjuncts to nonpharmacologic treatments.

Deciding whether a patient's anxiety is endogenous or exogenous is the key to choosing the best treatment. Whether or not the patient has reason to be worried, the astute clinician can usually help alleviate anxiety symptoms. □

Schizophrenic Disorder

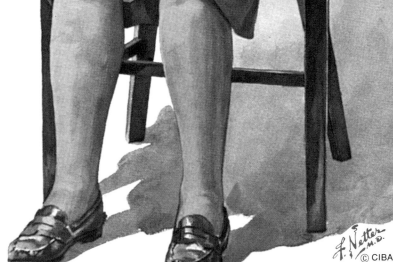

Schizophrenic Disorder

"I know that my head aches because they're putting wires in my brain. The voices control all my thoughts and try to drive me crazy"

Schizophrenia is a concept that has occupied physicians since the eighteenth century, although the name itself was not introduced until 1911. The most recent diagnostic criteria of the American Psychiatric Association are found in the third edition of the *Diagnostic and Statistical Manual of Mental Disorders*. These criteria are classified into six categories, all of which are important in making a diagnosis of schizophrenic disorder.

The first category includes those symptoms that indicate *psychosis*, including various kinds of delusions, auditory hallucinations, incoherence, loosely associated or illogical thinking associated with flat or inappropriate affect, and catatonic or disorganized behavior. Although the diagnosis of schizophrenic disorder of necessity includes at least one psychotic symptom during some phase of the illness, the presence of one or more of these symptoms does not necessarily indicate a diagnosis of schizophrenia.

Psychosis can be a symptom of all types of organic brain problems, drug intoxication, certain seizures, or other mental illnesses such as mania or depression. Therefore, the diagnosis of schizophrenia currently requires that there has been deterioration in the previous level of functioning and continuous signs of the illness for at least 6 months at some time during the patient's lifetime (including an active phase with or without a carefully defined prodromal or residual phase). The onset of the prodromal or active phase must be before age 45. In addition, the full depressive or manic syndrome, if it is manifested, must have developed after the psychotic symptoms or must have been much more brief than the psychotic symptoms. The final criterion is that the symptoms are *not* due to any organic mental disorder or mental retardation.

The terms "disorganized," "catatonic," "paranoid," "undifferentiated" and "residual" are used to describe types of schizophrenia. Each type has its own additional diagnostic criteria. When a similar illness has a duration of less than 6 months or an onset after age 45, it can be called a "schizophreniform disorder," but not schizophrenia.

Clearly, if the label of schizophrenia is reserved for illnesses that meet the diagnostic criteria, two objectives can be met. First, a number of other, sometimes reversible, problems will not be included under the rubric of schizophrenia, with its overtones of grave prognosis and progressive functional decline. Brief reactive psychoses, affective disorders, hallucinogen and amphetamine use, partial complex seizures, psychotic symptoms in degenerative brain disease, or unacceptable behavior in patients with personality disorders have all been misdiagnosed as schizophrenia at times in the past.

Second, the use of accepted criteria allows greatly improved research. Despite enormous research effort, the cause of schizophrenic disorders remains elusive. The neurochemical hypothesis that involves increased dopaminergic activity in parts of the brain has had great heuristic value, but clearly is not an adequate explanation for all the phenomena grouped in the schizophrenia concept.

Schizophrenia offers many challenges. The diagnosis itself often requires collaboration to exclude other disorders. In addition, treatment may cause complications, other disorders may be superimposed, and somatic delusions must be differentiated from new organic complaints. Acute and chronic movement disorders are common and may be associated with the syndrome or, more commonly, with treatment with antipsychotic medications. These problems affect the chronic management of schizophrenia and require expert collaborative psychopharmacologic and long-term psychosocial interventions. □

Compulsive Personality Disorder

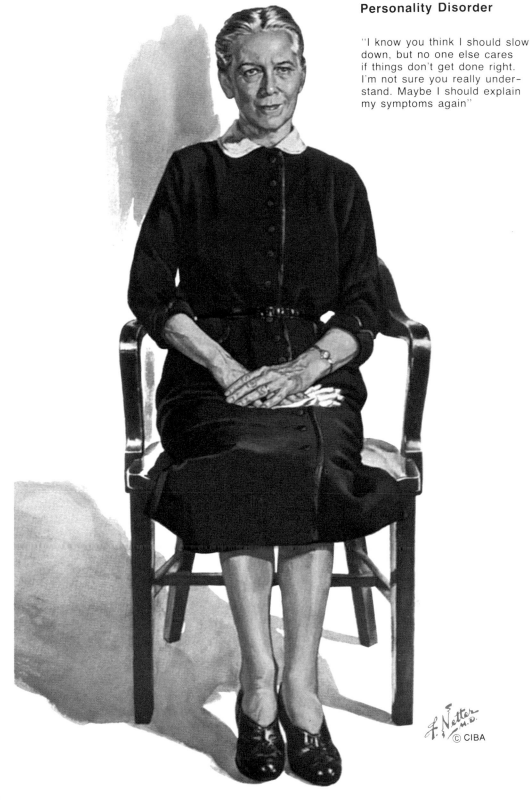

**Compulsive
Personality Disorder**

"I know you think I should slow
down, but no one else cares
if things don't get done right.
I'm not sure you really understand. Maybe I should explain
my symptoms again"

The neat and highly controlled patient shown in the illustration represents a stereotype of a person who might have a compulsive personality disorder. Such persons tend to be cold, formal, perfectionistic, work-addicted, judgmental, controlling of others, and indecisive because of their fear of making a mistake.

Patients with a compulsive personality might complain of a number of psychosomatic problems related to the impact of the personality disorder on their life and relationships. However, even when there is a clear-cut organic disorder in such a person that requires physician intervention, the personality disorder significantly affects the quality of the doctor-patient relationship. This is true of patients with any type of personality disorder. Thus, a basic understanding of the concept of personality disorder may be useful to all clinicians.

A normal person exhibits characteristic and preferred, but not exclusive, ways of thinking, acting and feeling. A personality disorder is characterized by traits that are limited in scope, rigid and maladaptive. When such narrowly focused, inflexible styles of perception, relationships and thinking significantly impair social or occupational functioning or lead to personal discomfort, a personality disorder can be diagnosed.

The third edition of the *Diagnostic and Statistical Manual of Mental Disorders* from the American Psychiatric Association lists diagnostic criteria for 12 different personality disorders, divided into three categories. Odd, bizarre or eccentric behavior often falls into a category that includes paranoid, schizoid and schizotypal personality disorders. Persons with an overly dramatic, emotional, erratic or impulsive personality are included in the histrionic, narcissistic, antisocial and borderline categories. Anxious or fearful behavior is classified with the avoidant, dependent, compulsive and passive-aggressive personality disorders.

Each disorder has distinct, descriptive diagnostic criteria. Atypical, mixed or other personality disorders may also be diagnosed, and a person may have more than one type of personality disorder. The superimposed diagnosis of personality disorder often explains some unusual presentation of other medical or psychiatric problems.

A personality disorder can affect the management of common neurologic problems. For example, the woman with the compulsive personality shown in the illustration could be expected to be very indecisive and hesitant about choosing treatment options for a vascular headache. She might insist on an extraordinary amount of explanation and information, but resist any attempt at advice for fear of losing control of the situation. Recognizing her needs while not resenting her perfectionistic judgment could allow a clinician to couch his advice in nonauthoritarian terms and leave much control to the patient.

Patients who are treated in a spinal cord injury center often display a personality disorder characterized by the dramatic and reckless or impulsive behavior that predisposed them to serious injuries. Understanding this aids in planning a rehabilitation program that requires certain kinds of motivated and cooperative patient behavior. In fact, understanding the characteristics of persons with any of the various personality disorders allows a personalized approach to each patient. Once it is established that a patient's problem behavior is characteristic, ie, fairly stable, expected and long-term, and is not some recent acute change due to another psychiatric or neurologic disorder, understanding personality disorders provides for a comfortable and effective doctor-patient relationship. □

Section VII

Degenerative Disorders of Central Nervous System

Frank H. Netter, M.D.

in collaboration with

Louis R. Caplan, M.D.   *Plates 1–8*
Roger C. Duvoisin, M.D.   *Plates 9–12*

Alzheimer's Disease: Clinical Manifestations, Progressive Phases

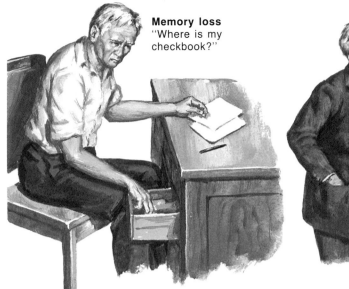

Memory loss
"Where is my checkbook?"

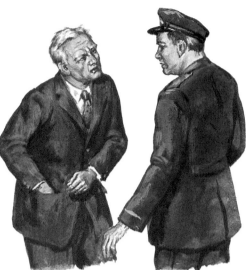

Spatial disorientation
"Could you direct me to my office? I have the address written down here somewhere, but I can't seem to find it"

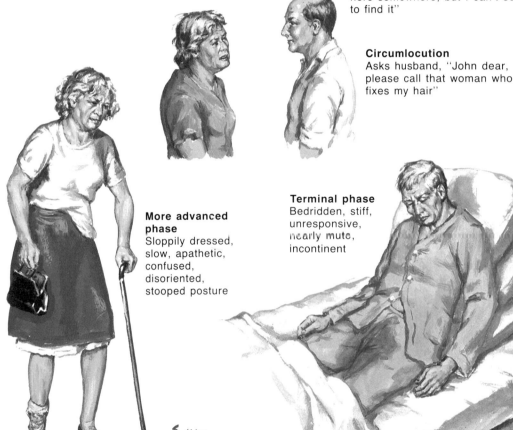

Circumlocution
Asks husband, "John dear, please call that woman who fixes my hair"

More advanced phase
Sloppily dressed, slow, apathetic, confused, disoriented, stooped posture

Terminal phase
Bedridden, stiff, unresponsive, nearly mute, incontinent

Although the clinical picture of all patients with Alzheimer's disease is not always the same, intellectual loss always precedes motor abnormalities. Posture, stance and gait are preserved until mental deterioration is extensive.

The *earliest stage* of Alzheimer's disease usually includes the following four abnormalities.

1. *Memory loss*. Patients cannot find objects that they have put away and forget details of recent conversations and events. When tested, they fail to recall events in a story, but may be able to correctly choose items in a series of alternative choices.

2. *Decreased language facility*. Written and verbal communications are less precise than normally and contain more "filler" words and circumlocutory elements. Perseveration is common. Patients cannot recall names, especially of people and later of objects, but retain the ability to understand and repeat spoken language and do not make paraphasic errors, in contrast to patients with aphasia due to stroke.

3. *Visual spatial dysfunction*. Patients often cannot find the way to their parked car and lose their sense of direction when traveling by foot or car, especially if the route is not extremely familiar. They cannot use maps and have difficulty in following verbal or written routings. Testing shows inability to draw a clock or a bicycle or copy a complex diagram.

4. *Apraxia*. Some patients lose the ability to carry out everyday activities, such as unlocking a door with a key, starting a car, dressing or playing the piano.

Although most patients have some abnormality in each of these areas, in an occasional patient, the clinical picture is dominated by aphasia, amnesia or apraxia disproportionate to other findings. In this early phase of Alzheimer's disease, patients' appearance, dress, expressions, mannerisms and interpersonal behavior seem normal. Only in substantive conversation does the intellectual deficit become apparent. Patients have no insight into their problem, and are usually taken to the physician by concerned friends and relatives.

The *second stage* of the illness begins years after onset and is dominated by abnormalities resulting

from progressive atrophy of the frontal lobe. Patients become increasingly apathetic and less interested in others and in their environment. They also lose interest in reading, television and social gatherings, and seem content to sit listlessly for hours at a time. Less attention is paid to grooming and attire, and even formerly fastidious people allow their house, room and belongings to become untidy and disorganized. Conversation is slow and less spontaneous. Gait slows and becomes a shuffle of small steps, and patients often grasp nearby objects. Occasionally, agitated or belligerent behavior occurs. Computed tomography (CT) at this stage shows widened sulci and enlarged ventricles, and the electroencephalogram

(EEG) reflects generalized slowing. Results of cerebrospinal fluid examination (CSF) and cerebral angiography are normal.

In the *advanced stage* of Alzheimer's disease, patients cannot perform the simple activities of daily living. They remain in bed unless they are helped up, and require aid for dressing, eating and toilet functions. They cannot venture out alone and become lost even in their home. They confuse night and day, and incontinence develops.

The course of the disease is usually from 3 to 10 years. In the terminal phase, patients are bedridden, mute and stiff unless life is cut mercifully short by pneumonia, urosepsis or decubitus ulcers. □

Alzheimer's Disease: Pathology

Regional atrophy of brain with narrowed gyri and widened sulci, but precentral and postcentral, inferior frontal, angular, supramarginal and some occipital gyri fairly well preserved. Association cortex mostly involved

Alzheimer's Disease: Pathology

Contrary to popular belief, Alzheimer's disease, or senile dementia of Alzheimer type (SDAT), is not generalized brain atrophy and is not caused by cerebrovascular disease. Despite the frequent use of the phrase "hardening of the arteries" in referring to Alzheimer's disease, there is no evidence that this disorder is related to stroke or to vascular degenerative disease. Certain brain regions, eg, the precentral, postcentral and some occipital gyri and parasylvian regions are spared, whereas the prefrontal, superior parietal and inferior temporal gyri are severely atrophied. Initially, atrophy affects the posterior parietal, inferior temporal and hippocampal regions; later, the frontal lobe becomes severely atrophic. Regions concerned with basic functions such as vision, hearing, somatosensory perception and movement are preserved, although regions important for cognitive function but not necessary for primitive survival are damaged.

The regions most involved in Alzheimer's disease are also especially vulnerable to chemical and metabolic derangements in the body. Alcohol and some drugs slow the thought processes and cause drowsiness, but do not ordinarily cause brain damage that would result in blindness, deafness or paralysis. Perhaps solving the mystery of why certain regions of the brain are selectively vulnerable to degeneration and intoxication may help unravel the cause of Alzheimer's disease.

Cut section of the brain shows enlargement of the ventricles and widening of the sylvian fissure. Many convexal gyri are shrunken, and the sulci between these gyri are widened. The cerebral cortex may appear thin, and the basal ganglia are relatively small. Microscopic examination of the affected regions shows a loss of neurons and an increase in glial cells and fibers. Many neurons contain neurofibrillary tangles that have been compared to tennis rackets, pretzels or skeins of wool. Although these tangles are visible on hematoxylin and eosin staining, silver stain impregnation methods show that they are accumulations of paired helical filaments containing cross-linked polypeptides. Senile plaques consisting of a central core of argyrophil amyloid material surrounded by astrocytes and microglia are plentiful and are also seen in the thalami and putamen. Some cells, especially in the hippocampus, contain granulovacuolar inclusions.

Blood vessels do not show any distinctive pathologic changes. Although some patients have

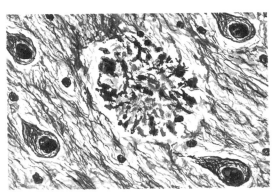

Senile plaque (center) made up of argyrophil fibers around core of pink-staining amyloid (Bodian preparation). Neurons decreased in number, with characteristic tangles in cytoplasm

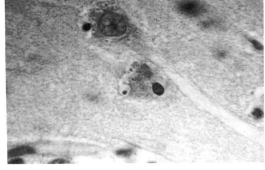

Section of hippocampus showing granulovacuolar inclusions and loss of pyramidal cells

Section of brain schematically demonstrating postulated normal transport of acetylcholine (ACh) from basal nucleus of Meynert (substantia innominata) to cortical gray matter

Basal nucleus

extensive atherosclerosis, with or without accompanying cerebral infarctions, in many patients, arteries are normal despite severe cerebral atrophy and dementia. Some patients with Alzheimer's disease also have vascular amyloid deposits stainable with Congo red.

Recent advances in chemical analysis have led to the assessment of the neurotransmitter and enzymatic composition of brain regions, which has helped define the chemical pathologic abnormalities in the various dementias. Biochemical data from study of biopsy specimens and autopsy findings in patients with Alzheimer's disease reveal an early decrease in *choline acetyltransferase* and *acetylcholinesterase*, indicating dysfunction in the neural pathways that use acetylcholine as a neurotransmitter. These chemical changes may precede obvious morphologic damage. In addition, the number of neurons is reduced in the basal nucleus of Meynert. Experimental studies show that loss of this region in animals results in a loss of acetylcholine markers in the cerebral cortex. Some investigators have also documented a loss of norepinephrine-containing cells in the locus ceruleus in patients with Alzheimer's disease. Cortical dysfunction could be the result of loss of basal corticopetal projections. Whether the origin of Alzheimer's disease is cortical or subcortical, its cause remains obscure and a major challenge for the future. □

Testing for Defects of Higher Cortical Function

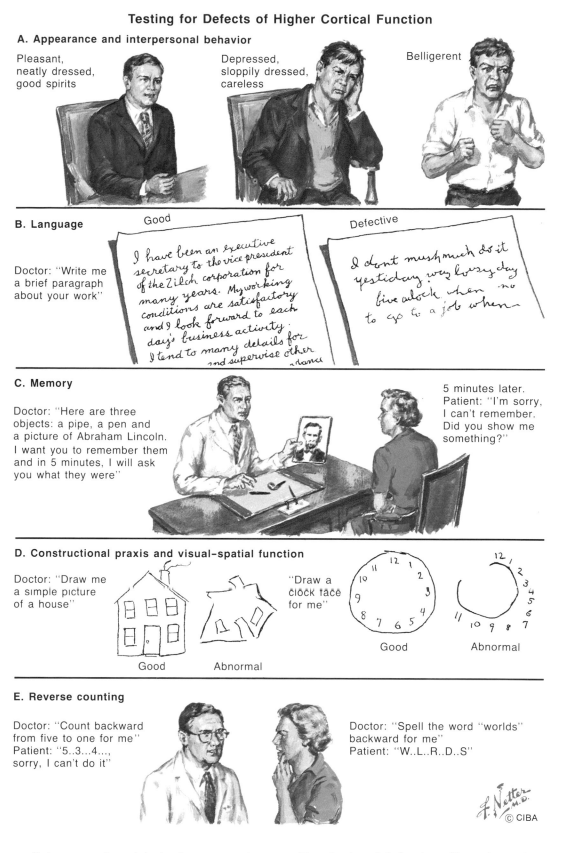

Testing for Defects of Higher Cortical Function

A. Appearance and interpersonal behavior

Pleasant, neatly dressed, good spirits

Depressed, sloppily dressed, careless

Belligerent

B. Language

Doctor: "Write me a brief paragraph about your work"

Good

Defective

C. Memory

Doctor: "Here are three objects: a pipe, a pen and a picture of Abraham Lincoln. I want you to remember them and in 5 minutes, I will ask you what they were"

5 minutes later. Patient: "I'm sorry, I can't remember. Did you show me something?"

D. Constructional praxis and visual–spatial function

Doctor: "Draw me a simple picture of a house"

Good   Abnormal

"Draw a clock face for me"

Good   Abnormal

E. Reverse counting

Doctor: "Count backward from five to one for me"
Patient: "5..3...4...,
sorry, I can't do it"

Doctor: "Spell the word "worlds" backward for me"
Patient: "W..L..R..D..S"

Only a small part of the human brain governs elementary sensory and motor functions; the greater portion of the brain is reserved for complex intellectual activity. It is the higher cortical function that determines how well a person relates to others, the environment, his work and society. Yet, evaluation of the very functions that differentiate man from beast is all too often omitted from the neurologic examination.

It is difficult to obtain an accurate quantitative assessment of intellectual function during a brief examination. Test results can be skewed by making questions too complicated when examining a patient with superior education who is suspected of having a deficit, or too simple when examining a patient with little education. Moreover, interests, experience and premorbid intelligence vary so widely that tests of general information, such as "Who are your local representatives or senators?" and "Who won the World Series last year?" are not helpful in detecting patients with brain disease. It is more important to test functions that can be localized to individual brain regions, since abnormalities on these tests reliably predict brain disease. For example, if a quantitative assessment is needed to use as a baseline for comparison with future tests or prior functioning, formal psychometric testing using the Wechsler-Bellevue intelligence scale or other standardized tests should be carried out.

Screening for disorders of higher cortical function can be done in 5 to 10 minutes, and should be carried out as follows.

Test language function. Ask the patient while in the waiting room to write a paragraph of introduction, giving his name, the date, nature of his work, and description of recent symptoms. No aphasic patient writes normally. Look for errors in spelling, grammar, use of words and repetitions, and note whether he has organized the paragraph coherently. Listen carefully to the use, rhythm and pronunciation of spoken language as the patient relates his history, and note whether he gives details of his symptoms. Ask the patient to read and interpret a paragraph, repeat aloud short phrases, and name common objects. Inability to perform any of these tasks indicates dysfunction of the parasylvian region of the dominant, usually left, cerebral hemisphere.

Test memory objectively. Usually, it is not possible to verify details from the patient's recent history or responses to questions such as "What did you have for lunch today?" or "What did you do yesterday?" Thus, it is important to test the patient's memory by asking him such things as to

recall the paragraph read during language testing. Other methods of testing memory are to ask the patient to identify pictures of three famous persons, to tell him a story and ask him to recall 5 to 10 facts from the story, or to ask him to recall three objects in the room, which were pointed out earlier. The most common abnormality of memory, "absentmindedness," is failure to concentrate. Thus, it is necessary to make certain that the patient repeats aloud the story or the list of objects and to emphasize that he later will be asked to recall them. Failure to perform satisfactorily tests of memory function may indicate local disease in the thalamus or medial temporal lobes or a generalized degenerative or metabolic process.

Test visual-spatial functions. Have the patient draw a clock, house, daisy or bicycle, and check for organization, angulation and asymmetry. Also ask the patient to copy a simple design. If the drawings indicate abnormal visual-spatial orientation, the patient may have a lesion in the right cerebral hemisphere.

Test ability to concentrate. Ask the patient to recite in reverse a series of numbers or to subtract 7s serially from 100. Also observe the patient's degree of alertness and orientation, manner of dress and grooming, and note whether the patient is happy, sad or indifferent and how he relates to others. Such objective observations are an important part of a complete neurologic examination. □

Dominant Hemisphere Language Dysfunction

Broca's aphasia • Global aphasia • Wernicke's aphasia • Conduction aphasia • Angular gyrus • Inferior temporal lobe • Occipital region

	Broca's aphasia	Wernicke's aphasia	Conduction aphasia	Angular gyrus	Inferior temporal lobe	Occipital region	Global aphasia
Pronunciation, speech rhythm	Dysarthria, stuttering, effortful	Normal, fluent, loquacious	Normal	Normal	Occasional pause in word finding	Normal	Very abnormal
Speech content	Missed syllables, agrammatical, telegraphic	Use of wrong or nonexistent words	Some wrong words	Often normal	Occasional circumlocution	Normal	Very abnormal
Repetition of speech	Abnormal but better than spontaneous	Abnormal	Abnormal	Normal	Normal	Normal	Very abnormal
Comprehension of spoken language	Normal	Very abnormal	Slightly abnormal	Normal	Normal	Normal	Very abnormal
Comprehension of written language	Not as good as for spoken language	Abnormal but better than for spoken	Often normal	Very abnormal	Normal	Very abnormal	Very abnormal
Writing	Clumsy, agrammatical, misspelling	Penmanship OK but misspelling and inaccuracies	Occasional spelling and language errors	Very abnormal, spelling errors	Normal	Normal	Very abnormal
Naming	Better than spontaneous speech	Wrong names	Occasional wrong names	Often abnormal	Very abnormal	Occasionally abnormal	Very abnormal
Other	Hemiplegia, apraxia	Sometimes hemianopsia and apraxia	Slight hemiparesis, neglect of right-sided stimuli	Slight hemiparesis, trouble calculating, finger agnosia, hemianopsia	——	Hemianopsia, color anomia	Hemiplegia

Slide 3431

Dominant Hemisphere Language Dysfunction

Aphasia, a disorder of language usage and comprehension, should be distinguished from *dysarthria*, impaired articulation and *mutism*, the absence of speech. Usually, the presence of aphasia accurately localizes dysfunction to the cerebral hemisphere concerned with speech.

To classify an aphasia, it is necessary to determine whether the patient can: (1) Speak fluently, with normal articulation and rhythm and without paraphasic, syntactical or grammatical errors or use of circumlocutory phrases. (2) Accurately repeat spoken sounds, words and phrases. (3) Understand spoken language, as evidenced by accurate responses to spoken questions and ability to follow spoken commands (failure to follow a command may be due to apraxia or paralysis and does not necessarily reflect poor comprehension). (4) Consistently name common objects, presented visually, verbally or tactilely. (5) Read aloud accurately and with comprehension. (6) Name words spelled aloud. (7) Write legibly and grammatically.

In *transcortical aphasia*, repetition of spoken language is preserved. *Transcortical motor aphasia* is characterized by inability to produce spontaneous speech, but ability to understand spoken language is retained. Failure to understand spoken language usually indicates a lesion deep in the basal ganglia or in the paramedian frontal lobe. Patients with Gerstmann's syndrome have difficulty with naming of fingers, left-right orientation, calculation, constructional drawing and writing. The lesion causing the disorder is usually located in the angular gyrus of the dominant hemisphere. □

Nondominant Hemisphere Higher Cortical Dysfunction

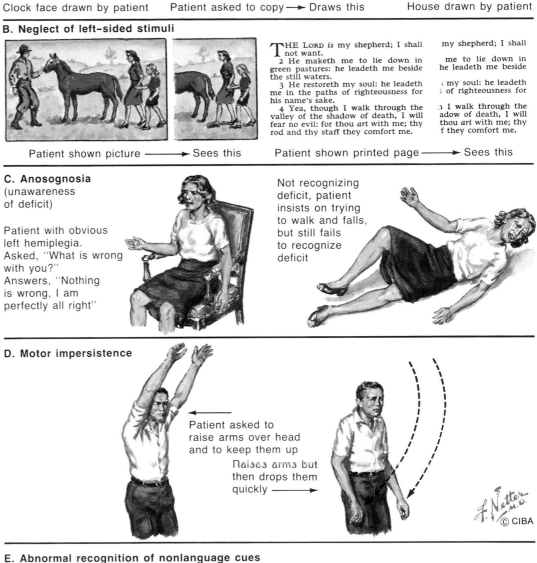

A. Constructional dyspraxia and spatial disorientation

Clock face drawn by patient   Patient asked to copy ⟶ Draws this   House drawn by patient

Nondominant Hemisphere Higher Cortical Dysfunction

B. Neglect of left–sided stimuli

Patient shown picture ⟶ Sees this   Patient shown printed page ⟶ Sees this

THE LORD *is* my shepherd; I shall not want.
2 He maketh me to lie down in green pastures: he leadeth me beside the still waters.
3 He restoreth my soul: he leadeth me in the paths of righteousness for his name's sake.
4 Yea, though I walk through the valley of the shadow of death, I will fear no evil: for thou *art* with me; thy rod and thy staff they comfort me.

my shepherd; I shall
me to lie down in
he leadeth me beside
, my soul: he leadeth
; of righteousness for
.1 I walk through the
adow of death, I will
thou *art* with me; thy
f they comfort me.

C. Anosognosia (unawareness of deficit)

Patient with obvious left hemiplegia. Asked, "What is wrong with you?" Answers, "Nothing is wrong, I am perfectly all right"

Not recognizing deficit, patient insists on trying to walk and falls, but still fails to recognize deficit

D. Motor impersistence

Patient asked to raise arms over head and to keep them up

Raises arms but then drops them quickly ⟶

F. Netter M.D.
© CIBA

E. Abnormal recognition of nonlanguage cues (facial expression, voice tone, mood)

Patient shown picture. Asked, "Which is the happy face?"

Patient answers, "I don't know, they are all the same"

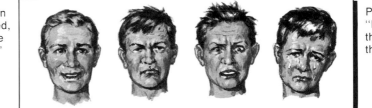

Patients with left-sided hemiplegia caused by damage to the nondominant right cerebral hemisphere do not recover as well as patients with similar left hemisphere lesions, despite the fact that they are not aphasic. Return to the work place and adequate home and family participation occur less frequently after a stroke causing left-sided hemiplegia. Although disturbances of higher cortical function and behavior in patients with right hemisphere disease are more subtle, they are equally or more functionally disabling than the more obvious aphasia caused by left hemisphere disease. Deficits in right hemisphere disease include the following.

Constructional Dyspraxia. The right cerebral hemisphere, especially its inferior parietal lobe, is specialized for visual-spatial functions. Parietal lesions compromise the patient's ability to draw and copy figures and diagrams, reproduce block designs or figures made with sticks or tongue blades, read a map, and follow or give directions to a given destination. Spontaneous drawings are complex and contain all appropriate details, but proportions, angles and picture relationships are inaccurate and the left half of the drawing often is omitted or minimized. Copying a figure does not significantly improve the performance.

Unilateral Spatial Neglect. Patients with right hemisphere lesions, especially those involving the frontal or parietal lobe or thalamus, often neglect objects, people or sounds on their left side. They may also fail to adequately dress the left side of their body. When asked to read a headline or paragraph or examine a picture, they do not appreciate words or objects on the left. When instructed to bisect all lines on a piece of paper, patients with right hemisphere damage often divide the right side of the line and fail to cross lines on the left side of the page. Similar spatial neglect of the right side after left hemisphere damage is unusual.

Anosognosia and Blunted Emotional Responses. Patients who have right hemisphere damage often fail to recognize or acknowledge an obvious left-sided hemiplegia. Not only do they verbally deny weakness or fail to localize it to one side, but they may fall when foolishly attempting to walk. Furthermore, even when they admit the deficit, these patients seem not to be appropriately concerned or distressed, and generally are not discouraged about their uncertain future.

Testing of patients with right hemisphere lesions also shows that they have difficulty in appreciating the tone, mood and emotional content of facial expressions or spoken language and miss nonlanguage cues. They also may be unable to invest their own voice or face with a given mood. Apathy and blunted recognition and transmission of emotional tone probably severely hamper rehabilitation and resumption of an active goal-oriented life.

Impersistence. Some patients with nondominant cerebral hemisphere damage are unable to persevere with a given task. A command that is quickly followed is just as quickly forgotten. When asked to keep their eyes closed, for example, or to

cross off all A's on a page, they begin the task correctly but soon abandon it. Questions are often answered before the query is complete. Impulsive behavior with little forethought and poor perseverance is also functionally disabling.

Other Dysfunctions. Damage to the right cerebral hemisphere can also affect either the ability to perceive rhythm, pitch or tonality or to read, write or play music. Some patients have difficulty in recognizing familiar faces (prosopagnosia), and may be unable to visualize from memory the appearance of an object or a person. Loss of topographical recall of places and errors of localization or distance concerning buildings or geographical landmarks also occur. □

Treatable Dementias

Mental decline is not an inevitable accompaniment of aging. Many elderly people remain mentally alert in their ninth and tenth decades. Moreover, the changes in mental function associated with many diseases that occur in the elderly are reversible.

Since Alzheimer's disease, or senile atrophy, is the most common cause of intellectual decline in later life (Plates 1–2), symptoms or signs that are unusual in Alzheimer's disease should particularly alert the physician to a different diagnosis and the possibility of reversing the dementing process. Such features include early age at onset; prominent headache; disturbances of gait or incontinence early in the course of the illness; epileptic seizures; fever; precipitous decline over a period of weeks or months; alteration of consciousness, especially sleepiness, stupor or delirium; history of head trauma; focal neurologic signs such as lateralized visual, motor or sensory abnormalities; accompanying dysfunction of peripheral nerves characterized by paresthesias and absent distal reflexes; and known systemic cancer, collagen vascular disease or endocrinopathy. The presence of any of these features should dictate further evaluation and consideration of the following treatable dementias.

Metabolic Disease With Encephalopathy. When intellectual decline is caused by systemic metabolic disease, there are usually four associated features: diminished alertness; asterixis; a global decrease in mental function, often with a flight of ideas; and variability of intellectual function during the day. The metabolic dysfunction can be either *endogenous* or *exogenous*. An endogenous abnormality indicates too much or too little of a substance or metabolite usually found in the body, such as calcium, sodium, thyroid hormone, sugar, etc.

Failure of the lungs, kidneys or liver is also in this category. Exogenous metabolic dysfunction is caused by a deficiency of a dietary substance, such as vitamin B_{12} or nicotinic acid, or by intoxication with a growing variety of agents, such as alcohol, barbiturates or narcotics.

Brain Tumors. Primary benign brain tumors such as meningiomas that affect the olfactory grooves and frontal lobes decrease mental function by pressing on brain tissue or by obstructing the ventricular system. Malignant primary metastatic tumors can also cause intellectual decline, usually with focal or multifocal signs and seizures.

Head Trauma. A history of head injury, sleepiness and slight lateralized weakness are clues, particularly to a subdural hematoma. The physician should be aware of this possibility, as many patients will have forgotten the inciting trauma by the time they seek medical attention.

Normal-Pressure Hydrocephalus. In most patients, this occult condition is unrecognized until the pathologic state causes overt symptoms (Plate 7).

Infection. An altered mental state, usually with headache and cerebrospinal fluid (CSF)

Treatable Dementias

Metabolic

- Hypothyroidism
- Hyperparathyroidism (hypercalcemia)
- Emphysema (CO_2 narcosis)
- Liver disease
- Pancreatic disease (hypoglycemia)
- Cortisol excess (Cushing's syndrome)
- Nutritional disorder (malabsorption, pellagra)
- Vitamin B_{12} deficiency (pernicious anemia)

Iatrogenic

Overmedication

Side effects

Surreptitious alcohol or drug abuse

Depressive pseudodementia

Subdural hematoma

Brain tumor

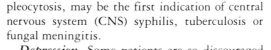

pleocytosis, may be the first indication of central nervous system (CNS) syphilis, tuberculosis or fungal meningitis.

Depression. Some patients are so discouraged and disinterested that they cannot and do not perform well. Called *depressive pseudodementia*, this condition often cannot be easily differentiated from true organic dementia except by the response to antidepressant therapy. To further complicate the diagnosis, many patients with Alzheimer's disease are depressed by their inabilities, and this depression further compromises their mental function.

Cerebrovascular Disease. Strokes can decimate the regions of the brain governing thought

processes. When this occurs, motor and reflex abnormalities usually parallel or exceed the degree of intellectual decline. Usually, the patient also has a history of an abrupt decline, as well as hypertension and coronary or peripheral vascular disease.

Diagnostic Studies. Screening of biochemical parameters, especially the vitamin B_{12} level and thyroid, renal, liver and lung function, is important in all demented patients. Computed tomography (CT), electroencephalography and CSF analysis also frequently detect unsuspected causes of dementia, and are indicated before a patient is institutionalized or given a diagnosis of irreversible dementia. □

Normal-Pressure Hydrocephalus

The "plumbing system" of the central nervous system (CNS) operates in a tenuous balance. Fluid produced in the choroid plexus of the lateral ventricles circulates through the third ventricle, cerebral aqueduct (of Sylvius) and fourth ventricle. After exiting from the roof of the fourth ventricle, the cerebrospinal fluid (CSF) circulates around the brain within the subarachnoid cisterns, and is ultimately absorbed by the arachnoid granulations into the circulation. If more CSF is produced than is absorbed, the ventricles and subarachnoid space distend with fluid. In the adult, this imbalance leads to enlargement of the ventricles, which then encroach on the normal cerebral white matter, especially frontally.

Conditions known to cause scarring of the pia-arachnoid membranes, such as meningeal infection, subarachnoid hemorrhage or bleeding from past trauma, can cause hydrocephalus by decreasing the effectiveness of CSF absorption. Altered resilience of white matter, as in patients with softening of white matter and basal ganglia resulting from hypertension, may contribute to ventricular enlargement. In most elderly patients, communicating hydrocephalus has no easily identifiable cause. The disorder develops insidiously. Although it could possibly result from senile degeneration of the arachnoid granulations and membranes, there has been little detailed study of the morphologic structure of the arachnoid in either normal persons or patients with hydrocephalus. Since the CSF pressure is usually high in obstructive hydrocephalus due to tumor and, for uncertain reasons, is within normal range in communicating hydrocephalus of the elderly, the latter disorder has been called normal-pressure hydrocephalus.

Normal-pressure hydrocephalus is a disease of the elderly. The condition usually develops over a period of 6 to 12 months, but at times progresses insidiously for a few years. Computed tomography (CT) shows markedly enlarged ventricles, often with little or no cortical atrophy.

Clinical Manifestations. Most symptoms relate to enlargement of the anterior (frontal) horns and loss of frontal lobe white matter. The three cardinal symptoms may be described as follows.

1. *Abnormality of gait.* The patient usually has difficulty arising from a chair, and cannot seem to initiate the first steps. Gait is slow and shuffling, with small steps.

2. *Dementia.* The patient shows decreased interest in the environment and seems apathetic. Speech becomes less spontaneous, and words are mumbled in a voice of lower volume than normal. Later, the patient may become mute. Despite the reduced amount of conversation, vocabulary and memory are preserved, and answers to questions, although terse, are usually correct.

3. *Incontinence.* The patient loses the ability to retain urine despite normal perception of the urge and need to urinate. The rapid course; prominence of apathy and early motor, gait and sphincter dysfunction; and slowness of preserved

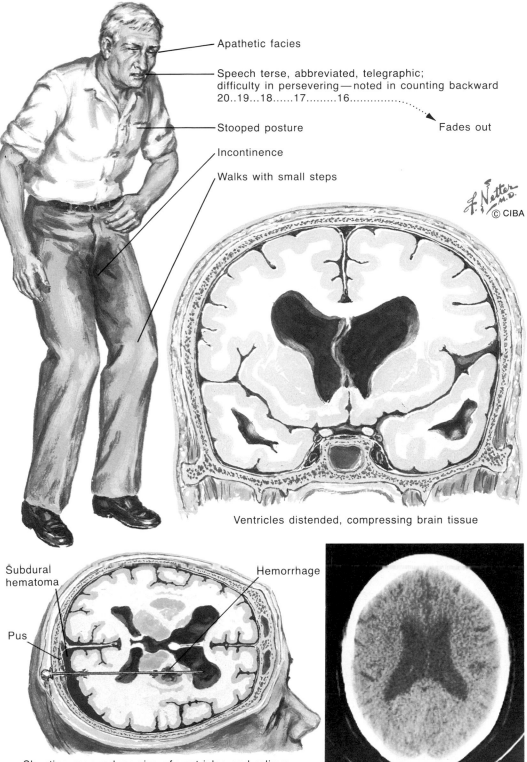

Apathetic facies

Speech terse, abbreviated, telegraphic; difficulty in persevering—noted in counting backward 20..19...18......17.........16.................
Fades out

Stooped posture

Incontinence

Walks with small steps

Ventricles distended, compressing brain tissue

Subdural hematoma

Hemorrhage

Pus

Shunting may reduce size of ventricles and relieve symptoms, but may cause hemorrhage along cannula tract, brain edema, subdural hematoma and infection

CT scan showing distended ventricles

memory function and vocabulary contrast with the findings in Alzheimer's disease, or senile dementia Alzheimer type (Plates 1–2).

Treatment. Spinal puncture with drainage of fluid can lead to temporary improvement in gait and alertness. Administration of *acetazolamide* reduces production of CSF and thus may improve the imbalance between production and absorption of CSF.

Cisternography after introduction of a radionuclide by lumbar puncture is of value in assessing abnormal CSF flow patterns. Unfortunately, however, there is no single definitive test that reliably predicts whether the patient will improve after surgical placement of a ventricular drain.

Ventricular shunts seem to be most effective in patients who have the classic triad of symptoms and in whom the course of the hydrocephalus has been short and a cause of the disorder, such as past subarachnoid hemorrhage, can be identified (see Section IV, Plate 10). Complications of ventriculoperitoneal shunts in adults include intracerebral or intraventricular hematoma during insertion of the tube; infection of the shunt and peritoneal space; oversiphoning of CSF, which causes subsequent brain swelling to take up the void; and collapse of the thin cerebral mantle, with tearing of bridging veins and formation of a subdural hematoma. The incidence of subsequent shunt infection is high. □

Chorea

The term "chorea" was originally selected because involuntary movements periodically interrupted gait and superficially resembled a dance. The term is now used to describe quick, complex and diverse adventitious movements affecting multiple regions of the body, particularly the distal limb muscles. Although choreiform movements may occur in many different conditions, Huntington's disease and Sydenham's chorea are common prototypes.

Huntington's Disease. This degenerative disorder of autosomal dominant inheritance is characterized by abnormal facial and limb movements, behavioral disturbances and progressive dementia. Onset is usually after age 40. Recent studies indicate that the marker for Huntington's disease probably involves the gene sequence on a single chromosome. Approximately half of the patient's progeny will be affected. However, if a person with an affected parent escapes the disease, so will all his children.

The patient often tries to hide the movements by incorporating them into purposeful patterns of movement, such as licking the lips after involuntary tongue protrusion or smoothing the hair after sudden arm flexion. However, in fully developed disease, grimacing, eyebrow elevation, tongue protrusion, lip and eyelid twitches, and flinging movements of limbs are sudden and dramatic. When walking, the patient may veer suddenly or exhibit abnormal posturing.

The earliest manifestations of mental deterioration are unwise, ill-considered, impulsive social or business behavior and uninhibited interpersonal relationships. Later, judgment, logic and ability to perform sequential tasks deteriorate. Although the movement disorder and dementia usually develop and progress together, one may precede the other by months or years. Rarely, the disease develops in childhood or early adult life.

Huntington's disease progresses inexorably during a 5- to 10-year period. Terminally, the patient is bedridden, mute and immobilized by severe rigidity. Autopsy reveals severe *shrinkage* of the *caudate nucleus* and *cortical atrophy*, especially frontally. Computed tomography (CT) documents prominent caudate atrophy.

Sydenham's Chorea. A major clinical manifestation of rheumatic fever, Sydenham's chorea is now uncommon. Abnormal flexion or abduction of single digits or joints produces characteristic "piano playing" movements of the outstretched limbs, giving the patient a "nervous" or "twitchy" appearance. Ataxia, weakness and reflex abnormalities may also occur.

Central nervous system (CNS) findings are probably related to rheumatic vasculitis or other immunogenically mediated damage to the *basal ganglia*. The disease is self-limited but is a marker for rheumatic disease, indicating need for prophylaxis against streptococcal infection.

Differential Diagnosis. In the absence of rheumatic fever or a family history of Huntington's disease, choreiform movements have diverse causes. Systemic and biochemical disturbances such as *intoxification with pharmacologic agents*, especially phenytoin, barbiturates, antihistamines or antipsychotic drugs, can cause chorea. Choreic

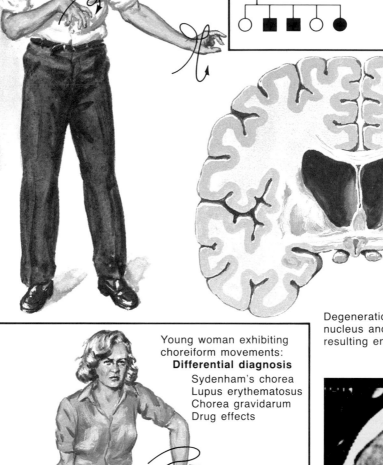

Huntington's disease
Middle-aged person: mental deterioration, grimacing, choreiform movements

Chorea

Genetic chart (example)

Young woman exhibiting choreiform movements:
Differential diagnosis
Sydenham's chorea
Lupus erythematosus
Chorea gravidarum
Drug effects

Degeneration and atrophy of caudate nucleus and cerebral cortex, with resulting enlargement of ventricles

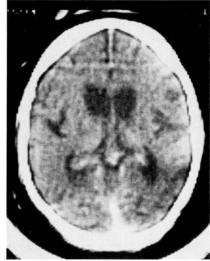

CT scan of brain: atrophy of caudate nucleus and enlargement of ventricles

movements without other CNS manifestations such as seizures, cerebrospinal fluid (CSF) pleocytosis or psychosis may develop in patients with *systemic lupus erythematosus*. A disorder referred to as *chorea gravidarum* affects pregnant women, and female patients who previously had Sydenham's chorea may have recurrences when pregnant or while taking contraceptives, indicating a sensitivity of chorea to female hormones. *Lacunar infarcts* in the basal ganglia can cause hemichorea.

Differential diagnosis must include consideration of: *athetosis*—slow, vermicular, almost sinusoidal alterations in limb postures; *ballism*—sudden flinging movements of the proximal limbs; *dystonia*—fixed, abnormal postures of the limbs and trunk; and *myoclonus*—sudden, often synchronized stereotyped single movements of a joint or limb. These organic movement disorders also must be distinguished from *hysterical* gyrations and psychogenic repetitive, stereotyped *tics*.

Differentiating the organic movement disorders is often difficult and arbitrary. In practice, most clinicians use pattern recognition for classification. Do the patient's abnormal movements resemble those in patients with known Huntington's disease or Sydenham's chorea or are they more like athetosis caused by perinatal cerebral damage? All these abnormal movements, with the exception of myoclonus, reflect damage to extrapyramidal structures. □

Parkinsonism

Parkinsonism is primarily a patho-physiologic state resulting from dysfunction of brain dopaminergic systems. The dysfunction may be caused by involvement of the pigmented dopaminergic neurons of the substantia nigra by various disease processes, loss of the striatal neurons receiving dopaminergic input from the substantia nigra, or metabolic disorders or pharmacologic agents that impair dopaminergic neurotransmission in the basal ganglia. Thus, parkinsonism is clinically a syndrome of diverse causes.

Various types of parkinsonism can be differentiated according to etiologic factors, associated features and pathologic findings, and can be classified as follows: Parkinson's disease, postencephalitic parkinsonism, iatrogenic parkinsonism, parkinsonism as part of a widespread degenerative process, symptomatic parkinsonism and pseudoparkinsonism.

Parkinson's Disease (Idiopathic Parkinsonism, Paralysis Agitans). This prototypical form of parkinsonism is by far the most common type, affecting about 1% of the population over age 50. The disease begins insidiously and slowly progresses at a variable rate for 10 to 20 years or more before culminating in severe invalidism.

The basic disease process in untreated patients can be divided into five stages (Plates 10–11).

Stage 1: mild, usually unilateral disease. The most common initial symptom is a tremor of one upper limb at rest. Vague prodromal aches and pains may precede the tremor by a year or more.

Examination reveals other abnormalities, even though the patient may complain only of tremor. A slight lateral tilt of the trunk away from the side affected by tremor may be noted. The patient tends to carry the involved upper limb in a position of slight abduction at the shoulder and flexion at the elbow (Plate 10). Use of the arm in gesturing and swing of the arm while walking are diminished. Mild rigidity, evidence of akinesia, and impairment of rapid alternating movements (dysdiadochokinesia) and finger dexterity are apparent on further examination. The movements are slow and deteriorate rapidly on repetition. If the dominant upper limb is involved, handwriting shows characteristic changes, including micrographia, tremulousness and poorly formed loops (Plate 9).

Ipsilateral facial hypomimia mimicking a central facial paresis is often present. On the affected side, the palpebral fissure may be narrowed, and the nasolabial fold and normal wrinkles of the forehead may be less pronounced. Seborrhea of the forehead is occasionally present.

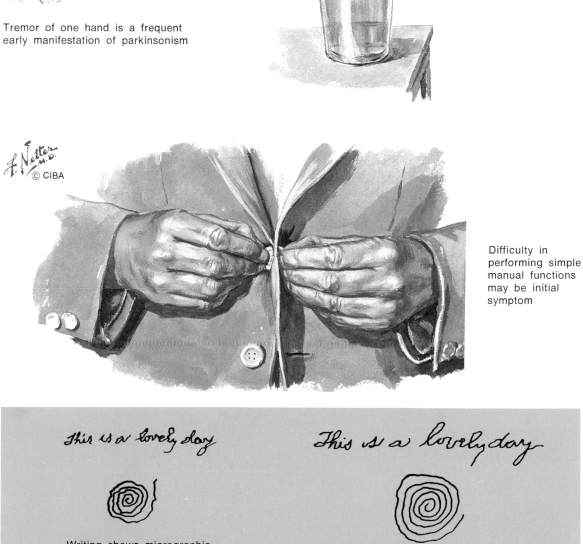

Tremor of one hand is a frequent early manifestation of parkinsonism

Tremor often improves or disappears with purposeful function

Difficulty in performing simple manual functions may be initial symptom

Writing shows micrographia and effects of tremor

Improvement after levodopa therapy

The classic triad of parkinsonism (tremor, rigidity and akinesia) and mild edema of the foot and ankle may also be seen in the lower limb of the affected side; yet, the patient may be quite unaware of any disability.

In this early stage of Parkinson's disease, the signs and symptoms are largely, although not completely, confined to one side, and the patient is said to have "hemiparkinsonism." In most patients, the disease becomes bilateral within 1 or 2 years. Often, however, the side first affected remains more severely affected throughout the course of the illness.

Stage 2: bilateral involvement with early postural changes. As the clinical manifestations of Parkinson's disease gradually become bilateral, the patient assumes a stooped posture on standing and walking. The trunk is inclined forward, and the vertebral column, hips, knees and ankles are slightly flexed.

The fingers tend to remain adducted at rest, with the metacarpophalangeal and distal interphalangeal joints slightly flexed and the proximal interphalangeal joints extended. The wrist is dorsiflexed. The foot tends to assume a slight varus position, with some clawing of the toes.

All movements gradually become slower (bradykinesia) and more deliberate. The patient may complain of fatigue, weakness and lethargy, but usually is unaware of the slowness. Later,

Parkinsonism
(*Continued*)

when bradykinesia becomes well established, the patient may admit that simple tasks require undue time and effort (Plate 9). Movements normally performed unconsciously, such as swinging the arms when walking, facial expressions, etc, become diminished. Walking is reduced to a slow, shuffling gait (Plate 10). Changes in direction are executed with deliberation.

The patient is eventually compelled to retire from regular employment. At this time, many patients begin to withdraw gradually from social activities and abandon interests. Reactive depression often develops. However, physical disability is still minimal.

Stage 3: pronounced gait disturbances and moderate generalized disability. The onset of retropulsion and propulsion reflects increasing impairment of postural reflexes and marks the beginning of the third stage in Parkinson's disease (Plate 10). Retropulsion occurs initially; propulsion tends to develop somewhat later. The patient's steps become progressively faster and shorter, and the trunk inclines further forward. Retropulsion and propulsion eventually become severe and begin to cause falls. Walking becomes slower and more hesitant. Other movements are hesitant and may be arrested suddenly. As bradykinesia progresses and movement becomes extremely slow, the disabled patient begins to accept occasional assistance in dressing and in minor tasks.

Stage 4: significant disability. After a variable number of years and further progression of Parkinson's disease, the patient requires frequent assistance in completing the activities of daily living and is no longer able to live alone. Tremor may be less marked than in earlier stages; however, rigidity and bradykinesia are disabling, and all movements become slow and uncertain. Standing is unsteady; a slight push precipitates severe retropulsion, culminating in a fall if the patient is not caught. The gait is festinating; propulsion and retropulsion are severe, and the patient falls frequently if left unattended.

Finger dexterity is also usually impaired. Tasks requiring fine motor control are difficult or impossible. Eating utensils can still be managed, but food must be specially prepared and served in small pieces.

Stage 5: complete invalidism. Eventually, the patient becomes severely bradykinetic and rigid and is a complete invalid (Plate 11). Tremor is no longer significant, but little, if any, voluntary motor function remains. The patient cannot stand, and walking is impossible.

Stage 1: unilateral involvement; blank facies; affected arm in semiflexed position with tremor; patient leans to unaffected side

Stage 2: bilateral involvement with early postural changes; slow, shuffling gait with decreased excursion of legs

Stage 3: pronounced gait disturbances and moderate generalized disability; postural instability with tendency to fall

In bed, the patient lies supine and motionless; the head is rigidly flexed on the trunk. The legs, slightly flexed at the hips, are adducted and held tightly together, and the feet are plantar flexed and adducted. Both arms are slightly abducted and flexed, the wrists are dorsiflexed, and the fingers are deformed. Dystonic posturing of the limbs is often fixed by contractures.

Speech is a soft, barely intelligible monotone but is surprisingly rapid. The face is expressionless, and blinking is infrequent. Retraction of the upper eyelids gives the appearance of intense staring. The mouth is constantly open, and, because of dysphagia and reduced spontaneous swallowing, drooling is present. Feeding now becomes

difficult and time-consuming; dehydration and cachexia often result.

The clinical picture is further complicated by the ever-present danger of infection from diminished thoracic excursion and ineffectual cough, neurogenic bladder dysfunction, and constant confinement to bed. Despite the most heroic therapeutic efforts, the patient eventually succumbs to an intercurrent infection.

Postencephalitic Parkinsonism. This disorder represents almost exclusively the sequelae of encephalitis lethargica (von Economo's disease), which occurred in scattered epidemics throughout the world from 1916 to 1926. Recovery from the acute phase of this disease was followed by the

Parkinsonism
(Continued)

gradual development of a parkinsonian syndrome distinguished from Parkinson's disease by the youth of the patients; by a predominance of bradykinesia and rigidity; and by many additional features, notably behavioral disorders and oculogyric crises. A transient parkinsonian syndrome may occur during the acute and convalescent phases of various types of viral encephalitis.

Iatrogenic Parkinsonism. A condition closely resembling Parkinson's disease may be induced by various agents that interfere with dopamine metabolism. These include drugs inhibiting dopamine synthesis, such as alpha methylparatyrosine and, rarely, methyldopa; drugs causing depletion of brain dopamine (eg, reserpine); and the numerous dopamine receptor blocking agents (eg, the major tranquilizers).

Parkinsonism in Degenerative Disorders. Brain dopaminergic neural systems may be involved, along with other systems, as a part of a more widespread degenerative disorder, such as olivopontocerebellar atrophy, striatonigral degeneration, progressive supranuclear palsy, the Parkinson-dementia complex and the Shy-Drager syndrome. Wilson's disease, a major cause of juvenile parkinsonism, may also be included.

Symptomatic Parkinsonism. Various congenital, traumatic, neoplastic and inflammatory lesions may rarely involve the substantia nigra and thus cause a parkinsonian syndrome. Although unilateral lesions causing contralateral hemiparkinsonism are extremely rare, they have contributed to the understanding of the pathophysiology of parkinsonism.

Pseudoparkinsonism. Arteriosclerosis with multiple small cerebral infarctions; gait apraxias of varied cause, including normal-pressure hydrocephalus; and, rarely, hypoparathyroidism all mimic parkinsonism, and differentiation may be difficult.

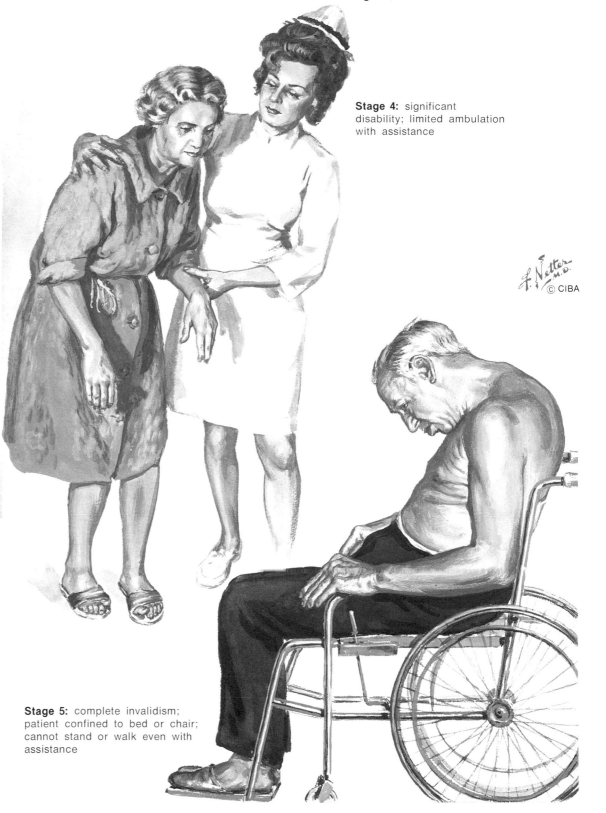

Stage 4: significant disability; limited ambulation with assistance

Stage 5: complete invalidism; patient confined to bed or chair; cannot stand or walk even with assistance

Pathology

At postmortem examination, the degeneration of the substantia nigra in Parkinson's disease is evident as a loss of the normal black pigmentation. Microscopic examination shows loss of neuronal cells and mild reactive gliosis, notably in the substantia nigra, locus ceruleus, substantia innominata and certain reticular nuclei. The amount of pigment in surviving neurons is decreased. Many neurons contain small eosinophilic granular bodies and distinctive cytoplasmic inclusions known as Lewy bodies, which are also eosinophilic, spherical and usually laminated; three or four of these inclusions may be seen in a single neuron. Lewy bodies are found mainly in the substantia nigra and locus ceruleus. They are

highly characteristic of Parkinson's disease and are believed to be a metabolic product rather than a virus or virion, but their origin and chemical nature remain largely unknown.

Atrophy, cell loss and neurofibrillary tangles are also found at autopsy in the cerebral cortex in over half of the patients with Parkinson's disease. Cerebral cortical degeneration is the pathologic basis for the progressive dementia that may occur in patients with advanced parkinsonism. In patients with postencephalitic parkinsonism, progressive supranuclear palsy or the parkinsonism-dementia complex, neurofibrillary tangles are characteristic in the substantia nigra. These tangles are similar to those of Alzheimer's

disease; they appear as bands or coils of argyrophil material that largely replaces the cytoplasm of the neurons (Plate 2).

The nigral degeneration in parkinsonism was rendered significant by the discovery that these neurons were dopaminergic and projected principally to the neostriatum, where the dopaminergic nerve fibers form a dense network throughout the caudate nucleus and putamen.

In Parkinson's disease, the loss of striatal dopamine correlates with the degree of neuronal cell loss in the substantia nigra. Studies have shown that drugs that interfere with dopamine metabolism or neurotransmission, such as reserpine, induce a "chemical" form of parkinsonism.

Parkinsonism
(Continued)

Dopamine is believed to act as a neuro-modulator in the striatum, reacting with specific receptor sites on striatal neurons.

Treatment

The goal in treatment of parkinsonism is to replenish striatal dopamine stores. Dopamine cannot cross the blood-brain barrier; therefore, therapy consists of administering its metabolic precursor, levodopa, which can cross the barrier.

Orally administered levodopa is absorbed into the circulation principally from the proximal small intestine. Most of it is promptly converted to dopamine by the enzyme aromatic L-amino-acid decarboxylase (dopa decarboxylase), which is present in the walls of blood vessels throughout the body. Levodopa can be detected in the blood for several hours following an oral dose, peak levels being found 2 to 3 hours following ingestion. Presumably, about 1% of the oral dose penetrates the cerebral capillaries to diffuse through the brain parenchyma, where it is picked up and converted to dopamine in the remaining dopaminergic neurons, probably throughout the length of the nerve fibers. Dopamine probably is then stored in neurosecretory vesicles for subsequent release from the neuronal varicosities into the striatal neuropil (Plate 12). It is rapidly deactivated, principally to homovanillic acid, and nearly all the levodopa administered orally is excreted as this metabolite.

Levodopa is the most effective treatment currently available for Parkinson's disease. It is also useful in postencephalitic parkinsonism and in some patients in whom parkinsonism is part of a widespread degenerative process. However, levodopa is not helpful in pseudoparkinsonism or in the iatrogenic syndrome induced by dopamine receptor blockers, such as the phenothiazines and related drugs used as major tranquilizers.

Dopa decarboxylase plays a crucial role in levodopa therapy. If the activity of this enzyme is enhanced in peripheral tissues, the rate of conversion of levodopa to dopamine is increased, and less levodopa remains to cross the blood-brain barrier. For example, pyridoxine (vitamin B_6), a cofactor for dopa decarboxylase, enhances the enzyme's activity. As a result, coadministration of pyridoxine markedly antagonizes or totally abolishes the effect of levodopa. By contrast, if the activity of dopa decarboxylase in peripheral tissues is inhibited, more levodopa is available for uptake by dopaminergic neurons in the brain. Among the

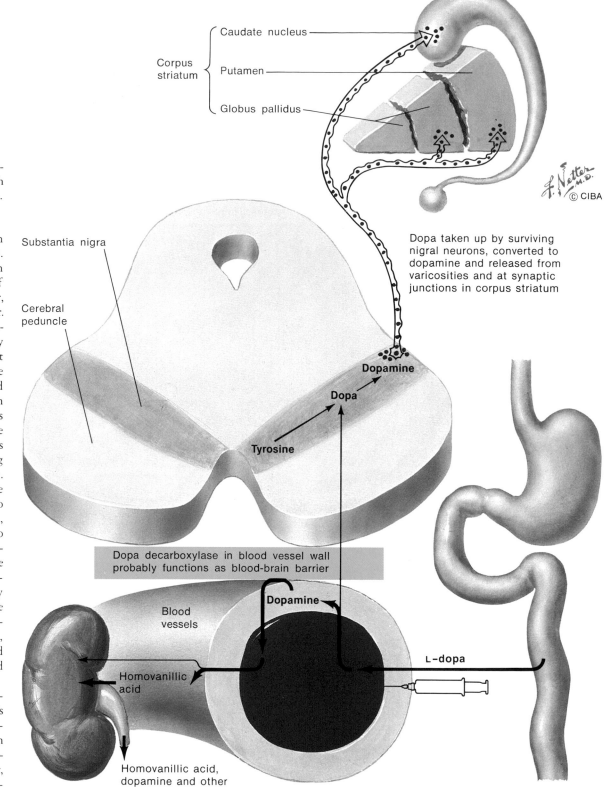

Corpus striatum
- Caudate nucleus
- Putamen
- Globus pallidus

Dopa taken up by surviving nigral neurons, converted to dopamine and released from varicosities and at synaptic junctions in corpus striatum

Substantia nigra

Cerebral peduncle

Dopamine

Dopa

Tyrosine

Dopa decarboxylase in blood vessel wall probably functions as blood-brain barrier

Blood vessels

Dopamine

Homovanillic acid

Homovanillic acid, dopamine and other metabolites

L-dopa

drugs that inhibit peripheral dopa decarboxylase activity are alpha-methyldopa, benserazide and alpha-methyldopa hydrazine. Of these, alpha-methyldopa hydrazine is approved in the United States for use in conjunction with levodopa. It is usually used in a ratio of 1 part alpha-methyldopa hydrazine to 10 parts levodopa.

The chief *side effects* during the initial phases of treatment are *anorexia, nausea* and *vomiting*, reflecting a central emetic action. However, the use of levodopa combined with a dopa decarboxylase inhibitor largely eliminates these side effects; presumably, the inhibitor blocks the conversion of levodopa to dopamine in the medullary vomiting center and prevents activation of the center.

The major dose-limiting side effect of levodopa therapy is *adventitious involuntary movements*, usually choreiform, in about 80% of patients. Most frequently seen are head nodding, grimacing, alternate opening and closing of the mouth, tongue protrusion, exaggerated gestures, exaggerated arm swinging when walking, and increased respiratory movements. These adventitious movements subside when the dosage of levodopa is decreased. Thus, the physician must seek the dosage that yields the best compromise between the involuntary movements and relief of the parkinsonism. This "seesaw" relationship between parkinsonism and chorea appears to be inherent in the pathophysiology of parkinsonism. □

Section VIII

Infectious Diseases

Frank H. Netter, M.D.

in collaboration with

Ann Sullivan Baker, M.D.   *Plates 1–5, 7*

William S. Fields, M.D.   *Plate 6*

Martin S. Hirsch, M.D.   *Plates 12–13*

H. Royden Jones, Jr., M.D.   *Plates 8, 11*

Albert B. Sabin, M.D.   *Plates 9–10*

Bacterial Meningitis

Pathophysiology. Infection of the lepto-meninges within the subarachnoid space, or meningitis, is usually caused by spread of an infectious agent via the bloodstream from an infective focus elsewhere in the body, such as otitis media, naso-pharyngeal infection, pneumonitis or, less commonly, a skin infection. Contiguous spread of infection from the paranasal sinuses or mastoid or via a perforating head or spinal injury or congenital dural defect is a less frequent cause of meningitis.

The identity of the infecting organism may be suspected by considering the patient's age group. In neonates, gram-negative organisms such as *Escherichia coli* account for more than 50% of cases, and group B streptococci account for about 20% (Plate 1). These organisms are acquired during passage through the birth canal. The organism that most commonly causes meningitis in children from age 2 months to 3 years is *Haemophilus influenzae*. *Neisseria meningitidis* is seen most frequently in meningitis in young adults and especially in outbreaks in overcrowded areas. *Streptococcus pneumoniae* is isolated most often in adults with meningitis, usually in association with upper respiratory infections, pneumonitis, otitis or bacteremia. Other conditions predisposing to pneumococcal meningitis in adults include cerebrospinal fluid (CSF) rhinorrhea, head trauma, sinusitis, sickle cell anemia, alcoholism, cirrhosis of the liver and defects in host defenses such as immunoglobulin deficiencies and asplenia.

During the past 2 decades, the number of cases of meningitis caused by *S pyogenes* has decreased, while cases caused by *Listeria* and gram-negative bacilli have increased. *L monocytogenes* is a rare cause of meningitis in the newborn, but is increasingly more common in immunocompromised adults. Meningitis caused by gram-negative bacilli (*E coli, Proteus, Pseudomonas, Serratia, Klebsiella* and *Citrobacter*) is more frequently found in the immunocompromised host or in the patient who has sustained previous trauma or undergone neurosurgical procedures, or both.

Staphylococcal meningitis is associated with penetrating trauma, previous neurosurgery and staphylococcal bacteremia. Meningitis associated with ventricular shunts may be caused by coagulase-negative staphylococci (*Staphylococcus epidermidis*) or *S aureus*.

Clinical Manifestations. The onset of acute bacterial meningitis is rapid, over several days. Clinical symptoms include generalized headache, fever, vomiting, lethargy, stiff neck and confusion. Malaise and backache are common.

Diagnosis. A thorough history relative to otitis media, trauma, etc, is imperative in evaluating the patient with presumed bacterial meningitis. Physical examination may show that the patient is

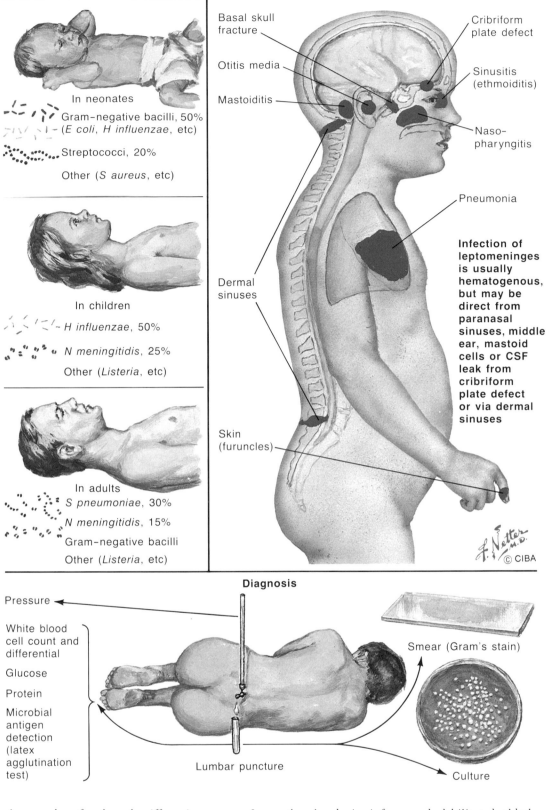

Bacterial Meningitis

Most common causative organisms

In neonates
Gram-negative bacilli, 50% (*E coli, H influenzae*, etc)
Streptococci, 20%
Other (*S aureus*, etc)

In children
H influenzae, 50%
N meningitidis, 25%
Other (*Listeria*, etc)

In adults
S pneumoniae, 30%
N meningitidis, 15%
Gram-negative bacilli
Other (*Listeria*, etc)

Sources of infection

Basal skull fracture
Otitis media
Mastoiditis
Dermal sinuses
Skin (furuncles)
Cribriform plate defect
Sinusitis (ethmoiditis)
Naso-pharyngitis
Pneumonia

Infection of leptomeninges is usually hematogenous, but may be direct from paranasal sinuses, middle ear, mastoid cells or CSF leak from cribriform plate defect or via dermal sinuses

Diagnosis

Pressure
White blood cell count and differential
Glucose
Protein
Microbial antigen detection (latex agglutination test)
Lumbar puncture
Smear (Gram's stain)
Culture

sleepy and confused; neck stiffness is common. In true nuchal rigidity, an attempt to move the neck in any direction is resisted. Evidence of inflamed meningeal coverings of the lumbosacral nerve roots can be demonstrated by testing for Kernig's and Brudzinski's signs (Plate 2). Kernig's sign is elicited by flexing the patient's hip to a 90° angle and then attempting to passively straighten the leg at the knee. Pain and tightness in the hamstring muscles prevent the completion of this maneuver. The sign should be positive bilaterally for the diagnosis of meningitis. Brudzinski's sign is positive if the patient's hips and knees flex automatically when the examiner flexes the patient's neck while the patient is supine. On the other hand, in infants and debilitated elderly patients with meningitis, these signs of meningeal irritation may not always be present.

Presence of a rash is helpful in determining the cause of meningitis. A maculopapular or petechial/purpuric rash usually indicates *N meningitidis* infection. The macular-petechial rash of aseptic meningitis caused by echovirus may be confused with meningococcal infection. This viral exanthem commonly involves the face and neck early in the infection, unlike the rash in meningococcal infection, which is more common on the trunk and extremities. Rarely, purpuric lesions may be found in the patient with fulminant pneumococcal bacteremia and meningitis.

Bacterial Meningitis
(Continued)

Mania and delirium occur more frequently in patients with meningococcal meningitis.

Diagnostic Studies. The presence of lethargy raises the possibility of increased intracranial pressure, and computed tomography (CT) should precede lumbar puncture in order to rule out a focal mass lesion with brain shift. Physical signs of increased intracranial pressure include coma, papilledema, hypertension and bradycardia. The application of a 20- to 22-gauge needle helps avoid a dural leak.

CSF analysis provides conclusive proof of bacterial infection of the subarachnoid space. CSF evaluation should include a smear and culture. Gram's stain reveals the morphology of the organism involved in about 80% of the cases. This allows selection of appropriate antibiotic therapy before definitive culture and sensitivity data are obtained. *Pneumococcus* is the most likely bacterial agent when gram-positive diplococci are seen in the CSF.

In meningitis, the CSF pressure is frequently elevated and the fluid is turbid. The white blood cell count and differential of the CSF are important in assessing the type of meningitis. The CSF may be separated into predominantly polymorphonuclear cells (purulent or bacterial meningitis) versus a lymphocytic pattern. The purulent pattern comprises mainly polymorphonuclear leukocyte pleocytosis, with a low glucose level and elevated protein level, a typical pattern in most bacterial meningitides. In more than 50% of patients with bacterial meningitis, the CSF glucose level is less than 60% of the blood glucose level (less than 40 mg/100 ml). The CSF glucose level is also low in *Listeria*, cryptococcal or tuberculous meningitis, whereas lymphocytosis and a normal glucose level are more common in viral meningitis or encephalitis.

CSF protein levels in patients with purulent meningitis are often above 100 mg/100 ml. A protein level of 1,000 mg/100 ml or greater indicates an impending subarachnoid block.

In patients with parameningeal foci, such as a brain abscess or epidural abscess (Plate 3), the CSF protein level is also elevated.

Finally, demonstration of antigen by counterimmunoelectrophoresis or the latex agglutination test may be helpful in the early diagnosis of meningitis, especially when the Gram's stain is negative or when the culture remains negative because of previous antibiotic therapy.

Treatment. The patient with presumed bacterial meningitis should receive, for a minimum of 10 days, a course of high-dose intravenous antibiotics that cross the blood-brain barrier. The three major types of bacterial meningitis may be treated with antibiotics that achieve bacterial levels in the CSF (such as penicillin and chloram-

Bacterial Meningitis (continued)

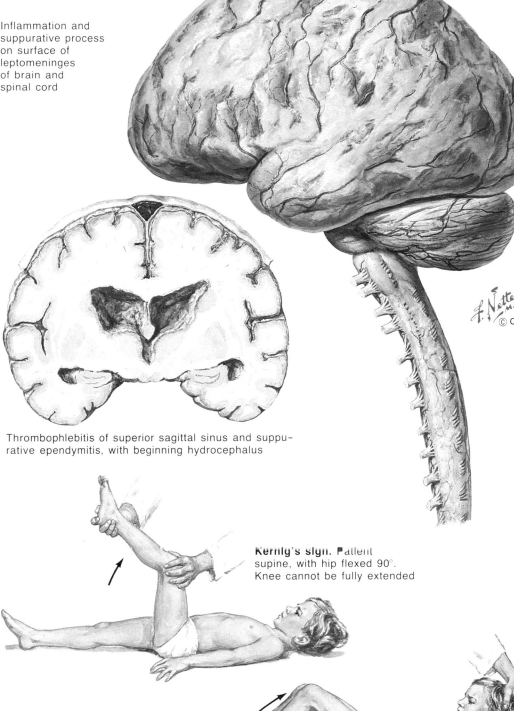

Inflammation and suppurative process on surface of leptomeninges of brain and spinal cord

Thrombophlebitis of superior sagittal sinus and suppurative ependymitis, with beginning hydrocephalus

Kernig's sign. Patient supine, with hip flexed 90°. Knee cannot be fully extended

Neck rigidity (Brudzinski's neck sign). Passive flexion of neck causes flexion of both legs and thighs

phenicol). Penicillin is the drug of choice for pneumococcal and meningococcal meningitis; intravenous therapy should continue for 10 to 14 days. Chloramphenicol or ampicillin is used in meningitis caused by *H influenzae*; ampicillin resistance should be evaluated. Third-generation cephalosporins such as cefotaxime and moxalactum are effective against gram-negative bacilli other than *Pseudomonas*. Agents such as clindamycin or first-generation and second-generation cephalosporins do not cross the blood-brain barrier and are not effective in bacterial meningitis.

Complications. Neurologic complications include seizures, focal cerebral signs and acute cerebral edema. Dysfunction of cranial nerves III, IV, VI and VII occurs in about 15% of patients. Sensorineural hearing loss may follow, most often after meningococcal infection. Hemiparesis, dysphasia and hemianopsia also occur in about 15% of patients; persistence of these findings suggests cerebral arteritis, thrombophlebitis or a mass lesion.

Chemoprophylaxis with rifampin is recommended only for persons who are in close contact with a patient who has meningococcal meningitis (ie, household members). The risk of secondary disease with *H influenzae* is age-dependent. If a child less than 4 years of age lives in the household where an index case has been identified, all household members should receive rifampin. □

Parameningeal Infections

Brain Abscess. One of four mechanisms usually causes brain abscess: (1) direct extension from a contiguous focus such as a middle ear or sinus infection; (2) in association with congenital heart disease, with a right-to-left or pulmonary arteriovenous shunt; (3) by hematogenous spread from distant sites of infection; or (4) by direct introduction of bacteria following penetrating head injuries. The cardinal symptom of a brain abscess is headache, relentless and progressive, which is usually followed by focal neurologic manifestations. Fever is present in only two thirds of patients. Papilledema and other signs of increased intracranial pressure are common later in the course.

Streptococci, Enterobacteriaceae and staphylococci are the most common aerobic bacteria. Anaerobic microorganisms are present in at least one third of brain abscesses, and multiple organisms in more than one quarter.

Early diagnosis is possible with computed tomography (CT). Lumbar puncture should be avoided, to prevent herniation or rupture of the abscess into the ventricular system.

The abscess may be aspirated and medical therapy started with penicillin and chloramphenicol. Surgery may not be necessary if follow-up CT scans show the abscess has decreased in size. Brain edema associated with acute brain abscess necessitates use of steroids and mannitol, as well as phenytoin to prevent convulsions.

Subdural Empyema. A purulent collection in the potential space between the dura mater and the arachnoid, subdural empyema usually results from extension of the infection in the paranasal sinuses, especially the frontal sinuses. Infection can also be directly introduced through operative or traumatic wounds. Streptococci account for more than one half of the cases; *Staphylococcus aureus*, gram-negative bacteria and *Bacteroides* are also found frequently.

Subdural empyema is most often preceded by sinusitis or mastoiditis. Swelling, erythema and local tenderness of the site overlying the primary infection may become evident. In the early stages, pain or headache may be localized or moderate. As the illness progresses, the headache becomes generalized and severe, and high fever, vomiting and nuchal rigidity develop. Seizures, hemiparesis, visual field defects and papilledema may occur. The cerebrospinal fluid (CSF) contains 1 to 1,000 white blood cells; the protein level is increased and the glucose level is normal. The CT scan reveals a low-absorption extracerebral mass. A thin, moderately dense margin may be visualized with contrast medium.

Subdural empyema is a life-threatening infection requiring prompt surgical drainage and intensive antimicrobial therapy. The initial choice of antibiotics should include intravenous semisynthetic penicillin and an agent to cover gram-negative bacilli, such as chloramphenicol. Prophylactic use of anticonvulsants and corticosteroids is also helpful.

Spinal Epidural Abscess. A purulent or granulomatous collection within the spinal epidural space may lie over or encircle the spinal

Brain abscess

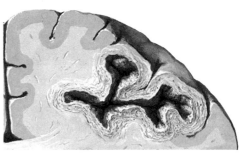

Multiple abscesses
of brain

Scar of healed brain abscess, with
collapse of brain tissue into cavity

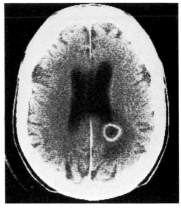

CT scan shows brain abscess
with thin enhancing rim and
central necrosis

Subdural abscess

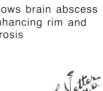

Osteomyelitis of skull, with
penetration of dura to form
subdural "collar button" abscess

Epidural abscess

Fat in epidural space

Anterior spinal
artery

Dura

Arachnoid

Venous
plexus

Dura

Posterior spinal arteries

Abscess in epidural space
compressing spinal cord
and its blood supply

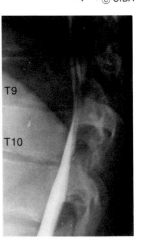

Myelogram: block at
T9–10 due to spinal
epidural abscess

cord, nerve roots and nerves. Infection is usually localized within 3 to 4 vertebral segments, although it may rarely extend the length of the spinal canal.

S aureus is the most common organism found in spinal epidural abscess, but streptococci, gram-negative organisms and, rarely, anaerobic or mixed organisms from dental or upper airway infections have also been isolated.

The most common focus for hematogenous spread to the epidural space is a skin infection, especially a furuncle. Antecedent hematogenous vertebral osteomyelitis accounts for about 40% of spinal epidural abscesses. Dental and upper respiratory infections are also frequent sources.

Heusner in 1948 described the clinical picture of an epidural abscess as a progression from spinal ache to nerve root pain to weakness and, eventually, paralysis. The ache starts at the level of the affected spine.

The CSF shows a white blood cell count of 0 to 1,000/mm³, an elevated protein level and a normal glucose level. The patient with back pain, fever and localized tenderness should have radiographs of the spine and a careful spinal puncture, with slow insertion of the needle and intermittent aspiration to ensure that epidural pus is detected. If a block or epidural mass is found on myelography, laminectomy should be done and parenteral antibiotics given for 3 to 4 weeks. □

Infections in Immunocompromised Host

Organisms such as *Streptococcus pneumoniae* and anaerobic bacteria are the usual cause of central nervous system (CNS) infections in the immunocompromised host. However, *Listeria* and *Cryptococcus* frequently cause meningitis, and *Nocardia*. *Cryptococcus* and *Toxoplasma* are important considerations in the etiology of brain abscess.

Nocardiosis

Nocardia are present in the soil and decaying vegetable matter. The respiratory tract is the site of entry of *N asteroides* in most cases of brain abscess, even though the pulmonary focus may not be prominent. The initial pulmonary focus is suppurative and not well localized, thus allowing infection to spread to the brain. Meningitis is infrequent in the absence of a contiguous abscess.

Brain biopsy is the most reliable diagnostic technique. *Nocardia* organisms are weakly acid-fast, and can be stained with the modified Ziehl-Neelsen method. They may be isolated on Sabouraud's medium or brain-heart infusion agar, but growth may not be visible for 2 to 4 weeks.

Sulfonamides are the drugs of choice in treating nocardiosis. Therapy should continue for at least 3 months or several weeks after clinical disappearance of the lesion.

Cysticercosis

Infection with the larval form of the porcine tapeworm *Taenia solium* is the cause of cysticercosis. Humans acquire the adult tapeworm by eating undercooked pork, and also may become infected with the larval stage (cysticercus) by accidental ingestion of tapeworm eggs. The eggs hatch in the small intestine; burrow into venules; and are carried to distant sites.

The larvae are relatively large and may lodge in the subarachnoid space of ventricles. Symptoms may not occur until 4 to 5 years later, when larvae die and provoke an inflammatory response.

Cysts in the cerebrum may mimic a brain tumor; cysts in the subarachnoid space may result in a chronic meningitis and arachnoiditis; and cysts in the ventricular system may cause obstructing hydrocephalus. Eventually, old nonviable cysts calcify, simplifying detection.

The use of contrast-enhanced computed tomography (CT) increases the possibility of detecting CNS infection. Subcutaneous cysts; positive findings in a biopsy specimen, serum or cerebrospinal fluid (CSF) serologic study; or skeletal muscle calcifications support the diagnosis.

Praziquantel has been recently used in cysticercosis, with promising results. Steroids have been advocated to decrease inflammation.

Preventive measures include attention to hygiene and control of deposition of human excreta. Screening for eggs in the infected patient may also help decrease spread of the infection.

Listeriosis

Listeria is a widespread bacteria isolated from soil, animal feed, water and sewage. The species *L monocytogenes* causes listeriosis, or *Listeria* meningitis, which most often occurs in the neonatal

Nocardiosis

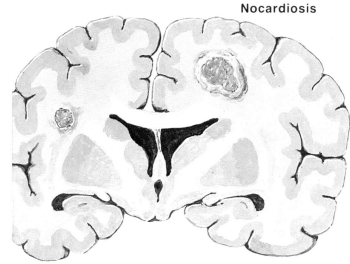

Multiple nocardial abscesses in brain

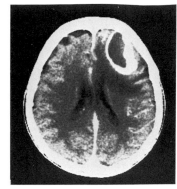

CT scan: thick-walled nocardial frontal lobe abscess in immunocompromised patient

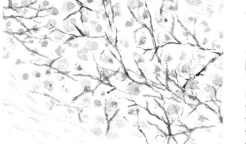

Branching hyphae of *Nocardia asteroides* in brain abscess (methenamine-silver stain)

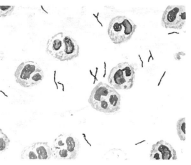

Modified acid–fast organisms as they may appear in pus, sputum or tissues. They may be mistaken for tubercle bacilli, but are actually fragmented nocardial hyphae

Cysticercosis

Ovum of *Taenia solium* (pork tapeworm); indistinguishable from that of *T saginata* (beef tapeworm)

Cysticercus (larval stage) of pork tapeworm. Fluid–filled sac (bladder) containing scolex (head) of worm

T solium ova hatch after ingestion by hogs; embryos migrate to hog tissues and form cysticerci. When humans eat infested pork, intestinal tapeworms develop. However, if humans ingest ova instead of larvae, or if ova reach stomach by reverse peristalsis from intestinal worm, human cysticercosis may occur

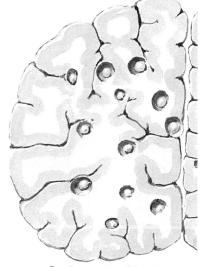

Cysticercosis of brain

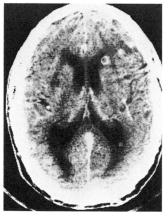

CT scan: punctate calcifications, cystic lesions (some with ring enhancement) and noncystic areas, which enhance

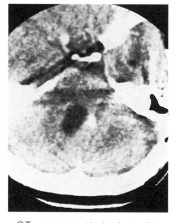

CT scan: cystic lesion with calcification in region of 4th ventricle, producing hydrocephalus

Listeriosis

Smear of CSF showing white blood cells and *Listeria* organisms, which appear as gram-positive rods. They may be very short, to resemble cocci, and they often orient in palisades suggestive of Chinese characters. They cause severe purulent meningitis, most commonly in immunocompromised patients or newborns

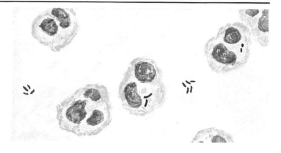

Infections in
Immunocompromised Host
(Continued)

setting and in immunocompromised adults. Symptoms include headache, fever, lethargy, seizures and focal neurologic deficits. Diagnosis is based on the CSF formula: elevated white blood cell count with a predominance of polymorphonuclear cells and a low glucose level. A Gram's-stained smear reveals small gram-positive bacilli resembling diphtheroids.

Intravenous administration of ampicillin and gentamicin is the suggested treatment.

Toxoplasmosis

Toxoplasma gondii is a parasite that infects most mammalian species. Humans may acquire *T gondii* infections by ingestion, transplacental transmission, blood transfusion or organ transplantation. Infection by the oral route results from ingestion of either *T gondii* cysts in undercooked food (pork, lamb) or *T gondii* oocysts, which are found in 1% of cat feces. Enzymes in the human intestinal tract liberate *T gondii* trophozoites, which cause clinical toxoplasmosis.

In the United States, serologic evidence of *Toxoplasma* infection is seen in about 50% of the population. Most infections are subclinical and are most often manifested by asymptomatic cervical lymphadenopathy.

Symptomatic toxoplasmosis can be divided into four major clinical syndromes: congenital, ocular, lymphadenopathic and that occurring in immunocompromised patients. In immunocompromised patients, *T gondii* can cause severe neurologic or disseminated disease; neurologic abnormalities predominate in at least 50% of these patients. The clinical picture may take the form of diffuse encephalitis, meningoencephalitis or a cerebral mass lesion. The CSF often shows mild lymphocytic pleocytosis and an elevated protein level; the glucose level remains normal.

The indirect fluorescent antibody test is the most widely used diagnostic procedure; the Sabin-Feldman dye test and an indirect hemagglutination test are also available. All three tests measure IgG antibodies; results become positive 1 to 3 weeks after infection. Because positive titers in these tests persist for years after infection, definitive diagnosis requires a four-fold rise in IgG titer, or a single high IgM titer.

Chemotherapy should be considered in patients with CNS involvement. Pyrimethamine and sulfadiazine are the most active agents. Treatment is continued for 4 to 5 weeks.

Cryptococcosis

This chronic, subacute or, rarely, acute CNS infection is caused by *Cryptococcus neoformans*, a yeastlike fungus that has been isolated worldwide from soil, fruits and matter contaminated by pigeon excreta. The organism probably enters the body through the lungs, from which it may disseminate to all organs. Mild, self-limited infections are common. Clinical disease may develop in healthy persons, as well as in immunocompromised patients.

Toxoplasmosis

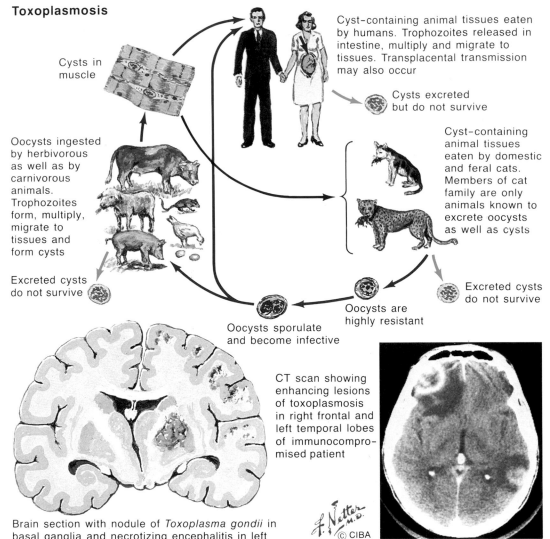

Cysts in muscle

Cyst-containing animal tissues eaten by humans. Trophozoites released in intestine, multiply and migrate to tissues. Transplacental transmission may also occur

Cysts excreted but do not survive

Oocysts ingested by herbivorous as well as by carnivorous animals. Trophozoites form, multiply, migrate to tissues and form cysts

Cyst-containing animal tissues eaten by domestic and feral cats. Members of cat family are only animals known to excrete oocysts as well as cysts

Excreted cysts do not survive

Excreted cysts do not survive

Oocysts are highly resistant

Oocysts sporulate and become infective

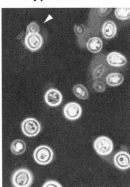

Brain section with nodule of *Toxoplasma gondii* in basal ganglia and necrotizing encephalitis in left frontal and temporal corticomedullary zones

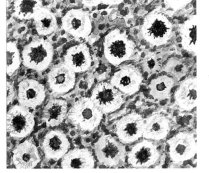

CT scan showing enhancing lesions of toxoplasmosis in right frontal and left temporal lobes of immunocompromised patient

Cryptococcosis

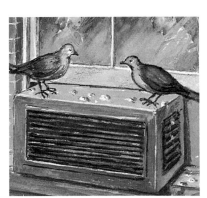

Infection is by respiratory route. Pigeon dung and air conditioners may be factors in dissemination

India ink preparation showing budding and capsule

Accumulation of encapsulated cryptococci in subarachnoid space (PAS or methenamine–silver stain)

Meningeal involvement is the most common form of cryptococcosis, the onset of which is usually insidious. Symptoms may be present for months, and complaints may be nonspecific, such as headache, nausea, irritability, somnolence and clumsiness. Cranial nerve involvement is seen in 20% of patients and may cause decreased visual acuity, diplopia and facial numbness. Patients are often afebrile, and most have minimal nuchal rigidity. Papilledema is noted in about 33% of patients. Direct involvement of the brain by the infection may cause dementia.

The CSF examination reveals an elevated opening pressure, decreased glucose in 50% of patients, increased protein concentration and 40

to 400 white blood cells, with lymphocytes predominating.

The organism can be defined in India ink preparations, but isolation of *C neoformans* by culture is the single best diagnostic test. Cultures of urine are positive in about 33% of patients. Less commonly, diagnosis is made by culturing or identifying the organism with PAS or methenamine-silver stain in a specimen from the CNS. Latex agglutination for detection of cryptococcal capsular antigen is also available; antigen can be detected in 94% of patients.

Treatment consists of a combination of amphotericin B, intravenously, and flucytosine, orally, for approximately 6 weeks. □

Neurosyphilis

The *Treponema pallidum*, the organism that causes syphilis, is a delicate, spiral parasite whose size, shape and activity are best visualized by dark-field microscopy of a preparation from a primary venereal lesion. Syphilis of the central nervous system (CNS) occurs in less than 20% of patients with a primary infection. The response of the meninges, brain and spinal cord to the spirochetal parasite is a chronic inflammatory process of cellular and interstitial tissues that produces mainly small lymphocytic cells, epithelioid cells and giant cells. Eventually, the granulomatous process produces endarteritis and degenerative and gummatous lesions.

Neurosyphilis can occur in several forms. *Syphilitic meningitis* usually develops during the early weeks after a primary infection, often during the period of the secondary rash. The symptoms are nocturnal headache, malaise, stiff neck, fever and cranial nerve palsies. The cerebrospinal fluid (CSF) contains an increase in lymphocytes and an elevated total protein; the serum VDRL is usually positive.

Meningovascular syphilis is a rare, more chronic disorder occurring 2 to 20 years after the primary lesion, with a prominent inflammatory disorder. Cranial nerve palsies, cerebrovascular accidents, seizures or paraplegia follow infarction of brain or spinal cord. Argyll Robertson pupils, which do not constrict reflexly to light but do respond to accommodation, are also present.

Tabes dorsalis predominates in males between 25 and 45 years of age and develops 10 to 20 years after the primary infection. Direct invasion by the spirochete and an immunologic reaction may both occur, leading to degenerative and sclerotic changes in the posterior nerve root fibers of the spinal cord, spinal ganglia cells, long fibers of the posterior columns of the spinal cord, optic nerves and oculomotor nuclei. The symptoms of lightning nerve root pains, gastric crisis, spastic gait, failing vision, and urinary and sexual disturbances vary in order of appearance and intensity. The optic nerves show progressive primary atrophy, and the pupils are small and irregular, with Argyll Robertson characteristics. Vibration sense is impaired. Romberg's sign is positive, and ataxia is present. Knee and ankle jerks are absent. The VDRL in the blood and CSF is positive in only 59% of patients.

Dementia paralytica, also called *general paresis*, predominates in males between 40 and 45 years of age. There is direct invasion of neural tissue by the spirochete, in addition to meningitis. Degen-

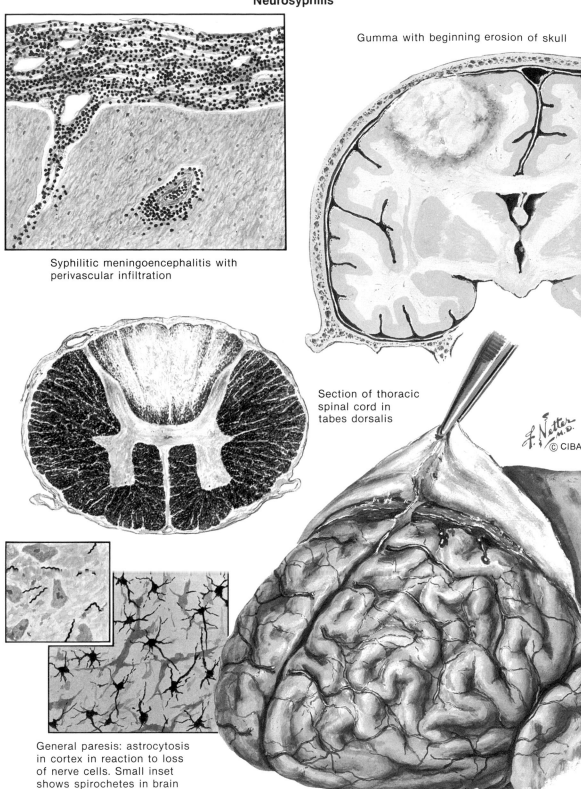

Syphilitic meningoencephalitis with perivascular infiltration

Gumma with beginning erosion of skull

Section of thoracic spinal cord in tabes dorsalis

General paresis: astrocytosis in cortex in reaction to loss of nerve cells. Small inset shows spirochetes in brain

General paresis: atrophy of brain and chronic subdural hematoma

erative and sclerotic changes result in a thickening of the dura mater, chronic subdural hematoma, atrophy of the cortical cells (giving a worm-eaten appearance on microscopy), and proliferation of astrocytes. This process has a particular affinity for the frontal lobes.

Progressive simple dementia is initially seen in 60% of patients. Other predominant symptoms of the insidious disease are headaches, insomnia, personality change, delusions of grandeur, impaired judgment, disturbed emotional responses, slurred speech and tremors. Argyll Robertson pupils are characteristic of this condition. VDRL in serum and CSF are positive in 90% to 98% of patients.

Gumma of the brain or spinal cord is rare indeed. Initial symptoms indicate an expanding CNS lesion. Surgical removal of the gumma, with penicillin therapy, gives excellent results.

Diagnosis. CSF analysis shows a modest increase in cells, mainly lymphocytes. The total protein is moderately elevated and the glucose is normal.

Serologic tests show VDRL in serum, and CSF analysis is the optimal screening test. The specific fluorescent treponemal-antibody absorption (FTA-ABS) test should be used for confirmation.

Treatment. Penicillin is the antibiotic of choice for all forms of neurosyphilis. Prolonged therapeutic blood and CSF levels are necessary for cure. □

Tuberculosis of Brain and Spine

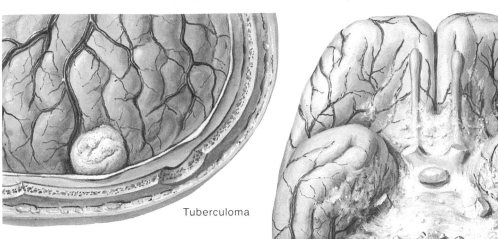

Tuberculoma

Tuberculous basilar meningitis

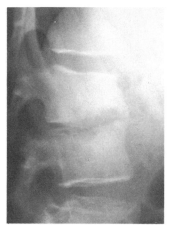

X-ray film: destruction of disc space and adjacent end plates of vertebrae

CT scan: paraspinous abscess in addition to bony destruction

Tuberculous Meningitis. In the United States, tuberculous meningitis tends to affect adults, although its incidence has markedly decreased. In populations in which tuberculosis is more common, tuberculous meningitis more frequently affects children as part of the primary infection. (For a complete discussion of the pathophysiology, evaluation and treatment of tuberculosis, see CIBA COLLECTION, Volume 7, pages 199–207.)

Although tuberculous meningitis may result from contiguous spread from a tuberculoma or parameningeal granuloma with rupture into the subarachnoid space, it is more often caused by hematogenous meningeal seeding during the primary infection. In this event, tubercle bacilli may discharge directly into the subarachnoid space from a local caseous focus in the meninges, brain or spinal cord. These foci are assumed to have been present since the time of hematogenous seeding during the primary infection, usually in childhood. The infection then spreads along the perivascular spaces into the brain. The intense inflammatory reaction at the base of the brain leads to occlusive arteritis with thrombosis of small vessels and resultant infarction of the brain, direct compression of cranial nerves and obstruction of the free flow of cerebrospinal fluid (CSF) at the foramina of the fourth ventricle or the basal cisterns, resulting in subarachnoid block and cerebral edema.

The clinical course of tuberculous meningitis is rapidly progressive, with headache, fever and meningismus followed by cranial nerve deficits, especially sixth cranial nerve palsy. Focal deficits are followed by alterations in the sensorium and coma. Death ensues within weeks if the disease is not treated.

Examination of the CSF is crucial in establishing the diagnosis of tuberculous meningitis. Classically, the CSF glucose level is less than two thirds that of serum glucose; the CSF protein is elevated above 50 mg/ml; and the cell count is elevated, with lymphocytes predominating.

Acid-fast smears may be positive only 25% of the time. To establish the diagnosis, let the CSF stand for a few hours so that a pellicle forms, then stain this fibrin web for acid-fast organisms.

For presumed tuberculous meningitis, antituberculous therapy should be instituted immediately with isoniazid, rifampin and ethambutol. Isoniazid and rifampin are essential, as both cross the blood-brain barrier. Corticosteroids may be

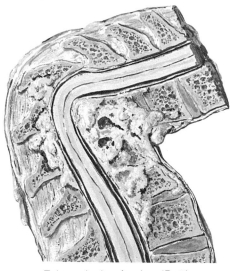

Tuberculosis of spine (Pott's disease) with marked kyphosis

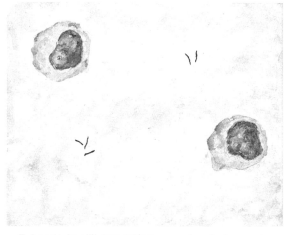

Tubercle bacilli appearing as red rods in smear of CSF (Ziehl-Neelsen stain)

added for the patient with cerebral edema or subarachnoid block, or both.

Tuberculoma. Cerebral tuberculomas, less common than tuberculous meningitis, may arise from successive attempts at encapsulation. Such lesions are often calcified and are usually found in the posterior fossa (cerebellum). Antituberculous therapy should be attempted before surgery is undertaken.

Vertebral Tuberculosis (Pott's Disease). In adults, skeletal tuberculosis occurs in joints most subject to trauma. The spine is involved in about 50% of such cases. Tuberculosis of the spine may involve the disc space and adjacent vertebral bodies and/or the epidural space.

Back pain and fever may be followed by progressive spinal cord compression caused by unrecognized epidural infection, or fracture, collapse or angulation of vertebral segments in bone infection. Plain x-ray films of the spine reveal infection of the disc space, with spread to the adjacent vertebrae. A myelogram is helpful in evaluating presumed epidural infection. If possible, bone biopsy or aspiration should be performed to obtain adequate material for culture and pathologic study.

Treatment includes administration of isoniazid plus rifampin and ethambutol for approximately 2 years. If spinal cord compression occurs, surgical decompression is necessary. □

Tetanus

The motor unit of the peripheral nervous system is particularly vulnerable to each of the three bacteria-produced toxins known to affect humans. Each toxin acts at a different level: tetanospasmin, on the motor neuron; diphtheria toxin, on the peripheral nerve, mimicking the Guillain-Barré syndrome; and botulin, on the neuromuscular junction (see Section XI, Plates 15, 34).

Clostridium tetani is a widespread organism. Its hearty spore is found in soil, dust and feces (particularly equine). It may enter the body through wounds, blisters, burns, punctures from hypodermic needles (particularly when contaminated with a powder used in heroin mainlining), insect bites, surgical procedures such as abdominal operations, abortions and circumcisions, and skin ulcers. When introduced into an area of devitalized tissue and low partial pressure of oxygen, the spore is converted to the toxin-producing anaerobic gram-positive rod, and two types of toxin are elaborated.

Tetanospasmin, the neurotoxin derived from *C tetani*, is second in strength only to botulin, the neurotoxin produced by *C botulinum*. It irreversibly binds to the presynaptic termination of the inhibitory Renshaw cell axon on the motor neuron cell in the anterior horn of the spinal cord. The absence of the inhibitory transmitters gamma aminobutyric acid and glycine, produced by the Renshaw cell, results in increased firing of the motor neuron. Tetanospasmin also acts on the neuromuscular junction, muscle cell and sympathetic neuron. Tetanolysin, the other toxin of *C tetani*, produces a clinically inconsequential local hemolysis.

The incubation period of *C tetani* may vary from a few days to several months. When the incubation period is long, the original wound may have been forgotten.

Clinical Manifestations. Early symptoms of tetanus include restlessness, localized stiffness and soreness, low-grade fever, and, sometimes, hemorrhage at the wound site. Occasionally, the disease arrests focally and is characterized by hypertonic muscles in the affected extremity or face. Repetitive voluntary movements often elicit a recruitment spasm. Although focal tetanus mimics various diseases, careful examination for the presence of minimal trismus may provide a clinical clue to the appropriate diagnosis.

Initial symptoms of generalized tetanus are nonspecific—irritability, insomnia and headache. Eventually, tonic contractures supervene secondary to the continuous activity of multiple muscle groups. Nuchal rigidity, risus sardonicus, trismus and the boardlike abdomen result.

The most minute sensory stimulation produces acute, explosive, painful massive muscle spasms. The patient may assume a decorticate or opisthotonic posture. Laryngospasm may lead to respiratory compromise, with a potential for asphyxia or heart failure, or both. These spasms usually last only a few seconds, but they vary in duration and occasionally may be repetitive. Manifestations of sympathetic hyperactivity include wide swings in blood pressure, tachyarrhythmias, sweating, and

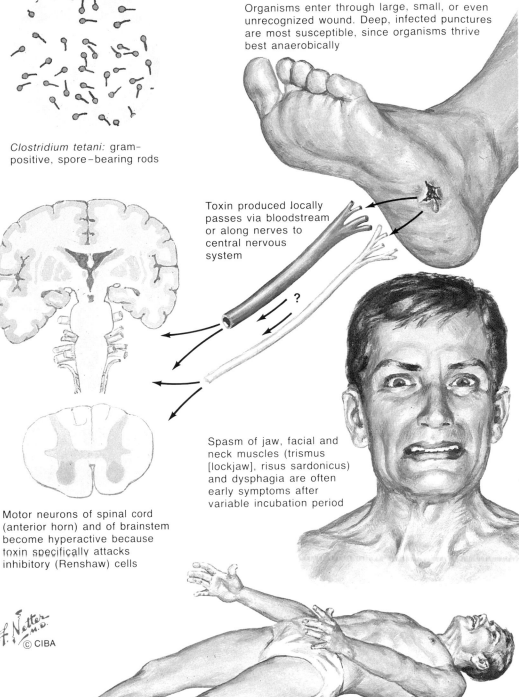

Clostridium tetani: gram-positive, spore–bearing rods

Motor neurons of spinal cord (anterior horn) and of brainstem become hyperactive because toxin specifically attacks inhibitory (Renshaw) cells

Tetanus

Organisms enter through large, small, or even unrecognized wound. Deep, infected punctures are most susceptible, since organisms thrive best anaerobically

Toxin produced locally passes via bloodstream or along nerves to central nervous system

Spasm of jaw, facial and neck muscles (trismus [lockjaw], risus sardonicus) and dysphagia are often early symptoms after variable incubation period

Complete tetanic spasm in advanced disease. Patient rigid in moderate opisthotonos, with arms extended, abdomen boardlike. Respiratory arrest may occur

vasoconstriction with pallor and cyanosis. Late in the course, a paralytic state sometimes occurs, which is thought to be secondary to the effects of the toxin on the neuromuscular junction.

Cerebrospinal fluid (CSF) is essentially unremarkable. A special electromyography test, the jaw jerk, fails to demonstrate the normal silent period.

Differential Diagnosis. Infectious diseases such as meningitis and encephalitis, a bite from a black widow spider, and strychnine poisoning should be considered in the differential diagnosis. The stiff-man syndrome is a more chronic process, and is characterized by painful spasms, a normal jaw jerk response and lack of trismus. Trismus

may result from dental abscess or phenothiazine drugs.

Treatment. The best treatment is prophylaxis, with immunization in the newborn and every 10 years thereafter. In active tetanus, wound debridement and administration of either procaine penicillin or tetracycline suppresses toxin production. Antitoxin is then given to block any toxin still in the nerve, the circulation or the wound. Spasm is best treated by a combination of diazepam and either barbiturates or phenothiazines, or both. Curarization or tracheostomy, or both, is sometimes necessary.

The recuperative period may be 2 to 4 months, and mortality is 25% to 75%. □

Poliomyelitis

Poliomyelitis begins as an acute febrile systemic illness. In a small proportion of infected persons, it progresses within 1 or more days to a lower motor neuron type of paralysis (usually asymmetric) of muscles innervated by spinal and cranial nerves. The paralysis is sometimes accompanied by respiratory and vasomotor disturbances caused by neuronal lesions in the medulla.

Etiology

Poliovirus (types 1, 2 and 3), Coxsackie virus (types A7, A9, B2 to B5), echovirus (types 1, 2, 4, 6, 7, 9, 11, 16, 18 and 30), and other enteroviruses (types 70 and 71) can all cause this distinctive paralytic disease. However, about 85% of cases of persistent paralysis in the prevaccine era and most epidemics have been caused by type 1 poliovirus, and the remainder, predominantly by types 2 and 3. The incidence of paralytic poliomyelitis caused by the other enteroviruses is not known.

Pathogenesis

The viruses enter the body through the mouth and are excreted in the feces (Plate 9).

Different strains of viruses differ in their capacity to multiply outside the alimentary tract and thus to produce the viremia that accompanies clinically apparent human infections. Extensive multiplication in the alimentary tract alone, with consequent invasion of intestinal lymph nodes, which occurs with the orally administered attenuated vaccine strains of poliovirus, leads to little or no demonstrable viremia or any clinical manifestations of illness.

The degree of neurovirulence of the infecting virus determines its capacity first to invade the sensory neurons in the peripheral ganglia (giving rise to early pain, hyperesthesia and paresthesia), then to multiply there sufficiently to permit axonal spread to motor neurons, and finally to multiply sufficiently to destroy enough motor neurons to produce clinical paralysis.

Pathology

The early signs of central nervous system (CNS) involvement, ie, nuchal and spinal rigidity and occasional hyperesthesias and paresthesias, as well as subsequent paralytic manifestations, are associated with neuronal lesions in the sensory ganglia, spinal cord and medulla. Destruction of neurons is primary, and the inflammatory reaction is secondary. The sequence of events in the complete destruction of a motor neuron is shown in Plate 10. Polymorphonuclear leukocytes, which initially phagocytose the destroyed neurons, are quickly replaced by mononuclear cells, and ultimately the foci of neuronophagia disappear completely. In addition, perivascular infiltration by mononuclear cells and interstitial infiltration by various glial cells are present. The inflammatory cells in the meninges represent an overflow of cells from the perivascular spaces. The anterior roots show secondary disintegration of the axis cylinders and inflammatory reaction; neuronal destruction, neuronophagia and interstitial cellular infiltration are seen in the sensory ganglia.

Since individual muscle fibrils are innervated by multiple neurons from different levels of the spinal cord, the extent and persistence of paralysis depend on the number and location of completely destroyed motor neurons. These factors are influenced by the neural pathways that first brought the virus into the CNS and the duration of the disease. The relative distribution of neuronal lesions found post mortem in primary spinal and primary bulbar paralysis is shown in Plate 10. Neuronal lesions in the medulla are located in the nuclei of various cranial nerves, in the vestibular nuclei and in the reticular formation.

Neuronal lesions also occur in the cerebellum (roof nuclei and vermis), midbrain (periaqueductal gray matter, tectum and tegmentum), thalamus, hypothalamus, globus pallidus and motor cortex. This distribution of lesions differentiates poliomyelitis from the human encephalitides produced by many different viruses, in which the lesions are much more diffuse.

Clinical Manifestations

Most infections produced by naturally occurring polioviruses are clinically inapparent. The types of recognizable disease are as follows.

Abortive minor illness has no signs of CNS involvement and is manifested by fever, headache, sore throat, anorexia, nausea, vomiting and abdominal pain lasting from a few hours to several days. *Nonparalytic illness*, with signs of CNS involvement, includes the clinical signs of abortive minor illness, often in more severe form, plus pain and stiffness in the neck, back and legs (positive tripod, kiss-the-knee, Kernig's and Brudzinski's signs); hyperesthesias and paresthesias; and an increased number of leukocytes in the cerebrospinal fluid (CSF). *Paralytic illness* develops 1 or more days after the clinical signs seen in the first two types.

The paralysis is flaccid, with loss of deep tendon reflexes. Paralysis of the intercostal and diaphragmatic muscles is life-threatening. Irregularities in rhythm, depth and rate of respiration, as well as vasomotor disturbances resulting from neuronal damage in the respiratory and vasomotor centers of the medulla, are also life-threatening. The mortality of 5% to 25% for paralytic disease varies with the availability and efficacy of treatment of intercostal and diaphragmatic paralysis.

In survivors, paralysis reaches a peak during the first few days or weeks after the temperature returns to normal. Patients with mild paralysis can recover completely within 2 months, which occurs more often when the disease is not caused by polioviruses. In patients with severe paralysis during the acute phase, some improvement occurs during the first 2 years, but not thereafter. Atrophy of paralyzed muscles begins within 8 weeks. When extensive paralysis occurs early in life and is untreated or inadequately treated, normal growth of the affected areas is arrested, and severe deformities develop in the limbs, chest, back and shoulders.

Treatment

During the acute phase, the following special treatment is required. *Disturbances in swallowing* are treated by postural drainage, mechanical suction and, when necessary, tracheostomy to prevent secretions from blocking the airway. For *paralysis of vocal cords, ineffective cough* and *laryngeal stridor*, tracheostomy is necessary, preferably before bouts of choking and cyanosis appear. *Intercostal and diaphragmatic respiratory paralysis* is treated with use of a negative-pressure or special chest respirator. *Respiratory failure of medullary origin associated with paralysis of deglutition* is treated by tracheostomy, with humidified oxygen supplied by a negative-pressure or positive-pressure respirator.

After the acute phase, appropriate physiotherapy and orthopedic intervention can help the patient achieve the maximum possible return of muscle function and prevent the tragic crippling deformities.

Epidemiology

Polioviruses and related fecal-borne enteroviruses are maximally disseminated during hot weather. In temperate climates, before successful vaccination programs, epidemics appeared during the summer and autumn months and usually ended with the advent of cold weather. Under conditions of poor sanitation and hygiene, these viruses spread extensively in early life, and the disease was predominantly infantile—hence the term "infantile paralysis." As the standard of living improved, virus dissemination diminished in early life to a point where infection and paralysis first appeared in ever larger proportions of older children, young adults and adults.

In tropical and subtropical economically less developed countries, fecal-borne viruses are disseminated so extensively throughout the year that most children become infected very early in life. Because paralytic disease occurs mostly during the first 2 years of life, it often is unrecognized during the acute phase and is recognized only when muscle atrophy, lameness and various deformities become apparent as the child begins to walk. The former belief that *paralytic* poliomyelitis is rare in the tropics and is an important public health problem only in countries with a high standard of living has now been shown to be a fallacy. Even in the absence of recognized epidemics, the estimated incidence of paralytic poliomyelitis in rural and urban tropical regions is as high or higher than in the United States before vaccine was available.

Prevention

Natural infection with polioviruses provides lifelong immunity to paralytic disease caused by polioviruses. This naturally acquired immunity is associated with partial or complete resistance of the intestinal tract to reinfection in all persons and with demonstrable levels of neutralizing antibody in the majority. Each resistant intestinal tract breaks one link in the chain of transmission of polioviruses.

Formalin-inactivated poliovirus vaccine (Salk type), administered subcutaneously in adequate and repeated doses, produces neutralizing antibodies that protect against paralytic disease but afford insufficient or no resistance to infection in the intestinal tract. Accordingly, although the inactivated poliovirus vaccine (IPV) can greatly reduce the incidence of paralytic disease in repeatedly inoculated subjects, it does not break the chain of human transmission of the virulent polioviruses.

Poliomyelitis

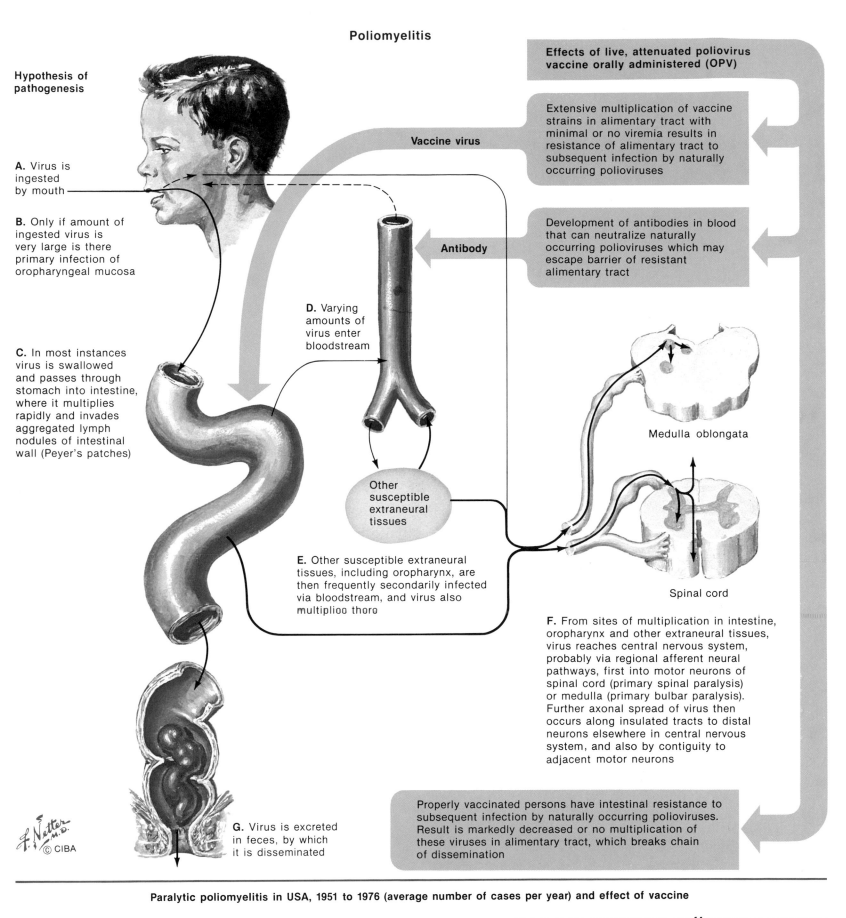

Hypothesis of pathogenesis

A. Virus is ingested by mouth

B. Only if amount of ingested virus is very large is there primary infection of oropharyngeal mucosa

C. In most instances virus is swallowed and passes through stomach into intestine, where it multiplies rapidly and invades aggregated lymph nodules of intestinal wall (Peyer's patches)

D. Varying amounts of virus enter bloodstream

E. Other susceptible extraneural tissues, including oropharynx, are then frequently secondarily infected via bloodstream, and virus also multiplies there

G. Virus is excreted in feces, by which it is disseminated

Vaccine virus

Antibody

Other susceptible extraneural tissues

Medulla oblongata

Spinal cord

Effects of live, attenuated poliovirus vaccine orally administered (OPV)

Extensive multiplication of vaccine strains in alimentary tract with minimal or no viremia results in resistance of alimentary tract to subsequent infection by naturally occurring polioviruses

Development of antibodies in blood that can neutralize naturally occurring polioviruses which may escape barrier of resistant alimentary tract

F. From sites of multiplication in intestine, oropharynx and other extraneural tissues, virus reaches central nervous system, probably via regional afferent neural pathways, first into motor neurons of spinal cord (primary spinal paralysis) or medulla (primary bulbar paralysis). Further axonal spread of virus then occurs along insulated tracts to distal neurons elsewhere in central nervous system, and also by contiguity to adjacent motor neurons

Properly vaccinated persons have intestinal resistance to subsequent infection by naturally occurring polioviruses. Result is markedly decreased or no multiplication of these viruses in alimentary tract, which breaks chain of dissemination

Paralytic poliomyelitis in USA, 1951 to 1976 (average number of cases per year) and effect of vaccine

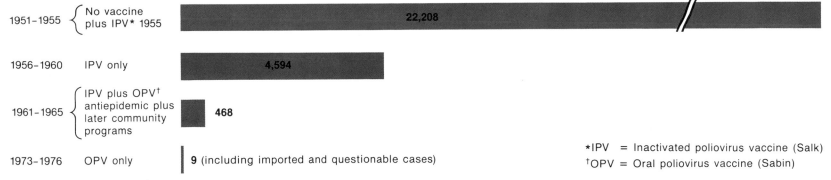

1951–1955	No vaccine plus IPV* 1955	22,208
1956–1960	IPV only	4,594
1961–1965	IPV plus OPV† antiepidemic plus later community programs	468
1973–1976	OPV only	9 (including imported and questionable cases)

*IPV = Inactivated poliovirus vaccine (Salk)
†OPV = Oral poliovirus vaccine (Sabin)

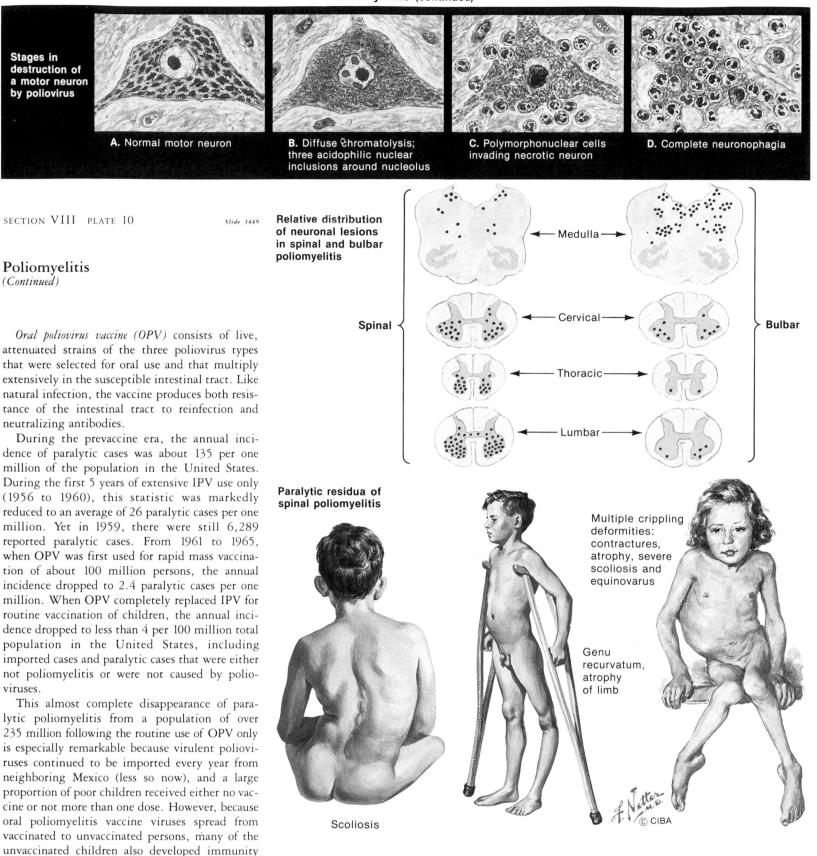

Stages in destruction of a motor neuron by poliovirus

A. Normal motor neuron

B. Diffuse Chromatolysis; three acidophilic nuclear inclusions around nucleolus

C. Polymorphonuclear cells invading necrotic neuron

D. Complete neuronophagia

SECTION VIII PLATE 10   *Slide 3449*

Poliomyelitis
(Continued)

Oral poliovirus vaccine (OPV) consists of live, attenuated strains of the three poliovirus types that were selected for oral use and that multiply extensively in the susceptible intestinal tract. Like natural infection, the vaccine produces both resistance of the intestinal tract to reinfection and neutralizing antibodies.

During the prevaccine era, the annual incidence of paralytic cases was about 135 per one million of the population in the United States. During the first 5 years of extensive IPV use only (1956 to 1960), this statistic was markedly reduced to an average of 26 paralytic cases per one million. Yet in 1959, there were still 6,289 reported paralytic cases. From 1961 to 1965, when OPV was first used for rapid mass vaccination of about 100 million persons, the annual incidence dropped to 2.4 paralytic cases per one million. When OPV completely replaced IPV for routine vaccination of children, the annual incidence dropped to less than 4 per 100 million total population in the United States, including imported cases and paralytic cases that were either not poliomyelitis or were not caused by polioviruses.

This almost complete disappearance of paralytic poliomyelitis from a population of over 235 million following the routine use of OPV only is especially remarkable because virulent polioviruses continued to be imported every year from neighboring Mexico (less so now), and a large proportion of poor children received either no vaccine or not more than one dose. However, because oral poliomyelitis vaccine viruses spread from vaccinated to unvaccinated persons, many of the unvaccinated children also developed immunity and helped to break the chain of transmission of virulent polioviruses brought into the community.

Paralytic poliomyelitis was rapidly eliminated from the temperate climate regions of America, Europe, Asia, Australia and New Zealand by an initial mass campaign with OPV, which was carried out in 1 or 2 days for each type of poliovirus or each dose of trivalent vaccine, with intervals of 6 to 8 weeks between each dose. This was followed by routine vaccination of children as part of their regular health care. To date, the immunity induced by OPV is as long-lasting as after natural infection.

Relative distribution of neuronal lesions in spinal and bulbar poliomyelitis

Medulla

Spinal — Cervical — Bulbar

Thoracic

Lumbar

Paralytic residua of spinal poliomyelitis

Multiple crippling deformities: contractures, atrophy, severe scoliosis and equinovarus

Genu recurvatum, atrophy of limb

Scoliosis

f. Netter M.D. © CIBA

The same procedure reduces but does not eliminate the amount of paralytic poliomyelitis in tropical and subtropical less developed countries, because (1) the combination of hot climate, poor sanitation, poor hygiene and overcrowding is responsible for a much higher prevalence of paralyzing polioviruses and other intestinal viruses in the community throughout the year; (2) single (even well-organized) mass campaigns are therefore less effective in interrupting the transmission of the larger number of paralyzing polioviruses, except for brief periods of 12 to 18 months, by which time large numbers of new babies have been

born; and (3) ongoing routine vaccination programs reach only a small proportion of children.

Paralytic poliomyelitis can be eliminated from less developed countries by annual, well-organized mass vaccination of *all children under 3, 4 or 5 years of age* (depending on the age by which 90% or more of the reported cases occur in the region), regardless of how many doses of OPV they may have had previously. Two days should be allowed for the administration of each of two doses, with a 2-month interval between them. Repetition of such mass campaigns every year is essential. □

Herpes Zoster

Only a small number of infectious diseases affect the peripheral nervous system, in contrast to the many and varied types of central nervous system (CNS) infections. The most common infection of the peripheral nervous system in industrialized nations is herpes zoster. In the United States, the annual incidence is 0.3% to 0.5% of the population.

Known to the layman as "shingles," herpes zoster is an acute neuralgia confined to the distribution of a specific spinal nerve root or cranial nerve. It is associated with a characteristic vesicular rash and occurs more often in the immunocompromised host. About 10% of all patients with lymphoma contract herpes zoster, the highest incidence (25%) occurring in those with Hodgkin's disease. The physician should take a complete history and conduct a physical examination and routine laboratory studies in any patient with recent onset of herpes zoster, because 1 in 25 of these patients may be harboring a previously undetected carcinoma or lymphoma. Other patients at high risk of herpes zoster include those on corticosteroid therapy or therapeutically immunosuppressed patients such as transplant recipients.

Pathology. The dorsal root ganglion is the primary site of infection. It is thought that the responsible DNA-type virus, varicella-zoster virus, is the same virus that causes chickenpox in children. Current theories suggest that the virus, which is also similar to herpes simplex virus, migrates up the peripheral nerve to the dorsal root ganglion subsequent to an attack of chickenpox in childhood. The virus then lies dormant for many years until the proper immunologic milieu develops and allows it to become active again. When this occurs, the dorsal root ganglion may be destroyed by an acute inflammatory reaction. Concomitantly, the virus spreads down the nerve root and peripheral nerve to the skin, producing the characteristic rash. It also spreads centrally into the spinal cord, causing an occult focal poliomyelitis in the anterior horn cells.

Clinical Manifestations. The clinical picture depends on the level at which the spinal cord is involved. Usually, only a single sensory ganglion is affected, although contiguous ganglia are involved at times, and rarely a generalized rash develops. Although the rash seems to occur most often in the distribution of the lower thoracic dermatomes, any spinal segment may be implicated. In the same way, a few cranial nerves, namely, the trigeminal (gasserian) ganglion and geniculate ganglion, are predominantly affected.

The rash is reminiscent of chickenpox but confined to a radicular or cranial nerve distribution. Its onset is often heralded by a few days of either severe localized pain or nonspecific discomfort in the affected area. The vesicles appear 72 to 96 hours later. They have an erythematous base with a tight, clear bubble that eventually becomes opaque and dries and crusts over after 5 to 10 days. The pain usually ceases in 1 to 4 weeks. However, in 15% to 25% of patients, the pain may persist for 1 to 2 years and is particularly disagreeable.

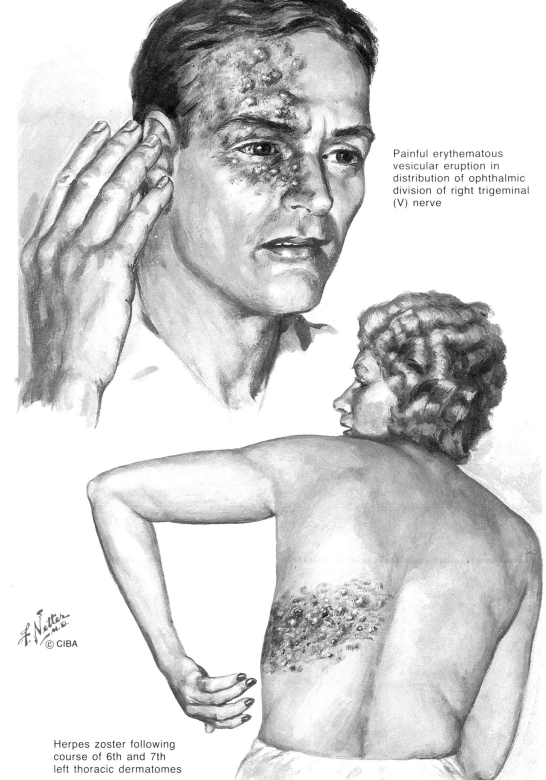

Painful erythematous vesicular eruption in distribution of ophthalmic division of right trigeminal (V) nerve

Herpes zoster following course of 6th and 7th left thoracic dermatomes

Ophthalmic herpes zoster is fairly common and carries the risk of corneal anesthesia and consequent scarring. Occasionally, the oculomotor (III), trochlear (IV) and abducens (VI) nerves may be affected. Rarely, vasculitis may develop in the contiguous carotid artery and cause a cerebral infarct (see Section III, Plate 17).

The Ramsay Hunt syndrome is secondary to herpes zoster of the facial (VII) nerve, which affects the geniculate ganglion. It is usually associated with vesicles in the external ear, and sometimes causes tinnitus, vertigo and deafness.

Rarely, some patients with radicular involvement of the arm or leg may have concomitant loss of motor function. Even more rarely, the spinal cord involvement becomes severe enough to produce generalized meningoencephalitis, which may have a variable prognosis.

Treatment. For uncomplicated herpes zoster, treatment is primarily symptomatic, with cool, wet compresses for the rash and analgesics for the pain. Occasionally, phenytoin and/or carbamazepine may relieve pain. Recently, trials with levadopa or cimetidine, or both, have been beneficial in a few patients. However, this treatment must be used in large series of patients before its effectiveness can be determined. Although pain may persist, it eventually disappears. Patients with ophthalmic herpes zoster should be referred to an ophthalmologist. □

Herpes Simplex Encephalitis and Rabies

Herpes Simplex Encephalitis

Herpes simplex encephalitis (HSE) is the most common sporadic acute viral disease of the brain in the United States. It affects both sexes and all age groups in every season. The mortality is high (about 70%), and survivors often have significant neuropsychiatric sequelae.

After the neonatal period, nearly all HSE results from infection with herpes simplex virus type 1 (HSV-1). Although pathogenic pathways have not been fully clarified, spread into temporal lobes via the olfactory tract or trigeminal (V) nerve has been postulated. Encephalitis can result from either primary or reactivation infection, and most often involves the medial temporal and frontal lobes. Hemorrhagic necrosis, inflammatory infiltrates, and cells containing intranuclear inclusions characterize the histologic picture.

The most common clinical findings are fever and alteration of consciousness. Headache, personality changes, speech difficulties and seizures occur in the majority of patients. Physical examination or diagnostic tests usually reveal focal findings suggesting temporal lobe involvement. Electroencephalography may show spike and slow waves localized to the involved area, while computed tomography (CT) demonstrates localized edema, low-density lesions, mass effects, contrast enhancement or hemorrhage. Cerebrospinal fluid (CSF) findings are nonspecific, but often include a lymphocytic pleocytosis, with slight elevation of the protein level.

The diagnosis in most patients can best be confirmed by biopsy of involved areas of the brain. Biopsy specimens are examined for histopathologic changes, for HSV antigens by immunofluorescence, and for infectious virus by appropriate culture techniques. Among disorders that can mimic HSE are vascular disease, bacterial abscess, cryptococcal infections, toxoplasmosis, tuberculosis, tumor and other forms of viral encephalitis.

Within recent years, it has become clear that the mortality and morbidity associated with HSE can be substantially reduced by early antiviral therapy. Acyclovir reduces mortality 20% to 30%, and is most effective in persons less than 40 years of age who are treated before coma or semicoma develops. Unfortunately, the number of survivors without neurologic sequelae remains unacceptably low, and the search for better alternative treatment continues.

Rabies

An acute viral disease of the central nervous system (CNS), rabies is caused by an RNA virus of the rhabdovirus family. It is usually transmitted to humans through a wound contaminated by the saliva of a rabid animal, although rare airborne transmission has been noted in bat-infested caves. Transmission by corneal transplants has also been reported. Dog and cat bites account for 90% of

Herpes Simplex Encephalitis

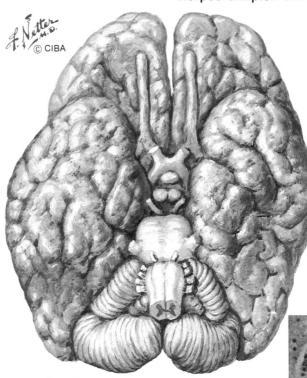

Swelling and patchy hemorrhagic areas, most marked in right temporal lobe

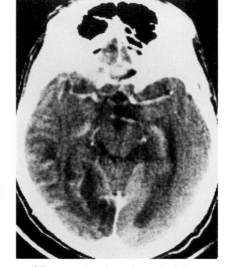

CT scan showing characteristic low absorption in temporal lobes

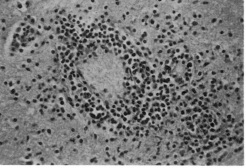

Perivascular infiltration with mononuclear cells in disrupted brain tissue

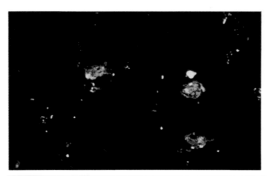

Immunofluorescent staining shows presence of herpesvirus antigen in neurons

Rabies

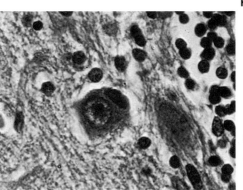

Negri inclusion body in Purkinje cell of brain

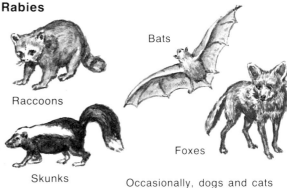

Raccoons

Bats

Skunks

Foxes

Occasionally, dogs and cats

Common animal disseminators

human rabies cases, although in developed countries, wild animals (raccoons, skunks, foxes, bats) are a greater threat.

The virus travels by nerve routes into the brain where it disseminates widely. Thereafter, it travels centrifugally along nerves to multiple organs, such as the salivary glands and the skin. Immunofluorescence of hair follicles taken from skin in the neck for evidence of rabies antigen is a rapid and reliable diagnostic test. Incubation periods range from 15 days to over 1 year.

The disease begins with a prodrome of anxiety, fever and headache, often with paresthesias at the bite site. Two to 10 days later, delirium, seizures, nuchal rigidity, paralysis and excitability develop.

Stimulus-sensitive spasms of the pharynx, esophagus or neck muscles may occur. When this stage has been reached, patients have not survived.

Clinical manifestations contrast strikingly with neuropathologic findings. Only mild congestion and perivascular inflammation are noted. The Negri body, a neuronal cytoplasmic inclusion of 1 to 7 μm with a dark central inner body, is pathognomonic.

Recent improvements in the use of vaccine grown in human cells and human anti-rabies globulin have made early postexposure prophylaxis safe and effective. However, no effective treatment is available once clinical illness develops. □

Slow Virus Infections

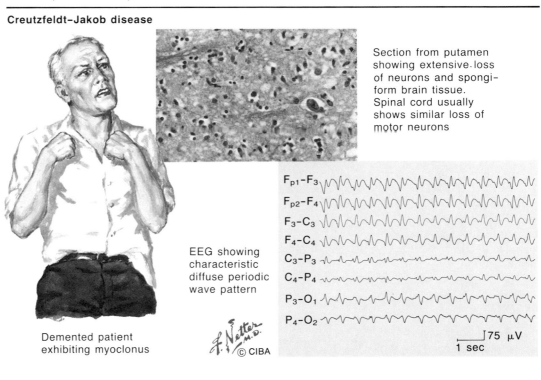

Progressive multifocal leukoencephalopathy (PML)

Coronal section of brain showing many minute demyelinating lesions in white matter, which have coalesced in some areas to form irregular cavitations

Section from edge of demyelinated focus showing abnormal oligodendrocytes with large hyperchromatic nuclei (H and E stain)

Electron micrograph showing giant glial nucleus with inclusion bodies

Electron micrograph showing papovavirus virions isolated from brain

Creutzfeldt–Jakob disease

Section from putamen showing extensive loss of neurons and spongiform brain tissue. Spinal cord usually shows similar loss of motor neurons

Demented patient exhibiting myoclonus

EEG showing characteristic diffuse periodic wave pattern

$F_{p1}-F_3$
$F_{p2}-F_4$
F_3-C_3
F_4-C_4
C_3-P_3
C_4-P_4
P_3-O_1
P_4-O_2

75 μV
1 sec

Chronic neurologic syndromes resulting from a viral infection sometimes develop many years after the initial infection. Such conditions may arise from a variety of different mechanisms, depending on the pathogenicity of the virus and the immunologic integrity of the host. These disorders are generally progressive, relentless and fatal; to date, there are no effective treatments.

Infection with the JC papovavirus often occurs asymptomatically at an early age. Thereafter, the virus probably remains latent until a time of prolonged intense T lymphocyte immunosuppression, as in certain organ transplant recipients, in patients with cancer, or in *acquired immunodeficiency syndrome (AIDS)*. At such times, the virus may reactivate and cause a patchy demyelinating disease called *progressive multifocal leukoencephalopathy (PML)*. Alternatively, primary infection with JC papovavirus at a time of maximum immunosuppression may be responsible for PML. Clinical findings include mental deterioration, paralysis, visual loss and sensory loss. Patients are afebrile, and the cerebrospinal fluid (CSF) shows no abnormalities. Computed tomography (CT) may demonstrate multiple radiolucent areas in white matter, but histologic examination of brain tissue is required for definitive diagnosis. Histologic features include bizarre morphologic changes in astrocytes and oligodendrocytes, with virus-filled intranuclear inclusions in the latter.

Subacute sclerosing panencephalitis (SSPE) is probably caused by reactivation of a measleslike virus that has been dormant for many years after early childhood infection. The mechanisms leading to latency and subsequent reactivation after a period of approximately 7 years are unclear. The disease appears more common in males living in rural areas. Onset is usually insidious, and over a period of months to years, the disease progresses from behavioral problems to disturbed motor function to stupor and autonomic instability. The CSF is

normal except for elevated measles antibody titers, and an electroencephalogram (EEG) may show a burst-suppression pattern. Histologic studies reveal leptomeningitis and gliosis, with eosinophilic intranuclear inclusions containing measles antigen. Measles virus can be isolated from brain tissue by appropriate tissue culture techniques, and use of measles virus vaccine has been accompanied by a marked reduction in cases of SSPE.

Spongiform encephalopathies occur in a variety of species, including sheep, mink and humans. The responsible transmissible agents are very small and unlike any other animal viruses in their biophysical properties.

The two human diseases caused by these agents are *kuru* and *Creutzfeldt-Jakob disease*. Both diseases are characterized by neural loss, absence of inflammatory infiltrates, neuronal vacuolation and astrocytosis. Kuru has been localized in the New Guinea highlands and was spread by cannibalistic practices, which are now dying out. Creutzfeldt-Jakob disease has a worldwide distribution, although certain families or populations may be particularly susceptible. The clinical hallmarks are progressive dementia and myoclonus. The EEG shows a characteristic pattern of periodic discharges, and the CSF is normal. The disease progresses to death, usually within 15 months after onset. □

Section IX

Demyelinating Disorders of Central Nervous System

Frank H. Netter, M.D.

in collaboration with

Jose A. Gutrecht, M.D.   *Plates 2–3*

H. Stephen Kott, M.D. and H. Royden Jones, Jr., M.D.   *Plates 1, 4*

Michael J. Moore, M.D. and Vincent P. Sweeney, M.D.   *Plate 5*

Multiple Sclerosis: Clinical Manifestations

Visual manifestations

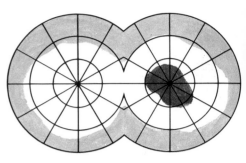

Sudden unilateral blindness, self-limited (usually 2 to 3 weeks). Patient covering one eye, suddenly realizes other eye is partially or totally blind

Visual fields reveal central scotoma due to acute retrobulbar neuritis

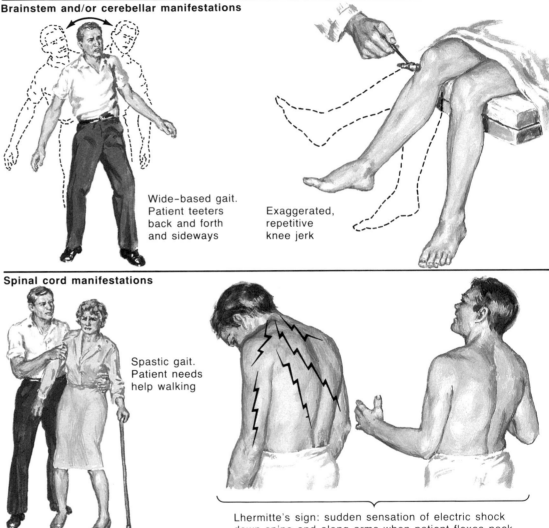

Brainstem and/or cerebellar manifestations

Wide-based gait. Patient teeters back and forth and sideways

Exaggerated, repetitive knee jerk

Spinal cord manifestations

Spastic gait. Patient needs help walking

Lhermitte's sign: sudden sensation of electric shock down spine and along arms when patient flexes neck

Multiple sclerosis is probably the most common neurologic illness affecting young adults in Canada and the northern sections of the United States and Europe. The prevalence is about 40 to 60 per 100,000 in high-risk areas, in contrast to 4 per 100,000 in Japan, Africa and South America. Studies indicate that with population migration from a high-risk to a low-risk area, immigrants' children less than 15 years of age are subject to the prevalence in the low-risk region. These data suggest an *environmental agent* in the pathogenesis of this disease.

A virtual epidemic of multiple sclerosis occurred in the Faroe Islands following occupation by British soldiers during World War II, which suggests an *infectious pathogenic agent*.

Among Caucasian patients with multiple sclerosis, 60% to 70% carry the HLA-Dw2 antigen. The risk of multiple sclerosis in a relative of a patient with the disease is 15 to 25 times that in the general population. However, the risk that an individual family member will contract the disease is only 1% to 2%. These statistics suggest a *genetic etiologic factor*.

Clinical Manifestations. The symptoms and signs of multiple sclerosis depend on the number and location of plaques. Early symptoms include visual disturbances, paresthesias, gait disturbances and brainstem syndromes.

Optic neuritis is a common early sign, occurring in 25% to 40% of all patients. The patient experiences photophobia, pain on movement of the globe, and decrease in vision. Demyelination at the nerve head causes papilledema. When the lesion is retrobulbar, the only finding may be a central or paracentral scotoma. Later, optic atrophy may become apparent. While optic neuritis suggests the diagnosis of multiple sclerosis, it should be remembered that only 20% to 30% of optic neuritis is caused by this disease.

Brainstem lesions are common and occur early. Diplopia is usually caused by disruption of the abducens (VI) nerve. Vertigo (5% of all cases) may be difficult to differentiate from labyrinthitis. Nystagmus (20% to 40%) is a common sign but is usually asymptomatic. Trigeminal neuralgia and peripheral facial weakness are sometimes confused with idiopathic tic douloureux and Bell's palsy, respectively.

Internuclear ophthalmoplegia is a classic sign of multiple sclerosis and indicates involvement of the medial longitudinal fasciculus. Examination reveals paresis of adduction on lateral gaze, and associated nystagmus in the abducting eye. Conversion may be preserved.

Sensory symptoms signifying posterior column demyelination often occur early and include paresthesias, dysesthesias and Lhermitte's sign. Examination may reveal a decrease in two-point discrimination, along with diminished vibration and position sense. A positive Romberg sign indicates sensory ataxia of posterior column origin.

Corticospinal tract dysfunction causes muscle fatigue, stiffness, spasticity and weakness. Hyper-

reflexia, clonus and the Babinski sign are frequently elicited. Urinary frequency and urgency suggest a hyperreflexic neurogenic bladder.

Cerebellar ataxia occurs in about 50% of all patients, but is usually not an early sign. Symptoms include poor balance, intention tremor, dysarthria and titubation. Cerebellar symptoms tend to be progressive and severely disabling.

Mental changes are noted in a large percentage of patients, but are initially subtle. Mood changes are common, and include depression and frontal lobe disinhibition. Seizures occur in 5% of patients, and significant dementia may also appear.

Clinical Course. Multiple sclerosis occurs predominantly in patients between 20 and 40

Clinical Manifestations

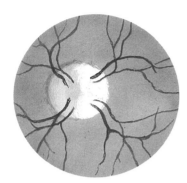

Temporal pallor in optic disc, caused by delayed recovery of temporal side of optic (II) nerve

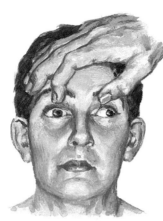

Eyes turned to left, right eye lags

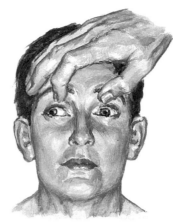

Eyes turned to right, left eye lags (to lesser degree)

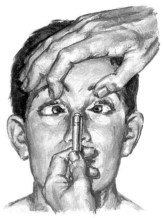

Convergence unimpaired

Internuclear ophthalmoplegia

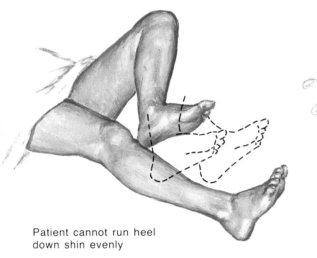

Patient cannot run heel down shin evenly

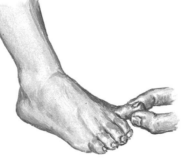

Intention tremor. Hand unsteady on attempting to hold glass, write, etc

Finger-to-nose test. Patient cannot direct finger accurately with eyes closed

Neurogenic bladder, with urinary urgency and dribbling

Loss of position sense

Paraplegia, partial or complete. Patient in wheelchair

years of age. Onset in persons younger than 10 or older than 50 accounts for only 2% to 5% of all cases. The clinical picture in late-onset disease is usually that of a progressive myelopathy with spastic paraparesis. Approximately 65% of the patients with gradually progressive myelopathy have either positive visual evoked potentials or oligoclonal bands in the cerebrospinal fluid (CSF).

Multiple exacerbations and remissions mark the usual course of the disease. Although exacerbations tend to remit completely in the early stages, later relapses heal incompletely and contribute to progressive disability.

Relapses are often acute in onset, but may progress over days or weeks, the average attack

persisting for several weeks. The patient may experience symptoms for only a few minutes or a few hours. Heat, infection, fatigue and tension may trigger diplopia, paresthesia and visual blurring. However, these episodes should not be considered exacerbations, since they are probably caused by conduction delay in partially demyelinated tracts.

The course appears benign in some patients, with few exacerbations and very little progressive disability. One study showed that 80% of patients who had remissions had no restrictions 10 years after onset of disease. Many such patients continue to do well for several years, and the overall survival rate at 25 years is at least 50%.

Some patients may have only a few scattered lesions, and the disease may remain subclinical. The incidence of silent multiple sclerosis has been estimated to vary from 5% to an astonishing 20% of all cases.

Treatment. Currently, there is no effective treatment for multiple sclerosis. ACTH or prednisone is often used to treat exacerbations. However, although these steroids may decrease inflammation and edema in the acute plaque, they are ineffective in preventing gliosis or exacerbations. At the present time, trials are under way with interferon and cyclophosphamide immunosuppression in the hope of arresting the progression of the disease. □

Multiple Sclerosis: Diagnostic Tests

Visual evoked response (VER)

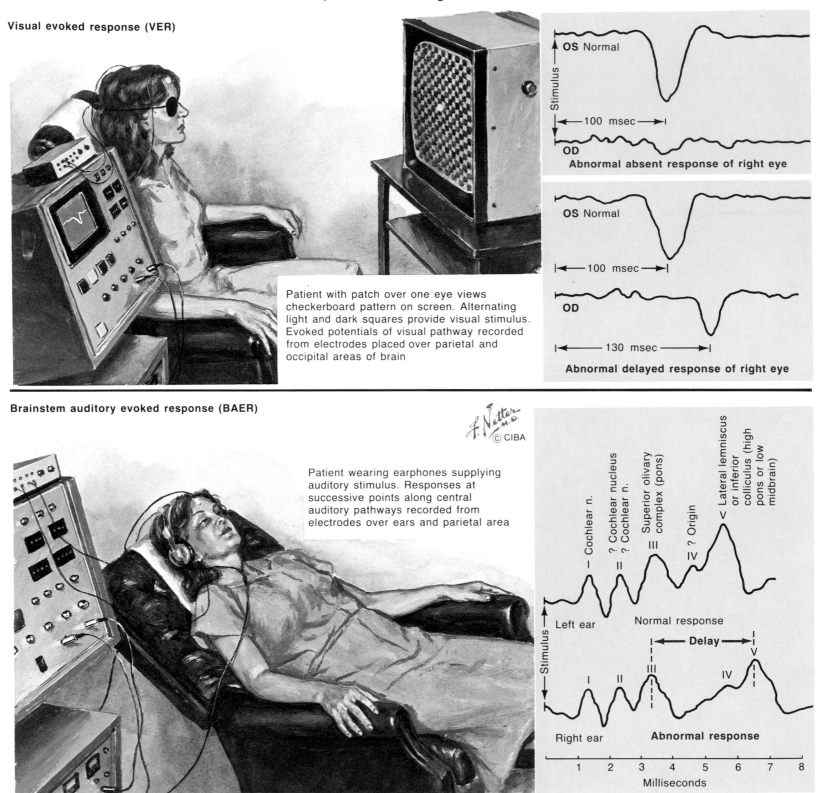

Patient with patch over one eye views checkerboard pattern on screen. Alternating light and dark squares provide visual stimulus. Evoked potentials of visual pathway recorded from electrodes placed over parietal and occipital areas of brain

OS Normal

100 msec

OD

Abnormal absent response of right eye

OS Normal

100 msec

OD

130 msec

Abnormal delayed response of right eye

Brainstem auditory evoked response (BAER)

Patient wearing earphones supplying auditory stimulus. Responses at successive points along central auditory pathways recorded from electrodes over ears and parietal area

I Cochlear n.

II ? Cochlear nucleus ? Cochlear n.

III Superior olivary complex (pons)

IV ? Origin

V < Lateral lemniscus or inferior colliculus (high pons or low midbrain)

Left ear — Normal response

Right ear — **Abnormal response**

Delay

1 2 3 4 5 6 7 8
Milliseconds

Multiple Sclerosis: Diagnostic Tests

Accuracy in the diagnosis of multiple sclerosis has been improved with the development of refined electrophysiologic testing. In particular, *evoked potential* studies have allowed recognition of previously unsuspected lesions, often in areas remote from each other.

Stimulation of receptors or sensory fibers generates electrical activity along their peripheral and central pathways, as well as in specific receptive areas in the brain. The stimulus is generally physiologic and responses are recorded to allow evaluation of their pathways.

Visual Evoked Responses (VER). A reversing checkerboard pattern is presented to each eye separately (Plate 2). Responses are recorded from midline electrodes in the parietal and occipital regions. The normal response (P_{100}) is a major positive wave of approximately 10 μV in amplitude and 100 msec in latency, which originates in the receptive visual cortex. Unilateral abnormalities suggest prechiasmatic lesions, whereas bilateral delays are much less specific.

Prolonged latencies are often seen in about 66% of patients, many of whom have no clinical evidence of optic neuritis. In more severe cases, no response is elicited. Compressive lesions of the anterior visual pathways also produce an abnormal P_{100}, but decreased amplitude is more common than prolonged latency.

Brainstem Auditory Evoked Responses (BAER). Clicks are presented to each ear and recording is done from the ear lobes, mastoid areas or external auditory canal. Normal responses consist of five distinct waves of different latencies (Plate 2). Wave I reflects activity of the vestibular nerve; wave II, the vestibular nerve or perhaps the cochlear nucleus; and wave III, the superior olivary complex. Wave V is probably generated somewhere in the high pons or lower midbrain. Sometimes, waves VI and VII are seen. With the

Multiple Sclerosis: Diagnostic Tests (continued)

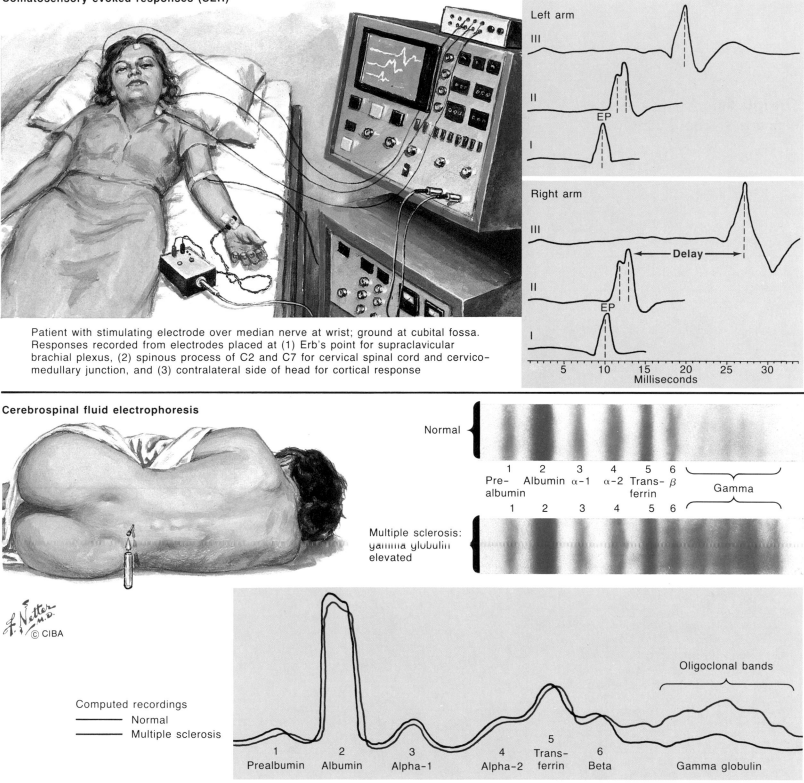

Somatosensory evoked responses (SER)

Left arm

III

II

EP

I

Right arm

III

Delay

II

EP

I

5   10   15   20   25   30
Milliseconds

Patient with stimulating electrode over median nerve at wrist; ground at cubital fossa. Responses recorded from electrodes placed at (1) Erb's point for supraclavicular brachial plexus, (2) spinous process of C2 and C7 for cervical spinal cord and cervico-medullary junction, and (3) contralateral side of head for cortical response

Cerebrospinal fluid electrophoresis

Normal

1   2   3   4   5   6
Pre-   Albumin α-1   α-2 Trans- β   Gamma
albumin   ferrin

1   2   3   4   5   6

Multiple sclerosis: gamma globulin elevated

Oligoclonal bands

Computed recordings
——— Normal
——— Multiple sclerosis

1   2   3   4   5   6
Prealbumin Albumin   Alpha-1   Alpha-2 Trans-   Beta   Gamma globulin
                                         ferrin

SECTION IX   PLATE 3   *Slide 3455*

Multiple Sclerosis: Diagnostic Tests

(Continued)

possible exception of wave V, these waves are assumed to arise in pathways ipsilateral to the stimulated ear.

Almost 50% of patients with multiple sclerosis exhibit abnormal brainstem auditory evoked responses, eg, decreased amplitudes, absence of wave V or prolonged interwave latencies.

Somatosensory Evoked Responses (SER). Peripheral nerves in the upper or lower limbs are

stimulated and responses are recorded from electrodes over (1) the brachial plexus at the supraclavicular space for the arm, and the cauda equina at the lumbar spine for the leg, (2) the spinous processes of high cervical vertebrae, and (3) the contralateral sensory cortex (Plate 3).

Abnormalities in amplitude or latencies of the responses at Erb's point and at the lumbar point suggest peripheral nerve involvement. Asymmetry of response amplitude or delays in latencies thereafter suggest central sensory pathway involvement. These abnormalities occur in almost 66% of all patients, but are not pathognomonic for multiple sclerosis and have been described in a variety of other conditions.

Cerebrospinal Fluid (CSF) Analysis. Even though the CSF may be normal, some of its components may be abnormal in multiple sclerosis (Plate 3). Total white cell count is elevated in about 25% of patients, but rarely above 25 mononuclear cells per mm³. The total protein concentration is slightly elevated in 33% of patients. In 40% to 60% of patients, the gamma globulin (IgG) fraction is elevated above 13% of the total CSF protein, reflecting an increased production of IgG within the demyelinated areas in the central nervous system (CNS). Oligoclonal bands in the IgG sector of the protein electrophoretic pattern may be detected in almost 90% of all cases. CSF pressure and glucose content are normal. □

Multiple Sclerosis: Central Nervous System Pathology

Although the pathogenesis of multiple sclerosis is still unknown, recent interest centers around the possibility that it is a demyelinating *slow-virus illness* or an *autoimmune process*. No virus has been isolated from tissue affected by the disease; however, several naturally occurring animal infections have some features in common with multiple sclerosis.

Both cellular and antibody phenomena have been demonstrated in experimentally induced disease and in patients with multiple sclerosis. Helper T cells appear to be predominant in the outer margin of the multiple sclerosis plaque, and suppressor T cells are decreased in number during many acute relapses of the disease. Despite the apparent role of immune processes, it is still not known what mechanisms are responsible for remission of an attack, exacerbations or chronic progressive demyelination.

Despite the fact that the cause of multiple sclerosis remains an enigma and the pathophysiologic mechanisms are still speculative, the structural pathologic processes of this disease have been carefully described.

The primary process appears to be inflammatory. Initially, lymphocytes and macrophages respond to some unknown immunologic stimulus, penetrate the blood-brain barrier, and cause focal destruction of myelin while sparing axons. Oligodendroglia disappear from involved foci, and it is not clear whether these cells are attacked coincidentally with myelin or whether demyelination is secondary to oligodendroglial damage.

Microglia proliferate and help in the phagocytosis of myelin, while astrocytic processes infiltrate the area, producing a glial scar. Areas of demyelination with variable degrees of scar formation are known as *plaques*. Charcot recognized that these lesions are the hallmark of the disease and called the process *sclérose en plaque*.

Plaques are scattered randomly throughout the white matter of the brain and spinal cord, but they tend to be close to cerebrospinal fluid (CSF) pathways. Common areas of involvement include the cervical posterior columns, optic (II) nerve and chiasm, corpus callosum, periventricular white matter, brainstem and floor of the fourth ventricle, and pyramidal tract. Plaques also occur frequently in gray matter in the subpial regions of the cerebral gyri. Neurons in gray-matter plaques are preserved.

Study of plaques in acute attacks shows that the inflammatory activity may begin as a perivenous infiltration of lymphocytes, macrophages and plasma cells. Edema is present, and the borders of the lesion are indistinct. Oligodendroglia are swollen, and myelin is digested in macrophages

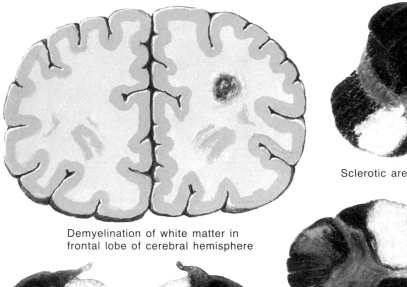

Demyelination of white matter in frontal lobe of cerebral hemisphere

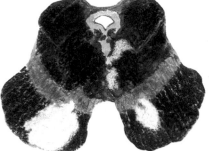

Sclerotic areas in cerebral peduncle

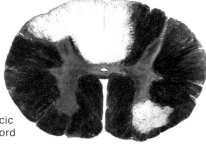

In cervical spinal cord

In medulla

In thoracic spinal cord

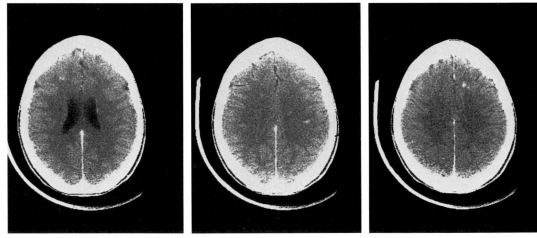

CT scans with contrast medium showing multiple foci of demyelination, evidenced by focal enhancing lesions of varying size, located primarily in white matter

and microglia. Staining methods show binding of IgG to microglia and astrocytes, and this staining is much more intense in plaques in acute attacks.

As the lesion matures, edema and the inflammatory response subside, and demyelinated and normal tissue are more clearly delineated. Gliosis imparts a gray, rubbery, homogenous appearance to the plaque. Although axons traversing the area are still seemingly unaffected, some are damaged by the scarring process.

Remyelination attempts, which are characteristic of multiple sclerosis, may occur at the margin of the plaque. In some foci, incomplete myelin staining signifies the presence of thinly myelinated axons. Electron microscopy has shown

surviving oligodendroglia elaborating the abnormally thin myelin layers that surround the axons. These areas have been called *shadow plaques*.

The number and location of plaques determine the clinical symptoms and signs, while the time interval between the appearance of new lesions determines the clinical course. Postmortem studies may show hundreds of lesions of variable age. Each focus is usually smaller than 1.5 cm in diameter, but coalescence may occur. When plaques are numerous in the cerebral white matter, ventricular dilatation may be striking.

Shrinkage secondary to plaque formation may also be responsible for areas of focal atrophy or diffuse thinning of the spinal cord. ☐

Acute Disseminated Encephalomyelitis (ADEM)

Acute Disseminated Encephalomyelitis and Acute Hemorrhagic Leukoencephalopathy

CT scan without contrast medium (left) shows several areas of low density in frontal and parietal lobes, primarily involving periventricular white matter. CT scan with contrast medium (right) shows gyral enhancement

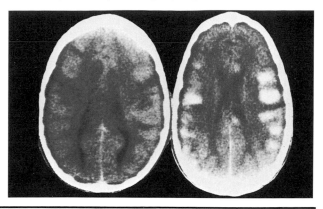

Acute Hemorrhagic Leukoencephalopathy (AHL)

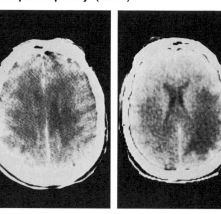

Fatal case of AHL confirmed at autopsy. CT scans with contrast medium show widespread low-density changes in white matter of both hemispheres. Right lateral ventricle compressed, with midline shift to left. Patchy enhancement seen over both cortices

Nonfatal case of AHL treated with high-dose steroids. Initial CT scan (left) shows low-density areas in frontal and parietal areas, as well as in occipital lobes. CT scan at right shows improvement in white matter abnormalities after steroid treatment and clinical improvement. Complete clinical recovery, with normal CT scan, was confirmed on follow-up

Acute Disseminated Encephalomyelitis (ADEM)

This acute demyelinating disease is an uncommon inflammatory disorder, which may occur following exanthems (rubeola, variola, varicella); vaccination for rabies, smallpox or pertussis; or, occasionally, *Mycoplasma* infections. A causative organism has never been isolated from patients with ADEM. However, the association with a preceding illness or immunization and the latency period strongly suggest an immunologic process.

The incidence of ADEM varies, depending on location, season and possible genetic predisposition. The overall mortality in the disease is unknown, but it has been as high as 30% in the postvaccinal form and has varied from 11.5% to 32% following measles. In those who survive ADEM, permanent neurologic deficits can occur, and a large proportion of patients have mild to severe psychiatric complications.

The clinical manifestations of all types of ADEM are similar. The disease begins with fever, headache, malaise and signs of meningeal irritation such as pain on flexion of the neck, which are soon followed by encephalitic features such as focal weakness, numbness, aphasia, ataxia, seizures, delirium, stupor and coma.

The duration of symptoms varies; some nonfatal, mild cases last a few days to a month, while fatal cases may last several days to a year. The clinical sign that correlates most closely with prognosis is the level of consciousness.

Coronal section of cerebral hemispheres at level of corpus striatum showing punctate hemorrhagic lesions in subcortical white matter

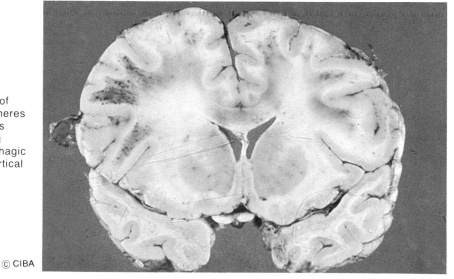

© CIBA

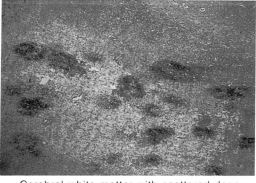

Cerebral white matter with scattered deep hemorrhages in pale, edematous areas. (H and E stain, × 10)

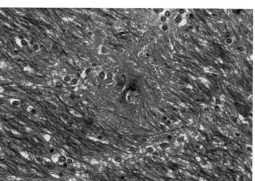

Cingulate gyrus white matter showing area of perivenous demyelination. (Luxol-fast blue-Holmes, × 100)

Acute Disseminated Encephalomyelitis and Acute Hemorrhagic Leukoencephalopathy
(Continued)

The cerebrospinal fluid (CSF) is sometimes normal, although the opening pressure may be elevated. Leukocytosis is commonly present, with many neutrophils in the early stages that later convert to lymphocytes, varying from a few to several hundred cells. The gamma globulin level is frequently elevated in ADEM, especially following antirabies vaccination. The electroencephalogram (EEG) shows diffuse slowing, and computed tomography (CT) may show patchy areas of contrast enhancement bilaterally in the cerebral and cerebellar cortex.

The differential diagnosis of ADEM includes the various acute aseptic meningoencephalitides and acute multiple sclerosis. The characteristic pathologic lesions, found predominantly in the white matter of the central nervous system (CNS), consist of perivenous mononuclear cell infiltration associated with demyelination within the cellular cuff.

The course of ADEM is self-limited, and therapeutic measures are aimed at general medical supportive care. However, the use of high-dose intravenous steroids is probably of value in decreasing intracranial pressure and suppressing the immune response that is thought to underlie progression of the disease.

Acute Hemorrhagic Leukoencephalopathy (AHL)

An acute and fulminating form of ADEM, AHL is a demyelinating disease characterized by a rapid and dramatic onset, short clinical course, and usually fatal outcome. In the hypothetical spectrum of demyelinating diseases, AHL is the most acute and severe form, while multiple sclerosis is the most chronic. There is now some evidence to support this association, because typical multiple sclerosis has subsequently developed in patients who have recovered from AHL. Because the diagnosis of AHL is usually made at autopsy, few patients have been available for clinical study. A viral illness usually precedes the development of this disease by several days to weeks, although many other types of predisposing conditions, including pneumonia, vaccination and surgery, have been described.

The early symptoms of AHL are malaise, fever and headaches, which rapidly progress to produce focal signs of CNS disease. Hemiparesis, dysphasia, sensory loss and seizures are common. Confusion and decline in the level of consciousness to coma invariably occur.

Laboratory investigations show that the peripheral white blood cell count is elevated (12,000 to 20,000/mm³). Analysis of CSF typically shows a slight increase in pressure; a moderate increase in protein, with levels of up to 1,000 mg/100 ml being reported occasionally; and pleocytosis of 10 to 1,000 cells per mm³. Initially, polymorphonuclear leukocytes predominate, but lymphocytosis develops within a few days. CSF glucose level is normal, which helps to differentiate this condition from bacterial meningitis. Red blood cells are often seen in the CSF. The EEG shows diffuse slow-wave activity, and serial CT scans show low-density white matter changes throughout both hemispheres, which correlate with clinically involved areas. Angiographic findings may suggest a space-occupying lesion, minor abnormalities, or may be normal.

The pathologic findings in AHL are unique and to date have been the only means of making a definitive diagnosis. The white matter of the cerebral hemispheres shows widespread edema, ball and ring hemorrhages, perivascular exudates, and perivenous foci of microglial proliferation. Zones of demyelination are seen around vessels.

The cause of this disease is unknown, although it is thought to result from an abnormal immune process, with involvement of both cell-mediated and humoral responses. A trial of steroids has been suggested on theoretical grounds because of the suspected autoimmune nature of the illness. In at least one case, high-dose steroids seemed to be of benefit. Since AHL is usually fatal or causes severe neurologic deficit, the clinical picture, together with the distinctive changes seen on the CT scan, should lead to the early institution of high-dose steroid treatment. □

Section X

Disorders of Spinal Cord, Nerve Root and Plexus

Frank H. Netter, M.D.

in collaboration with

Richard A. Baker, M.D.   *Plates 7, 12–13*

Stephen R. Freidberg, M.D.   *Plates 5–6, 14–15*

Stephen R. Freidberg, M.D. and H. Royden Jones, Jr., M.D.   *Plate 17*

William A. Friedman, M.D.   *Plate 11*

John R. Hayes, M.D.   *Plate 16*

H. Royden Jones, Jr., M.D.   *Plates 1–4, 18–19*

H. Stephen Kott, M.D. and H. Royden Jones, Jr., M.D.   *Plates 8–10*

Spinal Cord Dysfunction

A spinal cord lesion should be considered in any patient who has numbness or weakness of one or more extremities, particularly if there is pain in the neck or back and sphincter dysfunction. Various combinations of symptoms and signs point to: (1) extradural extramedullary, (2) intradural extramedullary or (3) intradural intramedullary spinal cord lesions.

Motor Impairment

The degree of motor dysfunction depends on the extent of the spinal cord lesion. *Complete lesions* destroy all function below the affected level. *Incomplete lesions* cause partial weakness, atrophy and hyporeflexia at the affected level, usually in combination with a distal upper motor neuron lesion, which may predominate and cause a varying degree of weakness, spasticity and hyperreflexia. A search for subtle signs of a distal upper motor neuron lesion is imperative in any patient who has an apparently isolated spinal nerve root lesion, particularly in the cervical region.

In contrast to a complete peripheral nerve lesion, in which motor function is completely destroyed in the distribution of that nerve, a complete nerve root lesion usually causes a partial, although sometimes severe, paresis but not total paralysis of the various muscles innervated by that nerve root. This is because each muscle is innervated by multiple nerve roots arising from more than one spinal level (Plate 1).

The diaphragm is predominantly innervated by segment C3, 4; therefore, a lesion high in the cervical spinal cord threatens respiratory function. Shoulder abduction is a good test of C5 function. In the presence of normal function of the deltoid muscle, weak elbow flexors, predominantly the biceps brachii muscles, suggest a C6 lesion. The elbow and wrist extensors, subserved primarily by the triceps brachii and extensor carpi radialis and ulnaris muscles, are innervated by C7. Function of the pronator teres muscle is also helpful in identifying a lesion at C7.

Lesions at C8 predominantly affect the intrinsic muscles of the hand, which are also innervated by T1. The abdominal musculature can be tested clinically for lesions that affect thoracic nerves; a positive Beevor sign indicates weakness below T9 or T10.

The hip flexors and adductors are innervated by L2 and predominantly by L3. The quadriceps femoris muscle is a good marker of L4 function. L5 innervates the ankle dorsiflexors and great toe extensors, while the ankle plantar flexors are

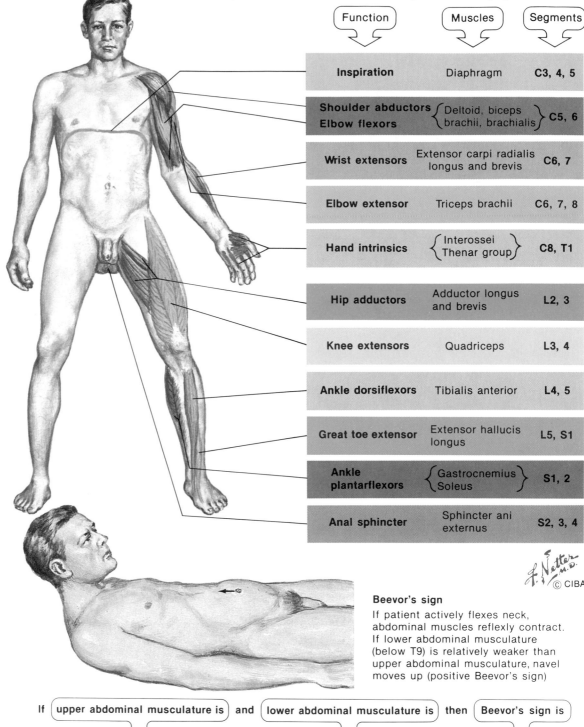

Motor Impairment Related to Level of Spinal Cord Injury

Function	Muscles	Segments
Inspiration	Diaphragm	C3, 4, 5
Shoulder abductors / **Elbow flexors**	Deltoid, biceps brachii, brachialis	C5, 6
Wrist extensors	Extensor carpi radialis longus and brevis	C6, 7
Elbow extensor	Triceps brachii	C6, 7, 8
Hand intrinsics	Interossei / Thenar group	C8, T1
Hip adductors	Adductor longus and brevis	L2, 3
Knee extensors	Quadriceps	L3, 4
Ankle dorsiflexors	Tibialis anterior	L4, 5
Great toe extensor	Extensor hallucis longus	L5, S1
Ankle plantarflexors	Gastrocnemius / Soleus	S1, 2
Anal sphincter	Sphincter ani externus	S2, 3, 4

Beevor's sign

If patient actively flexes neck, abdominal muscles reflexly contract. If lower abdominal musculature (below T9) is relatively weaker than upper abdominal musculature, navel moves up (positive Beevor's sign)

If upper abdominal musculature is	and lower abdominal musculature is	then Beevor's sign is
Normal	Normal	Negative
Normal	Weak or nonfunctioning	Positive
Weak	Nonfunctioning	Positive
Nonfunctioning	Nonfunctioning	Negative

innervated by S1 and S2. The lowest segments of the spinal cord (S2, 3, 4) control the anal sphincter.

Sensory Impairment

Sensory examination often provides the most significant information in localizing a spinal cord lesion. However, if results of the examination are normal, the patient's symptoms may be the most important clue. The segmental distribution may be most useful in diagnosis when both the nerve root and spinal cord are involved, as seen in a dumbbell tumor, or neurilemmoma (Plate 6).

The sensory dermatomal pattern shown in Plate 2 provides a useful guide. The C1 root has

no significant sensory component; thus, a lesion high in the cervical spinal cord at its most proximal limit affects C2, which involves the posterior part of the scalp. Since the descending spinal tract of the trigeminal (V) nerve extends into the upper cervical spinal cord, lesions at this level may produce changes in pain and temperature sensation over the temple and forehead, possibly with a diminished corneal reflex.

Segments C5, 6, 7, 8 and T1 innervate the arm and hand, with the deltoid muscle supplied by C5. The thumb is a good marker for C6, the index and middle fingers for C7, and the ring and little fingers for C8. T1 innervates the medial upper arm adjacent to the axilla. The nipple line

Spinal Cord Dysfunction
(Continued)

is innervated by T4, and the area over the abdomen at the umbilicus by T10.

In the lower extremities, L3 and L4 segments innervate the anterior thigh and pretibial regions, respectively. The first three toes are innervated by L5, while S1 innervates the fourth and fifth toes and S2 the posterior medial thigh. The saddle area of the buttocks is innervated by segments S3, 4, 5.

Paresthesias in the buttocks are an important sign of possible spinal cord dysfunction. Since segments S3, 4, 5 are the lowest and most peripheral segments in the spinal cord, an *extramedullary lesion* at any level may first compress these fibers and affect pain and temperature sensation. If the saddle area of the buttocks is not examined for pain and temperature sensation, an early spinal cord lesion may not be suspected. In contrast, if an *intramedullary lesion* is present, the buttocks region is the last to be affected, with resultant sacral sparing. Demonstration of this condition in a patient alerts the radiologist performing myelography to pay careful attention to the possibility of an intramedullary lesion.

Because the various ascending spinal tracts decussate at different levels of the spinal cord, several relatively specific patterns of dissociated sensory loss may be recognized clinically. The *Brown-Séquard syndrome* implies a hemisection or unilateral lesion of the spinal cord. This is characterized by ipsilateral diminution of touch, vibration and position sense and contralateral loss of pain and temperature sensation. Because the descending motor fibers decussate at the distal medulla, damage to these nerve fibers causes ipsilateral loss of function, with associated weakness and hyperreflexia.

The *anterior spinal artery syndrome* affects the anterior two thirds of the spinal cord bilaterally, causing loss of pain and temperature sensation at approximately one to two segments below the level of the lesion associated with paraplegia. However, because the posterior columns are preserved, bilateral touch, vibration and position sense is normal.

Intramedullary lesions, such as those seen in *syringomyelia*, affect decussating spinothalamic fibers in the central gray matter of the spinal cord. This produces a capelike loss of pain and temperature sensation, with preservation of posterior column function. Pain and temperature sensation is preserved below the involved levels, because the lateral spinothalamic tract is not affected by this central spinal cord syndrome. A concomitant lower motor neuron lesion commonly causing atrophy and fasciculations of the hands and arms is usually seen at the level of the dysfunction.

Autonomic Impairment

In addition to its somatic components, the spinal cord also contains autonomic nerve fibers, carried in the intermediolateral columns. A lesion at any level may cause sphincter dysfunction. Spinal cord lesions in general damage the upper motor neuron pathways that control the bladder and rectum. Incontinence does

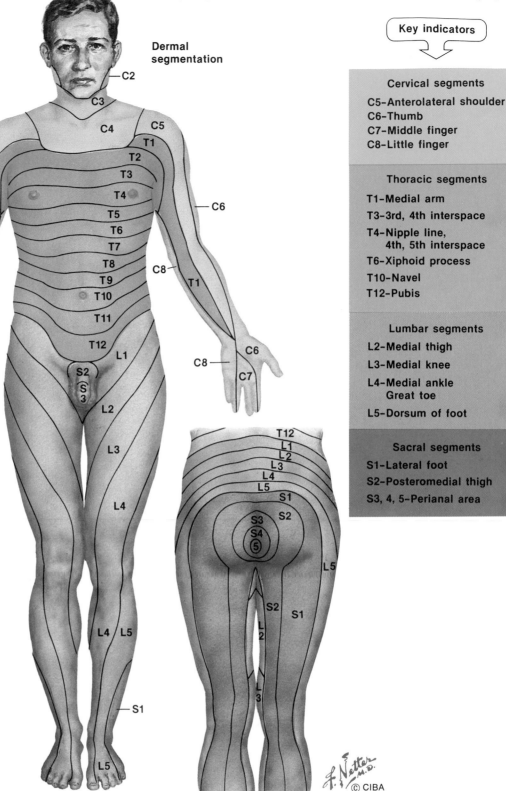

Sensory Impairment Related to Level of Spinal Cord Injury

Dermal segmentation

Key indicators

Cervical segments
C5-Anterolateral shoulder
C6-Thumb
C7-Middle finger
C8-Little finger

Thoracic segments
T1-Medial arm
T3-3rd, 4th interspace
T4-Nipple line, 4th, 5th interspace
T6-Xiphoid process
T10-Navel
T12-Pubis

Lumbar segments
L2-Medial thigh
L3-Medial knee
L4-Medial ankle Great toe
L5-Dorsum of foot

Sacral segments
S1-Lateral foot
S2-Posteromedial thigh
S3, 4, 5-Perianal area

not develop unless there is a severe bilateral lesion. Narcotics and tranquilizers can cause sphincter dysfunction and should not be given to a patient with a suspected spinal cord lesion.

Other signs of autonomic dysfunction include *sexual impotence; changes in sweating*, with anhidrosis below the level of the lesion; and *Horner's syndrome*, which includes ipsilateral miosis, ptosis and decreased facial sweating secondary to damage to sympathetic fibers at C8–T1.

Café au lait spots may suggest the presence of a *meningioma* or a *neurofibroma*. A tuft of hair or dimple in the midline, particularly in the lower spine, may point to an underlying *congenital vertebral defect* (see Section I, Plate 8). In rare cases,

a cutaneous angioma may overlie a spinal cord or *arteriovenous malformation*.

Although *scoliosis* is usually idiopathic, it rarely is the first sign of an evolving spinal cord tumor. *Pes cavus* may be seen with distal spinal cord lesions. A *short neck* may suggest the Klippel-Feil syndrome, which is sometimes associated with other cervical spine lesions.

Spinal cord dysfunction can be identified early if the patient's history and the results of neurologic examination are carefully assessed, with particular attention to the distribution of motor, reflex and sensory changes associated with autonomic dysfunction and the presence of various skeletal and cutaneous changes. □

Acute Spinal Cord Syndromes

The appropriate recognition of disease processes that can cause acute spinal cord damage is one of the major neurologic emergencies. If the disorder is diagnosed early, some patients with spinal cord damage can be successfully treated. However, when the subtleties of the clinical picture are not recognized, the course may be disastrous, often culminating in lifelong paraplegia (Plate 3).

The common mechanism in the patient with a potentially reversible condition is the presence of a mass lesion that has reached a critical size. Because the spinal cord lies within the bony spinal canal, an obstructive extradural or intradural extramedullary process causes compression of the cord and its vessels. If treatment can be initiated prior to the development of severe damage to spinal cord tissue, which is manifested by total paraplegia, an effective recovery is quite possible.

The acute onset of *back pain* in any patient, and particularly in a patient with cancer, should alert the physician to the potential for an impending spinal disaster. Often, however, the patient is not seen until further symptoms have also developed.

Predisposing Causes

Metastatic Carcinoma. The most common cause of an acute spinal cord syndrome, particularly in patients in the middle to late decades of life, is metastatic carcinoma. Most patients have had a known malignancy, but a spinal metastatic lesion may be the first indication of a primary tumor elsewhere, particularly carcinoma of the lung and lymphoma (Plate 5).

Infarction. Occlusion of the anterior part of a spinal artery affects the anterior two thirds of the spinal cord (Plate 4). Spinal cord infarction is usually precipitous. The clinical findings in this uncommon syndrome include paraparesis or paraplegia in combination with dissociated sensory loss, ie, loss of pain and temperature sensation, with preservation of position and vibration sense. Back pain, often at a segmental level, may be present.

Although some spinal cord infarctions appear to be idiopathic, a number of vascular lesions may be implicated, including an aortic dissection that compromises the artery of Adamkiewicz (major anterior radicular artery) and emboli from aortic atheroma. Postoperative sequelae of cardiac or aortic surgery and various types of arteritis also may be implicated.

Myelography is indicated to exclude other lesions, including the rare spontaneous epidural hematoma. Treatment is determined according to the underlying mechanism involved. Prognosis is usually poor.

Epidural Abscess. This lesion has a fairly characteristic clinical setting (Plate 4). The vast majority of patients are febrile, and most are acutely ill, sometimes becoming disoriented but always complaining of severe back and nerve root pain. Examination demonstrates an exquisite tenderness on percussion over the affected spinal process and signs of spinal cord impairment.

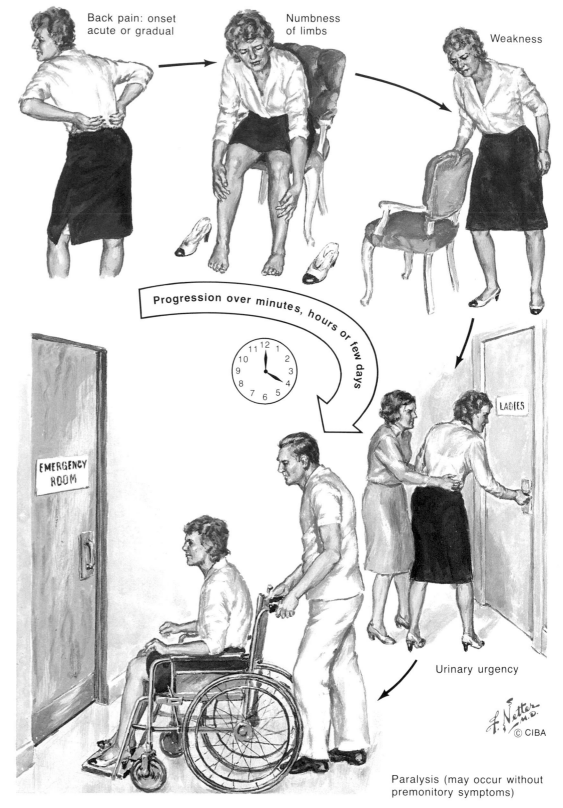

Back pain: onset acute or gradual — Numbness of limbs — Weakness — Progression over minutes, hours or few days — Urinary urgency — Paralysis (may occur without premonitory symptoms)

There is an apparent predisposing source of infection, with staphylococci and gram-negative bacilli as the predominant causative organisms.

Radiographs of the back should be immediately followed by myelography. Surgery should be done expeditiously to open and drain the area. Antibiotic therapy is administered according to the pathogen isolated in cultures.

Transverse Myelitis. This syndrome of acute spinal cord dysfunction (Plate 4) appears to be a demyelinating disorder similar to acute disseminated encephalomyelitis (see Section IX, Plate 5). Initial symptoms include leg weakness, loss of all sensation, and sphincter involvement. Nerve root pain and back pain are common findings. Early

in the course, deep tendon reflexes are either depressed or absent. Spasticity and optic neuritis (Devic's syndrome) develop in some patients.

The diagnosis is one of exclusion in a patient who has a complete acute spinal cord syndrome and in whom myelographic findings are normal. Involvement of all sensory modalities in acute transverse myelitis differentiates this disorder from spinal cord infarction, in which dissociated sensory loss is present. Despite the apparent underlying pathophysiologic mechanism of demyelination, these patients do not appear to have multiple sclerosis. Often, definite but incomplete recovery occurs and permits a relatively independent life. ☐

Acute Spinal Cord Syndromes: Pathology, Etiology and Diagnosis

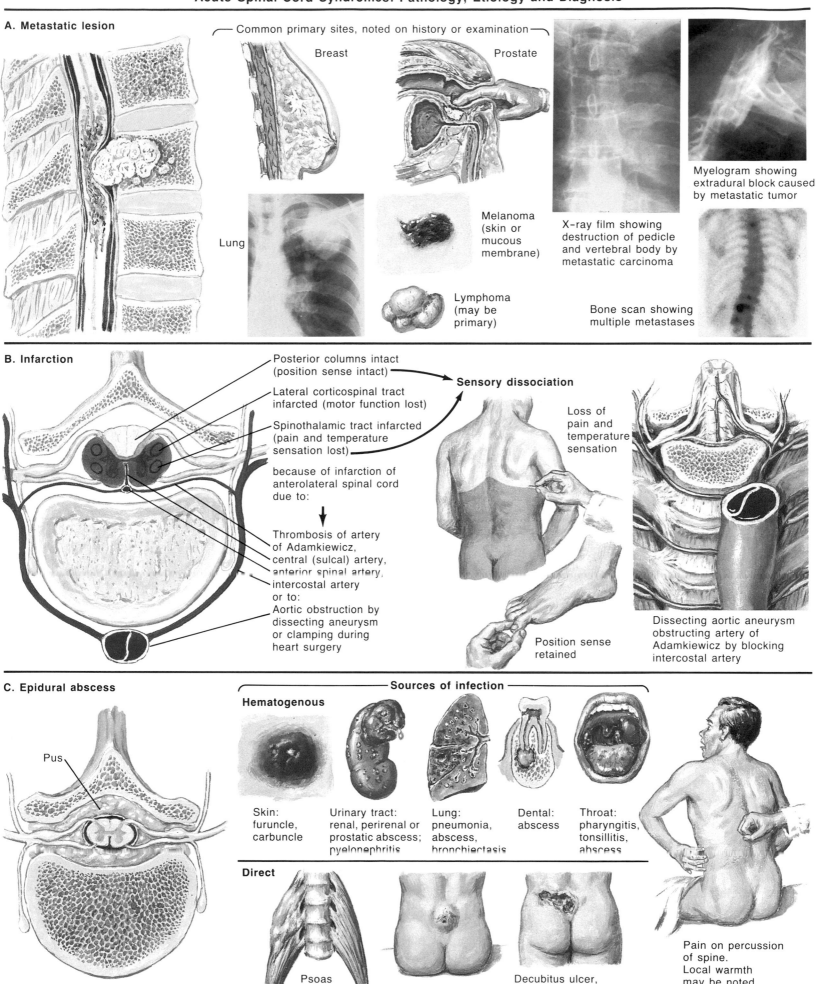

A. Metastatic lesion

Common primary sites, noted on history or examination

Breast

Prostate

Lung

Melanoma (skin or mucous membrane)

Lymphoma (may be primary)

Myelogram showing extradural block caused by metastatic tumor

X-ray film showing destruction of pedicle and vertebral body by metastatic carcinoma

Bone scan showing multiple metastases

B. Infarction

Posterior columns intact (position sense intact)

Lateral corticospinal tract infarcted (motor function lost)

Spinothalamic tract infarcted (pain and temperature sensation lost)

Sensory dissociation

Loss of pain and temperature sensation

Position sense retained

because of infarction of anterolateral spinal cord due to:

Thrombosis of artery of Adamkiewicz, central (sulcal) artery, anterior spinal artery, intercostal artery or to:

Aortic obstruction by dissecting aneurysm or clamping during heart surgery

Dissecting aortic aneurysm obstructing artery of Adamkiewicz by blocking intercostal artery

C. Epidural abscess

Pus

Sources of infection

Hematogenous

Skin: furuncle, carbuncle

Urinary tract: renal, perirenal or prostatic abscess; pyelonephritis

Lung: pneumonia, abscess, bronchiectasis

Dental: abscess

Throat: pharyngitis, tonsillitis, abscess

Direct

Psoas abscess

Dermal sinus

Decubitus ulcer, direct or hematogenous

Pain on percussion of spine. Local warmth may be noted

D. Transverse myelitis

Cause and specific pathologic process undetermined

Diagnosis by exclusion of other causes

Slide 3462

Spinal Tumors

Tumors involving the spine are usually classified as either extradural or intradural. The intradural tumors are further divided into extramedullary and intramedullary lesions, and an additional category, lumbar intradural tumors, should be added. The anatomic location of the tumor provides a clue to the pathologic diagnosis, but accurate diagnosis is based on histologic studies.

Extradural Tumors

Extradural tumors are usually *metastases* to the vertebrae that subsequently invade the epidural space (Plate 5). Almost any neoplasm can spread to the spine, but spinal metastases most commonly occur from a primary tumor in the lung, breast or prostate. The tumor metastasizes through the arterial circulation or Batson's venous plexus, although direct extension from lung cancer or lymphoma is possible. Primary bone tumors such as *osteogenic sarcoma* and *giant-cell tumor* are also seen, as is benign *hemangioma* of bone. In most cases, pain is the first symptom of a vertebral tumor. Spinal cord compression, with associated symptoms, usually develops late and may be slowly progressive, but a rapidly growing tumor may cause acute neurologic deterioration secondary to infarction of the spinal cord.

A patient with a known primary cancer in whom spinal pain develops must be assumed to have a metastasis. A bone scan reveals a lesion earlier than does a plain x-ray film. However, when neurologic symptoms are present, myelography is mandatory.

Epidural tumors must be treated before serious spinal cord dysfunction develops, but treatment is controversial. High-dose corticosteroids should be administered, and the lesion irradiated if the primary lesion is known. If there is no known primary tumor, if the tumor is known not to be radiosensitive, or if the neurologic status is rapidly deteriorating, surgical decompression should be done. Radiation therapy is usually administered postoperatively.

Intradural Tumors

not diagnosed u...
cit becomes evident...
helpful in diagnosis u...
caused widening of the i...
extending through it in th...
Myelography demonstrates ...
an intradural extramedullar...
These tumors can be complete...
roots in the thoracic region ma...
provide better exposure, but dan...
arteries must be avoided.

Intramedullary tumors may invol...just a short segment of the spinal cord or extend almost to its full length. They are the most difficult tumors to diagnose and treat. Plain x-ray films may show a widening of the interpediculate distance. Results

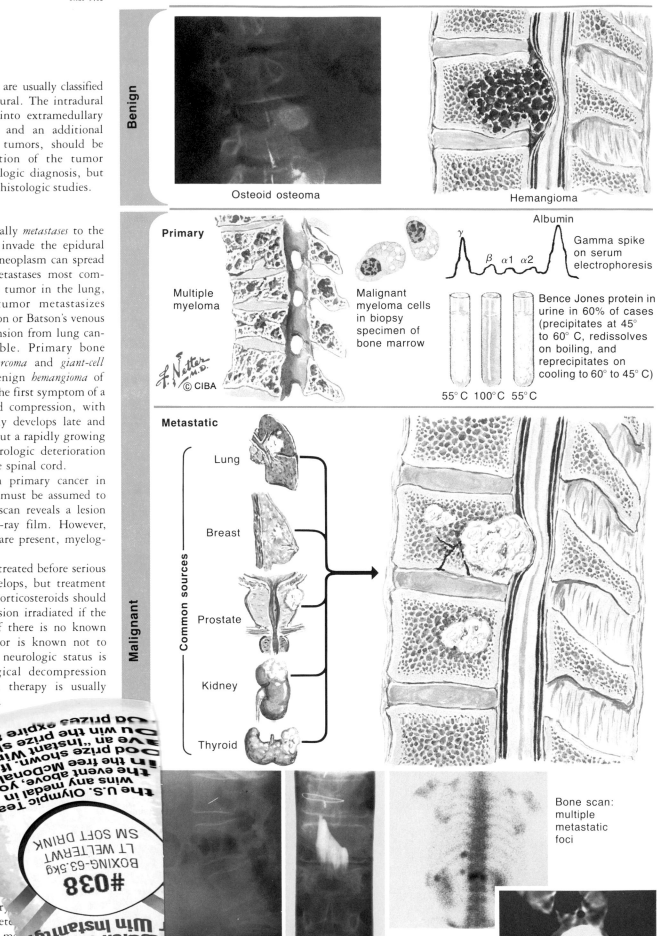

Tumors of Spinal Column

Benign

Osteoid osteoma

Hemangioma

Primary

Multiple myeloma

Malignant myeloma cells in biopsy specimen of bone marrow

Gamma spike on serum electrophoresis

Albumin

Bence Jones protein in urine in 60% of cases (precipitates at 45° to 60° C, redissolves on boiling, and reprecipitates on cooling to 60° to 45° C)

55°C 100°C 55°C

Metastatic

Malignant

Common sources:
Lung
Breast
Prostate
Kidney
Thyroid

Bone scan: multiple metastatic foci

Bone lesions in spine (lateral view)

Myelogram evidencing CSF obstruction (AP view)

CT scan of spine demonstrating destruction of vertebral body by metastatic tumor

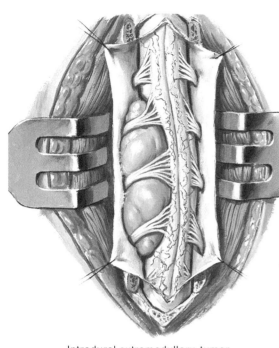

Intradural extramedullary tumor (meningioma) compressing spinal cord and deforming nerve roots

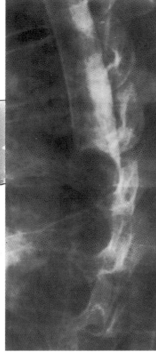

Myelogram of meningioma at level of T4 demonstrating classic capping of tumor by contrast material

Dumbbell tumor (neurilemmoma) growing out along spinal nerve through intervertebral foramen. (Neurofibromas of von Recklinghausen's disease may act similarly)

Intramedullary tumor and myelogram showing widening of spinal cord

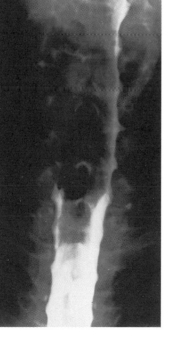

Tumor of filum terminale compressing cauda equina. Enlarged vessels feed tumor

Ependymoma of cauda equina. Myelogram with complete block of contrast material from above and widening of interpediculate distance due to pressure

SECTION X   PLATE 6   *Slide 3463*

Spinal Tumors
(Continued)

of myelography in early cases may be equivocal, although metrizamide myelography combined with computed tomography (CT) shows the enlarged spinal cord (Plate 6). However, demonstrating a swollen spinal cord with even the most sensitive radiographic studies does not confirm the diagnosis of intramedullary tumor. If the diagnosis is in doubt and the patient is deteriorating, the spinal cord should be explored surgically.

The two most common intramedullary tumors are the *astrocytoma* and the *ependymoma*. The astrocytoma is infiltrative, and total excision is not possible; however, there is frequently a well-demarcated plane around the ependymoma, and excision of the tumor is possible.

Surgery on the spinal cord demands the most meticulous technique. The operating microscope and bipolar coagulation must be used. If the tumor is not completely excised, radiation therapy is indicated.

Intradural tumors of the lumbar spine involve the conus medullaris, filum terminale and cauda equina. Both the ependymoma and astrocytoma arise from the conus medullaris. These tumors produce early deficit of sphincter and sexual function, and are difficult to remove without incurring significant neurologic deficit. The ependymoma of the filum terminale causes pain, often without significant neurologic findings, and can be cured by surgical excision.

The diffuse myxopapillary ependymoma, which involves the roots of the cauda equina, is difficult to excise and should receive postoperative radiation therapy. A neurilemmoma or a meningioma can be successfully removed. Lipoma of the cauda equina arises from fetal rests and is associated with spina bifida occulta. Excision of this tumor is difficult, but meticulous microsurgery can reduce the tumor and preserve neurologic function. □

Extradural tumors

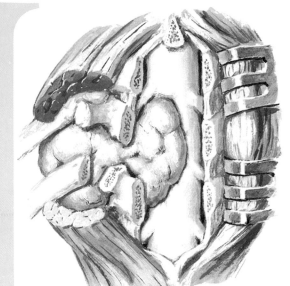

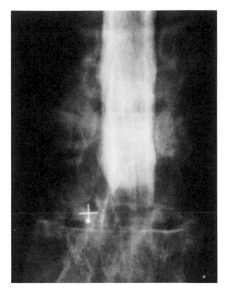

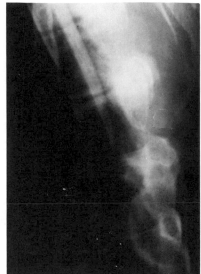

Lymphoma invading spinal canal via intervertebral foramen, compressing dura mater and spinal cord

Frontal (left) and lateral (right) metrizamide myelograms show complete obstruction just above T6-7. Spinal cord displaced forward and to right, with similar displacement of arachnoid, which suggests that mass is extradural

Intradural extramedullary tumors

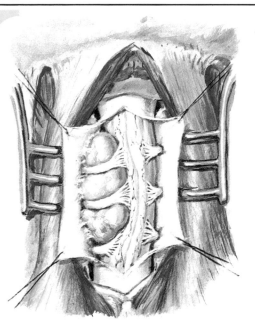

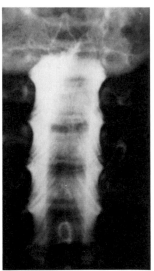

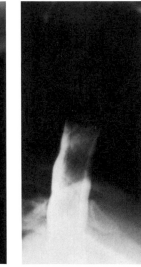

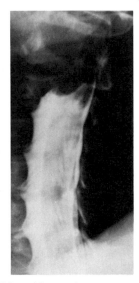

Meningioma compressing spinal cord and distorting nerve roots

Frontal (left), lateral (center) and oblique (right) metrizamide myelograms show right lateral displacement of spinal cord and complete obstruction. Frontal view shows injection from above; lateral and oblique views show inferior margin of intradural mass, separate from spinal cord, defined by injection from below

Intramedullary tumors

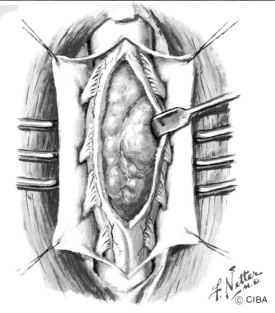

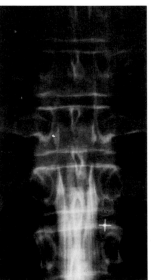

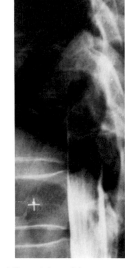

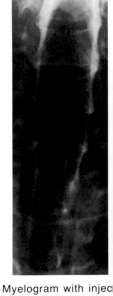

Astrocytoma exposed by longitudinal incision in bulging spinal cord

Frontal (left) and lateral (right) metrizamide myelograms with injection from below show high-grade stenosis caused by nearly symmetric expansion of spinal cord beginning at T12

Myelogram with injection from above show extension of tumor to upper cervical level

Myelographic and CT Characteristics of Spinal Tumors

Radiographic studies are an important means of detecting, defining and localizing the various pathologic disorders that may affect the spine, including tumors, congenital abnormalities, infection and vascular lesions.

Plain radiographs and, especially, radionuclide bone scans demonstrate processes that affect bone, such as infection; metastatic tumor; or primary bone disorders, such as Paget's disease. Nonetheless, myelography and computed tomography (CT) remain the most definitive diagnostic modalities. In addition to demonstrating a lesion, these procedures should localize the disease process as being: (1) primarily of bone, or outside the dura mater (extradural); (2) inside the dura mater but not primarily involving the spinal cord (extramedullary); or (3) involving the spinal cord (intramedullary).

This precise anatomic localization is important in determining the likely cause of the problem and in guiding further diagnostic efforts and appropriate treatment. □

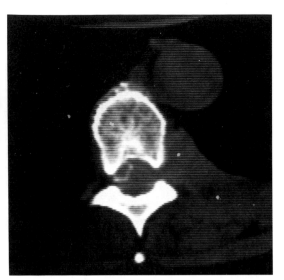

CT scan more graphically displays left and posteriorly situated soft-tissue mass within spinal canal and its extension through left intervertebral foramen. Absence of bony involvement confirmed

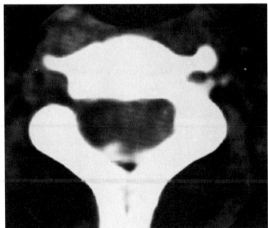

CT scan at C2 shows only small amount of contrast medium posteriorly. Tumor is more dense than spinal cord, which is displaced to right and severely deformed and compressed

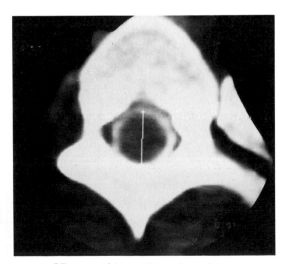

CT scan of lower thoracic region showing rounded, expanded spinal cord that is nearly twice normal sagittal diameter

Classification of Myelographic Abnormalities

Extradural	Intradural Extramedullary	Intramedullary
Disc disease	Neurinoma	Syringomyelia
Tumor	Meningioma	Tumor
Metastatic		Ependymoma
Lymphoma	Intracranial tumor seeding	Glioma
Sarcoma	Ependymoma	Hemangioblastoma
Plasmacytoma	Medulloblastoma	
Primary bone	Glioma	
Scar	Cauda equina lesions	Myelitis
	Scarring	
Abscess	Hypertrophic neuropathy	Edema
Hemangioma		Lipoma
Rare lesions	Rare lesions	Rare lesions
Hemorrhage	Lymphoma	Abscess
Neurilemmoma	Metastasis	Hematoma
Meningioma	Hemangioblastoma	Varix with AVM
Chordoma	Lipoma	Lymphoma
	Dermoid	Neuroblastoma
	Epidermoid	Metastasis
	Cyst	
	Clot	

Dermoid or epidermoid, teratoma, lipoma and cysts are often associated with spinal dysraphism. In this setting, many tumors are intradural, although they may involve all three areas.

Syringomyelia

Syringomyelia is a condition in which a tubular cavity, or syrinx, in the central area of the spinal cord gradually expands and produces neuronal and tract damage.

The syrinx develops most frequently in the cervical and upper thoracic segments. Serial sections of pathologic material show that it arises as a diverticulum from the central canal of the spinal cord. It may then dissect into the dorsal or ventral gray matter on one side, or enlarge symmetrically into a large, fluid-filled cavity, which in turn causes transverse enlargement of the spinal cord. Anterior horn neurons and pain and temperature fibers crossing in the central gray matter are destroyed. Long tracts, first the pyramidal and lastly the posterior column, may be compressed.

In some cases, the syrinx extends from the cervical area into the posterolateral medulla, producing syringobulbia. Lumbar extension is rare.

Pathogenesis. The pathogenesis of syringomyelia is poorly understood. Initially, the condition was considered degenerative or developmental. Indeed, almost all patients have an associated type I Arnold-Chiari malformation, which may in itself produce symptoms of medullary or upper cervical compression (see Section I, Plate 8). Other associated developmental defects include basilar impression, the Dandy-Walker syndrome, and atresia of the foramen of Magendie.

Gardner felt that the presence of the Arnold-Chiari malformation meant that flow of cerebrospinal fluid (CSF) from the fourth ventricle is diminished, and that increased pressure forces fluid into the central canal, producing a gradually expanding syrinx. However, it is now apparent that some patients with an Arnold-Chiari malformation do not have a connection between the central canal and the fourth ventricle. Thus, a different pathogenetic factor must be at work.

Some cavities appear to be caused by spinal cord trauma and may develop months or even years after injury. Spinal arachnoiditis and intramedullary tumors are also associated with syrinx formation.

Clinical Manifestations. Syringomyelia is rare, with a prevalence of 8/100,000 persons. Symptoms appear late in the second decade through the fifth. Average age at onset is 30 years. The disease progresses at a variable rate; some patients become quadriplegic in 10 years, while others have a more benign course with long periods of stabilization. In 20 years, however, probably 50% of patients are wheelchair-bound.

The classic sign of syringomyelia is *dissociated anesthesia*, or loss of pain and temperature sensation in a capelike distribution, with preservation of light touch sensation and proprioception. Fibers carrying pain and temperature sensation cross in the central gray matter near the central canal and then form the spinothalamic tract in the ventrolateral portion of the spinal cord. These fibers are damaged near the central canal or in the dorsal horn before they cross. Fibers carrying light touch and proprioception information do not cross and course rostrally in the posterior columns.

Trophic changes occur, and the appearance of Charcot's joints is not uncommon. When the cavity expands into the anterior horn, atrophy and

motor weakness become apparent. Fasciculations may be seen, and kyphoscoliosis resulting from paraspinal muscle weakness is common.

As the lesion expands further, it compresses the corticospinal and spinothalamic tracts. Progressive spastic paraparesis with a sensory level becomes apparent.

Diagnosis. Syringomyelia is readily diagnosed with the use of metrizamide myelography and computed tomography (CT) to establish widening of the spinal cord and presence of the Arnold-Chiari malformation. The CT scan is repeated 6 hours later, when the metrizamide has diffused into the spinal cord and concentrated in the syrinx. In the near future, magnetic resonance

imaging (MRI) will be helpful in differentiating a syrinx from an intramedullary tumor (see Section V, Plate 17).

Treatment. The cause of the syrinx dictates the appropriate treatment. In most cases, an Arnold-Chiari malformation is present, and decompression of the area with suboccipital craniectomy and upper cervical laminectomy may be sufficient. In patients with no cervicomedullary abnormality, syringostomy may be considered. A plastic tube is placed into the syrinx cavity to provide communication to the subarachnoid space. If the tube remains patent, the process may stabilize. Symptomatic hydrocephalus is treated with ventriculoperitoneal shunting. □

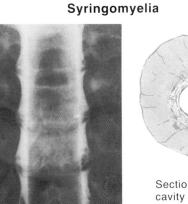

Syringomyelia

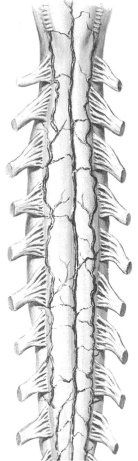

Bulging of spinal cord due to syrinx

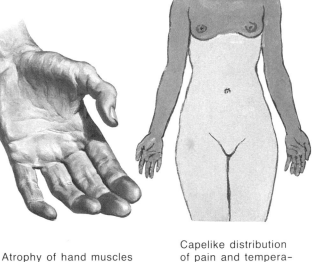

Myelogram showing subtle widening of cervical spinal cord

Section of cervical spinal cord showing cavity of syrinx surrounded by gliosis

Diagram demonstrating interruption of crossed pain and temperature fibers by syrinx. Uncrossed light touch and proprioception fibers preserved

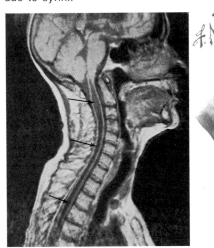

Magnetic resonance image: area of diminished signal within cervical and upper spinal cord (arrows) is fluid-filled syrinx. Cerebellar tonsil extends below foramen magnum

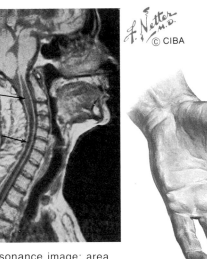

Atrophy of hand muscles due to neurotrophic deficit

Capelike distribution of pain and temperature sensation loss

Subacute Combined Degeneration

Subacute combined degeneration of the spinal cord refers to degeneration of the posterior and lateral spinal columns resulting from vitamin B_{12} deficiency. Although many terms have been used to describe this condition, in recent years, the term "B_{12} neuropathy" seems to have gained favor.

Pathogenesis. Most cases of subacute combined degeneration are the result of Addisonian *pernicious anemia*, with atrophy of gastric parietal cells and absence of intrinsic factor. The same neurologic picture may appear in any condition in which vitamin B_{12} absorption is impaired or its dietary intake is insufficient. Cases have been reported in strict vegans and in patients who have sprue, Crohn's disease, fistula of the small intestine, or fish tapeworm infestation, or who have had a bowel resection or gastrectomy.

Pathology. The earliest neuropathologic lesion in this disorder is myelin swelling in the thoracic and lower cervical posterior columns. Later, demyelination and axonal destruction occur, and still later, the lateral columns and spinocerebellar tracts are involved. Ascending secondary degeneration may be seen in the posterior columns, and descending degeneration may be seen in the corticospinal tract. Small foci of demyelination are scattered throughout the cerebral white matter and optic (II) nerve. Secondary degeneration of association tracts may be present. Mild changes occur in peripheral nerves, and damage to cortical neurons has been described.

Clinical Manifestations. Fatigue, weight loss, abdominal distress, diarrhea and sore tongue are the most common general symptoms of pernicious anemia. Examination reveals glossitis and a lemon-yellow tint to the skin.

The most common neurologic symptoms relate to *involvement of the posterior columns.* Tingling, burning and numbness of the distal extremities are the earliest symptoms. Depending on the site of initial demyelination, the feet or hands may be involved first, or paresthesias may occur simultaneously in all four extremities. Occasionally, Lhermitte's sign is present. Due to proprioceptive loss, imbalance, which worsens in the dark, may be an early sign.

Stiffness is often the first sign of *lateral column dysfunction*, but usually occurs after the onset of paresthesias. Later, overt spasticity develops, and if the disease remains untreated, paraplegia with bowel and bladder incontinence ensues.

Mental symptoms may be noticed at any stage of the disease. Early manifestations are subtle and include fatigue, irritability and mild depression. Delirium and paranoid psychosis are the most common major cerebral manifestations. Rarely, seizures or visual blurring occur.

The cardinal neurologic sign is diminution of vibration sense. Position sense is affected to a lesser degree, but the Romberg sign is often positive. Involvement of the posterior column and spinocerebellar tract may cause severely disabling sensory ataxia.

With extensive spinal cord damage, a sensory level may be noted, usually in the middle or lower

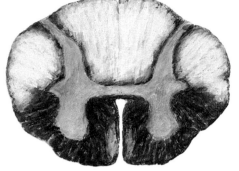

Degeneration of posterior columns, and corticospinal and direct spinocerebellar tracts, chiefly in midthoracic spinal cord

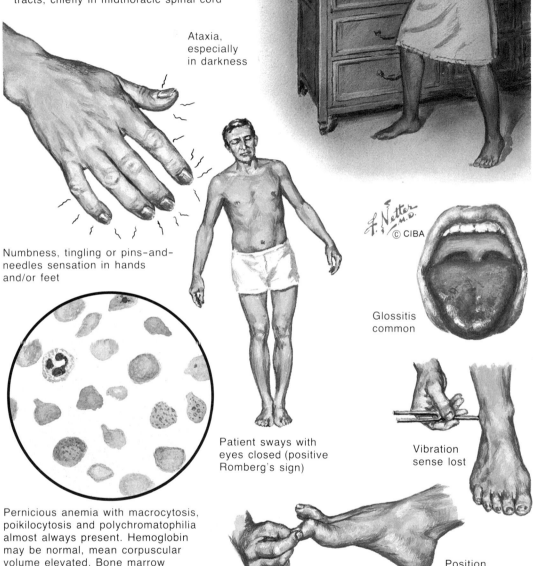

Ataxia, especially in darkness

Numbness, tingling or pins-and-needles sensation in hands and/or feet

Pernicious anemia with macrocytosis, poikilocytosis and polychromatophilia almost always present. Hemoglobin may be normal, mean corpuscular volume elevated. Bone marrow characteristically abnormal

Patient sways with eyes closed (positive Romberg's sign)

Glossitis common

Vibration sense lost

Position sense lost

thoracic segment. A glove-and-stocking anesthesia, although uncommon, is a reflection of peripheral neuropathy.

Hyperreflexia, spasticity, clonus and the Babinski sign signify lateral column damage. A hyperactive bladder may be an associated finding. In severe untreated cases, paraplegia with flexor spasms may develop.

Diagnosis. Subacute combined degeneration is diagnosed clinically by recognition of posterior and lateral column involvement. Determination of the serum vitamin B_{12} level and the Schilling test are usually sufficient for confirmation. It has long been recognized that neurologic signs and symptoms may precede the appearance of anemia.

The red blood cell count and the mean corpuscular volume, however, are often abnormal in the face of normal hemoglobin and hematocrit values.

Treatment. A loading dose of parenterally administered vitamin B_{12}, followed by a maintenance dosage of at least 100 μg/month for life, is the accepted treatment for subacute combined degeneration. Since irreversible axonal damage occurs shortly after demyelination, early diagnosis is mandatory.

Mild paresthesias and mental changes of recent onset may completely resolve with treatment, but when symptoms have been present for several months, there is little hope for complete recovery. □

Cervical Spondylosis

The pathologic process in cervical spondylosis is a gradually progressive degeneration of intervertebral discs, with subsequent changes in vertebrae and meninges. Disc degeneration may result from dessication of the nucleus pulposus that begins in the fifth decade and progresses rapidly thereafter. At the same time, the annulus fibrosus may weaken to allow bulging of the nucleus pulposus. Disc material extrudes when portions of the annulus rupture.

Osteophytes appear on the margins of the vertebral bodies and articular cartilages, probably as a result of trauma and disc degeneration. If osteophytes or discs project posteriorly or posterolaterally, they may compress the spinal cord or cervical nerve roots. Osteophytes growing from zygapophyseal joints can compromise neuroforamina or the spinal canal. As discs degenerate and bulge posteriorly, so-called spondylitic bars may be formed, which also may compress the spinal cord or neuroforamina.

Finally, as disc spaces narrow secondary to degeneration, the cervical spine shortens. This can produce infolding of the ligamentum flavum, which narrows the anteroposterior diameter of the spinal canal. The vertebral column shortens, but the length of the spinal cord remains unchanged, resulting in traction on the lower cervical nerve roots.

The anteroposterior diameter of the spinal canal may be critical to the development of spondylitic myelopathy. The average sagittal diameter is about 17 mm, while the average spinal cord diameter is 10 mm. In most patients, large cervical bars are necessary to produce spinal cord compression. However, patients with spondylitic myelopathy often have an associated congenital narrowing of the spinal canal.

When spinal cord compression occurs, pathologic examination shows flattening and distortion. Several indentations may be present, depending on the number of spondylitic bars. Demyelination of the lateral and posterior columns, and neuronal damage at the points of compression, are the primary microscopic findings.

Clinical Manifestations. The onset of spondylitic myelopathy is usually insidious. *Paresthesias* of the hand may occur early, and the patient may experience numbness and tingling in a radicular distribution, as well as *nerve root pain.* Weakness and atrophy in the upper extremities vary, depending on the spinal cord segments or nerve roots compressed. Since the fifth and sixth cervical segments are most frequently compressed, reflexes in the biceps and triceps, respectively, may be diminished.

In the lower extremities, the typical picture is *spastic paraparesis*; however, one leg may be more severely involved than the other. Vibration and

Cervical Spondylosis

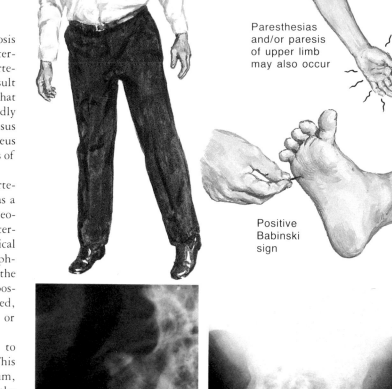

Weakness of lower limb evidenced by circumduction of leg in walking

Paresthesias and/or paresis of upper limb may also occur

Ankle clonus

Positive Babinski sign

Loss of vibration sense

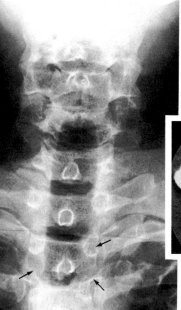

Cervical myelogram showing severe spondylosis with multiple extradural compression sites (arrows)

X-ray film showing stenosis secondary to cervical spondylosis. Ridging of vertebral bodies produces cervical bar (arrows) and narrows AP diameter of vertebral canal

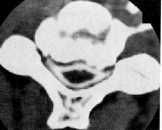

Metrizamide myelogram with CT scan showing spinal cord compression secondary to severe cervical spondylosis

position sense may be diminished in the feet. Sphincter disturbances and sensory levels are seen only in later stages.

Spastic paraparesis may be slowly progressive in some cases; in others, muscle fasciculations, atrophy and weakness of the upper extremities may develop in conjunction with spastic paraparesis. The latter cases may be difficult to differentiate from motor neuron disease.

Diagnosis. The diagnosis of spondylitic myelopathy may be suspected when x-ray films show an anteroposterior sagittal diameter of 11 mm or less in any area of the cervical spine. However, myelography is required to establish the presence of spinal cord compression. Cerebrospinal fluid

(CSF) is normal or shows a mild to moderately elevated protein content.

Treatment. Although most nerve root syndromes subside spontaneously, spondylitic myelopathy, if progressive, requires *surgical intervention.* Some patients improve following surgery, but only stabilization can be realistically expected.

Spinal cord decompression may be done through either an anterior or a posterior approach. If the process is localized to one or two segments and the remaining canal is of normal diameter, the anterior approach may be preferred. If multiple or scattered areas of involvement are present or if the canal is congenitally narrow, a posterior laminectomy is advised. ☐

Cervical Disc Herniation

Cervical disc disease is a common disorder, accounting for 1% to 2% of all hospital admissions in the United States. Unlike lumbar disc disease, which is approximately 6 times more common, cervical disc disease is rarely caused by trauma. In fact, severe degenerative cervical disc disease (spondylosis) often develops in indolent patients.

Etiology. The cause of cervical disc disease is clearly multifactorial. With age, the nucleus pulposus of the disc dehydrates, placing more stress on the annulus fibrosus (outer lining). Tears in the annulus may permit a sudden herniation of the nucleus—a *ruptured disc.* Alternatively, chronic annular bulging or nuclear herniation may incite a bony reparative process, leading to the formation of extensive bony spurs (osteophytes). These spurs are generally located along the anterior portion of the disc interspace or posteriorly, within the nerve root foramen. For unknown reasons, some patients are predisposed to a severe degree of this degenerative process.

Osteophytes or ruptured discs produce symptoms only if they compress the spinal cord or nerve roots against posteriorly located structures, including the posterior nerve root foramen and ligamentum flavum.

Symptoms. The first manifestation of cervical disc disease is often cervical radiculopathy, with symptoms and signs referable to compression of a cervical nerve root. The cervical nerve roots exit above the vertebral body of the same number, with the exception of C8, which emerges at the C7–T1 interspace. Thus, a lesion of the C5–6 disc produces C6 radiculopathy. Spondylosis is implicated in cervical nerve root compression about 3 times more often than acute disc rupture, and most frequently involves the C6 and C7 nerve roots. The C5 and C8 nerve roots are involved less often, and the T1 root only rarely.

Cervical and unilateral arm pain is a common symptom of cervical disc disease, and patients often complain of numbness or weakness in the involved arm. Occasionally, pain also involves the shoulder, occiput or anterior chest. Cervical tenderness is present, and range of motion in the neck is decreased. Hyperextension and rotation of the neck (Spurling's maneuver) decrease the diameter of the nerve root foramen and often exacerbate radicular symptoms.

Diagnosis. Neurologic examination, with careful attention to motor, reflex and sensory findings in the upper extremities, often reveals a diagnostic constellation of signs. *C5* radiculopathy usually causes weakness of the infraspinatus, supraspinatus and deltoid muscles, with decreased biceps reflex and hypalgesia over the shoulder. *C6* radiculopathy leads to weakness of the elbow flexors and extensor carpi radialis. The biceps reflex is usually decreased or absent, and sensation over the thumb and index finger is characteristically diminished.

In *C7* radiculopathy, weakness is noted in the triceps brachii and extensor muscles of the wrist

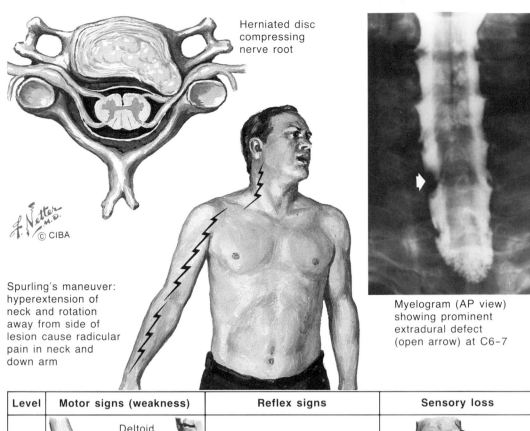

Herniated disc compressing nerve root

Spurling's maneuver: hyperextension of neck and rotation away from side of lesion cause radicular pain in neck and down arm

Myelogram (AP view) showing prominent extradural defect (open arrow) at C6–7

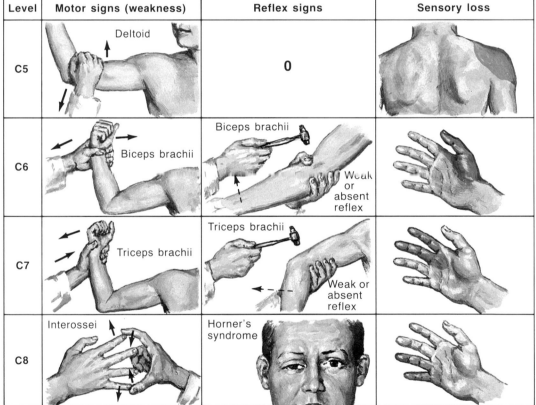

Level	Motor signs (weakness)	Reflex signs	Sensory loss
C5	Deltoid	0	
C6	Biceps brachii	Biceps brachii — Weak or absent reflex	
C7	Triceps brachii	Triceps brachii — Weak or absent reflex	
C8	Interossei	Horner's syndrome	

and finger. The triceps reflex is usually decreased or absent, and sensation over the index and middle fingers is often decreased. *C8* radiculopathy causes weakness primarily of the intrinsic muscles of the hand. The triceps reflex may be decreased and Horner's syndrome (ptosis, miosis and anhidrosis) may be present. Sensation may be diminished over the ring and little fingers. The rare *T1* radiculopathy is associated with weakness of the intrinsic muscles of the hand and Horner's syndrome, which results from disruption of the sympathetic outflow to the face and eye via the root of C8 or T1, or both.

Treatment. The majority of patients who have appropriate symptoms and signs of cervical radiculopathy respond to *conservative treatment*, including use of a soft cervical collar to immobilize the neck, mild analgesics, and muscle relaxants as required. Many believe that cervical traction is also helpful. If symptoms persist after 2 weeks, further testing, including cervical myelography, is indicated. If the radiographic findings show compression of the clinically appropriate nerve root, *surgical therapy* is undertaken. Some neurosurgeons strongly advocate the anterior approach, and others, the posterior approach in the surgical treatment of this disease. In skilled hands, either route should lead to excellent relief of symptoms in over 90% of patients (see Section IV, Plates 22–24). □

Cervical disc herniation

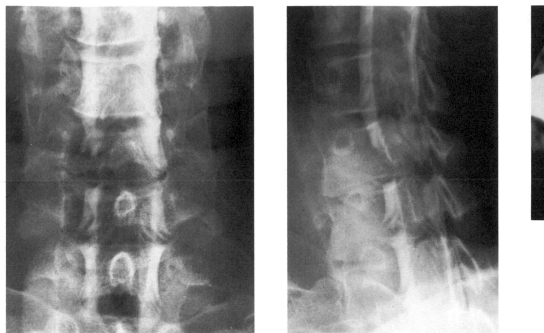

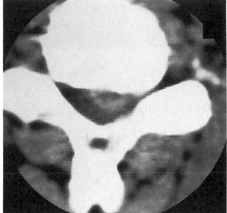

CT scan of different patient shows large area of density greater than that of spinal cord and occupying major portion of left cervical spinal canal

AP (left) and lateral (right) myelograms show axillary sleeve of left C6 distorted by disc fragment that extends to touch spinal cord

© CIBA

Cervical spinal stenosis and spondylosis

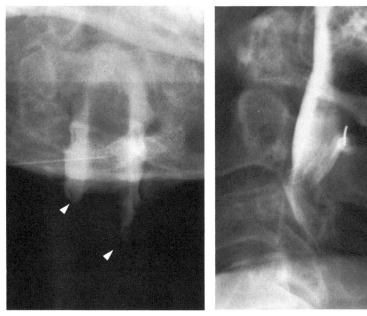

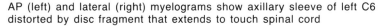

CT evaluation after myelography, shows large osteophyte associated with left uncinate process, which accounts for asymmetry of block (arrowheads)

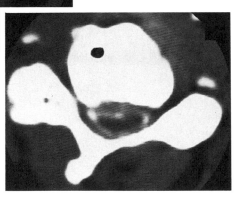

AP (left) and lateral (right) cervical myelograms with injection from above show high-grade stenosis at C3, higher on left (arrowheads). Obstruction was eventually overcome by voluntary forced flexion of neck

Spinal cord compression secondary to spondylosis and disc protrusion is confirmed at C3-4

SECTION X PLATE 12   *Slide 3469*

Radiographic Diagnosis of Radiculopathy

Herniation of an intervertebral disc, alone or in combination with spondylosis, is the most common cause of surgically remediable lumbar and cervical radiculopathy. In patients with signs and symptoms of radiculopathy, the clinician can often localize the problem to within one or two spinal segments. However, when conservative management has failed or when excruciating, unrelenting pain or severe weakness with or without loss of sphincter control forces consideration of surgery, precise anatomic localization of the disc herniation is necessary. Computed tomography (CT) and myelography are the most reliable diagnostic procedures.

CT effectively demonstrates the bony architecture of the spine, the contours of the intervertebral disc, the paraspinal soft tissues, and to some extent, the contents of the spinal canal. The contours of the dural sac, the axillary sleeves and neural ganglia are best delineated in the lower lumbar region, where they contrast against the lower density, epidural fat. A herniated portion of disc distorts the epidural fat, dural sac or axillary sleeve. In addition, the herniated fragment is usually more dense than the normal structures of the spinal canal and is sometimes calcified.

The *cervical region* has little, if any, epidural fat, and frequently only a small fragment of disc is enough to cause severe nerve root compression. Because of the lack of epidural fat and the small size of disc herniations, CT is less effective than myelography for diagnosing cervical radiculopathy. In disc herniation, myelography commonly demonstrates displacement of the dural sac, impaired filling or displacement of an axillary sleeve (Plate 12), or nerve root swelling.

Radiographic Diagnosis of Lumbar Radiculopathy

Lumbar disc herniation

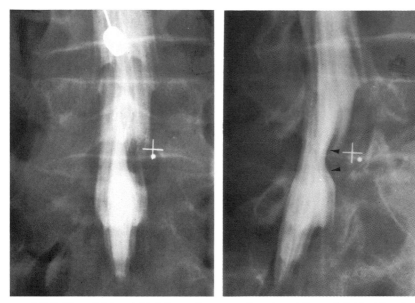

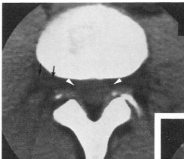

CT scan shows that spinal canal is normal just above L3-4. Dural sac outlined by fat (arrowheads). Portions of a distal nerve root seen laterally (small arrows)

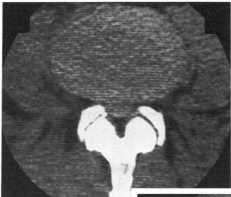

AP (left) and lateral (right) myelograms show herniation of right side of L5-S1 disc on dural sac, displacing S1 root posteriorly (arrowheads)

Mass slightly more dense than dural sac fills right anterolateral recess and distorts that side of dural compartment (arrows). More medial dark area is gas formed in degenerating disc

Lumbar spinal stenosis and spondylosis

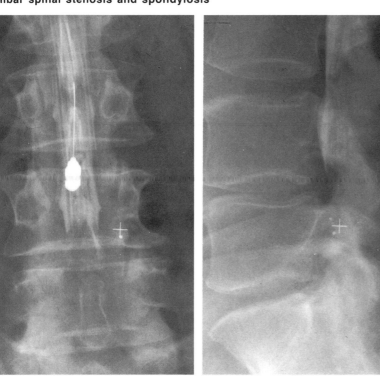

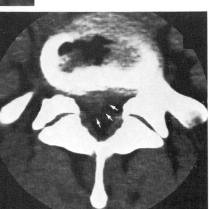

CT scan at L3-4 graphically confirms marginal canal and thick posterior arch

© CIBA

AP (left) and lateral (right) myelograms confirm marginally narrow spinal canal totally obstructed just above L4-5

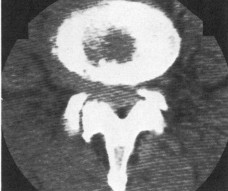

Degenerative involvement of facets and bulging annulus at level of block. These changes are difficult to distinguish from subarachnoid space. Surgery revealed that synovial and ligamentous hypertrophy accounted for much of narrowing

---

SECTION X PLATE 13   *Slide 3470*

Radiographic Diagnosis of Radiculopathy
(Continued)

When either CT or myelography fails to suggest a clear-cut diagnosis, the other procedure should be considered. Myelography may be more effective in patients with a small spinal canal or in large patients, in whom the quality of CT is

compromised. Myelography is also indicated when the clinical localization or characterization of the disorder is unclear.

CT is especially valuable for the disc herniation that is too far lateral to affect the dural sac or axillary sleeves. It is also more effective than myelography for evaluating the paraspinal region, spinal canal and sacrum.

In the cervical region, CT and myelography are complementary. The combination of both studies clearly shows the nature and degree of spinal cord distortion, which is valuable in determining the proper treatment.

Clinical localization of *cauda equina compression* may be difficult. In this case, myelography is

helpful in localizing the compressive lesion. The degree of myelographic block is a familiar method for quantitating the severity of neural compression and can be monitored in several different patient positions (Plate 13). Myelography, therefore, should usually precede CT.

Myelographic localization and characterization in conjunction with the clinical picture may be sufficient for planning surgery. In many instances, however, CT may supplement myelography and is ideally done immediately following myelography with injection of water-soluble contrast medium to provide the added perspective of the axial image and further delineate the extradural, bony and paraspinal tissues. □

Back Pain and Lumbar Disc Disease

Lumbar disc disease causing low back and nerve root pain is one of the most common problems affecting modern industrial society.

The *relevant anatomy* includes the five lumbar vertebrae and the sacrum. The adjacent vertebrae are joined by strong ligaments at the articular facets and at the vertebral bodies. Cartilage lines the articular surfaces of the vertebral bodies. The disc fills the space between the cartilaginous end plates and is normally a tough fibrocartilaginous structure. The dural sac contains the nerve roots of the cauda equina and extends through the spinal canal. As they exit the spinal canal at each segment, the nerve roots course caudad to the facet before passing through the intervertebral foramen. With aging, the disc degenerates, fragments and loses its adherent properties. Thus, appropriate mechanical forces can cause the fragment to move, usually posterolateral at the point of least ligamentous resistance, where the nerve root exits the spine. Pressure on the nerve root may produce pain and neurologic deficit.

As a result of abnormal movement at the facet joint, a hypertrophic, osteoarthritic process known as spondylosis develops. Enlargement of the facet joints by this spondylolytic process narrows the intervertebral foramen, which may cause mechanical pressure on the exiting nerve root. In some persons, the anteroposterior diameter of the spinal canal is narrow, with deep lateral recesses. Thus, the spondylolytic process produces spinal stenosis, which causes pressure on the dural sac and cauda equina.

Clinical Manifestations

Lumbar spine disease may be manifested by pain in the low back, a monoradicular syndrome, an acute cauda equina syndrome or spinal stenosis. As an isolated symptom, low back pain is usually self-limited and responds to conservative measures.

Initially, only a detailed history and physical examination may be necessary (Plate 14). However, a different pain pattern must be investigated further. Gradually increasing pain with or without neurologic symptoms in a person who has systemic symptoms raises the question of a destructive lesion.

The monoradicular syndromes are the classic syndromes of a ruptured disc. Most disc ruptures occur at L5–S1 and L4–5. The herniated disc at L5–S1 usually compresses the S1 root as it passes the interspace on its way beneath the S1 facet. In the same manner, the L4–5 disc compresses the L5 root, and the L3–4 disc compresses the L4 root. Rarely, the disc extrudes laterally into the intervertebral foramen, and then the L5–S1 disc

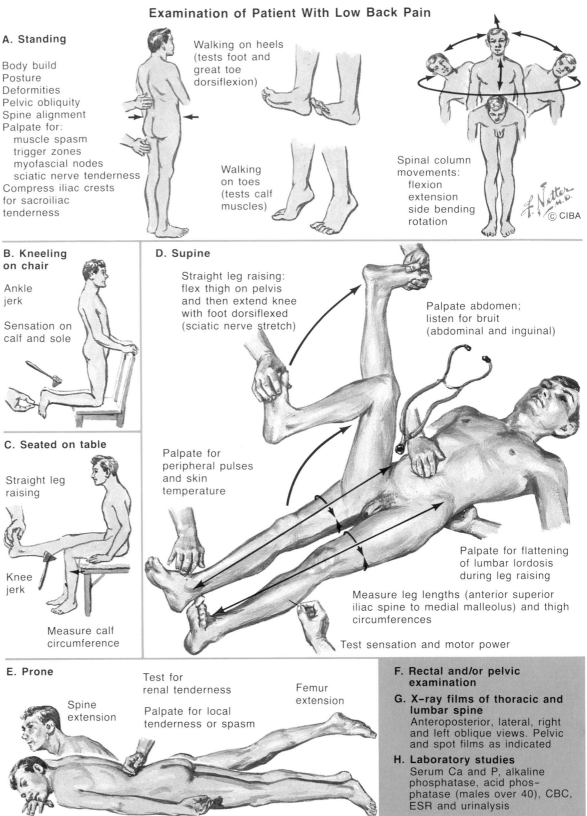

Examination of Patient With Low Back Pain

A. Standing

Body build
Posture
Deformities
Pelvic obliquity
Spine alignment
Palpate for:
  muscle spasm
  trigger zones
  myofascial nodes
  sciatic nerve tenderness
Compress iliac crests for sacroiliac tenderness

Walking on heels (tests foot and great toe dorsiflexion)

Walking on toes (tests calf muscles)

Spinal column movements:
  flexion
  extension
  side bending
  rotation

B. Kneeling on chair

Ankle jerk

Sensation on calf and sole

C. Seated on table

Straight leg raising

Knee jerk

Measure calf circumference

D. Supine

Straight leg raising: flex thigh on pelvis and then extend knee with foot dorsiflexed (sciatic nerve stretch)

Palpate abdomen; listen for bruit (abdominal and inguinal)

Palpate for peripheral pulses and skin temperature

Palpate for flattening of lumbar lordosis during leg raising

Measure leg lengths (anterior superior iliac spine to medial malleolus) and thigh circumferences

Test sensation and motor power

E. Prone

Spine extension

Test for renal tenderness

Palpate for local tenderness or spasm

Femur extension

F. Rectal and/or pelvic examination

G. X-ray films of thoracic and lumbar spine
Anteroposterior, lateral, right and left oblique views. Pelvic and spot films as indicated

H. Laboratory studies
Serum Ca and P, alkaline phosphatase, acid phosphatase (males over 40), CBC, ESR and urinalysis

produces an L5 root syndrome; the L4–5 disc, an L4 root syndrome; and the L3–4 disc, an L3 root syndrome. Failure to diagnose these problems accurately results in inadequate treatment.

The *S1 root syndrome* includes sciatic pain from the buttock to the posterior thigh, to the calf, and into the foot. Weakness, if present, is in plantar flexion of the ankle and foot. The ankle jerk is absent. Sensory symptoms are present on the lateral aspect of the foot, the sole and the heel.

The sciatic pain of the *L5 root syndrome* is indistinguishable from that of the S1 root syndrome. Dorsiflexion of the foot and eversion and inversion of the ankle may be weak. The ankle and knee jerk are normal, but the internal hamstring reflex

may be diminished or absent. Sensory change develops in the dorsal and medial aspects of the foot and great toe. In the less common *L4 root syndrome*, pain radiates to the lateral and anterior thigh. The quadriceps muscle is weak and atrophied, and the knee jerk is lost. Sensory change occurs in the anterior thigh and pretibial regions. The clinical manifestations of herniation at L4–5 and L5–S1 are summarized in Plate 15.

Treatment

Eighty percent of all monoradicular syndromes, even those with mild neurologic deficit, respond to bed rest for up to several weeks and a subsequent exercise program. For patients with a definite

Back Pain and Lumbar Disc Disease
(Continued)

diagnosis of radiculopathy secondary to a herniated disc who do not improve, options are limited. Some choose more prolonged rest, while some with mild symptoms may choose to return to activities of daily living despite the pain.

In patients in whom further treatment is necessary because of pain or neurologic deficit, surgery must be considered and must be preceded by radiographic examination of the lumbosacral spine to rule out a destructive lesion or an anomaly such as spondylolisthesis. The important tests are myelography, with a water-soluble contrast medium, and computed tomography (CT). Magnetic resonance imaging (MRI) is becoming more available, and is potentially the preferred diagnostic test (see Section V, Plate 17).

If no destructive lesion is present and test results show that the pain and neurologic deficit are caused by the herniated disc, surgery is indicated. The surgeon must keep in mind that the important structure is the nerve root. Adequate exposure is essential to expose the root cephalad and caudad to the extruded fragment and to the lateral margin of the spinal canal. This allows maximal exposure of the disc and nerve root, which can be minimally manipulated. The extruded disc is removed and foraminotomy is done. The root is then retracted medially, the annulus is exposed, and the disc is removed from the interspace to reduce the chance of recurrence.

With this technique, the entire evaluation can be done on an outpatient basis. The patient is discharged 1 to 3 days postoperatively and can return to a sedentary job in 2 weeks. Discectomy, with use of the operating microscope, is also a satisfactory procedure if done at the correct level to adequately expose the root. The use of chymopapain should be avoided because of the high rate of serious complications.

The *midline disc herniation* is a much more serious problem. The entire cauda equina can be compressed at the level of the rupture. The patient has bilateral radicular pain and varying bilateral neurologic signs and symptoms, which may include sphincter dysfunction and perineal sensory change. Because of the danger of irreversible neurologic damage, bilateral sciatica demands more urgent evaluation than unilateral sciatica. Any suggestion of sphincter disturbance should be considered emergent. Myelography or CT, or both, and a full, wide laminectomy with disc removal should be done.

The patient who does not improve after surgery should be reevaluated to rule out a recurrent disc fragment and to establish that surgery was done at the correct level. If no surgical lesion is found, the patient should be encouraged to exercise and to return to work and attempt to live with the symptoms. Analgesic drugs, especially narcotics and tranquilizing medications, should be avoided. Pain clinics have been helpful in rehabilitating some of these patients. Those with persistent lumbar disc signs but no clinical or radiographic findings should not have any type of surgery. Rehabilitation should be attempted. □

Lumbar Disc Herniation: Clinical Manifestations

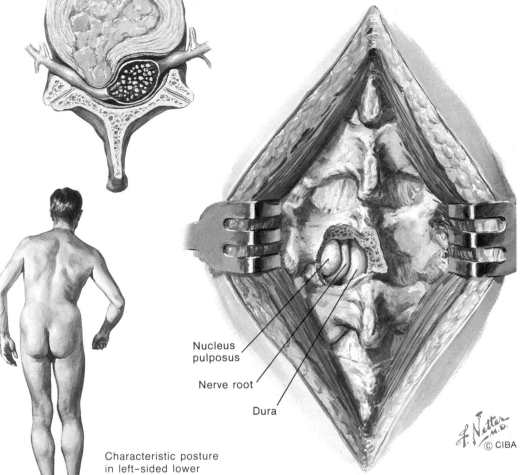

Schematic cross section showing compression of nerve root

Nucleus pulposus

Nerve root

Dura

Characteristic posture in left-sided lower lumbar disc herniation

Surgical exposure of lower lumbar disc herniation

Clinical features of herniated lumbar nucleus pulposus

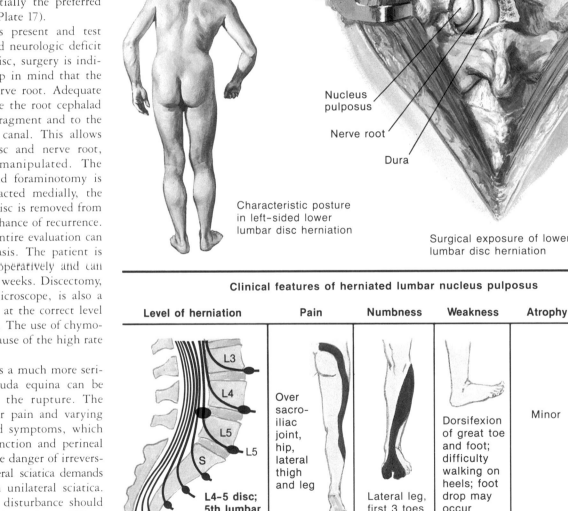

Level of herniation	Pain	Numbness	Weakness	Atrophy	Reflexes
L4–5 disc; 5th lumbar nerve root	Over sacro-iliac joint, hip, lateral thigh and leg	Lateral leg, first 3 toes	Dorsiflexion of great toe and foot; difficulty walking on heels; foot drop may occur	Minor	Changes uncommon in knee and ankle jerks, but internal hamstring reflex diminished or absent
L5–S1 disc; 1st sacral nerve root	Over sacro-iliac joint, hip, postero-lateral thigh and leg to heel	Back of calf, lateral heel, foot and toe	Plantar flexion of foot and great toe may be affected; difficulty walking on toes	Gastrocnemius and soleus	Ankle jerk diminished or absent

Psychosomatic Back Complaints

Psychologic problems can be major etiologic factors in patients with back pain. Furthermore, patients who have different types of psychosomatic back problems may have the same complaints. The most common mistake in the treatment of such patients is inadequate attention to the differential diagnosis. Specific diagnosis is necessary to determine an effective program of treatment. Generic labels such as "hysteric," "functional," "psychologic overlay" or "crock" rarely lead to a resolution of clinical problems. The differential diagnosis for psychiatric problems that may be manifested by back pain includes somatic delusions in schizophrenia, depression, psychophysiologic disorder, conversion disorder, hypochondriasis/somatization disorder, factitious disorder/malingering and chronic pain syndrome.

The physical complaints associated with schizophrenia, depression and anxiety disorders are discussed in Section VI. Failure to recognize and treat these psychiatric problems in patients with spinal complaints causes much needless frustration for both physician and patient.

Psychophysiologic disorders imply maladaptive stress responses. These patients have muscle tension/pain syndromes and usually have associated physical findings. They do well with treatments such as biofeedback, relaxation training, cognitive psychotherapy, and judicious use of minor tranquilizers and/or muscle relaxants during periods of high stress.

Patients with *conversion disorder* have unconsciously mediated symptoms that serve to "convert" unacceptable psychic conflicts into physical symptoms. The symptoms solve the conflict (primary gain) and may precipitate a supportive environmental response (secondary gain). Hypnosis, psychotherapy and brief behavioral interventions can eliminate symptoms of conversion disorder and often preclude a recurrence under future stress.

Hypochondriasis and *somatization disorder* are diagnoses that respectively apply to patients who are overly concerned about their health and to those for whom illness is the major focus of daily existence. Attempts to cure such patients result only in a "tug-of-war," since symptoms are psychologically needed. Good management supports increased functioning by the patient without insisting that symptoms be completely abandoned. Minimization of tests, surgery, appliances and medications can help patients immensely and assure physicians that they are doing the right thing despite the persistence of symptoms.

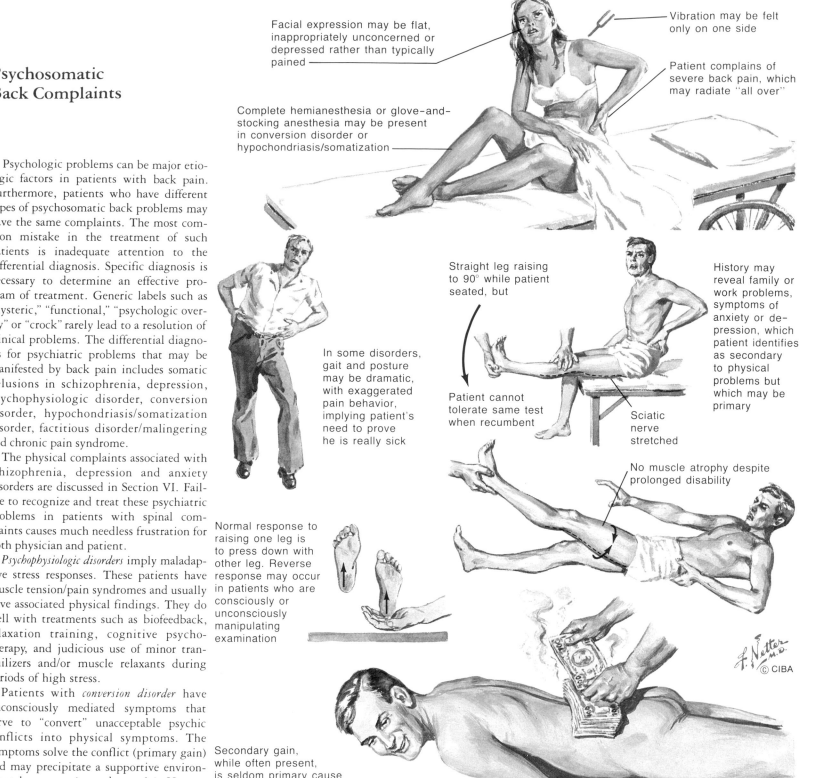

Facial expression may be flat, inappropriately unconcerned or depressed rather than typically pained

Vibration may be felt only on one side

Patient complains of severe back pain, which may radiate "all over"

Complete hemianesthesia or glove-and-stocking anesthesia may be present in conversion disorder or hypochondriasis/somatization

In some disorders, gait and posture may be dramatic, with exaggerated pain behavior, implying patient's need to prove he is really sick

Straight leg raising to 90° while patient seated, but

Patient cannot tolerate same test when recumbent

Sciatic nerve stretched

History may reveal family or work problems, symptoms of anxiety or depression, which patient identifies as secondary to physical problems but which may be primary

No muscle atrophy despite prolonged disability

Normal response to raising one leg is to press down with other leg. Reverse response may occur in patients who are consciously or unconsciously manipulating examination

Secondary gain, while often present, is seldom primary cause of pain and disability

Outright *malingering* for material gain is usually fairly apparent and should simply be confronted. More problematic than simple malingerers are patients with *factitious disorders*. Their acts of pain, while conscious, are not for material gain but for complex psychologic gain. Factitious illness behavior is often an expression of serious underlying personality problems. Even in these difficult cases, making the diagnosis and confronting patients with a caring attitude and a psychiatric treatment plan result in some treatment successes and preclude expensive and sometimes dangerous misuse of medical services.

For some patients, classification into any one of the categories described seems impossible. Their pain complaints take on an identity of their own and last for several months or years. They exhibit elements of anxiety, depression, psychophysiologic components and conversion of frightening anger about their plight. They adopt a "sick role" resembling somatization disorder. Financial, legal, insurance and compensation issues raise the specter of malingering. *Chronic pain syndrome* is a diagnostic concept that includes elements of all the other psychosomatic categories. Treatment programs that are flexible and provide attention to all the various treatment modalities discussed in the other categories have been strikingly successful in many patients who have chronic pain. □

Spinal Stenosis

Spinal Stenosis

In contrast to patients with a herniated disc, which is usually symptomatic at the level of just one spinal nerve root, some patients sustain compression of the lumbosacral nerve roots at several levels. In many of these patients, the spinal canal is narrowed at multiple levels, particularly L3–5. With aging, when spondylosis occurs, the resulting overgrowth of facets, laminae and vertebral bodies produces a relatively distinct clinical syndrome of spinal stenosis.

The majority of patients with spinal stenosis are men, and most are in at least their sixth decade of life. However, spinal stenosis may occur early in life in patients with certain developmental bony abnormalities such as achondroplasia, osteochondrodystrophy and mucopolysaccharidosis.

Clinical Manifestations. Initially, the symptoms in these patients often seem to mimic those of intermittent claudication associated with arteriosclerotic occlusive disease of the legs. The common denominator in both is the precipitation of symptoms with exercise, especially walking. This "pseudoclaudication" type of pain is more dysesthetic, in contrast to the aching, squeezing pain of arterial disease or the searing pain of nerve root disease. However, the distribution in the hips, thighs and buttocks is similar to that in arterial disease. True sciatica is often absent, and coughing and sneezing do not exacerbate the symptoms.

In contrast to arterial disease, in which the specific distance exercised necessary to precipitate symptoms becomes quite constant, the distance necessary to produce the symptoms of spinal stenosis is variable. This may relate to the patient's posture, as these patients often find that assuming a flexed simian posture prevents or delays onset of symptoms. For example, unlike patients with arterial disease, patients with spinal stenosis can pedal long distances on a bicycle as long as they maintain a fully flexed position.

Another illustration is the difference between walking uphill and downhill. When walking downhill, the normal tendency is to hyperextend the spine, with increasing lordosis, and with this posture, spinal stenosis may precipitate symptoms. The usually more difficult uphill climb may not be associated with any symptoms. This apparent paradox should alert the physician to the possibility of spinal stenosis. Later in the course in some of the more severely affected patients, even the seated posture may precipitate some discomfort.

Diagnosis. Results of examination of the patient with spinal stenosis may be relatively benign, especially in comparison with results in patients in whom a herniated nucleus pulposus produces nerve root disease. At rest, these patients are usually comfortable and have no back pain, muscle spasm or loss of lumbar lordosis. Straight leg raising does not aggravate symptoms, as it does in disc disease. In contrast, in spinal stenosis, hyperextension of the spine precipitates

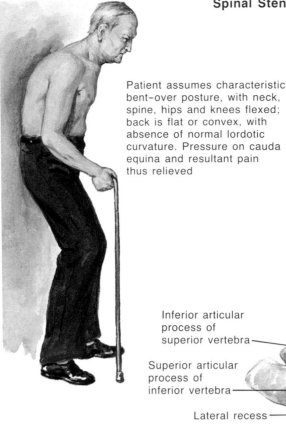

Patient assumes characteristic bent–over posture, with neck, spine, hips and knees flexed; back is flat or convex, with absence of normal lordotic curvature. Pressure on cauda equina and resultant pain thus relieved

Metrizamide myelogram with CT scan showing severe compromise of spinal canal, with compressed dural compartment

Inferior articular process of superior vertebra

Superior articular process of inferior vertebra

Lateral recess

Central spinal canal narrowed by enlargement of inferior articular processes of superior vertebra. Lateral recesses narrowed by subluxation and osteophytic enlargement of superior articular processes of inferior vertebra

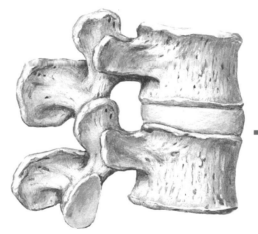

Properly spaced lumbar vertebrae, with normal thickness of intervertebral disc

Vertebrae approximated due to loss of disc height. Subluxated superior articular process of inferior vertebra has encroached on foramen. Internal disruption of disc shown in cut section

symptoms, which may be relieved by forward flexion. At times, the physician does not consider the patient's symptoms to be serious, because testing of strength, reflexes and sensation often fails to reveal any deficit. When exercise fails to elicit changes in pulses, the unwary physician may cease the evaluation.

The precise mechanism that produces spinal stenosis is not clear. It has been postulated that interaction occurs between mechanical compression and exercise-precipitated nerve root ischemia.

Plain radiographs of the spine demonstrate spondylosis. Myelography and computed tomography (CT) usually show high-grade obstruction or complete block. Frequently, multiple levels are

involved, usually L2 or L3–5. In contrast to acute disc rupture, L5–S1 is rarely involved.

Treatment. Wide laminectomy of the affected levels, with unroofing of the most symptomatic nerve roots, is the treatment of choice. The surgeon must search for extruded disc fragments. Postoperatively, pseudoclaudication is fully relieved in most patients, allowing them to lead much fuller lives. It should be stressed that in contrast to midline disc herniation, which can also produce bilateral paresthesias, surgery is not urgent. Rather, the patient and surgeon may wish to follow a conservative course of observation until the symptoms produce significant discomfort and interfere with normal leg patterns. □

Diabetic Radiculopathy

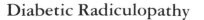

Diabetic Radiculopathy

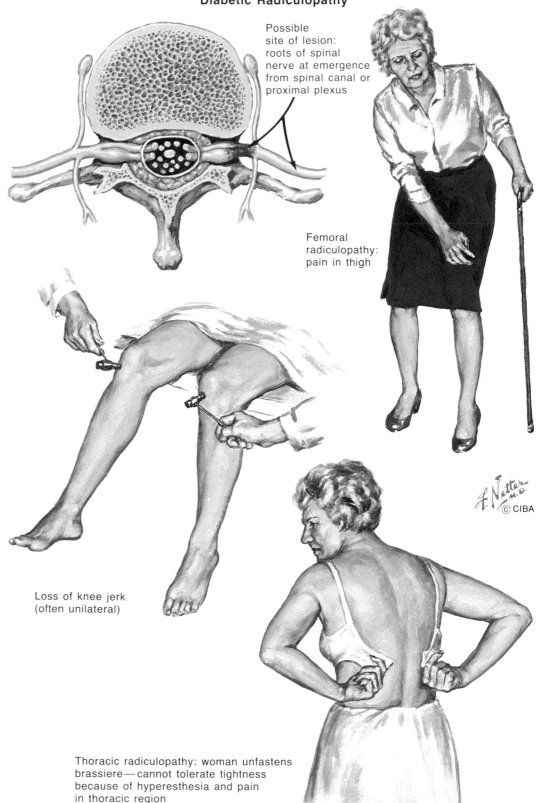

Possible site of lesion: roots of spinal nerve at emergence from spinal canal or proximal plexus

Femoral radiculopathy: pain in thigh

Loss of knee jerk (often unilateral)

Thoracic radiculopathy: woman unfastens brassiere—cannot tolerate tightness because of hyperesthesia and pain in thoracic region

Patients who have diabetes mellitus are predisposed to a variety of disorders of the peripheral nervous system, the most common of which is the insidiously progressive, predominantly sensory symmetric distal polyneuropathy (see Section XI, Plate 11). In addition, a variety of other neuropathic disorders may develop, including an asymmetric neuropathy, ie, mononeuritis multiplex (see Section XI, Plate 14); an acute oculomotor nerve palsy, which mimics an aneurysm except for pupillary sparing; sensitivity to compression or entrapment neuropathies (see Section XI, Plate 10); and an acute radiculoplexopathy.

The most common of the diabetic radiculoplexopathies chiefly affects the distribution of the femoral nerve. A number of clinical terms have been applied to this syndrome, including diabetic amyotrophy, femoral neuropathy, asymmetric proximal motor neuropathy and lumbar plexopathy. Differences in terminology have basically reflected various opinions as to the primary anatomic site of the lesion rather than pathologic definition. In one well-documented case, Raff et al noted multifocal infarcts suggestive of an ischemic mechanism in the lumbar plexus and most proximal part of the obturator and femoral nerves. In fact, various sites may be involved (nerve root, plexus or peripheral nerve), but the clinical spectrum is fairly constant.

Clinical Manifestations. Frequently, initial symptoms are severe pain in the hip, buttock or anterior thigh and weakness of the thigh, often associated with weight loss. This constellation may suggest an underlying malignancy or a primary intraspinal lesion. Less commonly, symptoms may mimic involvement of sacral and thoracic nerve roots. The cervical dermatomes are not involved. Occasionally, homologous areas of the opposite side are affected later.

Although the onset of symptoms is often fairly acute or even precipitous, the course may be insidiously progressive in some patients. Pain is the most common initial complaint. In contrast to the patient with disc disease, who usually can find a comfortable position at night, the patient with diabetic radiculopathy often has nocturnal exacerbations. The pain frequently has a particularly dysesthetic quality, often evoked by touch or exacerbated by clothing, such as brassiere straps or garments fitting tightly over the thigh. When thoracic dermatomes are involved, the pain is sometimes severe enough to mimic an abdominal or cardiac crisis.

Weakness without sensory loss may be the first sign in some patients. Weakness of the quadriceps femoris muscle makes it difficult to stabilize the knee to walk downstairs. Concomitant weakness

of the iliopsoas muscle may compromise climbing stairs or arising from a squatting position.

Diagnosis. Physical examination confirms the radicular or plexus pattern of motor loss. Unilateral loss of reflexes, particularly the knee jerk, is often present. Sensory loss may be difficult to define, although the area of hyperpathia may sometimes mimic a nerve root distribution. A moderate number of patients show signs of coexisting mild symmetric distal polyneuropathy. In patients with diabetes, back pain is usually conspicuously absent, and results of the straight leg-raising test are normal.

Nerve conduction velocities may be slightly to mildly decreased. Needle examination demonstrates abnormal insertional changes in a specific nerve root or plexus distribution. When nerve roots are involved, the paraspinal muscles are particularly affected, often bilaterally, pointing to the nerve root level of the lesion. These findings may suggest the presence of a concomitant intraspinal lesion. Myelography is normal; however, cerebrospinal fluid (CSF) protein may be elevated.

Course and Treatment. Improvement usually occurs over a period of 6 to 18 months. Pain may require specific therapy. Phenytoin or carbamazepine is often effective in controlling the particularly annoying dysesthesias common to this syndrome. Relapse may eventually occur in approximately 1 in 5 patients. □

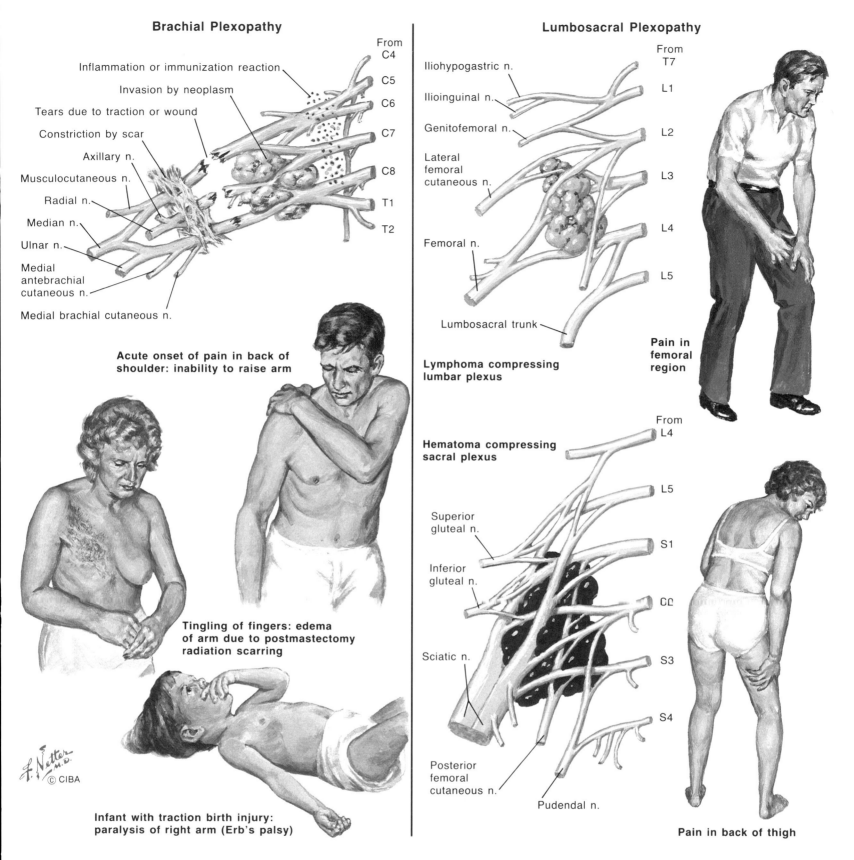

Brachial Plexopathy

Inflammation or immunization reaction

Invasion by neoplasm

Tears due to traction or wound

Constriction by scar

Axillary n.

Musculocutaneous n.

Radial n.

Median n.

Ulnar n.

Medial antebrachial cutaneous n.

Medial brachial cutaneous n.

From C4, C5, C6, C7, C8, T1, T2

Acute onset of pain in back of shoulder: inability to raise arm

Tingling of fingers: edema of arm due to postmastectomy radiation scarring

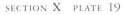

Infant with traction birth injury: paralysis of right arm (Erb's palsy)

Lumbosacral Plexopathy

Iliohypogastric n.

Ilioinguinal n.

Genitofemoral n.

Lateral femoral cutaneous n.

Femoral n.

Lumbosacral trunk

From T7, L1, L2, L3, L4, L5

Lymphoma compressing lumbar plexus

Hematoma compressing sacral plexus

Superior gluteal n.

Inferior gluteal n.

Sciatic n.

Posterior femoral cutaneous n.

Pudendal n.

From L4, L5, S1, S2, S3, S4

Pain in femoral region

Pain in back of thigh

Slide 3476

Plexopathies

The identification of damage in the brachial and lumbosacral plexuses may be initially confusing because of the seemingly disparate anatomic configuration of these structures. Generally, the anatomic distribution of deficit encompasses a territory beyond that supplying one specific peripheral nerve. Multiple pathophysiologic mechanisms can be implicated.

Brachial Plexopathy. *Trauma* is responsible for many acute brachial plexus lesions. The prognosis

depends on the portion of the plexus involved. Reinnervation is possible in upper lateral plexus lesions, but not usually in medial and lower plexus lesions, which result in a flail and numb hand. When the nerve roots are torn loose from the spinal cord, ie, evulsion, functional return is not possible.

Acute brachial plexitis may follow a viral illness or immunization. The lateral upper plexus is usually affected, causing poorly defined shoulder pain, inability to abduct the shoulder, and winging of the scapula. Recovery is usually gradual and relatively complete.

Chronic brachial plexus lesions commonly involve the medial lower portion of the plexus, producing

numbness and tingling in the fourth and fifth fingers of the hand. The clinician should carefully search for an underlying malignancy, a Pancoast tumor or lymphoma. In women, these lesions are frequently related to recurrent carcinoma of the breast or the effects of radiation therapy.

Lumbosacral Plexopathy. The lumbosacral plexus is relatively well protected, but severe blunt trauma can cause an acute lesion. Other types of acute lesions are uncommon, except in diabetics, in whom a midlumbar insult may mimic femoral neuropathy (Plate 18). Lymphomas and, less commonly, metastatic abdominal and genitourinary tumors may also invade the lumbosacral plexus and cause weakness. □

Section XI

Disorders of Motor Neuron, Peripheral Nerve, Neuromuscular Junction and Skeletal Muscles

Frank H. Netter, M.D.

in collaboration with

H. Royden Jones, Jr., M.D.   *Plates 1–2, 5–18, 20–34*

Thomas D. Sabin, M.D.   *Plate 19*

Ana Sotrel, M.D.   *Plates 3–4*

Diseases of Motor-Sensory Unit: Regional Classification

In his classic definition of the motor unit, the famous British neurophysiologist Sherrington conceptualized the motor neurons of the spinal cord and motor cranial nerves as the origin of the "final common path" through which all impulses are transmitted to the skeletal musculature via the axon and the neuromuscular junction.

Diseases of the motor-sensory unit must be differentiated clinically from central nervous system (CNS) lesions that affect primarily the spinal cord or the brain, or both. In general, *mental function* is not affected in motor-sensory unit diseases, but a mild degree of mental retardation may be present in both the Duchenne and the myotonic forms of muscular dystrophy.

Cranial nerve abnormalities, especially those producing *diplopia* or *ptosis*, or both, are frequent in diseases of the neuromuscular junction, particularly in myasthenia gravis, and may occasionally occur in the Fisher variant of the Guillain-Barré syndrome. *Dysphagia* or *dysarthria* may signal the onset of bulbar motor neuron disease, but extraocular muscles are not involved. Occasionally, dysphagia is also the first sign of myasthenia gravis or polymyositis.

Careful evaluation of *gait* is useful in differentiating lesions of the peripheral motor-sensory unit from those of the CNS. The patient with a peripheral neuropathy often has a painful gait, sometimes with characteristic foot slap, whereas the patient with a CNS lesion may have a circumducting spastic gait. The patient who has a myopathy may also give the examining physician a diagnostic clue when he pushes up with the arms in arising from a chair.

Muscle weakness is usually symmetric in most diseases that affect the motor-sensory unit; involvement of the *distal* musculature suggests a neuropathy, while involvement of the *proximal* musculature suggests a myopathy. Asymmetric involvement is most commonly seen in motor neuron disease and mononeuritis multiplex. Other important signs of motor-sensory unit dysfunction include *atrophy* and *fasciculations*.

In general, the *deep tendon reflexes* are either normal or suppressed in most disorders affecting the motor-sensory unit. Global areflexia is common early in the course of an acute Guillain-Barré syndrome, but in other neuropathies, distal reflexes are often absent and proximal reflexes are somewhat preserved. Pathologic reflexes should alert the examiner to the presence of a CNS lesion. A positive Babinski sign does not exclude a primary lesion of the motor-sensory unit, since this may also be present in amyotrophic lateral sclerosis, Friedreich's ataxia, pernicious anemia and metachromatic leukodystrophy. In each of

these illnesses, other specific clues point to the site of the primary lesion.

A simple but careful *sensory examination* is most important. In motor neuron disease, neuromuscular junction involvement or a primary myopathy, testing of both large and small fibers reveals normal sensation. In contrast, most peripheral neuropathies cause some degree of *distal sensory loss* in a stocking and, sometimes, glove distribution. A *dissociated sensory loss* such as isolated loss of pain and temperature sensation in the arms should raise a suspicion of an intraspinal lesion such as syringomyelia. However, dissociated sensory loss is also seen in some disorders affecting the peripheral nerves, such as hereditary sensory

neuropathy, diabetes or amyloidosis, which primarily affect the small, unmyelinated sensory fibers subserving pain and temperature.

Sphincter involvement usually indicates an intraspinal lesion. Rarely, it is a sign of a lesion in the motor-sensory unit, because of concomitant involvement of the autonomic nervous system. It may be seen particularly in diabetes mellitus and amyloidosis, rarely in the Guillain-Barré syndrome, and possibly in mercury poisoning.

With the exception of the burning dysesthesias symptomatic of peripheral neuropathy, the presence of neck or back pain points to an intraspinal lesion, particularly cervical or lumbar nerve root disease. □

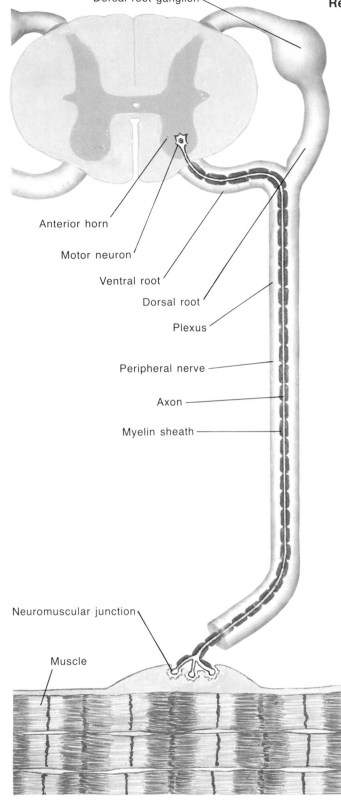

Diseases of Motor-Sensory Unit: Regional Classification

Motor neuron
Primary motor neuron diseases
Progressive muscular atrophy
Primary bulbar palsy
Amyotrophic lateral sclerosis
Werdnig-Hoffmann disease
Poliomyelitis
Tetanus

Dorsal root ganglion
Herpes zoster
Friedreich's ataxia
Hereditary sensory neuropathy

Spinal nerve (dorsal and ventral roots)
Disc extrusion or herniation
Tumor

Plexus
Tumor
Trauma
Idiopathic plexopathy
Diabetic plexopathy

Peripheral nerve
Metabolic, toxic, nutritional, idiopathic neuropathies
Arteritis
Hereditary neuropathies
Infectious, postinfectious, inflammatory neuropathies (Guillain-Barré syndrome)
Entrapment and compression syndromes
Trauma

Neuromuscular junction
Myasthenia gravis
Lambert-Eaton syndrome
Botulism

Muscle
Duchenne's muscular dystrophy
Myotonic dystrophy
Limb-girdle muscular dystrophy
Congenital myopathies
Polymyositis/dermatomyositis
Potassium-related myopathies
Endocrine dysfunction myopathies
Enzymatic myopathies
Rhabdomyolysis

Diagram labels:
Dorsal root ganglion
Anterior horn
Motor neuron
Ventral root
Dorsal root
Plexus
Peripheral nerve
Axon
Myelin sheath
Neuromuscular junction
Muscle

Slide 3478

Laboratory Studies in Neuromuscular Diseases: Electromyography and Serum Enzymes

Laboratory Studies in Neuromuscular Diseases: Electromyography and Serum Enzymes

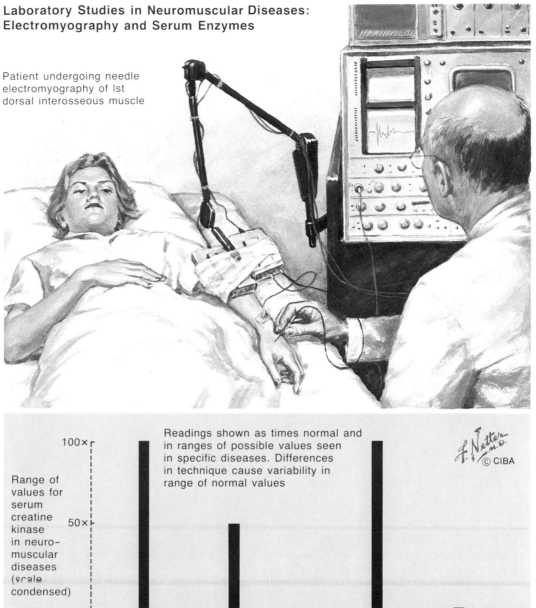

Patient undergoing needle electromyography of 1st dorsal interosseous muscle

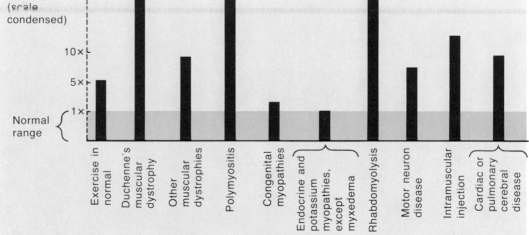

Range of values for serum creatine kinase in neuromuscular diseases (scale condensed)

Readings shown as times normal and in ranges of possible values seen in specific diseases. Differences in technique cause variability in range of normal values

Normal range

100×
50×
10×
5×
1×

Exercise in normal | Duchenne's muscular dystrophy | Other muscular dystrophies | Polymyositis | Congenital myopathies | Endocrine and potassium myopathies, except myxedema | Rhabdomyolysis | Motor neuron disease | Intramuscular injection | Cardiac or pulmonary cerebral disease

Careful clinical evaluation of the patient with a neuromuscular disease may provide sufficient clues to indicate the site of anatomic dysfunction in the motor unit. Asymmetric weakness, atrophy and fasciculations suggest *motor neuron disease*; symmetric distal weakness, hyporeflexia and sensory loss suggest *peripheral nerve disease*; fluctuating weakness, especially if it involves bulbar musculature, suggests a *neuromuscular transmission defect*; and weakness of proximal musculature suggests a *primary myopathic disorder*. There are significant exceptions to these clinical generalizations. Two types of laboratory investigation make possible anatomic and/or pathophysiologic definition of the precise site and type of abnormality.

Determination of levels of *serum enzymes*, including transaminases, aldolase and creatine kinase, are helpful in confirming the presence of a primary myopathic process (see CIBA COLLECTION, Volume 5, pages 92–93). Creatine kinase is the most important of these enzymes because it is active in normal muscles and, unlike the transaminases, is not present in the liver and erythrocytes. Creatine kinase may be strikingly elevated (10 to 100 times normal) in myopathic diseases such as Duchenne's muscular dystrophy, polymyositis, trichinosis, and conditions associated with myoglobinuria, including McArdle's disease, alcoholic myopathy and malignant hyperthermia. In contrast, creatine kinase may be elevated only slightly or not at all in congenital myopathies, in most endocrine myopathies (except myxedema), and in metabolic myopathies related to changes in serum potassium. The level of this enzyme may occasionally be 5 times normal in neurogenic diseases originating in the anterior horn cells, such as amyotrophic lateral sclerosis.

Because creatine kinase is derived from skeletal muscle, any recent trauma such as vigorous exercise, needle puncture for medications, or the needle portion of electromyography may produce false-positive test results. Thus, if determination of serum enzyme levels is a significant factor in the differential diagnosis of motor-sensory unit disease, the sample for analysis should be drawn before electromyography. False-positive results may occur in patients with myxedema, myocardial ischemia, pulmonary embolism, pneumonia or an acute cerebral insult.

Determining the *erythrocyte sedimentation rate* may also be helpful in evaluating motor-sensory unit diseases. It is particularly elevated (60 to 100 mm/hr) in an acute inflammatory disease such as polyarteritis nodosa, which causes mononeuritis multiplex. Although it is sometimes elevated in patients with polymyositis, it often is normal or only insignificantly increased.

Nerve conduction studies and *electromyography* are important physiologic diagnostic supplements to the neurologic examination. While performing the electromyography, the physician can select the combination of parameters that will best answer the questions raised by the clinical findings and the patient's symptoms.

Nerve conduction studies and electromyography are most helpful in defining the site of dysfunction in the motor-sensory unit, ie, (1) motor or sensory neuron; (2) peripheral nerve, whether nerve root, plexus, isolated single nerve, or symmetric or asymmetric multiple neuropathies; (3) neuromuscular transmission, either presynaptic or postsynaptic; or (4) muscle cell. These procedures are also helpful in determining the prognosis for recovery and possible need for surgery in traumatic peripheral nerve lesions. Also, the studies may demonstrate evidence of an organic disease in a symptomatic patient in whom results of neurologic examination were normal. Furthermore, they can prove the presence of an intact motor-sensory unit in a patient suspected of hysteria or malingering.

The timing of electromyography is important. For example, needle electromyography will not demonstrate the classic signs of denervation (fibrillation potentials and positive waves) until 14 to 21 days after damage.

The examining physician should always explain the purpose and nature of the procedure in order to gain the patient's confidence. Although they may experience mild discomfort, most patients tolerate electromyography very well. □

Muscle Biopsy: Technique, Freezing and Histochemical Studies

In addition to clinical, electrophysiologic and biochemical evaluation of a patient with a presumed skeletal muscle disorder, enzyme histochemistry and electron microscopy of the muscle biopsy specimen have become indispensable in establishing an accurate diagnosis.

Every muscle biopsy should be carefully planned and executed according to certain procedures agreed on by the clinician, the surgeon who will perform the biopsy, and the pathologist. From the pathologist's point of view, the following factors should be considered.

1. The tissue specimen most suitable for the study should be taken from a mildly involved muscle that has not been traumatized and was not used for the electromyographic tests preceding the biopsy procedure.

2. Routinely, biopsy specimens should be taken only from muscles for which normal age-matched and sex-matched controls have been established with respect to fiber size and distribution of fiber types (deltoid, biceps brachii, quadriceps and gastrocnemius muscles). Exceptions are allowed in diseases in which only certain parts of a muscle fiber need to be evaluated, for example, disorders of neuromuscular junction, when an external intercostal muscle would be the most suitable site for obtaining a biopsy specimen.

3. The surgeon who does the biopsy must be very well informed about the operative procedure and about the specific method of handling the tissue sample in order to minimize artifacts that can hinder adequate pathologic interpretation.

4. Specimens taken by needle biopsy are sufficient for studies of more advanced and diffuse pathologic changes, but are usually too small to be of use in a proper histochemical, ultrastructural and biochemical evaluation.

5. When the biopsy is carried out under local rather than general anesthesia, epinephrine should not be used, and the muscle itself must not be infiltrated with the anesthetic.

Procedure. A 1-in. surgical incision is made parallel with the long axis of the muscle fibers. The soft tissues are carefully dissected, and the muscle bellies are exposed through the incised fascia (Plate 3). The excised specimen intended for ultrastructural study (about $0.8 \times 0.3 \times 0.3$ cm) is removed in a clamp and promptly immersed in 4% phosphate-buffered glutaraldehyde to prevent excessive contraction of the tissue and to assure optimal fixation. The portion of the specimen needed for the histochemical study ($1.0 \times 0.5 \times 0.3$ cm) is excised without use of a stretching device. The surgeon should make certain that the sample remains properly oriented, so that the longitudinal axis of the muscle fibers is apparent. This tissue must not be fixed or immersed in saline solution; it should be kept wet by filter paper dampened with saline. The sample must be delivered in a fresh state to the pathology laboratory no later than about 30 minutes after removal, because it must be frozen as soon as possible to prevent the loss of enzymes.

Muscle Biopsy: Technique

If biopsy is done under local anesthesia, skin is infiltrated with anesthetic agent. Epinephrine is not used, and underlying muscle must not be infiltrated

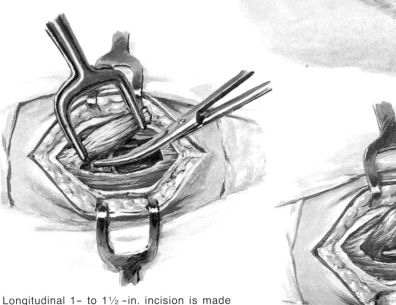

Longitudinal 1- to 1½-in. incision is made and fascia incised, exposing muscle belly. Thin cylinder of muscle for ultrastructural study is excised in clamp and promptly immersed in glutaraldehyde

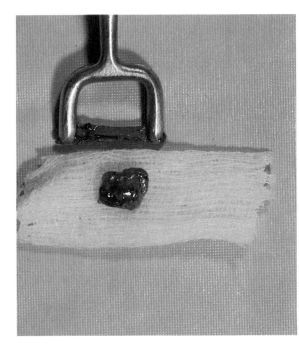

Another longitudinally oriented segment of muscle is excised for histochemical study, without use of stretching device. It is promptly placed on saline-soaked gauze, covered with filter paper dampened with saline without fixation, and delivered to laboratory within 30 min. Fascia is sutured with absorbable material and skin closed

Clamped portion of biopsy specimen must be promptly fixed in glutaraldehyde and processed for electron microscopy. Free portion on saline-soaked gauze must be frozen within 30 min, cryostat-sectioned and stained for histochemical study

Freezing Technique. Since both histologic and histochemical studies are performed on frozen tissue, it is essential that the specimen is frozen with utmost care to avoid artifacts. A simplified, reliable and inexpensive method of freezing muscle tissue with predictably good results is as follows.

A 250-cc glass beaker filled with isopentane is buried in dry ice within an insulated container and kept in a deep freezer ($-80°$ F) ready for use when the biopsy specimen arrives. The fresh muscle tissue should be trimmed to a cube approximately 0.5 cm in size and oriented in such a way that a transverse section can later be obtained from the frozen block. The specimen is then "glued" with a drop of frozen section-mounting media to the upper surface of the smaller limb of a 3.0×0.5 cm piece of index card that is bent at a 90-degree angle. The longer limb of the index card is held with a forceps, and the specimen is immersed in cold ($-70°$ F) isopentane. It should be kept there for only the optimal freezing period (about 30 seconds). If the freezing time is too short, tissue artifacts result, and if it is too long, the frozen blocks become friable. Frozen sections are placed in a cryostat kept at $-4°$ F (average temperature is $-4°$ F). They are then cut into sections 10 μm and 20 μm thick and stained with hematoxylin and eosin (H and E).

Histochemical Studies. Based on clinical information, as well as on the preliminary pathologic

Muscle Biopsy: Technique, Freezing and Histochemical Studies
(Continued)

findings obtained from the H and E-stained sections, a certain number of histochemical stains are applied to the cryostat sections, using the same staining techniques as those shown in Plate 4. The remaining frozen tissue can be used for biochemical analysis, if indicated, or it may be stored at −80° F for years without loss of histochemical activities. In addition to H and E and modified Gomori's trichrome stains, which are used for a general survey of the biopsy specimen, most of the other information required for accurate diagnosis can be obtained from applying the following histochemical reactions.

Myofibrillar *adenosine triphosphatase (ATPase)* at pH 9.4, pH 4.2 and pH 4.6 (reacts with myosin and actomyosin).

β-*nicotinamide adenine dinucleotide–reduced form (NADH)* (reacts with mitochondria, sarcoplasmic reticulum and T tubules).

Oil red O (reacts with neutral lipid droplets, normally present in the muscle).

Periodic acid Schiff (PAS) stain (reacts with glycogen if it is controlled by *alpha* amylase digestion).

If clinically or pathologically indicated, the following additional histochemical reactions may be of great diagnostic value.

Acid phosphatase (reacts with normal and abnormal lysosomes, which makes it indispensable in the diagnosis of lysosomal storage disorders).

Nonspecific esterase (strongly reacts with end plates).

Amylophosphorylase (reacts with glycogen-bound amylophosphorylase, the enzyme missing in McArdle's disease).

Alkaline phosphatase (stains some blood vessels and also certain abnormal muscle fibers).

Based on physiologic and histochemical criteria, skeletal muscle fibers are generally divided into two distinct groups.

Type I fibers are slow-twitch, fatigue-resistant, naturally darker, low in glycogen, high in oxidative enzymes, low in alkali-stable ATPase (pH 9.4), high in acid-stable ATPase (pH 4.2), and low in amylophosphorylase.

Type II fibers as a group share some physiologic and histochemical characteristics such as fast twitching and a higher amount of glycogen and amylophosphorylase. However, within this group, three different fiber subtypes, IIA, IIB and IIC, can be discerned by using other histochemical stains. Subtype IIC fibers are very rare and can be ignored in routine studies. While both IIA and IIB fibers are high in alkali stable ATPase (pH 9.4) and low in acid-stable ATPase (pH 4.2), type IIB fibers contain larger amounts of acid-stable ATPase (pH 4.6). Also, in contrast to IIB fibers, IIA fibers contain higher oxidative enzymes, are fatigue-resistant, and contain many large mitochondria.

In a normal adult muscle, the three fiber types (type I, IIA and IIB) are distributed at random in a checkerboard pattern, with each type usually accounting for about one third of the fibers.

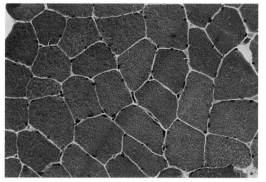

Cryostat section of normal adult muscle stained with hematoxylin and eosin. Muscle fibers are uniform in size and stain pink with eosin; their sarcolemmal nuclei are peripherally located and stain blue with hematoxylin

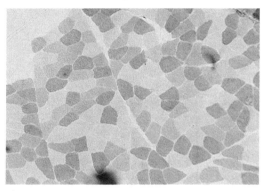

Cryostat section of normal muscle from adult male (ATPase stain, pH 4.6). Type II fibers, which contain low amounts of acid–stable ATPase, are subtyped into IIA (lightest) and IIB (intermediate) fibers. Type I (darkest) fibers contain largest amount of acid–stable ATPase. Each of these 3 fiber types amount to about ⅓ of total number

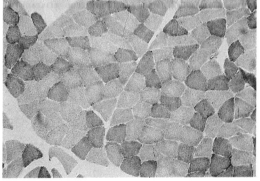

Cryostat section of normal adult muscle stained with NADH, an oxidative enzyme that reacts with mitochondria, sarcoplasmic reticulum and T tubules. Type I fibers stain more darkly

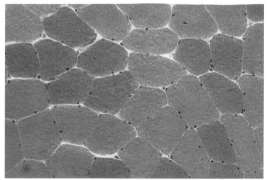

Cryostat section of normal adult muscle treated with modified Gomori's trichrome stain, which stains muscle fibers greenish blue and sarcolemmal nuclei dark red

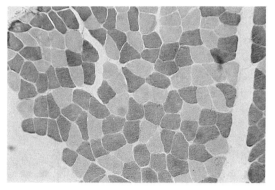

Cryostat section of normal muscle from adult male (ATPase stain, pH 9.4), showing typical checkerboard pattern with about twice as many type II fibers, which are high in alkali–stable ATPase and hence stain darkly

© CIBA

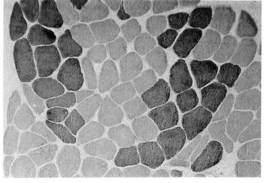

Cryostat section of reinnervated skeletal muscle stained with ATPase (pH 9.4), showing grouping of 2 fiber types: type I (lighter), type II (darker). Compare with normal section stained with ATPase (pH 9.4) above

However, the proportion of fiber types in different muscles may vary considerably.

Lower motor neurons determine the histochemical characteristics of muscle fibers in such a way that fibers innervated by one particular motor unit belong to the same type. Should another motor neuron take over, as in lower motor neuron disorders or peripheral motor neuropathies, all the reinnervated muscle fibers adopt the new characteristics. The end result is a loss of the checkerboard distribution pattern of the various fiber types and an appearance of grouping of the fiber types, which is regarded as pathognomonic of reinnervation. Another clear example that histochemical typing of muscle fibers is essential for

a correct diagnosis is seen in the congenital myopathy known as "fiber type disproportion," in which all type I fibers are uniformly smaller than type II fibers. Without histochemical stains, this could be mistaken for a large group atrophy and an erroneous diagnosis could be made.

The importance of other histochemical stains cannot be overemphasized. These include stains used to detect the lack of an enzyme such as phosphorylase and phosphofructokinase, the excessive storage of a material (neutral lipid with oil red O or glycogen with PAS), or the pathognomonic structural changes that may be too subtle for detection by ordinary stains (central cores with NADH). □

Primary Motor Neuron Disease

Primary motor neuron diseases have protean clinical manifestations. Recent estimates suggest that these diseases affect three to six of every 100,000 persons, with a male to female ratio of slightly less than 2:1. Onset is insidious and usually in middle to late life, although symptoms rarely begin late in the second or early in the third decade. About 8% to 10% of cases in adults are hereditary, primarily of dominant inheritance.

The pathology of primary motor neuron diseases is confined to motor neurons of the spinal cord, cerebral cortex and brainstem (with the exception of brainstem nuclei subserving eye movements), and to the associated corticospinal and corticobulbar tracts. Classically, these diseases are grouped into three categories, according to the predominant clinical manifestations at onset: (1) *progressive muscular atrophy* (primarily asymmetric lower motor neuron disease), (2) *primary bulbar palsy* (dysfunction of motor nerves originating in the brainstem), and (3) *amyotrophic lateral sclerosis* (upper motor neuron disease, ie, *corticospinal tract* involvement superimposed on primary muscular atrophy or primary bulbar palsy). The signs and symptoms characteristic of each of these diseases eventually blend in most patients.

Progressive Muscular Atrophy

Most patients with motor neuron disease initially report symptoms of progressive muscular atrophy, ie, clumsiness or weakness, sometimes associated with cramping. Most commonly, onset is asymmetric and in the distal musculature, beginning in either the upper or the lower extremity. Fine movements of the hands may be impaired, or a foot may become weak, mimicking foot drop (Plate 5).

In addition, patients may complain of "numbness," but a carefully elicited history rules out sensory loss per se. Patients with progressive muscular atrophy do not complain of back or neck pain, which is common in nerve root lesions of compressive origin, such as disc disease.

Initial complaints may be nonspecific, such as fatigue or cramping, with the latter sometimes occurring when the involved muscle is used. Patients may also note spontaneous twitching, or fasciculations, of muscles at rest.

Early involvement of the proximal musculature occurs in about 10% of patients. Those who have upper extremity involvement may erroneously conclude that they have a painless bursitis, demonstrated by the inability to raise their arms, while those who have lower extremity involvement may attribute their difficulty in climbing stairs to either hip or back problems.

It is important to emphasize that in patients with motor neuron disease who complain of muscle twitching, examination *always* reveals associated muscular weakness or atrophy, or both. Fasciculations alone, without associated weakness or atrophy, are benign and of indeterminate origin. Nevertheless, because they occur in motor neuron disease, patients experiencing fasciculations should undergo a complete neurologic examination, including electromyography. If

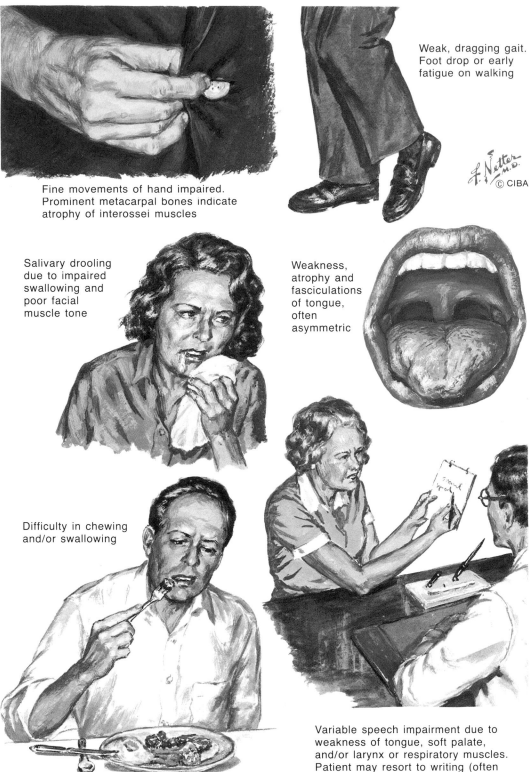

Fine movements of hand impaired. Prominent metacarpal bones indicate atrophy of interossei muscles

Weak, dragging gait. Foot drop or early fatigue on walking

Salivary drooling due to impaired swallowing and poor facial muscle tone

Weakness, atrophy and fasciculations of tongue, often asymmetric

Difficulty in chewing and/or swallowing

Variable speech impairment due to weakness of tongue, soft palate, and/or larynx or respiratory muscles. Patient may resort to writing (often also impaired) to communicate

results of neurologic tests are negative, these patients should be reassured that they have idiopathic benign fasciculations and are not at risk for development of motor neuron disease.

Primary Bulbar Palsy

In the early stages of motor neuron disease, symptoms may be related only to the motor nuclei of the brainstem, with the exception of the nuclei of cranial nerves III, IV and VI, which supply the extraocular muscles. In most patients, symptoms result from an involvement of the nuclei arising in the medulla. Progressive inability to move the tongue and failure of the palate to rise on phonation result in "mushy," breathy articulation. Early

pharyngeal involvement makes swallowing difficult, and subsequent involvement of the masseter muscles impedes chewing. The prognosis is most discouraging in patients who exhibit symptoms of brainstem dysfunction, because of the progressive risk of respiratory complications and aspiration pneumonia. Rarely, however, the course of the disease in these patients is relatively prolonged.

Amyotrophic Lateral Sclerosis

The manifestations of lower motor neuron dysfunction, as seen in progressive muscular atrophy and primary bulbar disturbances, may eventually converge with symptoms of degeneration of the

Primary Motor Neuron Disease
(Continued)

corticospinal or the corticobulbar tract, or both (Plate 6), to produce the classic picture of amyotrophic lateral sclerosis, known as "Lou Gehrig's disease" in nonmedical literature. Initial corticospinal tract involvement manifested only by a spastic gait, with later development of lower motor neuron dysfunction, is extremely unusual. If pseudobulbar palsy is the earliest clinical manifestation, the patient may develop a spastic, explosive type of speech and experience uncontrolled, inappropriate crying or laughing.

Differential Diagnosis

A diagnosis of motor neuron disease means helplessness and despair for the patient and his family, and frustration for the physician. Many diseases have similar characteristics, and the physician must carefully rule out all other possibilities before making a diagnosis.

Diseases of individual *peripheral nerves*, particularly of the ulnar or the peroneal nerve, are the disorders most commonly confused with early motor neuron disease. Motor involvement, including that of the bulbar musculature, may be a predominant sign in *Guillain-Barré disease*, although onset of this disease is usually rapid and symmetric and examination reveals marked hyporeflexia (Plate 15). Patients who have a chronic inherited peripheral neuropathy, particularly *hereditary motor-sensory neuropathy* type II, also have symmetric findings and usually a strong family history of the disease.

A localized *cervical spinal cord tumor* may be confused with motor neuron disease. Rarely, a lesion located high in the cervical spinal cord, particularly at the foramen magnum, produces the same signs as lower motor neuron disease (usually in muscles innervated by spinal nerves C8 to T1), namely, atrophy of the hands and concomitant spasticity of the lower extremities. However, neck pain is a common feature of a lesion at the foramen magnum.

Atrophy of the hand without sensory symptoms may sometimes be the initial complaint in a patient with *syringomyelia*. Careful sensory examination demonstrates a dissociated capelike loss of pain and temperature sensation (see Section X, Plate 8). Complete myelography through the foramen magnum may be necessary to exclude these possible lesions.

Patients always should be asked if they had *poliomyelitis* during childhood, as a small percentage of patients with a seemingly "complete" recovery from childhood poliomyelitis (see Section VIII, Plates 9–10) experience late-life deterioration that in all aspects mimics progressive muscular atrophy. However, the relatively rapid downhill course characteristic of motor neuron disease is unusual in these patients.

Rarely, the initial signs of a *brain tumor* at the frontal-central parasagittal level are a weak foot and spastic gait. Computed tomography (CT) of the brain can exclude this possibility. Diseases of the neuromuscular junction, such as *myasthenia*

Motor Neuron Disease
(continued)

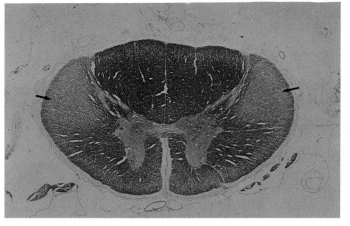

Cross section of spinal cord from patient with amyotrophic lateral sclerosis showing bilateral degeneration of corticospinal tracts (arrows)

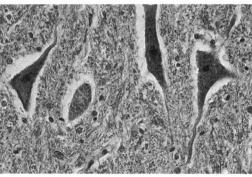

Anterior horn of spinal cord with normal motor neurons (luxol–fast blue with H and E stain)

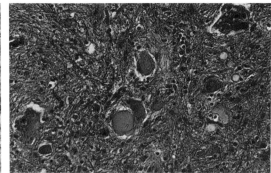

Degeneration of anterior horn cells in amyotrophic lateral sclerosis (same stain)

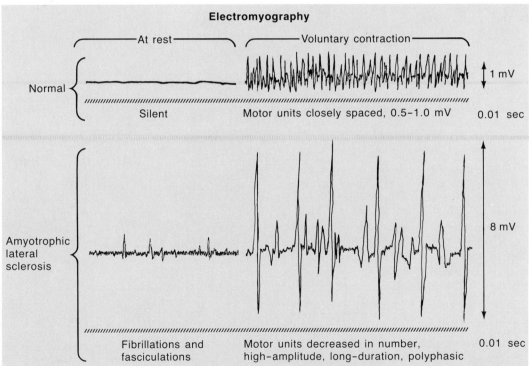

Electromyography

Normal — At rest — Silent — Voluntary contraction — Motor units closely spaced, 0.5–1.0 mV — 1 mV — 0.01 sec

Amyotrophic lateral sclerosis — Fibrillations and fasciculations — Motor units decreased in number, high–amplitude, long–duration, polyphasic — 8 mV — 0.01 sec

gravis (Plates 20–22) and the *Lambert-Eaton syndrome* (Plate 23) may be confused with primary bulbar palsy. However, signs of extraocular muscle involvement, such as diplopia and ptosis, are present in most patients with myasthenia gravis, while other clinical signs and electromyographic findings easily differentiate the Lambert-Eaton syndrome.

Primary myopathic disease does not commonly mimic motor neuron disease, although the serum creatine kinase level is variably elevated in both. Rarely, the myopathy associated with both *hyperthyroidism* and *hypothyroidism* may mimic motor neuron disease, and the serum creatine kinase level may also be mildly elevated in both diseases.

Disorders of calcium metabolism, such as *hyperparathyroidism* and *osteomalacia*, should be considered in the differential diagnosis. The physician should also remember that patients with *diabetic radiculopathy* may have acute, asymmetric signs of lower motor neuron involvement. Progressive muscular atrophy has been reported in patients with *paraproteinemia*; consequently, protein immunoelectrophoresis should be carried out in any patient in whom clinical signs clearly indicate a lower motor neuron disorder. A syndrome similar to motor neuron disease has also been reported in patients with Hodgkin's disease, but only after the diagnosis of this form of lymphoma has been established.

Primary Motor Neuron Disease
(Continued)

Diagnosis

Physical Examination. In a patient with symptoms of foot drop or an atrophied hand, the diagnosis usually considered is an isolated lesion of a peripheral nerve or nerve root. If such a lesion is the initial sign of early motor neuron disease, careful testing of other muscle strength often reveals more diffuse motor weakness. Fasciculations and widespread evidence of atrophy on examination are useful additional diagnostic signs. Atrophy and fasciculations of the tongue may be the first sign of cranial nerve involvement. Extraocular muscle function is always normal, no matter how advanced the disease.

Reflexes may vary from depressed to brisk. The Babinski sign may be extensor or plantar, depending on whether lower or upper motor neuron involvement predominates. Sensory examination must be thorough and detailed, and results should be normal if motor neuron disease is present.

Motor neuron disease is relatively easy to diagnose clinically in a middle-aged male who has asymmetric, widespread muscle weakness, atrophy and fasciculations (particularly fasciculations of the tongue), and in whom clinical examination shows no sensory changes.

Laboratory Studies. Electromyography and nerve conduction velocity studies are the most useful diagnostic techniques for confirming the diagnosis of motor neuron disease. Motor conduction may demonstrate no more than minimal slowing of conduction velocity and mild to moderate decrease in compound action potential amplitude. Sensory conduction is normal. Active neurogenic changes should be demonstrated in at least three extremities. When bulbar symptoms are present primarily, the edrophonium chloride (Tensilon) test and repetitive nerve stimulation should be done to exclude the possibility of myasthenia gravis (Plate 20). Rarely, a muscle biopsy specimen is taken to exclude inflammatory myopathy in the patient who has weakness of the proximal musculature, although electromyography is also helpful in differentiating this disorder.

When the diagnosis is not certain, careful clinical observation and follow-up are imperative, as the physician should never be in a rush to diagnose motor neuron disease unequivocally.

Treatment

Because the basic pathophysiologic mechanism of motor neuron disease is not yet understood, drug therapy has been empirical and, to date, universally unsuccessful. Symptomatic control and emotional support are the present therapeutic goals, since these diseases usually progress relentlessly to death in 2 to 10 years.

Cramping, which is occasionally a problem, can often be alleviated with diazepam, phenytoin or carbamazepine. Surgical ligation of the salivary duct may be necessary to prevent sialorrhea in the patient with bulbar involvement.

Feeding difficulties are frequently related to an inability to move food about in the mouth.

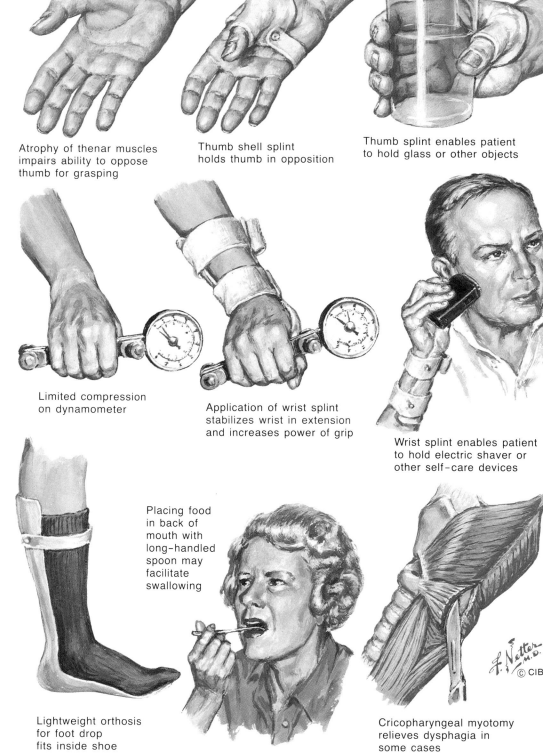

Atrophy of thenar muscles impairs ability to oppose thumb for grasping

Thumb shell splint holds thumb in opposition

Thumb splint enables patient to hold glass or other objects

Limited compression on dynamometer

Application of wrist splint stabilizes wrist in extension and increases power of grip

Wrist splint enables patient to hold electric shaver or other self-care devices

Placing food in back of mouth with long-handled spoon may facilitate swallowing

Lightweight orthosis for foot drop fits inside shoe

Cricopharyngeal myotomy relieves dysphagia in some cases

Careful placement of food in the posterior pharynx by means of a long-handled spoon may be helpful in this situation. Some patients may manage food prepared in a blender, while others may benefit from a feeding gastrostomy or esophagostomy or cricopharyngeal myotomy.

Lightweight plastic orthotic appliances may allow the patient with progressive atrophy of the extremities to regain function believed lost (Plate 7).

One of the many tragic consequences of motor neuron disease is the patient's loss of ability to speak understandably. A magic slate for writing messages can be helpful for the patient with bulbar involvement, and typing is a useful adjunct.

Early in the course of the illness, the patient should be warned against the use of respiratory depressants such as sedatives, particularly in combination with alcohol. Use of respiratory irritants such as tobacco should be discouraged, and the patient should be immunized against influenza and pneumococcal infections.

Most important is the physician's honest and compassionate approach to the total patient. It is important for the patient to know that the physician will continue to be concerned about him throughout the course of the illness. The physician should never destroy the patient's hope, but should provide symptomatic treatment and wise counsel whenever possible. □

Bell's Palsy

Acute lesions of the facial (VII) nerve are the most common of the mononeuropathies that affect the cranial nerves. The facial nerve is a mixed nerve consisting mainly of efferent motor nerve fibers of the ipsilateral facial muscles, autonomic nerve fibers to the lacrimal and salivary glands, special afferent sensory nerve fibers for taste (which supply the anterior two thirds of the tongue), and a minimal somatosensory component supplying the anterior portion of the ear canal. Bell's palsy is the most common disorder that affects the facial nerve.

Clinical Manifestations. Bell's palsy is an acute idiopathic lesion that occurs unilaterally and often develops overnight. The paralysis usually reaches a peak within a few hours. A family member often first notes that the patient cannot fully close one eye or has a grossly asymmetric smile. An attempt to close the eye on the affected side causes the eyeball to roll upward (Bell's phenomenon).

The patient may have noted pain behind or in the ear, or earlier difficulty in hearing. Hyperacusia is common and is characterized by an increased, unpleasant sensitivity to sound, which is particularly noticeable when using the telephone. This results from involvement of the nerve branch to the stapedius muscle. Involvement of the chorda tympani causes an unpleasant or distorted sense of taste. Sometimes, the patient notes an accompanying "numbness" in the face. However, examination fails to disclose an actual loss of sensation.

There is some indication that Bell's palsy more commonly affects young adults. It may also occur in diabetics and pregnant women. The mechanism is not clear. A familial occurrence has been noted in a small percentage of patients. Some patients have a peculiar constellation of findings known as the Melkersson-Rosenthal syndrome, ie, recurrent incomplete facial palsy, swelling of the lips and face, and so-called fissured tongue, or lingua plicata.

Differential Diagnosis. Peripheral facial lesions must be differentiated from *upper motor neuron lesions.* Because the frontalis muscle has bilateral cerebral innervation, an upper motor neuron lesion is characterized by weakness of only the lower two thirds of the face. In comparison, a peripheral lesion causes not only a weakness of mouth and eye closure, but also an inability to wrinkle the forehead.

Occasionally, Bell's palsy may be the first sign of a more diffuse disorder, such as the *Guillain-Barré syndrome* (Plate 15). However, in this setting, a contralateral lesion frequently follows. *Sarcoidosis* is another inflammatory lesion associated with bilateral facial nerve palsy, and *Hodgkin's lymphoma* may preferentially affect the facial nerve. The nerve is particularly vulnerable to *trauma* either at the stylomastoid foramen or to fracture across the petrous portion of the temporal bone.

Bell's Palsy

Course and distribution of facial (VII) nerve

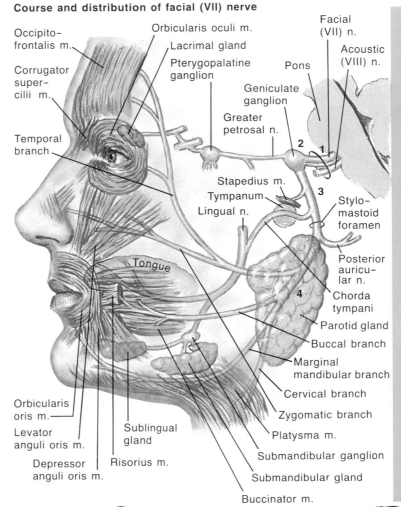

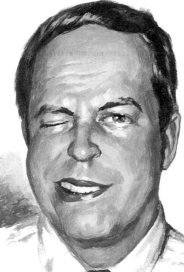

In patient's attempts to smile or bare teeth, mouth draws to unaffected side. Patient cannot wink, close eye, or wrinkle forehead on affected side

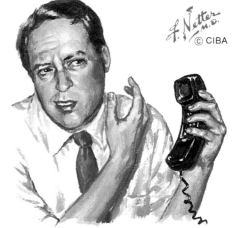

Hyperacusia: patient holds phone away from ear because of painful sensitivity to sound

Sites of lesions and their manifestations

1. Intracranial and/or internal auditory meatus. All symptoms of 2, 3 and 4, plus deafness due to involvement of eighth cranial nerve

2. Geniculate ganglion. All symptoms of 3 and 4, plus pain behind ear. Herpes of tympanum and of external auditory meatus may occur

3. Facial canal. All symptoms of 4, plus loss of taste in anterior tongue and decreased salivation on affected side due to chorda tympani involvement. Hyperacusia due to effect on nerve branch to stapedius muscle

4. Below stylomastoid foramen (parotid gland tumor, trauma). Facial paralysis (mouth draws to opposite side; on affected side, patient unable to close eye or wrinkle forehead; food collects between teeth and cheek due to paralysis of buccinator muscle)

Insidious onset and slow progression of symptoms in a patient without any autonomic, taste or hearing dysfunction should prompt careful peripheral examination. *Parotid tumors* are particularly suspect in this setting. More proximal tumors may involve the facial nerve. Among the more common are various lesions at the *cerebellopontine angle* (see Section V, Plate 11).

Treatment. Generally, treatment is nonspecific. Use of artificial tears and an eye patch at night to prevent corneal abrasions are useful adjuncts. There is some suggestion that, if begun at the onset of symptoms, a 7- to 10-day trial of prednisone may result in complete return of function. Although surgical decompression of the nerve canal has been advocated, this approach is generally not recommended.

Prognosis. The idiopathic lesion resolves satisfactorily in 75% to 80% of patients. However, in about 10% to 15%, incomplete or inappropriate reinnervation occurs. As the nerve regenerates, its branches may innervate muscles not previously supplied, resulting in so-called faulty reinnervation. Clinical manifestations of this anomaly are seen in the patient who may blink when attempting to smile, or form tears instead of salivating when tasting food. In a small percentage of patients, axonal regeneration is ineffective and leaves a facial paralysis that necessitates various repairs by plastic surgery. □

Carpal Tunnel Syndrome

The carpal tunnel syndrome, the most common example of a chronic entrapment peripheral neuropathy, is usually idiopathic in origin, with onset in midlife or later. Symptoms may occur earlier in persons who work extensively with their hands. Predisposing conditions include obesity, rheumatoid arthritis, eosinophilic fasciitis, diabetes mellitus, gout, myxedema, acromegaly and dysproteinemia. All these disorders increase the contents of the carpal tunnel, through inflammation, edema or protein deposits, and compress the median nerve. The carpal tunnel syndrome may occur during pregnancy, but almost always resolves spontaneously after delivery.

Clinical Manifestations. The patient usually awakens in the morning or during the night with the sensation that the hand is "asleep." Often, the location of the referred numbness or tingling cannot be pinpointed, and the patient may believe that all fingers are involved. At night, hanging the affected limb over the edge of the bed often relieves symptoms. During the day, certain activities, such as driving, sewing or hammering, precipitate symptoms. Eventually, a mild but persistent distal numbness develops in the first three and one-half digits. Later, paresthesias may spread into the forearm and, less commonly, the upper arm. Motor symptoms, with thenar atrophy or weakness, generally appear late in the course.

Differential Diagnosis. A classic carpal tunnel syndrome is not often confused with other lesions. However, unless the history is carefully elicited and a thorough examination performed, conditions can partially mimic this syndrome and other lesions may be missed. For example, the median nerve can be entrapped more proximally, particularly near the elbow in the vicinity of the pronator muscle. Entrapment here causes a syndrome in which involvement of the deep motor branch predominates and affects pinch function, and sensory symptoms are absent. Electromyography and studies of nerve conduction velocity have shown that most patients clinically diagnosed in the past as having a thoracic outlet syndrome actually have a carpal tunnel syndrome.

A *protruded disc* or, rarely, a *tumor* (eg, a neurilemmoma) at C7 or, less commonly, at C6, may cause numbness of the thumb and first two fingers but almost always is associated with neck or shoulder pain. Neurologic examination reveals weakness and depressed reflex of the triceps brachii muscle. Because of the large area of anatomic representation of the thumb and first digit in the sensory strip of the cerebral cortex, a *focal cerebral lesion* will rarely mimic the carpal tunnel syndrome, particularly in patients with transient

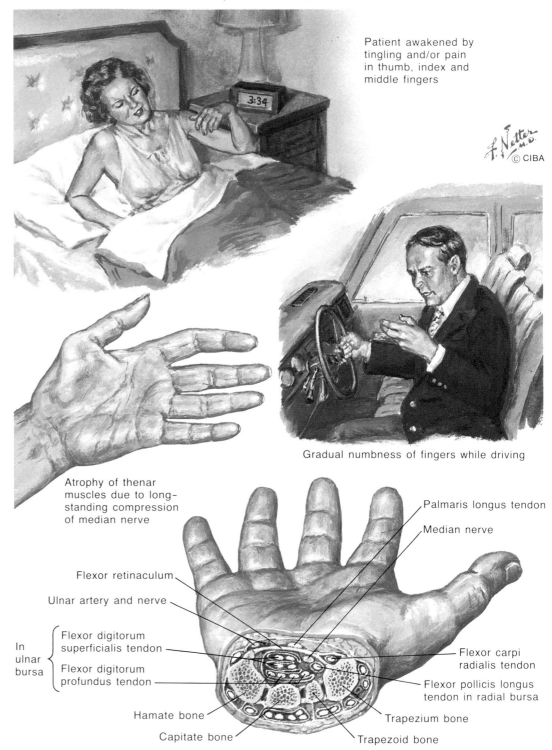

Carpal Tunnel Syndrome

Patient awakened by tingling and/or pain in thumb, index and middle fingers

Gradual numbness of fingers while driving

Atrophy of thenar muscles due to long-standing compression of median nerve

Palmaris longus tendon

Median nerve

Flexor retinaculum

Ulnar artery and nerve

In ulnar bursa {
Flexor digitorum superficialis tendon
Flexor digitorum profundus tendon
}

Flexor carpi radialis tendon

Flexor pollicis longus tendon in radial bursa

Hamate bone

Capitate bone

Trapezium bone

Trapezoid bone

Section through wrist at distal row of carpal bones shows carpal tunnel. Increase in size of tunnel structures caused by edema (trauma), inflammation (rheumatoid disease), ganglion, amyloid deposits or diabetic neuropathy may compress median nerve

ischemic attacks or, less often, in patients with sensory seizures.

Physical Examination. A thorough neurologic examination is necessary to exclude involvement of other peripheral nerves or lesions within the spinal cord or the central portions of the cerebral cortex. In most patients with a mild carpal tunnel syndrome, neurologic findings are minimal or absent. Perhaps the most helpful diagnostic clue is pain on percussion over the median nerve at the wrist (Tinel's sign).

Diagnostic Studies. Electrodiagnostic tests of motor-sensory conduction in the median nerve, particularly those that would show prolongation of the sensory and, sometimes, distal motor

latency, are most helpful in diagnosing the carpal tunnel syndrome. Appropriate studies should also be done to exclude any systemic illness that may predispose to an early carpal tunnel syndrome.

Treatment. Although discontinuation of activities that precipitate the carpal tunnel syndrome occasionally results in improvement, this is not a practical alternative for patients who do skilled work with their hands. Sometimes a splint to be worn at night is sufficient if the patient is seen early in the illness. Steroid injections into the carpal canal have also provided relief. However, simple surgical decompression has generally produced the best results, with a good long-term prognosis. □

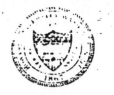

HOWARD UNIVERSITY HOSPITAL
2041 GEORGIA AVENUE N.W.
WASHINGTON, D.C. 20060

DATE _____

TO: _____
_____
_____

We should like to request a summary of your medical record on
patient named below. Our staff is interested in securing reports
of: laboratory findings, x-rays, operative procedures, final and
pathological diagnoses, and any other significant findings
including:

_____

_____

_____

Rose Mary Jones
NAME AT TIME CARE WAS RECEIVED

Capital Hill Rehab, Hosp.
ADDRESS AT TIME CARE WAS RECEIVED

12-28-36
DATE OF BIRTH

year 1995
DATE CARE WAS RECEIVED

PLEASE SEND REPLY TO:

_____

_____

_____

CONSENT:

Permission is hereby given to_____
to furnich information from (My record-My child's record) to
HOWARD UNIVERSITY HOSPITAL.

SIGNATURE _Rose Mary Jones_   DATE 10/27/96

WITNESS _Rhonda M. Lancaster_   DATE Oct 27, 96

Entrapment and Compressive Neuropathies

Although the carpal tunnel syndrome is the most common entrapment peripheral neuropathy, entrapment or compression of other peripheral nerves occurs with significant frequency. (See CIBA COLLECTION, Volume 1/I, pages 118–127.)

Tardy Ulnar Palsy. The common lesions of the ulnar nerve occur at the elbow. They involve either entrapment at the cubital tunnel or compression at the medial epicondylar groove. Patients note an insidious onset of numbness and tingling in the little finger and the medial half of the ring finger, with wasting of the interossei muscles. It is important to differentiate an ulnar nerve lesion from a medial plexus or C8 spinal root syndrome. Electrodiagnostic studies may show a nerve conduction block at the elbow. Although surgical decompression is usually advocated, carefully controlled follow-up studies are needed to confirm the value of this procedure.

Radial Nerve Palsies. Acute lesions of the radial nerve usually develop secondary to compression of the nerve in the upper arm (eg, Saturday night palsy in the alcoholic who falls asleep with one arm draped over the back of a chair frame).

Finger and wrist extensors are weakened, and the resulting wrist drop may mimic a stroke, particularly when the onset is acute. In contrast to the stroke patient, fine movements of muscles innervated by the median and ulnar nerves are not affected with radial nerve lesions. Recovery is in 8 to 12 weeks, providing there is little or no axonal damage.

Peroneal Nerve Palsy. The most common site of damage to the peroneal nerve is at the knee, where it courses around the fibular head.

Chronic compression is most commonly seen in asthenic or cachectic inactive persons who sit with their legs crossed, thus compressing the nerve against the bone of the opposite knee.

Patients note a tendency for the foot to slap, stemming from weakness of all the anterior compartment muscles. The clinician should make certain that the foot drop is not secondary to a nerve root lesion at L5, which is a main contributor to the peroneal nerve. The L5 nerve root also innervates the tibialis posterior muscle, which inverts the foot and is supplied by a branch of the posterior tibial nerve. It is important to test this muscle to differentiate an L5 root lesion from a peroneal nerve palsy. In addition, most patients with nerve root disease have associated back pain.

If electromyography documents a conduction velocity block of the peroneal nerve across the fibular head, indicating compression, the prognosis is good, providing the patient discontinues the activity causing the pressure. A foot-drop splint may be helpful while reinnervation develops.

Lateral Femoral Cutaneous Nerve Palsy. Meralgia paresthetica is a common sensory neuropathy caused by compression of the lateral femoral cutaneous nerve as it passes beneath the lateral end of the inguinal ligament. It is most commonly seen in obese patients wearing tight-fitting garments, and is often unilateral. Patients complain of burning dysesthesias or hypersensitivity on the lateral aspect of the thigh. The symptoms usually resolve spontaneously. □

Other Compressive or Entrapment Neuropathies

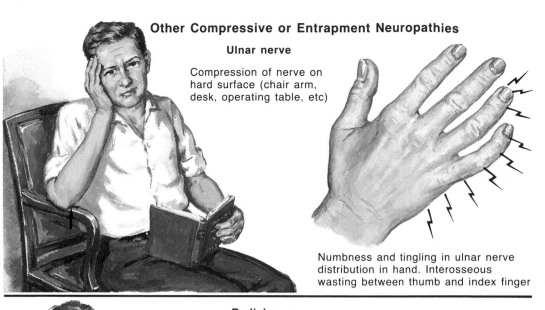

Ulnar nerve

Compression of nerve on hard surface (chair arm, desk, operating table, etc)

Numbness and tingling in ulnar nerve distribution in hand. Interosseous wasting between thumb and index finger

Radial nerve

Compression of nerve in axilla or upper arm in patient sleeping with arm over chair back, edge of bed, etc, or by crutch

Wrist drop

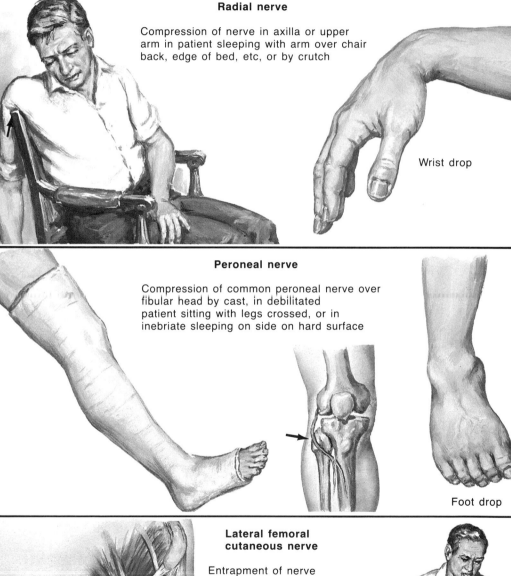

Peroneal nerve

Compression of common peroneal nerve over fibular head by cast, in debilitated patient sitting with legs crossed, or in inebriate sleeping on side on hard surface

Foot drop

Lateral femoral cutaneous nerve

Entrapment of nerve under inguinal ligament

Numbness and dysesthesias in lateral thigh

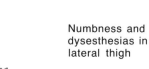

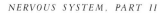

Peripheral Neuropathies: Metabolic, Toxic and Nutritional

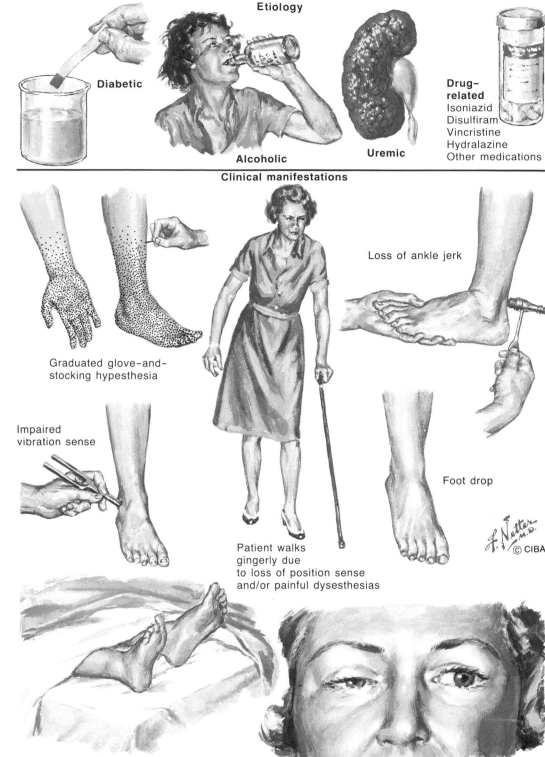

Etiology

Diabetic

Alcoholic

Uremic

Drug-related
Isoniazid
Disulfiram
Vincristine
Hydralazine
Other medications

Clinical manifestations

Graduated glove-and-stocking hypesthesia

Impaired vibration sense

Loss of ankle jerk

Foot drop

Patient walks gingerly due to loss of position sense and/or painful dysesthesias

Patient sleeps with covers off feet because of burning sensation

Diabetic third cranial nerve palsy

The most common of the neuropathies are chronic subacute, diffuse, symmetric disorders of the peripheral nerves associated with metabolic, toxic or nutritional conditions. No etiologic mechanism is identifiable in about 50% of neuropathies. However, in half of the remaining cases, a carefully elicited history and examination of family members indicate an apparent hereditary factor. In the majority of cases, onset of sensory symptoms is insidious. Typically, the patient complains of symmetric numbness, tingling, burning, tightness or bandlike constrictions or even a feeling that he is walking on sand or pebbles. In some patients, exercise exacerbates the symptoms, while in other patients, the symptoms are more severe at rest, particularly at night.

The physician should carefully question the patient about the onset of symptoms to exclude *mononeuritis multiplex*, an acute, asymmetric neuropathy initially confined to one peripheral nerve and then progressing to other peripheral nerves over a period of days to weeks (Plate 14).

Examination of the patient with a *symmetric polyneuropathy* usually demonstrates changes first evident in the legs and feet. There is a symmetric hyporeflexia, with distal weakness. On sensory examination, the patient typically reports that the degree of perception gradually improves along the limb in a stockinglike distribution.

In *metabolic* or *toxic neuropathies*, the more distal part of the peripheral nerve is affected and produces a so-called dying back effect, which is secondary to changes in the metabolism of the nerve cell and, perhaps, to changes in axonal flow.

Diabetes mellitus is one of the most common metabolic causes of generalized peripheral neuropathy. In some patients with diabetes mellitus, however, only a single nerve, most commonly the femoral or median nerve, is affected. Involvement of a cranial nerve, usually the oculomotor (III) nerve, is also common in diabetes, producing classic signs of third cranial nerve palsy, with pupillary sparing (see CIBA COLLECTION, Volume 4, page 118).

Uremia also causes distal axonal sensory peripheral neuropathy. Most affected patients have severe end-stage renal involvement, with a serum creatine level over 10 mg/100 ml. Nerve function is improved if dialysis is initiated early in the illness, but is not affected by later dialysis.

Hypothyroidism is the most common endocrine disorder predisposing to a neuropathy. The patient commonly has an unstable gait and may also have a superimposed carpal tunnel syndrome. Classically, reflexes are diminished, and the recovery phase is delayed, producing a so-called hung-up reflex.

Of the many *drugs* implicated as a cause of peripheral neuropathy, one of the most common is *vincristine*, used in the treatment of various hematologic malignancies. Other drugs predisposing to a neuropathy are isoniazid (secondary to vitamin B_6 deficiency), nitrofurantoin, disulfiram, gold, nitrous oxide, perhexiline and pyridoxine (when used in fad megavitamin diets). Heavy metals such as arsenic, lead and thallium may also affect nerve function (Plate 13).

Alcoholism is the most common *nutritional neuropathy* seen in Western countries. In many alcoholics, the neuropathy causes severe pain.

Rarely, a sensory peripheral neuropathy may be the first sign of an *occult malignancy*. About 5% of patients with carcinoma of the lung, particularly middle-aged or older patients, have evidence of a peripheral neuropathy. In some of these patients, the neuropathy is present as long as 3½ years before the malignancy becomes apparent.

Dysproteinemia (Amyloid Neuropathy)

Paraproteinemia, or dysproteinemia, manifested by a monoclonal protein spike on protein electrophoresis, is seen in approximately 10% of adult-onset peripheral neuropathies. However, this monoclonal gammopathy may not be evident unless immunoelectrophoretic techniques are used, because a relative amount of abnormal protein may be masked by normal protein on routine protein electrophoresis. Although monoclonal gammopathy may be found in up to 3% of the normal population over age 60, studies of large groups of patients with motor-sensory unit diseases have revealed that this disorder occurs primarily in patients with peripheral neuropathy.

The various peripheral nerve syndromes are best separated into those with either *benign* or *malignant plasma cell dyscrasias*. The benign dyscrasias are seen in amyloidosis, in other autoimmune diseases such as vasculitis, and in idiopathic monoclonal gammopathy.

Amyloidosis. In about 10% of patients with *primary systemic amyloidosis*, peripheral neuropathy is the cardinal manifestation. Incapacitating symmetric sensory symptoms often predominate. Burning, prickling numbness usually affects the feet and hands concomitantly, with stabbing pain occurring spontaneously. The dysesthesias are often incapacitating, and patients sometimes resort to narcotics. Motor symptoms, although present, are often less prominent. About 1 of 5 patients may initially have symptoms of a carpal tunnel syndrome (Plate 9).

Autonomic dysfunction is particularly suggestive of amyloidosis and is reflected in orthostatic hypotension, diarrhea or constipation, bladder dysfunction with incontinence, or decreased urinary force and impotence.

Systemic involvement is also common in primary amyloidosis and is often manifested by the nephrotic syndrome, congestive heart failure or sprue.

Laboratory studies show an axonal motor-sensory peripheral neuropathy on electromyography and a slight elevation in cerebrospinal fluid (CSF) protein. Demonstration of amyloid deposits in sural, rectal, or fat pad biopsy specimens confirms the diagnosis.

To date, there is no effective treatment for amyloidosis. Both the neuropathy and the systemic manifestations have a progressive course, with a 75% mortality rate within 3 years.

Two less common *hereditary varieties of amyloidosis* with prominent neural involvement usually have no associated dysproteinemia. The *Portuguese (Andrade) type* is of autosomal dominant inheritance, often with onset in the third or fourth decade. The *Indiana type* primarily affects the upper extremities.

Other Benign Monoclonal Gammopathies. Mononeuritis multiplex may be the first indication of a type of benign monoclonal gammopathy associated with autoimmune disease (Plate 14). Another type is characterized by peripheral neuropathy without concomitant systemic illness. The severe dysesthetic sensory symptoms and autonomic dysfunction seen in amyloid neuropathy are not present in this neuropathy. Nerve

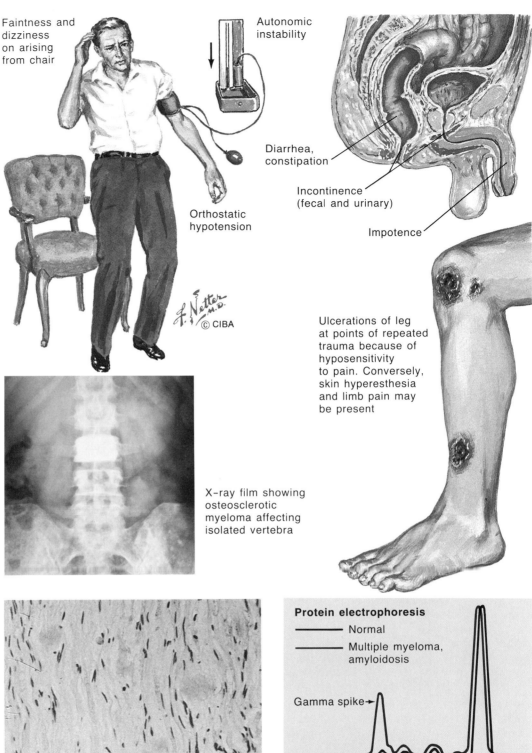

Faintness and dizziness on arising from chair

Autonomic instability

Orthostatic hypotension

Diarrhea, constipation

Incontinence (fecal and urinary)

Impotence

Ulcerations of leg at points of repeated trauma because of hyposensitivity to pain. Conversely, skin hyperesthesia and limb pain may be present

X-ray film showing osteosclerotic myeloma affecting isolated vertebra

Biopsy specimen of peripheral nerve: amyloid deposits displacing nerve fibers (Congo red stain)

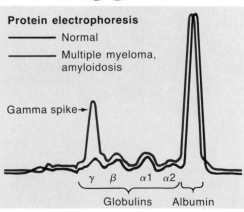

Protein electrophoresis
— Normal
— Multiple myeloma, amyloidosis

Gamma spike →

γ   β   α1   α2

Globulins   Albumin

conduction velocity studies demonstrate very slow velocities similar to those seen in demyelinating disease, and fluorescent techniques may show light-chain deposits in nerve biopsy specimens. Treatment with various combinations of corticosteroids, azathioprine, chlorambucil or cyclophosphamide may be effective.

Malignant Monoclonal Gammopathies. Malignancies that produce peripheral neuropathies and are associated with monoclonal gammopathies include multiple myeloma, plasmacytoma, Waldenström's macroglobulinemia, plasma cell leukemia and lymphomas.

The demyelinating peripheral neuropathy associated with osteosclerotic myeloma is particularly important. In any patient with what appears to be a chronic, predominantly motor, inflammatory peripheral neuropathy, careful evaluation should include a complete protein analysis in addition to radiographic survey of bone for metastases. Associated clinical findings of organomegaly, pituitary or adrenal dysfunction, and skin changes (including hyperpigmentation and hypertrichosis), are further indications for these studies. If bone survey shows a sclerotic or sclerotic lytic lesion, open biopsy should be performed. Tumoricidal irradiation of isolated lesions of osteosclerotic myeloma produces a satisfactory improvement in the peripheral neuropathy and eliminates the focus of the myeloma. □

Peripheral Neuropathy Caused by Heavy Metal Poisoning

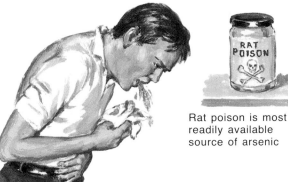

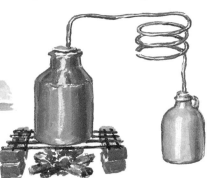

Rat poison is most readily available source of arsenic

History of nausea and vomiting may suggest arsenic poisoning in patient with peripheral neuropathy

Antique copper utensils (eg, still for bootleg liquor) and runoff waste from copper smelting plant may be sources of arsenic poisoning

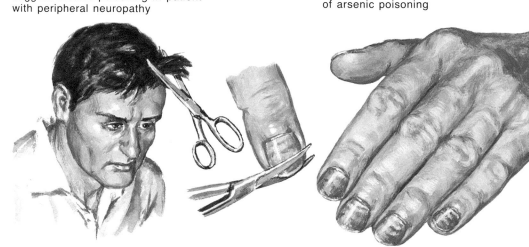

Although 24-hour urinalysis is best diagnostic test for arsenic, hair and nail analysis may also be helpful

Mees' lines on fingernails are characteristic of arsenic poisoning

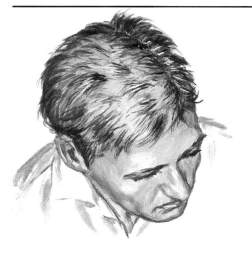

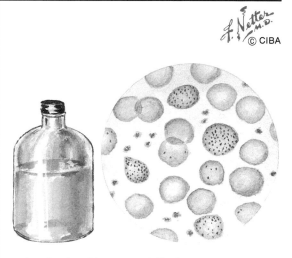

Spotty alopecia associated with peripheral neuropathy characterizes thallium poisoning

Lead poisoning, now relatively rare, causes basophilic stippling of red blood cells. 24-hour urinalysis is diagnostic test

The investigation of a peripheral neuropathy sometimes is like solving a mystery, especially when the physician searches for various toxic mechanisms. Nothing illustrates this better than the occasional patient exposed to a heavy metal.

Arsenical Neuropathy. Arsenic is the metal most likely to be implicated in toxic neuropathy. Although uncommon, arsenic poisoning should always be considered in the differential diagnosis of a peripheral neuropathy of recent onset. This is true even when the more usual mechanisms such as alcohol abuse or diabetes are obviously present, because unsuspected chronic arsenic intoxication is found occasionally.

Arsenic has a ubiquitous distribution in the environment, particularly as an impurity in copper ores. Although it is a means of notorious surreptitious homicide, the presence of excessive levels of arsenic in a patient should not immediately indicate a possible criminal cause. Arsenic contamination may be due to exposure to an agricultural environment, or to an industrial environment such as copper smelting. Other sources have included drinking water (eg, when a well has been inadvertently drilled in a former storage location of arsenic insecticides), an antique teakettle or copper still made of impure copper that leaches arsenic, and kelp, which concentrates arsenic and is used in large quantities by dietary faddists.

The *clinical manifestations* of arsenic poisoning may vary. Sometimes, a high degree of exposure may produce immediate gastrointestinal distress, with *nausea and vomiting* that may recur with each ingestion. A variety of systemic symptoms may also be present, including episodes of sweating, fevers, headaches, fatigue and blurred vision.

The peripheral nerves are particularly susceptible to damage from arsenic, and as the level increases, severe, motor-sensory *polyneuropathy* may develop. Occasionally, if the amount ingested is sufficiently large, growth arrest lines, so-called *Mees' lines,* may be seen in the fingernails. The triad of recurrent nausea and vomiting, peripheral neuropathy and Mees' lines is a conclusive indication of arsenic poisoning, although an anticancer agent may conceivably produce the same symptoms. Rarely, an organic encephalopathy may occur.

Normochromic anemia and leukopenia are sometimes associated findings. Nerve conduction velocity studies may demonstrate either an axonal or a demyelinating type of peripheral neuropathy.

Diagnosis is confirmed by analysis of a 24-hour urine sample, a more sensitive indicator than serum values. Samples of hair and nails may provide supporting evidence of arsenic exposure.

Treatment includes removing the source of the arsenic, and use of chelating agents such as penicillamine.

Neuropathies Caused by Other Metals. *Gold salts,* used in treating rheumatoid arthritis, have sometimes produced a distal motor-sensory peripheral neuropathy. Occasionally, patients receiving this treatment also report facial dysesthesias. The major consideration in the differential diagnosis is the neuropathy of arteritis secondary to rheumatoid arthritis. Improvement

in neuropathic symptoms after discontinuation of gold salts usually confirms an underlying toxic mechanism.

The anticancer agent *cisplatin* produces a severe motor-sensory neuropathy similar to the carcinomatous sensory neuropathy caused by the tumors for which it is used.

Ingestion of *thallium salts,* occasionally used in rodenticides and insecticides, causes a potentially severe motor-sensory neuropathy associated with development of alopecia 10 to 30 days after ingestion.

Exposure to *lead,* now seen infrequently, can cause a predominantly *motor neuropathy,* often initially involving wrist and finger extensions. □

Mononeuritis Multiplex With Polyarteritis Nodosa

The peripheral nerves are susceptible not only to various toxic, metabolic and genetic factors that produce the classic deficits of the motor-sensory unit manifested by a symmetric glove-and-stocking distribution, but also to a variety of lesions that may acutely compromise the circulation to a specific nerve. In the latter case, the lesion initially mimics an acute pressure palsy with no apparent mechanical cause. The patient may have noted an acute foot drop; ie, the foot tends to drag or slap because of an acute peroneal nerve lesion. Initial involvement of the femoral nerve produces an instability of the knee, which is especially noticeable when going downstairs.

In the arm and hand, the median, ulnar and occasionally the radial nerves may be separately involved. As the illness progresses, a second and then a third peripheral nerve may become affected, usually in an asymmetric fashion. If the basic disease state progresses acutely and rapidly, multiple nerves may be involved before the patient seeks medical attention. The findings on examination may then actually suggest a diffuse, symmetric polyneuropathy. However, careful questioning of the patient about the temporal profile of the illness should reveal separate acute insults to the extremities, which differ in both anatomic distribution and time of onset. This facet provides an important clinical clue.

At times, the acuteness of the initial lesion resembles a stroke. In fact, the patient has sustained a stroke, but the infarct involves the vasa nervorum of a peripheral nerve rather than a cerebral vessel. The clinician must carefully evaluate the distribution of the neurologic deficit. An acute lesion of the radial nerve may make the hand seem functionless. However, when the wrist and fingers are supported, it is apparent that musculature innervated by the median and ulnar nerves is totally intact. Similarly, a peroneal nerve infarct that causes an acute foot drop does not affect the muscles in the posterior compartment of the calf, which are innervated by the posterior tibial branch of the sciatic nerve.

Pathophysiologic Mechanisms. Once the clinical profile of the illness is apparent, the possible underlying pathophysiologic mechanisms should be considered. Acute lesions are most commonly caused by disorders affecting small-sized arterioles, which occur relatively often in *diabetes.* Only rare pathologic specimens of nerves have been available for study. The best example has been the oculomotor (III) nerve, in which an infarct was found that involved the most central fibers but spared the peripheral fibers. It has been assumed that similar lesions account for the acute peripheral mononeuropathy seen in occasional diabetics and which may be the initial sign of the disease. Many such patients slowly but definitely improve, in contrast to diabetics with a more predominant, painful, symmetric sensory polyneuropathy.

Polyarteritis nodosa should always be strongly considered in searching for the cause of mononeuritis multiplex. This disorder characteristically

Sudden occurrence of foot drop while walking (peroneal nerve)

Sudden buckling of knee while going downstairs (femoral nerve)

Pattern of diverse, asymmetric nerve involvement (nonsimultaneous in onset)
Unilateral ulnar n.
Unilateral radial n.
Unilateral femoral n.
Unilateral tibial n.
Bilateral peroneal nn.
(Lower limb more commonly affected)

Polyarteritis nodosa with characteristic multisystem involvement

Myalgia and/or arthralgia often associated with abdominal problems, anorexia, fever and weight loss

Nephropathy, a most serious effect. RBCs, WBCs and casts in urine; eventual renal failure

Hypertension common

Angiogram showing microaneurysm of small mesenteric artery

CNS involvement may cause headache, ocular disorders, convulsions, aphasia, hemiplegia and cerebellar signs

Inflammatory cell infiltration and fibrinoid necrosis of walls of small arteries lead to infarction in various organs or tissues

produces an inflammatory lesion, probably autoimmune in nature, which affects medium-sized arterioles throughout the body. In addition to myalgia and arthralgia, bowel, kidney and, rarely, cerebral infarcts may occur. The erythrocyte sedimentation rate is high in polyarteritis nodosa, with values up to 80 to 120 mm Westergren per hour. This test should always be carried out in the setting of mononeuritis multiplex. If values are elevated, histologic examination of a biopsy specimen of a muscle or nerve, or both, confirms the diagnosis. Clinical and laboratory findings in other arteritides, such as *systemic lupus erythematosus* or the *Churg-Strauss syndrome,* may mimic those in polyarteritis nodosa.

Very rarely, cardiac embolic lesions, such as *bacterial endocarditis* and *atrial myxoma,* cause mononeuritis multiplex. Other mechanisms rarely responsible include *vasculitis* secondary to amphetamine abuse, some of the *dysproteinemias* identified by analysis of immunoglobulins, and a yet-to-be explained remote effect of *carcinoma.*

Leprosy produces a slowly evolving sensory mononeuritis multiplex, which has a predilection for the cooler surfaces of the body such as the pinna of the ear, the tip of the nose, and digital nerves of the extremities. This is the most common cause of neuropathy and should always be considered in those who have emigrated from an area in which leprosy is endemic (Plate 19). □

Guillain-Barré Syndrome

The Guillain-Barré syndrome is an acute, rapidly progressive, symmetric polyradiculoneuropathy that predominantly affects motor function. Associated findings include total areflexia and elevated cerebrospinal fluid (CSF) protein. In about 50% of patients, a viral infection precedes the syndrome by a few weeks. Less commonly, the disease may follow an immunization or a surgical procedure, or may appear during the course of lymphoma or systemic lupus erythematosus.

Investigational studies suggest that the predominant lesion results from an attack on the myelin sheath by inflammatory cells, with concomitant myelin breakdown and, in severe cases, secondary axonal damage. The peripheral nerves may be affected at any level between the spinal nerve root and the distal ending of the nerve.

Clinical Manifestations. The majority of patients seek medical attention because of progressive symmetric paralysis, although cranial nerve dysfunction, particularly Bell's palsy, sensory ataxia, or pure autonomic dysfunction may be the initial disorder. Minimal distal paresthesias may also be the first symptom, although motor symptoms predominate in most patients. Early in the course, patients may also note inexplicable fatigue or difficulty in climbing stairs, getting out of a chair, and brushing their hair.

Physical Examination. Although examination reveals symmetric weakness, the degree of deficit may vary slightly from side to side. Areflexia is usually bilateral and universal. However, the more proximal reflexes may be less involved early in the course. Sensory loss is less conspicuous, even though two thirds of patients have some form of distal paresthesias. Evaluation reveals minimal to moderate glove-and-stocking hypesthesia. Proprioceptive sensation is often more severely affected. Involvement of posterior rather than anterior nerve roots may predominate, causing unsteady gait, ataxia and severe pain in a segmental distribution.

Cranial nerve dysfunction is much less common, although facial nerve palsy (sometimes asymmetric) is seen in up to 30% of patients, and extraocular muscles are affected in about 5%. Tongue and palate involvement is rare.

Autonomic abnormalities are frequent and labile, and may include supraventricular tachycardia or bradycardia, postural hypotension, swings in blood pressure, or other vasomotor

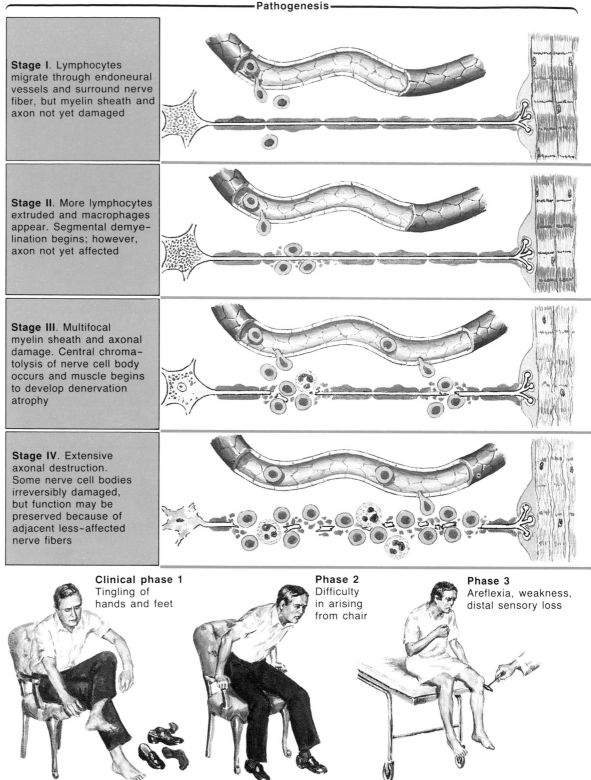

Pathogenesis

Stage I. Lymphocytes migrate through endoneural vessels and surround nerve fiber, but myelin sheath and axon not yet damaged

Stage II. More lymphocytes extruded and macrophages appear. Segmental demyelination begins; however, axon not yet affected

Stage III. Multifocal myelin sheath and axonal damage. Central chromatolysis of nerve cell body occurs and muscle begins to develop denervation atrophy

Stage IV. Extensive axonal destruction. Some nerve cell bodies irreversibly damaged, but function may be preserved because of adjacent less-affected nerve fibers

Clinical phase 1 Tingling of hands and feet

Phase 2 Difficulty in arising from chair

Phase 3 Areflexia, weakness, distal sensory loss

symptoms. A restrictive pulmonary insufficiency may develop secondary to weakness of the diaphragmatic and intercostal muscles.

Differential Diagnosis. Acute spinal cord lesions may be confused with the Guillain-Barré syndrome. These lesions also cause rapidly progressive paralysis, but sensory examination usually demonstrates a spinal cord level (see Section X, Plates 2, 4). Reflexes are commonly hyperactive, and are associated with a positive Babinski sign. Spinal cord lesions also typically cause early bowel and bladder dysfunction. Back pain may be a feature of either disorder, although it is common in spinal cord lesions and relatively rare in the Guillain-Barré syndrome.

Clinical findings in a number of *toxic, metabolic* or *infectious processes*, including arsenic poisoning, may be identical to those in the Guillain-Barré syndrome. A carefully documented history and appropriate laboratory studies usually point to the specific mechanism. Infectious diseases that should be considered include poliomyelitis and diphtheria. CSF pleocytosis with predominant polymorphonuclear response is seen in *poliomyelitis* (see Section VIII, Plates 9–10); a history of sore throat and, perhaps, bulbar palsy is characteristic of *diphtheria*. Acute intermittent *porphyria* may mimic the classic Guillain-Barré syndrome, and the patient should be questioned about use of any medication that could precipitate a porphyric

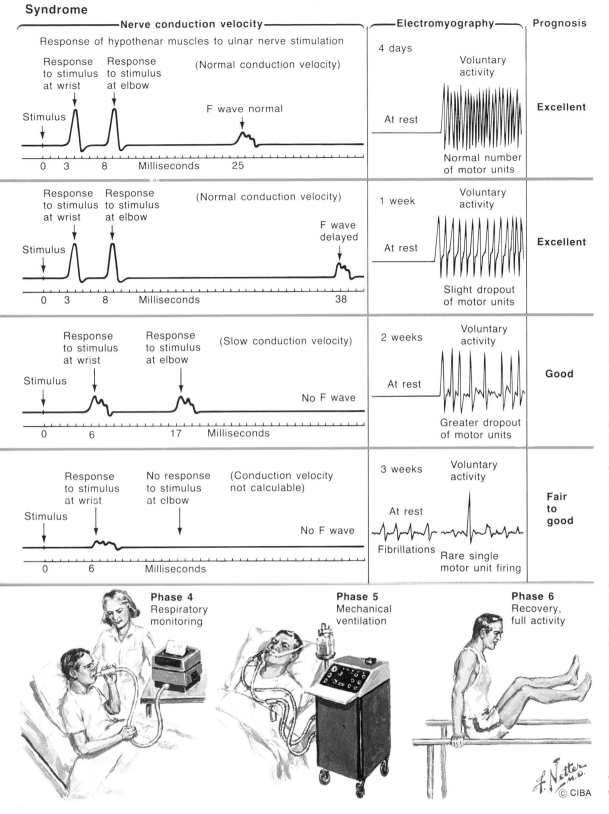

Nerve conduction velocity	Electromyography	Prognosis
Response of hypothenar muscles to ulnar nerve stimulation	4 days — Voluntary activity / At rest / Normal number of motor units	**Excellent**
Response to stimulus at wrist / Response to stimulus at elbow / (Normal conduction velocity) / F wave normal / Stimulus / 0 3 8 Milliseconds 25		
Response to stimulus at wrist / Response to stimulus at elbow / (Normal conduction velocity) / F wave delayed / Stimulus / 0 3 8 Milliseconds 38	1 week — Voluntary activity / At rest / Slight dropout of motor units	**Excellent**
Response to stimulus at wrist / Response to stimulus at elbow / (Slow conduction velocity) / No F wave / Stimulus / 0 6 17 Milliseconds	2 weeks — Voluntary activity / At rest / No F wave / Greater dropout of motor units	**Good**
Response to stimulus at wrist / No response to stimulus at elbow / (Conduction velocity not calculable) / No F wave / Stimulus / 0 6 Milliseconds	3 weeks — Voluntary activity / At rest / Fibrillations / Rare single motor unit firing	**Fair to good**

Phase 4 Respiratory monitoring

Phase 5 Mechanical ventilation

Phase 6 Recovery, full activity

crisis. The scalp should be carefully examined to exclude the presence of a tick that could produce *tick paralysis.*

Pupillary abnormality points to either diphtheria or *botulism,* both of which also have predominant bulbar symptoms (Plate 34). Associated facial palsy may suggest *sarcoidosis,* whereas bulbar symptoms may also be seen with *myasthenia gravis* (Plates 20–22).

Although acute onset of distal tingling of the extremities may be caused by *hyperventilation,* such a diagnosis should be established cautiously. Patients with this complaint should be reexamined in 24 hours, since it may be an early manifestation of the Guillain-Barré syndrome.

Laboratory Studies. Examination of CSF usually shows the classic albumino-cytologic dissociation (ie, essentially normal cellular response with elevated CSF protein). Characteristically, the elevation occurs early in the illness. In up to 20% of patients, values may be normal within the first week of illness, but serial determinations usually demonstrate a significant elevation in almost all patients. Persistently normal protein values almost rule out the diagnosis.

Although not imperative in the classic case, electrodiagnostic studies confirm the diagnosis. Any process destroying myelin significantly slows conduction velocity if the nerve is stimulated above and below the lesion. Conduction velocity

in the Guillain-Barré syndrome may be less than 60% of normal. However, because involvement of the individual nerves differs, conduction velocity may vary from markedly slow to normal. Slowing is most pronounced at common sites of nerve compression. The distal latency is often prolonged, and the compound action potential is dispersed.

Sensory conduction is also affected in many patients, but in up to 10% of subjects, values are persistently normal. A proximal lesion may be missed when routine conduction velocity studies are done in the more distal portion of the nerve. The introduction of F wave studies has made it possible to investigate these areas. The F wave is a late-evoked response occurring after the muscle action potential wave. Involvement at any point along the nerve prolongs F wave latency. Thus, nerves with proximal demyelination may show a prolonged F wave latency despite normal routine motor conduction velocity. Similarly, the H reflex, a monosynaptic circuit similar to the knee jerk and elicited only by stimulating the posterior tibial nerve, may also be prolonged.

Needle electromyography is used to demonstrate the muscle fiber's ability to fire motor units. The finding of abnormal insertion activity demonstrates the presence of axonal damage if this study is done at least 3 weeks after onset of illness.

The findings on electrodiagnostic studies mirror the degree of underlying pathologic changes in the four stages of the Guillain-Barré syndrome, as shown in the illustration.

Treatment. Most patients recover from the Guillain-Barré syndrome, but the course is not entirely predictable, and the efficacy of different therapeutic regimens is difficult to evaluate. Treatment with steroids, immunosuppressants and plasmapheresis is controversial, and only supportive measures are generally accepted. Careful monitoring of respiratory and autonomic dysfunction has significantly reduced mortality. Other complications that should be prevented or treated include deep vein thrombosis, pulmonary emboli and hyponatremia. Good nursing care minimizes pressure palsies and sores. Active physical therapy is also important.

Prognosis. The Guillain-Barré syndrome is self-limiting in most patients. The maximum deficit is usually seen in 2 to 4 weeks and improvement follows, with the course determined by the degree of axonal damage that accompanied demyelination. If axonal damage is severe, maximum recovery may take more than a year. □

Hereditary Motor-Sensory Neuropathies

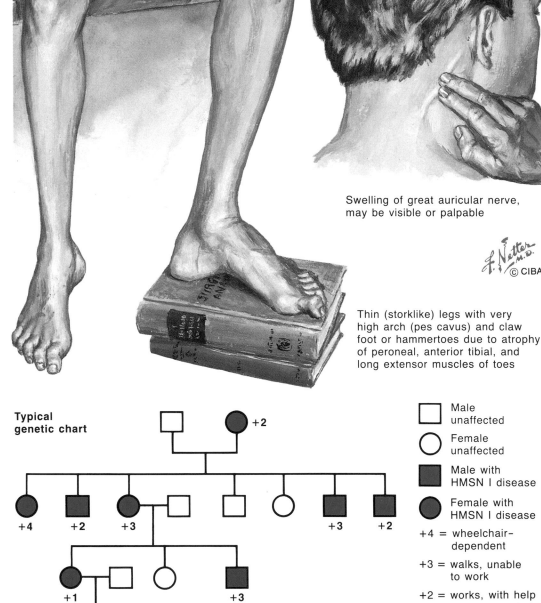

Swelling of great auricular nerve, may be visible or palpable

Thin (storklike) legs with very high arch (pes cavus) and claw foot or hammertoes due to atrophy of peroneal, anterior tibial, and long extensor muscles of toes

Typical genetic chart

Male unaffected

Female unaffected

Male with HMSN I disease

Female with HMSN I disease

+4 = wheelchair-dependent

+3 = walks, unable to work

+2 = works, with help

+1 = mild disability, no help required

About 50% of patients who seek medical attention because of symptoms that are typical of a chronic peripheral neuropathy have no manifestations of a common metabolic or a toxic causative mechanism. Previously, many of these patients were said to have idiopathic polyneuritis, but recent studies have shown that in about 25% to 30%, a carefully documented history of hereditary factors and evaluation of the patient's relatives point to a definitive diagnosis.

The classification of these disorders has been difficult since Charcot and Marie in France and Tooth in England first described them in 1886. However, careful studies by Dyck and others have delineated a spectrum of hereditary neuropathies. Whether the various clinical subdivisions proposed for these disorders actually represent separate nosologic entities is not clear, but certain generalizations appear to be valid. Peripheral neurons are symmetrically involved in all these disorders. Both motor and sensory fibers are usually affected, although in some variants, only motor or sensory neurons are involved.

These neuropathies appear to result from an as yet unidentified inborn error of metabolism. Each disease results in a chronic, slowly progressive clinical syndrome. Inheritance is variable.

The two most common types of hereditary motor-sensory neuropathy (HMSN) are type I, a demyelinating neuropathy (hypertrophic Charcot-Marie-Tooth neuropathy), and type II, a neuronal form of Charcot-Marie-Tooth disease. Type I and type II are both inherited as an autosomal dominant trait, whereas type III (Déjerine-Sottas disease) is an autosomal recessive disorder. The underlying biochemical defect has been demonstrated only in the rare type IV disorder (Refsum's disease), which causes a relative block in the degradation of phytanic acid and clinically mimics HMSN III in many respects.

Hereditary Motor-Sensory Neuropathy Type I and Type II

Clinical Manifestations. Although HMSN I and II closely resemble each other clinically, two basic differences can be demonstrated. In type I, the peripheral nerves are hypertrophic and certain nerves (eg, great auricular nerve) are easily palpable; in type II, the nerves are not hypertrophied. In addition, nerve conduction velocity studies demonstrate very slow conduction velocities in type I, whereas in type II, conduction velocity is generally normal.

Onset of HMSN I is usually in the second or third decade, although the disease may begin later in life, as does type II. Initial symptoms in both types include slight difficulty in walking. Teenage patients may tire easily during demanding athletic endeavors, and other patients may note excessive aching of muscles after exercise. These young people are gradually bypassed by their peers in a disproportionate fashion to that expected for their age. Eventually, they develop a clumsy, sometimes steppage, gait in which the knees are lifted abnormally high to get the feet off the ground.

Pes cavus or hammertoes become insidiously evident (Plate 16). Because of the disproportionate involvement of the intrinsic toe musculature, especially the dorsiflexors of the feet and toes, the long toe and foot flexors are unopposed. This results in the pes cavus posture and tight Achilles tendons. These deformities become more pronounced with age, being seen in up to 25% of children but in nearly 60% of adults.

Hereditary Motor–Sensory Neuropathy Type I: Motor Nerve Conduction Velocity

Hereditary Motor-Sensory Neuropathies
(Continued)

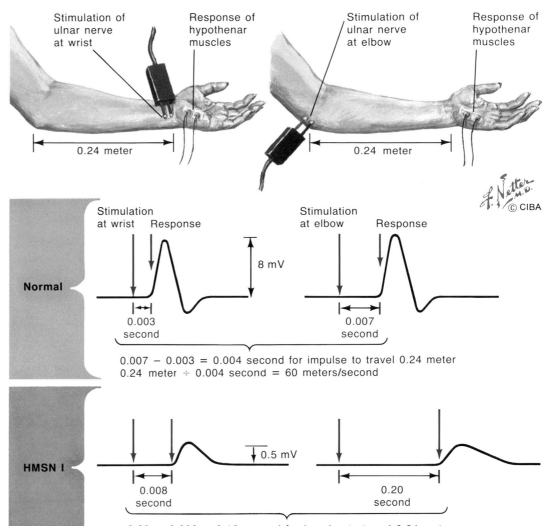

Atrophy becomes progressively more noticeable in the legs, particularly in the anterior tibial musculature. However, development of the so-called inverted champagne-bottle or storklike legs, as described in the more classic literature, appears to be relatively uncommon. Similarly, sensory complaints are unusual.

In a small percentage of patients, symptoms eventually develop in the upper extremities. Some lose fine motor control, while tremor develops in others. Tremor was originally described as a variant of this illness, the so-called Roussy-Lévy syndrome, but this differentiation has no apparent nosologic significance.

In addition to foot deformities, atrophy, hypoactive reflexes and slight distal sensory loss, careful examination may demonstrate, in about 25% of patients, the presence of thickened peripheral nerves, particularly in the upper extremity between the shoulder and the elbow, and in the great auricular nerve in the scalp. Nerve thickening at various anatomic loci known to predispose to nerve entrapment, such as the ulnar groove or the fibular head, is less significant.

Hereditary Motor-Sensory Neuropathy Type III

The clinical course of HMSN III differs from that in HMSN I and II. Onset of type III is earlier in life, sometimes in infancy, and the early course is characterized by remissions and exacerbations (see Section I, Plate 14).

Diagnosis. Nerve conduction velocity and electromyographic studies distinguish predominantly demyelinating diseases (HMSN I and III) from neuronal-axonal abiotrophic disorder, such as HMSN II. In the demyelinating varieties, conduction velocities are generally less than 60% of normal, and may be as low as 15% of normal (Plate 17). Normal motor conduction velocity ranges from 49 to 70 m/sec in the upper limbs, and 43 to 56 m/sec in the lower. In HMSN I and III, values can be as low as 15 to 30 m/sec in the upper extremities and 10 to 20 m/sec in the lower. The changes in velocity are usually quite symmetric. Distal latencies may be significantly prolonged. Motor unit compound action

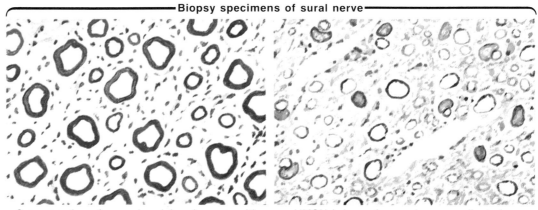

Cross section of normal peripheral nerve, with large and medium–sized myelinated fibers

HMSN I: loss of some large myelinated fibers and ongoing degeneration of myelin

potentials are diminished in amplitude but are not widely dispersed, as in the Guillain-Barré syndrome. Often, it is difficult to demonstrate the presence of a digital sensory evoked potential, despite the relatively minimal findings on clinical examination.

A nerve biopsy specimen demonstrates a decrease in the number of myelinated nerve fibers associated with an increased transfascicular area producing so-called onion bulbs, or circumferentially arranged Schwann cells (see Section I, Plate 14).

Treatment. Since the precise mechanism has not been defined, no specific therapy is available for these diseases. However, an optimistic

approach is warranted because the degree to which patients become handicapped varies considerably. Appropriate career guidance is important early in life. The patient should avoid any occupation that demands physical skills, fine manual dexterity, or long hours of standing or walking.

Care of the feet is important. Shoes should be sturdy but roomy enough, so that pressure sores are not likely to develop. Use of a lightweight plastic foot-drop brace may provide enough support to aid ambulation significantly. Surgery is usually not necessary, but occasionally arthrodesis stabilizes the foot. If this procedure is considered, both the patient and the physician should fully understand its limited objectives. □

Hereditary Sensory Neuropathy

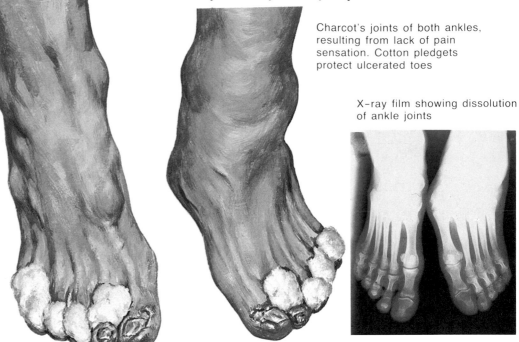

Hereditary Sensory Neuropathy

Charcot's joints of both ankles, resulting from lack of pain sensation. Cotton pledgets protect ulcerated toes

X-ray film showing dissolution of ankle joints

Hereditary sensory neuropathies form a rare but important spectrum of the various inherited disorders of the peripheral nervous system. Inheritance is usually autosomal dominant and onset is in early adulthood, although rarely, a syndrome of an autosomal recessive inheritance with onset in childhood is seen.

Pathology. The underlying pathologic disorder primarily affects the small unmyelinated nociceptive fibers responsible for pain and temperature sensation, and patients predominantly have dissociated sensory loss. Touch, vibration and position sense, subserved by larger myelinated fibers, are relatively well preserved. These findings mimic the dissociated sensory loss seen in syringomyelia. However, in contrast to a syrinx with primary involvement at the level of the central part of the spinal cord, the small neurons at the level of the dorsal root ganglion appear to be involved in hereditary sensory neuropathy.

Clinical Manifestations. Affected persons may notice mild neuropathic difficulties. Many have high arches similar to those seen in patients with hereditary motor-sensory neuropathy type I (HMSN I, Charcot-Marie-Tooth disease), frequent painless injuries, mild dysesthesias of early onset, and prominent calluses and corns of the toes and feet. Unfortunately, all too frequently the degree of discomfort is not significant enough to cause the patient to seek appropriate care at an early stage in the illness.

Because these patients do not perceive painful stimuli, and because appropriate preventive measures are not taken, their feet are subjected to repetitive trauma. With time, painless and seemingly minor ulcers develop over the sole of the foot, particularly at the metatarsal heads. These minor ulcers are often neglected, leading to chronic infection. A vicious cycle sets in as complications develop. The patient paradoxically seems to neglect good foot care because the ulcers fail to cause the discomfort that a person without sensory deprivation would feel. Chronic cellulitis results, and eventually concomitant osteomyelitis develops. If the osteomyelitis is not recognized, bone resorption occurs, joint problems ensue, and Charcot's joints, the deformity so typical of this neuropathy, develop.

Physical Examination. Detailed neurologic examination demonstrates a dissociated sensory loss, with loss of pain and temperature sensation but with minimal to no involvement of touch, vibration and position sense. Motor involvement is minimal, perhaps a very slight impairment of the intrinsic foot muscles. The deep tendon

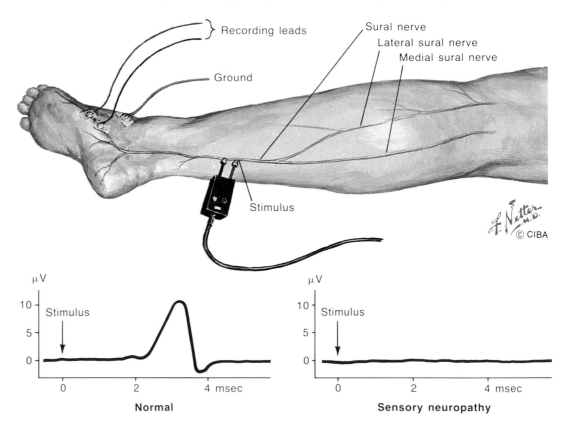

Testing of sensory (sural) nerve conduction (antidromic)

Recording leads — Sural nerve / Lateral sural nerve / Medial sural nerve — Ground — Stimulus

Normal — **Sensory neuropathy**

reflexes are hypoactive. Often, Charcot's joints are present asymmetrically or unilaterally.

Laboratory Studies. Electromyography and nerve conduction velocity studies confirm the loss of distal sensation if they are carried out late in the illness when all the modalities are involved. However, nerve conduction studies basically measure the conduction loss of the large myelinated group IA fibers, which primarily subserve position and vibration sense. Thus, if examined early in the illness, the patient with isolated involvement of unmyelinated pain fibers may have normal distal sensory conduction.

Treatment. Early clinical recognition of this disorder is most important for the prevention of

irremediable damage to the feet. Meticulous prophylactic foot care is essential to avoid development of ulcers. Patients should be made fully aware of the risk of chronic osteomyelitis and a possible need for amputation if they do not adhere to a stringent program of foot care, including meticulous care of toenails and calluses. Persons involved in occupations or athletic endeavors in which the feet may be traumatized should be advised to avoid activities that carry a high risk of injury to the feet.

Development of an ulcer demands careful orthopedic evaluation and cessation of all weight bearing until it resolves. Failure to adhere to these measures may result in loss of the foot. □

Slide 3495

Leprosy (Hansen's Disease)

Despite the availability of effective treatment, leprosy, or Hansen's disease, remains common in the world, although it is one of the least contagious of all contagious diseases. Most persons are immune to the disease, and among the 5% to 10% who can acquire it, the response to the invasion of *Mycobacterium leprae* varies remarkably.

Types of Leprosy. When resistance to invasion by *M leprae* is strong but not sufficient to ward off infection, *tuberculoid* leprosy develops. This form of leprosy is characterized by a single skin lesion or very few lesions that are usually hypopigmented and have an elevated border with insensitivity to pin, temperature and loss of sweating that is coterminous with the skin lesion. Nerve damage develops early in tuberculoid disease, because the nerves are damaged not by proliferation of the bacilli but by the vigorous response of tissue to the presence of a few bacilli. In tuberculoid disease, a biopsy specimen shows an epithelioid cell response with very few bacilli.

Lepromatous leprosy develops in those patients who have virtually no natural resistance to the invasion of *M leprae*. The bacilli in this form of the disease are abundant and widely disseminated by bacteremia, but survive and proliferate only in the cooler tissues of the body. Active proliferation is thus limited to the skin, superficial nerves, anterior third of the eyes, the upper respiratory tract as far down as the vocal cords, and the testes.

The histologic response to invasion of the bacilli is more "passive" in lepromatous leprosy, and packets of *M leprae* are seen in macrophages (Virchow cells). The widespread infiltration of the skin may be manifested by nodules, papules, macules or even bullae. Occasionally, infiltration is so diffuse that there are no obvious skin lesions at all! Since the proliferation of bacilli within the cutaneous nerves is controlled by temperature, the coolest areas of the body lose sensation first, and as the disease progresses, less cool areas become involved.

Superimposed on this pattern of sensory loss due to intracutaneous nerve involvement is the pattern of mixed motor-sensory nerve involvement related to invasion of the named nerves. These nerves are affected where they course closest to the surface of the body. Those commonly involved include the branches of the facial (VII) nerve to the orbicularis oculi, orbicularis oris, and medial parts of the corrugator supercilii muscles; the ulnar nerve over the 10 cm proximal to the ulnar groove to the cubital groove; the median nerve over the 5 or 6 cm proximal to the transverse carpal ligament; the peroneal nerve as it winds around the fibular head; and the posterior tibial nerve near the medial malleolus. Focal involvement of the nerves at these points does not disrupt any of the usually elicited deep tendon reflexes. The retention of deep tendon reflexes in the patient with extensive paralysis, enlarged nerves and sensory loss in lepromatous disease is highly diagnostic.

The wide spectrum of clinical and pathologic forms found between the polar tuberculoid and

Leprosy

World incidence
(rate/1,000)

☐	<0.1
▨	0.1 – 1.9
▨	2.0 – 20.0
■	>20.0

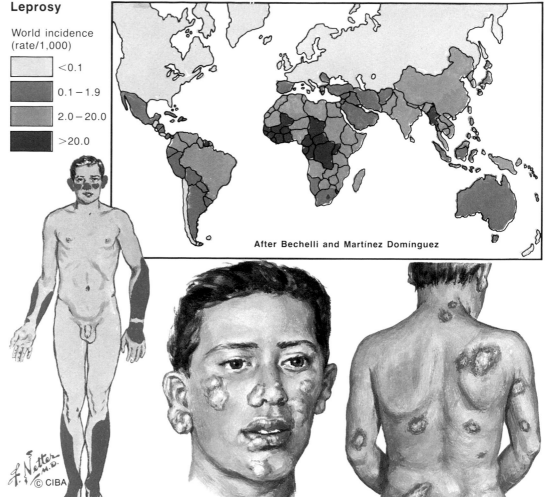

After Bechelli and Martínez Domínguez

Typical early pattern of sensory loss in leprosy (Hansen's disease) tends to affect cooler skin areas, not following either segmental or nerve distribution. Area kept warm by watchband not affected

Moderate lesions of face and ears

Skin lesions. Central healed areas tend to be hypesthetic or anesthetic (dimorphous leprosy)

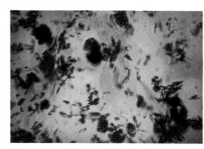

Biopsy specimen of nerve reveals abundant acid-fast lepra bacilli (*M leprae*)

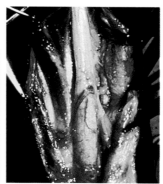

Median nerve appears normal when deep (top), grossly thickened and hyperemic when superficial (bottom)

Late-stage finger contractures with ulcerations due to sensory loss

the lepromatous form of leprosy is known as *dimorphous leprosy.* Some of the most extensive neurologic involvement is seen in the dimorphous disease, in which *M leprae* organisms become widespread but still evoke a vigorous tissue response that is sufficient to cause early and complete nerve dysfunction.

Complications. Leprosy is attended by several major complications. Secondary *amyloidosis* develops in a significant number of patients. Alterations in immune responses, known as *leprosy reactions*, may develop. These inflammatory disorders occur in all tissues invaded by bacilli and thus may add to the nerve damage produced by leprosy per se. The enlarged nerves are also

vulnerable to additional damage from *trauma* and *entrapment.* Some *deformity*, such as collapse of the nose, is caused by invasion by *M leprae*, while more serious deformities are caused by nerve involvement. Loss of pain and temperature sensation in the hands and feet is associated with cycles of painless trauma, skin breakdown and osteomyelitis, which cause extensive loss of the tissues with consequent deformity and disability.

The stigma of the disease can also be an important source of disability. Treatment thus consists not simply of eradicating bacilli but also of managing reactions and preventing and correcting deformity, as well as social and vocational rehabilitation. □

Slide 3496

Myasthenia Gravis

Myasthenia gravis is an acquired autoimmune disease characterized by the presence of binding antibodies to the principal immunologic region of the acetylcholine receptors at the postsynaptic portion of the neuromuscular junction. This antibody binding results in a complement-mediated destruction of junctional folds and an acceleration of the normal degradation of acetylcholine receptors, thus interfering with the transmission of nerve impulses (Plate 21). Myasthenia gravis is frequently associated with other autoimmune diseases such as rheumatoid arthritis, systemic lupus erythematosus and pernicious anemia. Thymic abnormalities occur in 80% of patients—10% having thymomas and 70%, germinal center hyperplasia.

Myasthenia gravis occurs worldwide and in all age groups; however, onset is most often in young adulthood, when the female to male ratio is 3:1, or in late middle or advanced age, when the sexes are equally affected. The incidence of new cases is about 1 in 300,000 persons, and the overall prevalence, about 1 in 50,000.

A variety of classification systems have been used to outline the clinical spectrum of myasthenia gravis. The five categories usually used are ocular, generalized, neonatal, congenital and drug-induced. The *ocular* form often progresses to generalized disease, but may be relatively benign if symptoms are still confined to the extraocular muscles 2 years after onset. The pupils are not involved. The *generalized* form is the most common type and is discussed in detail here. The *neonatal* form, manifested by the "floppy baby" syndrome (see Section I, Plate 11), is seen in 15% to 20% of infants born to affected mothers. The rare *congenital* type is usually present at birth. Although it is not related to the presence of acetylcholine receptor antibodies, it otherwise mimics autoimmune myasthenia gravis. The *drug-induced* form is caused by drugs such as penicillamine, phenytoin and trimethadione.

Generalized Myasthenia Gravis

Generalized myasthenia gravis may be mild, moderate, or acute and fulminating.

Clinical Manifestations. Early symptoms, which are related to a fluctuating bulbar palsy, include intermittent diplopia or ptosis, or both; slurring of speech, with a nasal twang; and difficulty in chewing and nasal regurgitation. The symptoms become more pronounced late in the day and are often temporarily relieved by rest. As the disease progresses, large muscle groups, particularly the muscles of the neck and arms, are affected. The patient may have to support his chin with his hand to keep his head from drooping, and a woman may find it difficult to fix her hair, particularly in the evening. Eventually, all muscle groups (both proximal and distal) may become affected.

The course fluctuates unpredictably. Infectious diseases, thyrotoxicosis, menstruation and

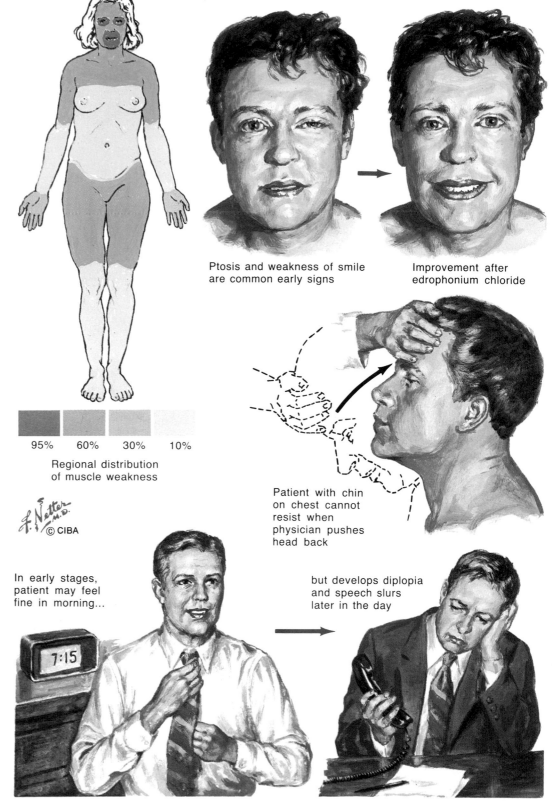

Myasthenia Gravis: Clinical Manifestations

Ptosis and weakness of smile are common early signs

Improvement after edrophonium chloride

95%   60%   30%   10%

Regional distribution of muscle weakness

F. Netter M.D.
© CIBA

Patient with chin on chest cannot resist when physician pushes head back

In early stages, patient may feel fine in morning...

but develops diplopia and speech slurs later in the day

pregnancy exacerbate the symptoms. Latent forms of the disease may be activated by various drugs, including certain neuromuscular blocking agents, central nervous system (CNS) depressants (eg, morphine and barbiturates), cardiac drugs (eg, quinine, quinidine, procaine and propranolol), glycoside forms of antibiotics that impair acetylcholine release, and potassium-depleting diuretics. The course may be relentlessly progressive or marked by intermittent exacerbations.

Physical Examination. Early in the course of generalized disease, abnormalities on physical examination are confined mainly to the cranial nerves, particularly those controlling the extraocular muscles. Asymmetric ptosis and diplopia

from paresis of extraocular muscles are common (Plate 20). Pupillary function remains normal. Fluctuating but progressive breathy dysarthria may become evident during the interview. The smile is almost transverse and snarling. The mouth may hang open as a result of weakening of the jaw muscles. Weakness of the neck flexor muscles is common. Weakness of the extremities may not follow a predictable pattern, although proximal muscles are usually more involved than distal muscles.

Differential Diagnosis. Many other diseases may mimic myasthenia gravis, but few cause such fluctuation of symptoms during the day. Early stages of the brainstem form of *multiple sclerosis*

Myasthenia Gravis
(Continued)

often resemble myasthenia gravis. Diplopia is common, but is usually associated with internuclear ophthalmoplegia, optic pallor and cerebellar changes.

Brainstem tumor, which causes symptoms of multiple tract involvement and, frequently, headache and altered levels of consciousness, should be ruled out. In older patients, abrupt onset and symptoms localized to an intracerebral artery usually indicate a *cerebrovascular accident* in the vertebrobasilar circulation. The Fisher variant of the *Guillain-Barré syndrome*, meningeal infiltration from *carcinomatosis*, and *poliomyelitis* should also be considered in the differential diagnosis, and *amyotrophic lateral sclerosis* should be ruled out in patients who have no signs of ptosis or diplopia.

Electrodiagnostic and antibody studies differentiate *ocular myopathies* and *dystrophies*. In addition, in the *ophthalmoplegia plus syndromes*, the course does not fluctuate and retinal pigmentation is frequently seen. In most myopathies, the extraocular muscles are not involved. Exceptions include thyroid myopathy, ocular myopathy with "ragged" red fibers, centronuclear myopathy in floppy babies, oculopharyngeal muscle dystrophy and, very rarely, polymyositis. *Sarcoidosis* may affect the cranial nerves but does not cause a defect in neuromuscular transmission. *Periodic paralysis* develops even more abruptly than myasthenia gravis but does not usually affect bulbar and respiratory functions.

The *Lambert-Eaton syndrome* (Plate 23) and *botulism* (Plate 34) may occasionally mimic myasthenia gravis. Other toxins that may cause symptoms mimicking myasthenia gravis are *diphtheria*, in which the pupils are affected and the reflexes are diminished, and some *insecticides* (eg, Parathion).

Diagnostic Studies. Although the combination of asymmetric ptosis, bulbar palsies and, perhaps, weakness of the neck flexor and the proximal muscles in myasthenia gravis is almost unique, it is necessary to localize the defect to the neuromuscular junction. Because a combination of chemical and electrical factors mediates transmission across this junction, both pharmacologic and electrodiagnostic studies are indicated.

The *edrophonium chloride (Tensilon) test* is reliable for office use. Edrophonium, an anticholinesterase, produces a rapid reaction of short duration. The test is most useful in patients in whom the disease is severe enough that the drug causes a quantifiable change in ptosis, diplopia or dysarthria. Weakness in the muscles of the extremities may be difficult to quantify, because muscle strength varies and is affected by the degree of individual effort.

A test dose of 2 mg edrophonium is given first, since 0.5% of patients may be hypersensitive to the drug. This is followed by a dose of 2 to 10 mg (0.2 to 1.0 ml) given intravenously. False-positive results have been reported in patients with brainstem glioma, parasellar meningioma or even an aneurysm. Instructions before the test must be

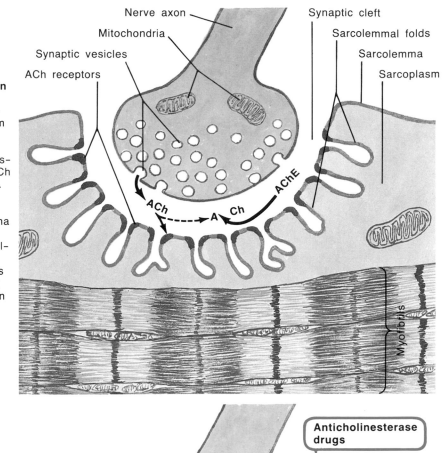

Normal neuro-muscular junction Synaptic vesicles containing acetylcholine (ACh) form in nerve terminal. In response to nerve impulse, vesicles discharge ACh into synaptic cleft. ACh binds to receptor sites on muscle sarcolemma to initiate muscle contraction. Acetylcholinesterase (AChE) hydrolyzes ACh, thus limiting effect and duration of its action

Myasthenia gravis Marked reduction in number and length of subneural sarcolemmal folds indicates that underlying defect lies in neuromuscular junction. Anticholinesterase drugs increase effectiveness and duration of ACh action by slowing its destruction by AChE

given carefully to avoid a false-positive response in a suggestible or hysterical patient.

Electromyographic studies localize the abnormality to the neuromuscular junction and differentiate a presynaptic defect and a postsynaptic defect (Plate 22). Normally, because of the functional reserve at the neuromuscular junction, successive skeletal muscle compound action potentials maintain a consistent amplitude with repetitive stimulation of a nerve (usually the ulnar, at 2 to 3 Hz). In contrast, in myasthenia gravis or other neuromuscular transmission defects, a voltage decrement similar to that caused by clinical fatigue is generally evident, reaching a maximum degree at the third to fifth stimulus (Plate 22).

A decrement of at least 8% to 10% between the initial and the fifth response is considered an abnormal response. In patients with primarily ocular disease, or even very mild bulbar lesions, results of repetitive stimulation studies may be normal.

Tests for serum antibodies to acetylcholine receptors and skeletal muscle are important. In about 70% to 90% of patients with generalized myasthenia gravis, the titer of acetylcholine receptor antibody is increased.

Radiography of the chest, including mediastinal tomography and computed tomography (CT), is required to exclude a thymoma. A benign lipoma and other anterior mediastinal masses may

Myasthenia Gravis
(Continued)

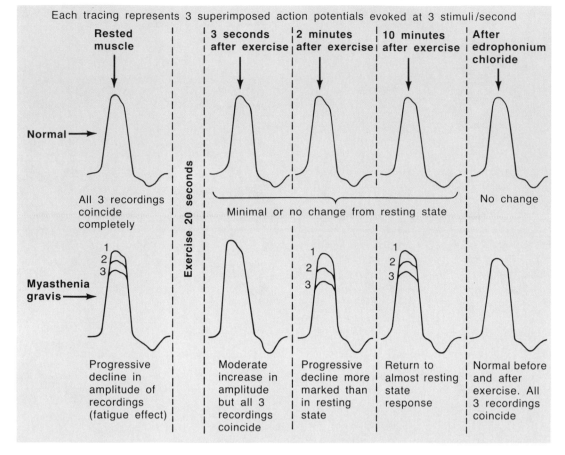

Each tracing represents 3 superimposed action potentials evoked at 3 stimuli/second

| | Rested muscle | 3 seconds after exercise | 2 minutes after exercise | 10 minutes after exercise | After edrophonium chloride |

cause a false-positive result on a CT scan. Calcium in the mediastinum is strong evidence of a tumor. Because 90% of patients with myasthenia gravis and thymoma have a positive skeletal muscle antibody titer, the absence of such a finding is good evidence that any questionable mass in the mediastinum is not a thymoma.

Treatment. The guiding principle in the multifaceted approach to treatment of myasthenia gravis is caution. The best approach cannot be dogmatically advocated, because controlled studies comparing the current therapeutic protocols have not been done.

Historically, anticholinesterases have been the mainstay of symptomatic therapy. In the United States, *pyridostigmine bromide* is administered initially. It is available in 60-mg tablets, in 180-mg slow-release tablets, and in syrup for patients who have difficulty in swallowing. Dosage must be titrated carefully to prevent cholinergic side effects. Nicotinic or muscarinic symptoms signal a cholinergic crisis. Cramping and fasciculations are characteristic nicotinic effects. Muscarinic symptoms include signs of gastrointestinal irritability (cramping and diarrhea), cardiovascular changes (palpitations and bradycardia), and neuroautonomic dysfunction (tearing and increased salivation, and bronchial secretions). When these symptoms develop, pyridostigmine bromide must be discontinued and the patient observed carefully.

Today, *steroids*, primarily *prednisone*, are the drugs of choice for symptomatic myasthenia gravis if no adequate response to pyridostigmine bromide occurs within 1 month. These medications are started in small dosages, usually in the hospital, and gradually increased to 60 to 120 mg/day until symptomatic control occurs. This may take place gradually. Eventually, the alternate-day doses are decreased over the next few months. As the steroid regimen is implemented, anticholinesterase medications should be gradually decreased. The remission rate in patients with moderate to severe disease is 60% to 90%. When maximal benefit has been achieved, further reduction of dosage is attempted. However, sudden exacerbations may require an upward adjustment of medication.

The immunosuppressive drug *azathioprine* inhibits the development of experimental allergic myasthenia gravis, tends to change the antibody binding to the acetylcholine receptor, and may be useful when pyridostigmine bromide and prednisone are ineffective.

Plasmapheresis provides short-term relief in patients with severe exacerbations, in whom the response to conventional therapy is delayed. This procedure is indicated in patients in myasthenic crisis or in those with progressively increasing weakness, particularly those with bulbar-related respiratory problems.

Thymectomy is valuable in autoimmune myasthenia gravis, except perhaps in the primary ocular form. Evidence indicates that better results are

Thymus gland abnormality in myasthenia gravis

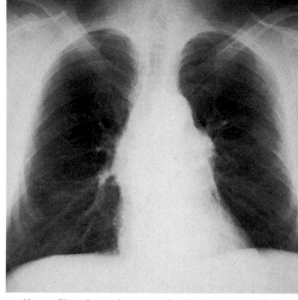

X-ray film shows large mediastinal tumor, which localized to anterior compartment (view not shown)

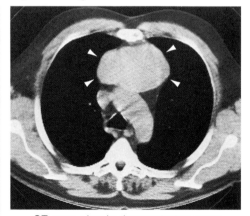

CT scan clearly demonstrates same large tumor anterior to aortic arch (arrowheads)

obtained when thymectomy is performed early in the course of the disease. When the condition has been stabilized and maximum benefit from medical therapy appears to have been achieved, thymectomy should be considered.

Comparison studies suggest that in patients who have had a thymectomy, remission is more likely, exacerbations are fewer, and the need for medications is decreased. The patient with the generalized form of myasthenia gravis may notice an improvement within a few years. Thymectomy is also indicated in any patient with suspected thymoma, but improvement is not as dramatic in those with thymoma as in those who do not have a malignant tumor.

Myasthenic Crisis. Although myasthenic crises were more common when patients were treated only with anticholinesterases, these sudden, severe exacerbations may still occur. Since they are more likely to occur during the summer months, patients should try to stay in an air-conditioned environment. Other contributing factors include administration of the drugs previously listed, alcohol ingestion, pregnancy and emotional stress. Severe exacerbation requires respiratory support, with endotracheal intubation and assisted ventilation. All medications should be discontinued. When the crisis has been controlled, steroids or plasmapheresis, or both, may be indicated. □

Lambert-Eaton Syndrome

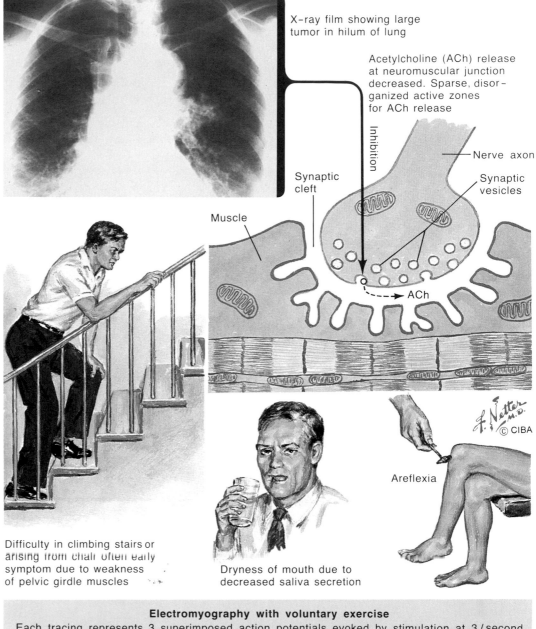

X-ray film showing large tumor in hilum of lung

Acetylcholine (ACh) release at neuromuscular junction decreased. Sparse, disorganized active zones for ACh release

Inhibition

Nerve axon

Synaptic vesicles

Synaptic cleft

Muscle

ACh

Difficulty in climbing stairs or arising from chair often early symptom due to weakness of pelvic girdle muscles

Dryness of mouth due to decreased saliva secretion

Areflexia

An underlying carcinoma is occasionally the inciting mechanism in various neurologic disorders, even though structurally apparent metastases that would account for the syndromes cannot be identified. Well-defined abnormalities of the motor-sensory unit that occur with greater frequency in patients with cancer include a pure sensory neuropathy, the Lambert-Eaton (myasthenic) syndrome and dermatomyositis. Among these disorders, the incidence of underlying cancer is highest in the Lambert-Eaton syndrome. A malignancy, most commonly oat-cell carcinoma of the lung, is present or eventually develops in 70% of patients with this syndrome. Occasionally, ovarian or gastrointestinal malignancies have been implicated.

Clinical Manifestations. Typically, a patient with the Lambert-Eaton syndrome complains of fatigue or weakness, or both. Although the weakness may be initially apparent to the examiner, on repetitive testing, muscle strength may be confusingly normal. The proximal musculature is generally affected, but occasionally the bulbar musculature is involved, as in myasthenia gravis. Additional diagnostic clues include vague paresthesias in the legs, dryness of the mouth, sexual impotence in the male, and the presence of generalized areflexia with complete absence of the deep tendon reflexes.

Diagnostic Studies. Results of basic laboratory studies, including those of muscle enzymes, are normal. Chest x-ray films should be carefully examined for a possible perihilar mass. No specific serum markers have been identified.

Electromyographic and nerve conduction studies are necessary for diagnosis. Muscle action potential induced by motor nerve stimulation is of abnormally low amplitude. Repetitive stimulation of the nerve at the rate of 2 to 3 Hz reveals evidence of a defect in neuromuscular transmission, which is characterized by a progressive decrease in the amplitude of each of the first three to four successive responses. However, this type of response is also seen in other diseases affecting neuromuscular transmission, such as myasthenia gravis, and occasionally in primary motor neuron disease. With maximal stimulation of the muscles by voluntary contraction for about 10 seconds, or an increase in the frequency of electrical stimulation to 50 Hz, an immediate facilitation of 200% or more can be demonstrated in patients with the Lambert-Eaton syndrome. This is a short-lived phenomenon and appears to explain the corresponding clinical observation that muscle strength returns to prestimulation level after

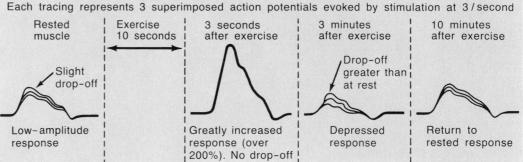

Electromyography with voluntary exercise

Each tracing represents 3 superimposed action potentials evoked by stimulation at 3/second

Rested muscle	Exercise 10 seconds	3 seconds after exercise	3 minutes after exercise	10 minutes after exercise
Slight drop-off			Drop-off greater than at rest	
Low-amplitude response		Greatly increased response (over 200%). No drop-off	Depressed response	Return to rested response

initial tests have indicated weakness, particularly in the proximal musculature. In contrast to myasthenia gravis or motor neuron disease, no significant improvement is noted with infusion of edrophonium chloride (Tensilon).

Pathophysiology. The type of defect seen in the Lambert-Eaton syndrome occurs at the presynaptic stage of neuromuscular transmission. The active zones for acetylcholine release at the nerve terminal are sparse and disorganized, resulting in a decreased uptake of calcium ions, which prevents release of acetylcholine quanta. It has been suggested that an autoimmune mechanism underlying this defect in presynaptic transmission may, in effect, be the mirror image of the mech-

anism that causes a defect in postsynaptic transmission, which results in myasthenia gravis.

Treatment. Corticosteroids may be the treatment of choice. Guanidine was used in the past because it potentiates presynaptic acetylcholine release, but it is used no longer because it proved to be toxic to the kidneys. Chemotherapy for oat-cell carcinoma may be the only treatment required, at least according to one report that documents clinical neurophysiologic recovery with chemotherapy alone. However, in patients in whom no tumor can be found, use of steroids would seem indicated to obtain symptomatic improvement. Careful follow-up in search of an occult malignancy is also warranted. ☐

Duchenne's Muscular Dystrophy

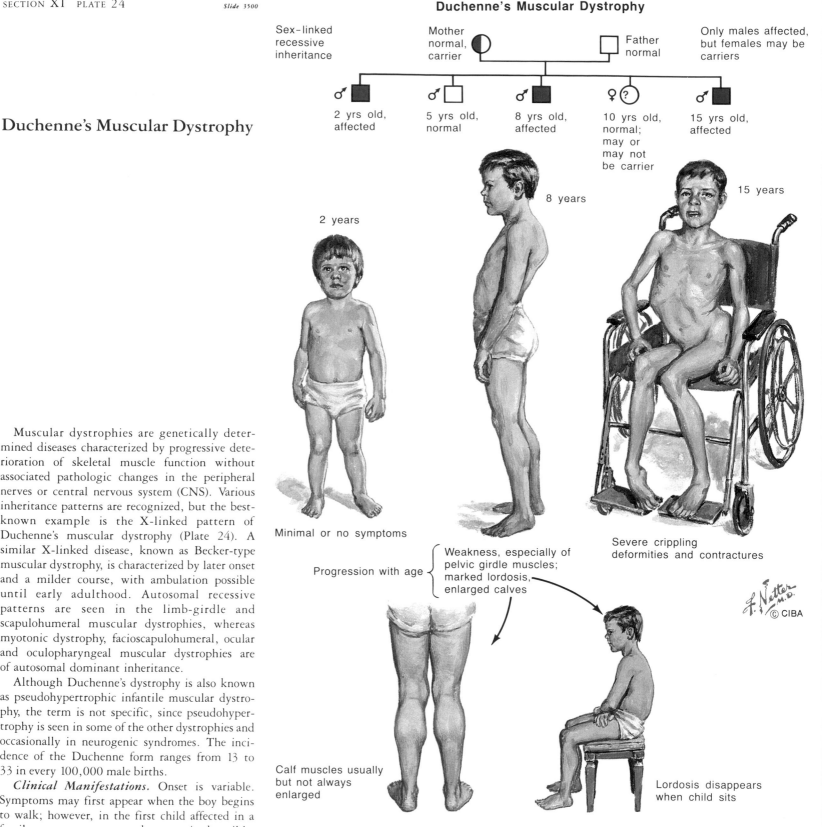

Sex-linked recessive inheritance

Mother normal, carrier

Father normal

Only males affected, but females may be carriers

♂ 2 yrs old, affected

♂ 5 yrs old, normal

♂ 8 yrs old, affected

♀ (?) 10 yrs old, normal; may or may not be carrier

♂ 15 yrs old, affected

2 years

8 years

15 years

Minimal or no symptoms

Severe crippling deformities and contractures

Progression with age { Weakness, especially of pelvic girdle muscles; marked lordosis, enlarged calves

Calf muscles usually but not always enlarged

Lordosis disappears when child sits

Duchenne's Muscular Dystrophy

Muscular dystrophies are genetically determined diseases characterized by progressive deterioration of skeletal muscle function without associated pathologic changes in the peripheral nerves or central nervous system (CNS). Various inheritance patterns are recognized, but the best-known example is the X-linked pattern of Duchenne's muscular dystrophy (Plate 24). A similar X-linked disease, known as Becker-type muscular dystrophy, is characterized by later onset and a milder course, with ambulation possible until early adulthood. Autosomal recessive patterns are seen in the limb-girdle and scapulohumeral muscular dystrophies, whereas myotonic dystrophy, facioscapulohumeral, ocular and oculopharyngeal muscular dystrophies are of autosomal dominant inheritance.

Although Duchenne's dystrophy is also known as pseudohypertrophic infantile muscular dystrophy, the term is not specific, since pseudohypertrophy is seen in some of the other dystrophies and occasionally in neurogenic syndromes. The incidence of the Duchenne form ranges from 13 to 33 in every 100,000 male births.

Clinical Manifestations. Onset is variable. Symptoms may first appear when the boy begins to walk; however, in the first child affected in a family, symptoms may not be recognized until he begins school. In retrospect, the child's parents may recall that his motor development was delayed. The course is similar in younger male siblings, but parents will have become aware of subtle abnormalities seen in the child just past the toddling stage. Most commonly, the child has a waddling or lurching gait, with a tendency to toe in. Occasionally, some children complain of pain in the calves, especially with exercise. Intellectual changes have also been documented in this illness. The mean IQ in children with Duchenne's muscular dystrophy is 85; however, 30% of these children have an IQ of less than 75.

Physical Examination. Many signs of weakness of the proximal musculature are evident

on examination. One of the best methods of demonstrating muscle weakness is to have the patient lie prone on the floor and perform the Gowers maneuver (Plate 25). Early in the illness, the boy may push up with his hands or with one hand placed on the thigh. As the illness progresses, he gradually pushes off with both hands and uses his hands successively from the floor to his knees to his thighs because of the involvement of the gluteal and spinal muscles. When finally erect, he stands in a lordotic posture, which often disappears when he is seated.

Facial and extraocular muscles are not affected. Although weakness in the arms is usually subclinical early in the illness, careful clinical examina-

tion generally demonstrates some degree of weakness in the deltoid muscles by age 6.

As the illness progresses, skeletal deformities become more apparent. Contractures of the gastrocnemii muscles may appear relatively early, with resultant tight heel cords causing the child to walk on his toes. The hip flexors also become contracted, and scoliosis eventually develops from weakness of the paraspinal musculature.

As atrophy commences, the calf muscles appear to retain their normal contour, producing so-called pseudohypertrophy. Most of these patients never learn to walk or run properly, which becomes obvious when they are asked to walk or run during physical examination.

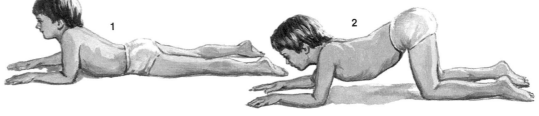

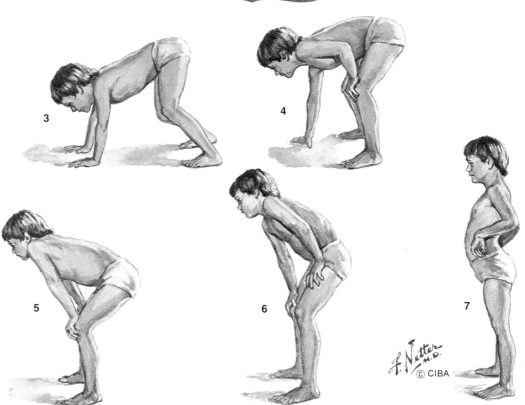

Characteristically, child arises from prone position by pushing himself up with hands successively on floor, knees and thighs, because of weakness in gluteal and spinal muscles. He stands in lordotic posture

Duchenne's Muscular Dystrophy
(Continued)

Diagnostic Studies. Early in this illness, the serum creatine kinase level is strikingly elevated, and may approach 50 to 100 times normal. These values gradually decrease with age. Levels less than 10 times normal suggest a more benign muscular dystrophy, a congenital myopathy or a chronic motor neuron disease.

Electromyography demonstrates classic myopathic features, including low-amplitude, short-duration polyphasic motor units recruited in increasing numbers, with minimal effort by the patient. Although these findings do not confirm a diagnosis of Duchenne's muscular dystrophy, they are helpful in differentiating a possible myopathic process from occult motor neuron disease.

Electrocardiographic abnormalities are noted despite the lack of symptoms. Increased R waves over the right ventricle suggest right ventricular strain, and Q waves are sometimes noted over the left ventricular leads. T waves may be inverted in the right precordial regions.

Muscle biopsy is the definitive diagnostic test. As with the enzyme changes, the findings in biopsy specimens depend on the clinical stage of the illness. Early in the course of the disease, variations in the size of muscle fibers reflect the various degrees of fiber degeneration and regeneration. Later, much of the normal muscle tissue is replaced by fat and fibrotic tissue.

Clinical Course. The illness progresses relentlessly, with increased muscle wasting and concomitant muscle contractures and skeletal deformities. By their teenage years, most patients are confined to a wheelchair. The majority of patients die during the late second or early third decade. Death may result from respiratory infections, in which even mild illnesses may be fatal due to pulmonary insufficiency caused by severely weakened chest muscles.

Treatment. Because no specific etiologic mechanism has been found to date, treatment is multidisciplinary and is directed toward slowing the progress of the disease and controlling the various complications. The child should be encouraged to lead as normal and active a life as possible. Unnecessary immobilization for a mild injury or illness may accelerate the rate of deterioration. Passive exercise decreases the degree of contractures, particularly in the gastrocnemii and hip flexor muscles. Ankle splints may be helpful at night. Caliper braces allow the child to stand alone, delaying his dependence on a wheelchair. Once he becomes wheelchair-dependent, he should be urged to keep his back in a vertical position to retard progressive scoliosis, which can lead to potentially fatal respiratory infections.

Carrier Detection. When Duchenne's muscular dystrophy is diagnosed in one member of a family, the physician is often questioned about

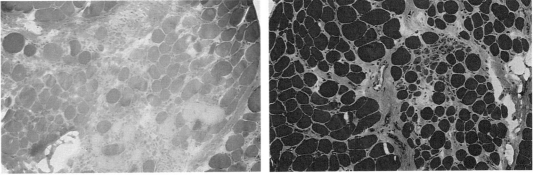

Muscle biopsy specimens showing necrotic muscle fibers being removed by groups of small, round phagocytic cells (left, trichrome stain) and replaced by fibrous and fatty tissue (right, H and E stain)

detection of possible carriers of the disease. Identification of carriers is difficult, because a totally reliable test is not yet available. Although the serum creatine kinase level is elevated in approximately 60% to 70% of carriers, the elevation may be minimal. In addition, exercise in the weeks before testing can cause postexertion elevation and a false-positive result.

Sometimes, electromyography may prove of value in detecting minimal changes in the duration of motor unit action potentials, which suggest a slight but definite myopathic process. Finally, because changes in the duration of action potential in a carrier may be too mild to be diagnostic, muscle biopsy specimens may be attempted;

however, these findings may also be difficult to interpret.

The mother of an affected child can be considered a definite carrier if a brother or maternal uncle had the disease. A mother who has had two or more affected sons but no other male relatives with the illness is a probable carrier. Possible carriers include a mother who has had one affected son but whose other sons are normal, a woman who has not yet had children but whose brother or maternal uncle has the disease, and the daughter of a proved carrier. In families in which one son has Duchenne's muscular dystrophy, there is a 50% chance that another son will have the disease and that a daughter will be a carrier. □

Other Types of Muscular Dystrophy

In addition to myotonic dystrophy and Duchenne's muscular dystrophy, there is a group of more benign muscular syndromes of undetermined cause that have a hereditary degenerative pattern in which no apparent abnormality of the anterior horn cell or its motor neuron has been defined. Results of nerve conduction velocity studies are normal, and needle electromyography demonstrates an abundant recruitment pattern of low-amplitude, short-duration action potentials most suggestive of a myopathic disorder. Muscle biopsy specimens have a nonspecific dystrophic appearance. Pseudohypertrophy does not occur in these disorders. Classification of these dystrophies is based on the clinical pattern of involvement and the associated genetic inheritance pattern.

Facioscapulohumeral Dystrophy. One of the more common muscular dystrophies, this type is second in incidence only to Duchenne's muscular dystrophy, and has an autosomal dominant inheritance pattern. Onset is usually in adolescence. Symptoms are loss of hearing, retinal telangiectasia and mental retardation (Coat's disease). Frequently, a family member is the first to note the insidious change in the patient's body habitus, particularly the "winging" of the scapulae.

At onset, facioscapulohumeral dystrophy may have a moderately asymmetric distribution. In some patients, the brachioradialis or the pectoralis major muscle may be congenitally absent.

Involvement of shoulder-girdle muscles is apparent on physical examination. The winged scapulae and the difficulty in raising the arms above the shoulders, which produce a characteristic picture of high-riding scapulae and prominent clavicles, are common. These findings are secondary to a disproportionate involvement of the lower portions of the trapezius muscle, as well as an involvement of the serratus anterior muscle, which normally connects the shoulder to the back.

Careful facial examination also reveals the patient's inability to sustain wrinkling the forehead, tightly closing the eyelids, and pursing the perioral muscles for whistling. Later in the course of the illness, some patients may also have more widespread muscle weakness, particularly of the pelvic-girdle or anterior tibial muscles, or both. Mild weakness of the erector spinae muscle may be manifested by a slightly increased lordosis.

The prognosis is relatively benign. At times, the clinical course seems stabilized. Most important, patients with this diagnosis should be assured that, in contrast to Duchenne's dystrophy, this disease will not prevent them from having a relatively normal life span.

Limb-Girdle Muscular Dystrophy. The lack of facial involvement differentiates primary limb-girdle dystrophy from facioscapulohumeral dystrophy. Pseudohypertrophy of various muscle groups may be noted. About one half of cases have an autosomal recessive inheritance affecting either sex, while the remainder are sporadic. Onset occurs in the second or third decade, with a significant variability of progression. In the worst eventuality, the patient may be confined to a wheelchair by the third or fourth decade.

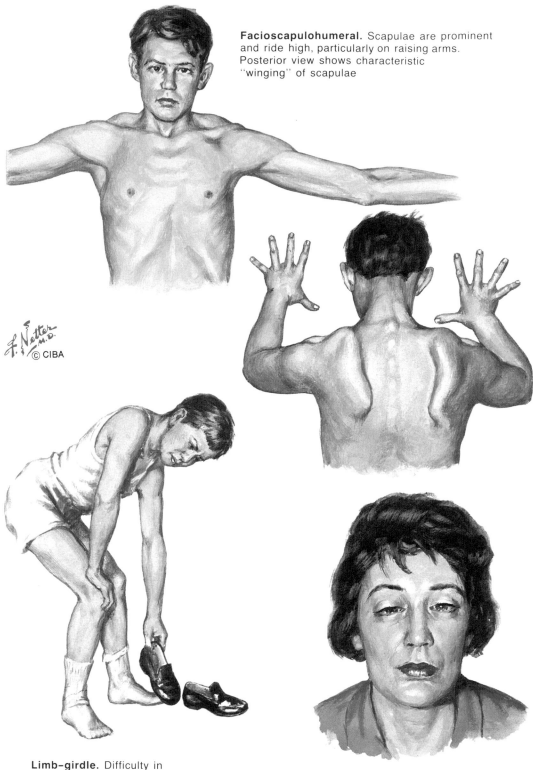

Facioscapulohumeral. Scapulae are prominent and ride high, particularly on raising arms. Posterior view shows characteristic "winging" of scapulae

Limb-girdle. Difficulty in arising from stooped position, lordosis, wide gait

Oculofacial. Ptosis, ophthalmoplegia, facial weakness

Oculofacial Muscular Dystrophy. This clinical spectrum, usually of autosomal dominant inheritance, probably represents a heterogeneous group of pathophysiologic mechanisms located variously between the brainstem nuclei and the specific extraocular muscles.

In patients with primary involvement in the extraocular muscles and eyelids, onset is usually in adolescence but may be delayed until middle age. These patients usually note a mild progressive ptosis secondary to involvement of the muscles used in elevating the eyelids. Early in the course, the affected patient may also start tilting the head back in order to overcome the effect of ptosis. A concomitant symmetric involvement of

the extraocular muscles eventually leads to total ophthalmoparesis, with the eyes assuming a neutral central position. The patient compensates by moving the head. Except for the disadvantages of a fixed-eye posture, the syndrome is relatively benign.

Oculopharyngeal Muscular Dystrophy. An onset later in life in some patients, particularly of French Canadian ancestry, may affect other bulbar muscles, particularly those used in swallowing. Dysphagia may be the first symptom. Ptosis may be prominent, but without associated paresis of the extraocular muscles. Mild facial, neck and proximal limb weakness may be noted in either oculofacial or oculopharyngeal dystrophy. □

Myotonic Dystrophy

Myotonic disorders are characterized by abnormalities of muscle relaxation, with _myotonic dystrophy (Steinert's disease)_ the most common example of these disorders. It has an autosomal dominant inheritance.

Clinical Manifestations. Myotonia, the hallmark of this illness, is the inability to immediately relax muscles after voluntary contraction. This defect is particularly apparent in the hands. Patients with a myotonic disorder frequently accept their deficit as normal and do not seek medical attention until other complications occur.

Occasionally, systemic complications may be the first manifestation of the illness. Early-onset cataracts are particularly prominent. Rarely, early involvement of smooth muscles produces dysphagia or constipation, or both.

Myotonic dystrophy most commonly occurs in early adulthood, although age at onset varies; rarely, it may manifest as a newborn floppy baby. Exposure to cold often exacerbates the myotonic phenomena, and patients working outdoors or in situations requiring manual skills may experience symptoms earlier in life.

The classic form of this illness is easily recognized. Occasionally, the diagnosis is apparent when the physician first shakes hands with the patient and notes the slow relaxation of grip. Percussion of the thenar eminence elicits the classic myotonic reaction. Normally, the thumb minimally contracts in opposition with prompt relaxation, or remains immobile, but in the patient with myotonic dystrophy, the thumb promptly opposes and only gradually returns to the neutral position. Release of the eyelids after they have been tightly closed may also be pathologically slow.

Evidence of weakness of the distal musculature is common. Weakness of the bulbar musculature, which includes ptosis, a droopy mouth, and wasting of the temporalis muscle, is also often seen. Other common findings include prominent frontal balding and signs of cataracts or a previous iridectomy. The associated atrophy in the temporalis and sternocleidomastoid muscles may produce a sharply angulated, hatchetlike facies. In males, testicular atrophy is often evident. Many patients have an asthenic habitus.

Differential Diagnosis. Although myotonic dystrophy is the most common cause of myotonia per se, classic myotonia is also seen in a few other clinical syndromes. _Myotonia congenita (Thomsen's disease)_, a more benign illness with none of the systemic manifestations of myotonic dystrophy, is a disease of either autosomal dominant or autosomal recessive inheritance. These patients often complain of stiffness and have trouble initiating movement, particularly after prolonged rest. They may fall on first attempting to walk after arising from a chair, or when they start to run. Gross muscle hypertrophy is often evident, producing an almost Herculean habitus.

Cold-precipitated myotonia may occur in _hyperkalemic periodic paralysis_. In the _Schwartz-Jampel syndrome_ (osteochondromuscular dystrophy),

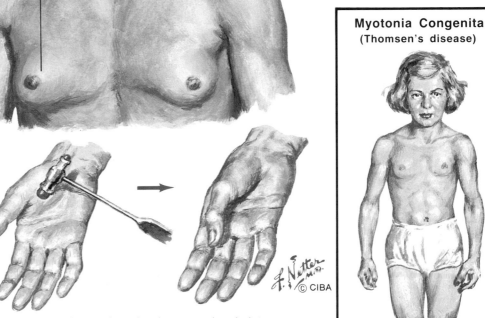

Myotonic Dystrophy

- Frontal balding
- "Hatchet" facies due to atrophy of temporalis muscle
- Ptosis and drooping mouth due to weakness of facial muscles
- Wasting of sternocleidomastoid muscle
- Cataracts
- Gynecomastia

Difficulty in releasing grasp

Percussion myotonic reaction: thumb moves sharply into opposition and adduction on percussion of thenar muscles and returns to initial position slowly

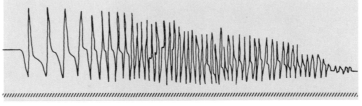

Electromyogram showing spontaneous myotonic discharge evoked by needle insertion

Myotonia Congenita
(Thomsen's disease)

Myotonia and muscular overdevelopment. Disease affects both males and females

myotonia is associated with dwarfism, bone disease and variable ocular and facial abnormalities.

Diagnostic Studies. Needle electromyography clearly demonstrates prolonged muscle contraction, which is characterized by the classic divebomber sound produced on audio amplification. Even minimal irritation on needle insertion may produce this muscle fiber discharge.

Careful investigation of the patient's family for similar disorders may be particularly enlightening when evaluating the patient with "no known family history."

There are no specific blood or urine abnormalities. As in any primary muscle disorders, serum creatine kinase levels may be mildly to moderately

elevated, usually 2 to 4 times the normal value. Findings in muscle biopsy specimens are not diagnostic.

Treatment. No medication reverses this illness. If myotonic symptoms are prominent, phenytoin may be useful, particularly in myotonia congenita. Death may result from cardiac or pulmonary insufficiency. Some patients appear to have increased cardiac sensitivity to anesthetics, particularly thiopental sodium. Malignant hyperthermia may be a common finding (Plate 33).

The most severely affected patients may become disabled and unemployable by midlife. Genetic counseling to prevent additional cases of myotonic dystrophy is essential. □

Polymyositis/Dermatomyositis

One of the most common of the diseases manifested by weakness of the proximal musculature is polymyositis. This disease is usually seen in middle-aged persons but occasionally develops in young children. It is thought to be an autoimmune disorder because it is sometimes associated with other connective-tissue diseases such as systemic lupus erythematosus, rheumatoid arthritis and systemic vasculitis. Rarely, polymyositis is associated with an underlying malignancy, particularly of the lung or breast. However, despite early reports to the contrary, the search for an occult neoplasm is usually fruitless in the patient with polymyositis.

Clinical Manifestations. Onset of polymyositis is usually insidious, although occasionally it may be almost precipitous. Symptoms are often nonspecific, such as malaise, fatigue or even a fever of unknown origin. The physician may have to ask specific questions to elicit a history of proximal muscle weakness. At times, family members may have noted that the patient has difficulty arising from a deep chair, often having to push up with the arms to overcome weakness in the proximal leg musculature, or that he may suddenly have found it difficult to climb stairs or high steps, as on a bus (Plate 28). Questions about bathroom activities may reveal that the patient has difficulty in getting out of the tub or arising from the toilet seat.

Although weakness of the shoulder girdle musculature does not usually predominate as an initial symptom, many patients have experienced difficulties in reaching up to a high shelf, combing their hair, or attempting to lift objects over their head. Rarely, the first sign may be inability to hold up the head, especially in elderly patients. Dysphagia may be present but usually is not an initial complaint. All symptoms commonly represent a symmetric loss of function. However, polymyositis rarely may have an asymmetric or even isolated focal muscular onset, affecting a few muscles in one extremity.

A significant percentage of patients have an accompanying rash; the combination of symptoms is known as *dermatomyositis*. The rash may be relatively subtle, and sometimes is unnoticed by both patient and physician until the patient is carefully examined. Occasionally, the rash may be the initial complaint, and an alert dermatologist may be the first to note minor signs of muscle weakness. Pain is quite uncommon. Other symptoms associated with inflammatory myopathy include dark urine due to myoglobinuria and the presence of Raynaud's phenomenon.

Differential Diagnosis. Diseases that should be considered in differential diagnosis include *polymyalgia rheumatica*, which produces muscular aching and stiffness without true muscle weakness. The erythrocyte sedimentation rate is characteristically quite high in this disease but only inconsistently elevated in polymyositis. However, the serum creatine kinase level and

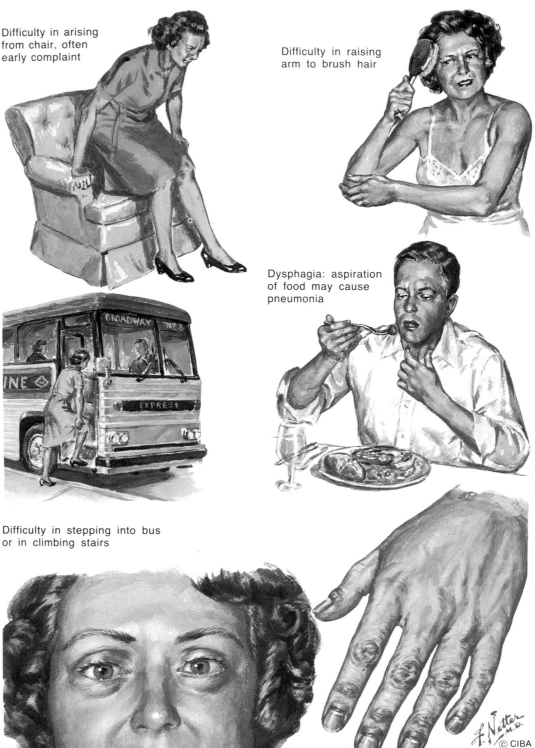

Difficulty in arising from chair, often early complaint

Difficulty in raising arm to brush hair

Dysphagia: aspiration of food may cause pneumonia

Difficulty in stepping into bus or in climbing stairs

Edema and heliotrope discoloration around eyes a classic sign. More widespread erythematous rash may also be present

Erythema and/or scaly, papular eruption around fingernails and on dorsum of interphalangeal joints

results of electromyography are normal in polymyalgia rheumatica, in contrast to the findings in polymyositis.

Chronic and acute *alcohol abuse* and, rarely, certain *drugs*, such as clofibrate, chloroquine, cimetidine, emetine, ϵ-aminocaproic acid, heroin, rifampin and steroids can also cause myopathy and should be considered.

Two storage diseases, *acid maltase deficiency*, a type II glycogenosis, and muscle *carnitine deficiency*, a lipid storage disease, may mimic all of the clinical and laboratory findings of polymyositis. Only studies of muscle biopsy specimens distinguish polymyositis from these disorders. Other diagnostic considerations include myopathies

induced by *endocrine dysfunction, potassium-related disorders* and the *Lambert-Eaton syndrome*.

A viral origin has been suspected but not proved in polymyositis. The only well-defined infectious diseases that may mimic classic polymyositis are *trichinosis* and *toxoplasmosis*.

Physical Examination. The first confirmation of a history suggestive of proximal muscle weakness may come when the patient pushes up with his arms in arising from the chair after physical examination. The patient should not be allowed any significant mechanical assistance, or subtle muscle weakness may not be noted. Shoulder abduction may not be possible. Weakness of the lower extremities is often most prominent in the

Slide 3505

Polymyositis/Dermatomyositis
(Continued)

hip flexors. Frequently, the patient is unable to maintain elevation of the flexed leg at the hip against resistance. Because the quadriceps femoris muscle is so powerful, early weakness is best elicited by having the patient attempt to squat and arise.

The physician should look for dermatologic changes, including a patchy, sometimes scaly, rash over the knuckles, elbows, knees or ankles, with hyperemia at the base of the nails or at the fingertips. A less common diagnostic dermatologic finding is the so-called heliotrope facial rash, a violaceous, lilac or purplish rash, which is usually seen over the upper eyelid and sometimes blends with a more erythematous rash that covers the face in a butterfly distribution. When severe, the rash encompasses the neck and anterior chest. Rarely, particularly in children, calcinosis is noted; this may be associated with ulcerations on prominent bony areas. At times, these lesions actually extrude calcium.

Diagnostic Studies. Diagnosis of an inflammatory myopathy is strongly supported by four major criteria: (1) recent onset of symmetric proximal muscle weakness, with or without the typical rash; (2) elevated serum levels of muscle enzymes, particularly creatine kinase; (3) consistent electromyographic changes; and (4) positive results of muscle biopsy. A *probable* diagnosis may be considered if three criteria are present, and a *possible* diagnosis if two criteria are present.

A hallmark of this illness is an elevated serum creatine kinase level. However, the degree of elevation varies, with the serum level often at 5 to 50 times normal. The diagnosis should not be excluded if the value is near or even within normal limits, particularly if the other three major criteria are present. In addition, a number of other possible causes for elevated serum creatine kinase should be considered (Plate 2).

Electromyography is particularly helpful in diagnosis. The percentage of active muscle fibers responding to a specific motor neuron is reduced, producing motor unit action potentials of short duration and low amplitude (Plate 29). To compensate, an increased number of normal motor neurons fires, with resultant rapid recruitment of a full interference pattern that may reach maximum with relatively minimal effort by the patient. The resting muscle commonly shows abnormalities on needle insertion, including fibrillation potentials, positive waves and complex repetitive discharges, changes that are most common in neurogenic processes. However, when seen in combination with low-amplitude, short-duration motor unit responses, these changes are highly suggestive of an inflammatory or, rarely, a metabolic myopathy such as acid maltase or carnitine deficiency.

Muscle biopsy is important (Plates 3–4). The most suitable biopsy site is indicated by electromyographic findings, with selection of the muscle that demonstrates the most active EMG changes. At times, the best sites may be the paraspinal muscles. Because needle insertion during electromyography can cause pseudomyopathic

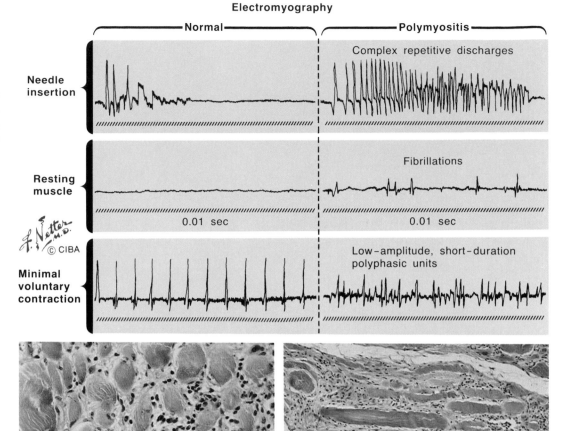

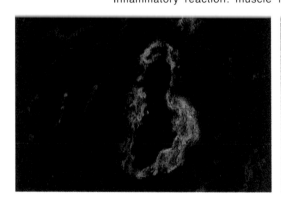
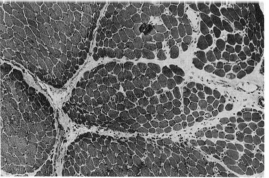

Transverse section ◄━━ **Muscle biopsy specimens** ━━► Longitudinal section
Inflammatory reaction: muscle fiber necrosis and regeneration

Anti–IgG immunofluorescence of frozen muscle section with positive–staining within blood vessel wall, indicating immunologic basis of dermatomyositis

Perifascicular muscle atrophy in child with dermatomyositis

changes in the biopsy specimen, the electromyographer should examine the patient with a suspected myopathic process on one side only, thus allowing the specimen to be taken from the contralateral homologue of the most affected muscle.

Changes commonly seen in biopsy specimens include necrosis, phagocytosis, regeneration, perivascular inflammation and perifascicular atrophy. Occasionally, the biopsy specimen is normal even in the presence of highly suspicious clinical findings. This may indicate a sampling error resulting from the nonuniform distribution of the affected muscle fibers. If clinical findings strongly suggest polymyositis, a subsequent biopsy specimen may prove diagnostic. If the second specimen

is also normal, other diagnostic possibilities should be considered.

Treatment. Steroids, especially prednisone, are the drugs of choice in treating polymyositis. Patients who appear refractory to steroids may benefit from an immunosuppressant drug, such as azathioprine or cyclophosphamide.

Prognosis. The prognosis for total recovery varies. The possibility of underlying carcinoma, although small, seems greatest in dermatomyositis. Overall mortality in polymyositis is 25% to 30%. Relapse occurs in about 20% of patients, particularly in younger patients. Two thirds of the survivors have little residual disability at 3-year follow-up. □

Myopathies Associated With Disorders of Potassium Metabolism

With the rare exception of hyperthyroidism, the majority of acute syndromes of generalized muscle weakness secondary to a myopathy appear to result from some form of metabolic dysfunction that produces either a depletion or an excess of serum potassium. One of the most dramatic of these disorders is the relatively uncommon syndrome of primary periodic paralysis. Secondary forms of potassium depletion are more common and are generally divided into those with inappropriate renal loss of potassium and those with potassium loss secondary to gastrointestinal disorders.

Secondary Hypokalemic Syndromes. Chronic urinary excretion of potassium may occur in hypertensive patients taking diuretics if they do not take appropriate potassium supplements. Excessive licorice ingestion, renal tubule disease and ureterosigmoidostomy also cause inappropriate renal excretion of potassium.

The threshold at which hypokalemia produces symptoms of muscular weakness varies. Usually, the level must drop below 2.5 mEq/L. However, patients with primary hypokalemic periodic paralysis may be more sensitive to diminution in the serum potassium level. Onset of weakness secondary to hypokalemia may be insidious and the course gradually progressive. However, in some persons, acute weakness may develop within a few hours.

Interestingly, although administration of steroids produces both a myopathic syndrome and hypokalemia, replacement of potassium alone does not improve either steroid-induced weakness or weakness in primary Cushing's syndrome. However, it does improve weakness in primary aldosteronism, an endocrinologic disease causing potassium depletion.

Primary Hypokalemic Periodic Paralysis. This illness of autosomal dominant inheritance usually begins in the first or second decade. Although the paralysis most often occurs at rest, precipitating factors are important. These include a period of rest after exercise or after eating a meal high in carbohydrate or salt. If the patient is awake and notices a premonitory feeling of heaviness, which often is first felt in the legs, the attack may be aborted with mild exercise. More severe attacks often commence during sleep, and the patient awakens with quadriparesis.

The severity of episodes of weakness is not predictable. Although the bulbar musculature used in speech is usually spared, in the most severe episodes, bulbar symptoms involving even the respiratory musculature may occur. Deep tendon reflexes are suppressed, but sensation is not affected. Most attacks gradually begin to subside in a few hours, but may not always totally clear up for 2 to 3 days, rarely persisting up to 1 week.

Acute primary hypokalemic periodic paralysis is treated with large oral doses of potassium. Acetazolamide given prophylactically is effective in preventing either hypokalemic or hyperkalemic primary periodic paralysis.

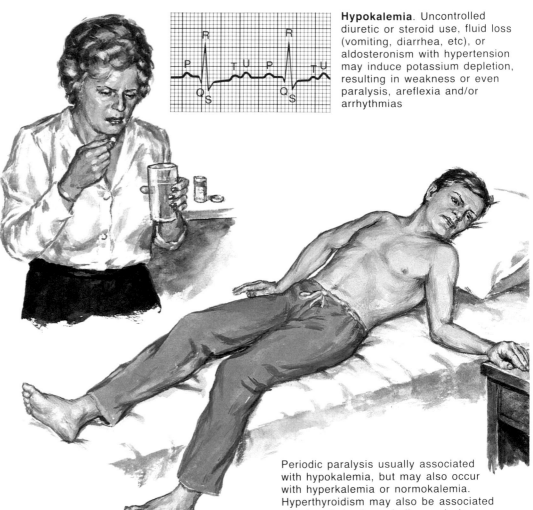

Hypokalemia. Uncontrolled diuretic or steroid use, fluid loss (vomiting, diarrhea, etc), or aldosteronism with hypertension may induce potassium depletion, resulting in weakness or even paralysis, areflexia and/or arrhythmias

Periodic paralysis usually associated with hypokalemia, but may also occur with hyperkalemia or normokalemia. Hyperthyroidism may also be associated with hypokalemic periodic paralysis

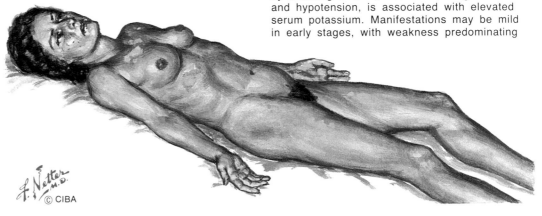

Hyperkalemia. Addison's disease (primary adrenocortical insufficiency), characterized by bronzing of skin, weakness, weight loss and hypotension, is associated with elevated serum potassium. Manifestations may be mild in early stages, with weakness predominating

Primary Hyperkalemic Periodic Paralysis. Primary and secondary forms of hyperkalemic periodic paralysis are less common than the hypokalemic forms. Onset of the hyperkalemic disorders is in the first decade. Potassium levels must be as high as 7.0 to 9.0 mEq/L to produce skeletal muscular weakness. Attacks of weakness are similar to those in hypokalemic paralysis; however, the hyperkalemic type is not precipitated by food. Hyperkalemic disorders may cause mild myotonia affecting the grip and in some cases may affect the bulbar musculature, particularly after exposure to cold.

Secondary Hyperkalemic Syndromes. Addison's disease is a rare but important secondary form

of hyperkalemic periodic paralysis. If there is no evidence of primary underlying renal failure on initial laboratory evaluation, the examining physician should consider the possibility of an impending adrenal crisis. In a suspected crisis, serum cortisol levels should be determined immediately and a large intravenous dose of steroids given.

Hyperkalemia must be rapidly controlled to prevent compromise of cardiac function. Calcium gluconate, chlorothiazide and sodium chloride have been given intravenously to treat acute episodes. If a secondary mechanism such as Addison's disease or renal disease cannot be detected, prophylactic therapy with acetazolamide usually is effective in preventing recurrent attacks. □

Myopathies and Other Neuromuscular Syndromes Secondary to Endocrine Disorders

Cushing's syndrome. Weakness (difficulty in rising from stooped position) and ecchymoses may be early manifestations. Other stigmata such as moon face and buffalo hump may be minimal. Osteoporosis may be present

Any primary process affecting the adrenal, thyroid, parathyroid or pituitary glands can cause dysfunction of the skeletal musculature. Thus, the possibility of an underlying endocrine disorder must be considered in the differential diagnosis of myopathic syndromes. Myopathy induced by endocrine dysfunction causes a slowly progressive weakness of the proximal muscles. Except in the patient with hypothyroidism, serum levels of muscle enzymes are often normal, as are results of nerve conduction velocity and electromyographic studies.

The most common myopathy of this type is an iatrogenic condition related to high-dose, usually long-term, *steroid therapy.* The degree of weakness may vary from subtle to so severe that the patient becomes wheelchair-dependent. Gradual reduction and, if possible, discontinuation of steroid therapy should lead to significant improvement.

Idiopathic *Cushing's syndrome* is much less common, but since fatigue and weakness may be early symptoms of this disorder, it should be considered in the differential diagnosis of any proximal muscle weakness. The classic findings of Cushing's syndrome, such as abdominal striae, truncal obesity and buffalo hump, may not have developed when muscle weakness becomes apparent. In some patients, however, careful inspection of the skin may demonstrate increased fragility and easy bruising.

A number of neuromuscular disorders are associated with various forms of thyroid dysfunction. *Hyperthyroidism (Graves' disease)* frequently causes proximal weakness of the pelvic girdle muscles, although other symptoms usually predominate. Rarely, the weakness is so profound that this disease may need to be considered in the differential diagnosis of motor neuron disease. When intermittent bulbar weakness is associated with Graves' disease, myasthenia gravis is a possibility. The incidence of hypokalemic periodic paralysis is increased in Orientals and in some Caucasians with hyperthyroidism. An infiltrative ophthalmo-

Hypothyroidism. Delayed or weak reflexes (biceps brachii) are characteristic. Other signs of myxedema, such as coarse features, dry scaling skin, edematous facies, thick lips, etc, may be striking

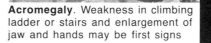

Acromegaly. Weakness in climbing ladder or stairs and enlargement of jaw and hands may be first signs

Enlargement of sella turcica and bony overgrowth of jaw and skull in acromegaly

myopathy accounts for the unilateral exophthalmos commonly seen.

Hypothyroidism may also be associated with a number of neuromuscular problems. The most common is the carpal tunnel syndrome. Other patients with myxedema have a broad, ataxic gait that should not be confused with the lordotic, waddling gait seen in some myopathies. Rarely, a syndrome of marked stiffness with associated significant slowing of muscular contraction and relaxation, known as *Hoffmann's syndrome,* is confused with Parkinson's disease. Delayed relaxation of deep tendon reflexes, particularly noticeable on percussion of the biceps or the ankle reflex, is often found in hypothyroidism.

Disorders of calcium metabolism may also affect the musculoskeletal system. Although findings of proximal muscle weakness are uncommon in *hyperparathyroidism,* the possibility should always be considered. Another disorder of calcium metabolism that may cause striking proximal muscle weakness is the *osteomalacia* associated with renal disease.

Acromegaly occasionally begins with neuromuscular symptoms, usually a carpal tunnel syndrome similar to that in myxedema, ie, infiltration of the transverse carpal ligament. Rarely, a patient with acromegaly first notices difficulty in climbing stairs, which may be secondary to an associated myopathy. ☐

McArdle's Disease and Other Types of Enzymatic Myopathies

Several uncommon forms of primary muscle disease are related to a lack of various enzymes that serve as important catalysts in energy metabolism. These diseases involve specific inborn errors of metabolism that may affect glucose (glycogen storage diseases) or lipids (carnitine palmityltransferase deficiency). The prototype of these disorders is type VI (type V of Cori), or myophosphorylase deficiency. The clinical syndrome was first described by McArdle, who also predicted the type of enzyme defect responsible for the patient's symptoms.

Symptoms in most of these syndromes are manifested only when the patient exercises—they do not inhibit routine daily activities. An exception to this rule is acid maltase deficiency (glycogen storage disease type II), which can be seen in infancy as a floppy baby, and in adulthood should be considered in the differential diagnosis of polymyositis, endocrine myopathies or the limb-girdle dystrophies.

McArdle's disease is characterized by the intramuscular accumulation of glycogen. Phosphorylase normally cleaves 1,4 linkages during the routine metabolism of glycogen. Absence of this enzyme impairs this process and prevents separation of glucose 1-phosphate from the glycogen molecule during exercise. The defect is chemically detectable when lactate production is below normal during ischemic exercise.

Clinical Manifestations. Patients with this disorder usually do not become symptomatic until late childhood. As a youngster expands his physical activities, he becomes dependent on a significant energy reserve. However, if this reserve is lacking because of an enzymatic defect, fatigue and cramping quickly develop. These symptoms often occur 6 to 10 minutes after exercise begins. If the defect is not too severe, symptoms abate about 15 to 20 minutes after commencing exercise, when lipid reserves become available for metabolism and provide an energy safety valve. At rest, these patients do not complain of symptoms such as lack of energy, general fatigue or tiredness, so often seen in the depressed or neurotic patient. Physical findings are almost invariably normal when patients are examined at rest.

Myoglobinuria may result if these patients engage in fairly strenuous exercise. If the degree of myoglobinuria is severe, renal damage and sometimes renal shutdown may result (Plate 33). Older adolescents who are subject to recurrent episodes of exercise-induced cramping and myoglobinuria, which suggest significant damage to the muscles, may well show evidence of a slight weakness of the proximal muscles on physical examination.

Diagnostic Studies. Results of routine blood studies may be normal if the patient has not been exercising before the blood sample is taken. However, if blood is drawn shortly after significant exertion, especially in symptomatic patients, very

McArdle's Disease

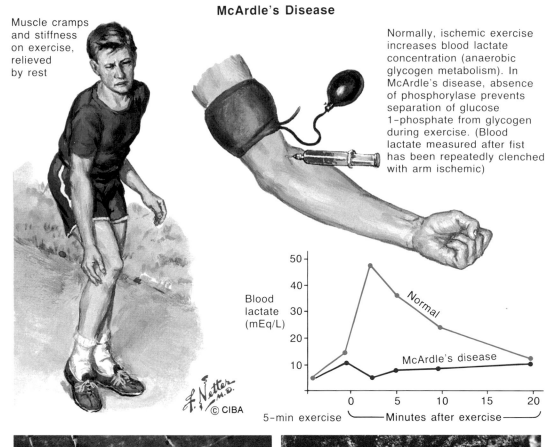

Muscle cramps and stiffness on exercise, relieved by rest

Normally, ischemic exercise increases blood lactate concentration (anaerobic glycogen metabolism). In McArdle's disease, absence of phosphorylase prevents separation of glucose 1-phosphate from glycogen during exercise. (Blood lactate measured after fist has been repeatedly clenched with arm ischemic)

Blood lactate (mEq/L)

Normal

McArdle's disease

5-min exercise — Minutes after exercise

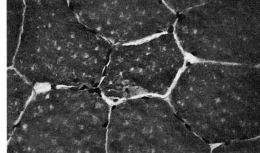

Frozen section of muscle tissue reveals "empty" subsarcolemmal vacuoles (H and E stain)

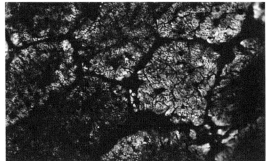

Frozen section of muscle tissue shows PAS-positive deposits of glycogen (PAS stain)

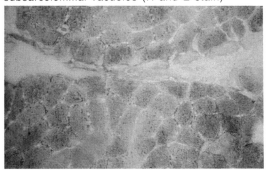

Positive staining for phosphorylase in normal muscle

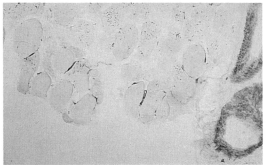

McArdle's disease: complete lack of staining for phosphorylase

high levels of skeletal muscle enzymes may be found. Levels of serum creatine kinase may approach 5,000 mU/ml or higher (normal, less than 110 mU/ml). Results of electromyographic and nerve conduction velocity studies are normal in most patients. However, electrically silent contractures have been reported in patients who exercise under ischemic conditions and undergo concomitant needle electromyography.

Ischemic exercise is the best method of detecting the lack of increased serum lactate production. If this is confirmed, a muscle biopsy should be carried out and the biopsy specimen studied with special stains to demonstrate phosphorylase or other specific enzymes involved in glycolysis.

In patients with McArdle's disease, staining demonstrates the absence of phosphorylase.

Differential Diagnosis. Two other rare forms of glycogen storage disease may mimic McArdle's disease, namely, *phosphofructokinase deficiency* and *phosphohexoisomerase deficiency.*

Occasionally, patients who have a classic history of poor exercise tolerance, cramping and myoglobinuria have normal lactate production during ischemic exercise. In this setting, another disorder of metabolism, *carnitine palmityltransferase deficiency* should be considered. These patients frequently become symptomatic if they exercise in a fasting state. Study of muscle biopsy specimens shows a significant accumulation of lipids. □

Myoglobinuric Syndromes, Including Malignant Hyperthermia

Myoglobin, the iron-containing protein found in skeletal and cardiac muscle, is responsible for oxygen transfer across membranes. Normally, this protein remains bound to muscles and is not found in serum. However, if a focal or diffuse process either physically or chemically impairs oxygen delivery to muscle, necrosis of the muscle results, and myoglobin is released and excreted in the urine. Abundant amounts of released myoglobin can produce renal damage and anuria.

Many different conditions may give rise to myoglobinuria. During times of military mobilization, exertional rhabdomyolysis, a muscular syndrome with marked myoglobinuria, may develop in physically untrained servicemen who are suddenly exposed to extremely strenuous exercise. The muscles become swollen, tender and weak, and the patient frequently becomes febrile. In hot climates, this syndrome may be confused with heatstroke. Serum creatine kinase levels are higher than in any other condition. Values may approach 2,500 times normal, compared with an elevation of 20 to 60 times normal in patients with acute polymyositis or Duchenne's muscular dystrophy.

In the general population, myoglobinuria may be a component of many different disorders, of which the most common relate to various *toxic substances*. Occasionally, acute myoglobinuria associated with acute weakness and tenderness of the proximal muscles and an elevated serum creatine kinase level is seen in alcoholics who indulge in "binge" drinking. Other toxins known to produce myoglobinuria include heroin, toluene, isopropyl alcohol, carbon monoxide, toxins from a wasp sting, or the bite of a Malayan sea snake.

Myoglobinuria may occur early in the course of severe *polymyositis*. There is also a familial syndrome of *idiopathic recurrent myoglobinuria*, with or without myopathy or underlying dystrophy. Other genetically determined diseases in which myoglobinuria may occur include some forms of *glycogen storage disease*, ie, phosphorylase deficiency (McArdle's disease) and phosphofructokinase deficiency, or carnitine palmityltransferase deficiency, *a lipid storage disease*.

Of the sporadic disorders rarely associated with myoglobinuria, the best known is *status epilepticus*. Other disorders to be considered include *ischemic syndromes*, such as the anterior tibial compartment syndrome; arterial occlusions in the leg; and compression from coma, particularly in drug overdose, when the individual may lie on one side crushing the muscles. Prolonged pressure from heavy falling objects as in building disasters, may also cause myoglobinuria. Use of heroin should be considered in any patient with symptoms of myoglobinuria.

Diagnostic confirmation of the myoglobinuria depends on identification of its pigment in the urine. Specific pigment identification can be obtained with use of electrophoresis, spectrophotometry, chromatography, or various antibody techniques.

Paroxysmal rhabdomyolysis

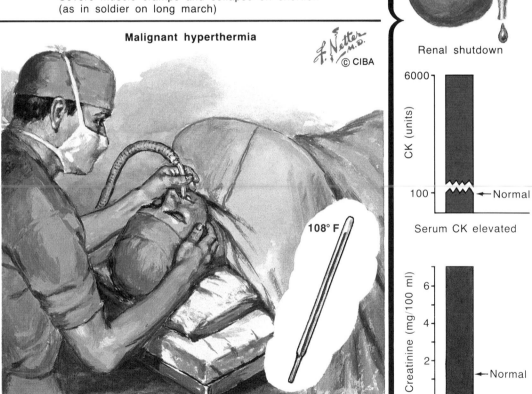

Severe muscle cramps and collapse on exertion (as in soldier on long march)

Malignant hyperthermia

Extreme temperature elevation in anesthetized patient

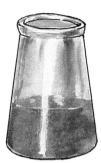

Urine brown, scanty (myoglobinuria)

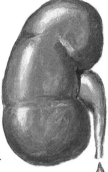

Renal shutdown

Serum CK elevated

Creatinine elevated

Treatment depends on the state of the patient's renal function and should be determined in consultation with an internist and a nephrologist.

Myoglobinuria is a serious complication of *malignant hyperthermia* secondary to the use of inhalation anesthetics, particularly halothane and succinylcholine chloride. It occurs in one of 15,000 children given a general anesthetic and in one of 50,000 adults. Clinically, after induction of the anesthetic agent, a rapidly fulminant picture develops, which includes a rigidity of the jaw and sudden tachycardia or other arrhythmia, followed by generalized muscle rigidity, shivering and extremely high fever, perhaps rising as fast as 1° C every 5 minutes.

If this autosomal dominant familial syndrome is not recognized shortly after its inception, mortality may be as high as 70%. Death results from cardiac arrhythmias or the malignant hyperthermic state alone. Immediate treatment is indicated. Dantrolene sodium reduces the degree of depolarization induced by the inhalation agents.

It has been suggested that the incidence of primary muscular disease, including Duchenne's muscular dystrophy, myotonic dystrophy and central core disease, is increased among these patients. The only test to determine patients at risk for malignant hyperthermia is an in vitro study of a muscle biopsy specimen treated with caffeine and halothane. □

Food-Borne Neurotoxins

Four distinct neuromuscular disorders result from ingestion of food-borne neurotoxin-producing organisms: botulism, trichinosis, ciguatera and shellfish (red tide) poisoning. The clinical hallmark of these disorders is severe gastrointestinal irritability manifested by nausea and vomiting, which usually precedes onset of neurologic dysfunction.

Botulism. The anaerobic organism *Clostridium botulinum* produces the most potent neurotoxin known to man. Although the spores of *C botulinum* are heat-resistant, boiling for 10 minutes (or at high altitudes, for 30 minutes at 80° C) inactivates the toxin. Because of the heat-resistant properties of the bacteria, home-processed foods may provide a perfect culture medium for the organism to grow and produce the neurotoxin. Rarely, commercially processed foods have also harbored this organism. Of the seven different types of *C botulinum*, types A, B, E and F, particularly types A and B, are the organisms that usually cause botulism. The different types cannot be distinguished on a clinical basis.

About two thirds of patients report *gastrointestinal irritability* (nausea, vomiting, abdominal cramps or diarrhea) before or shortly after onset of neurologic symptoms. The *bulbar musculature* is affected initially, particularly the extraocular muscles, producing diplopia or ptosis, or both. The pupils become nonreactive and widely dilated, and patients complain of blurred vision. Further signs of *cranial nerve dysfunction* include vertigo, dysphagia, and hoarseness or breathy nasal speech, or both. Neurologic dysfunction progresses rapidly and involvement becomes more widespread, producing paralysis of the extremities and the respiratory muscles.

Diagnosis is mainly on the basis of clinical manifestations. Although routine laboratory tests are not helpful, various immunologic techniques may be useful in identifying the type of organism involved.

Because the toxin inhibits the presynaptic release of acetylcholine at the neuromuscular junction, the Lambert-Eaton syndrome or diseases arising from defects in postsynaptic transmission, such as myasthenia gravis, should be excluded. This may be done clinically, as the pupil is not affected in either. The differential diagnosis should also include the Fisher variant of the Guillain-Barré syndrome, diphtheria, tick paralysis, and toxic reactions to various chemicals and drugs.

The effectiveness of treatment depends on very early diagnosis. *Trivalent (ABE) antitoxin* should be given initially, and type-specific antitoxin administered after the type of toxin has been identified. With improved respiratory intensive care, mortality from botulism has decreased, although it may still approach 50% in severe outbreaks.

Trichinosis. Ingestion of undercooked pork containing *Trichinella spiralis* organisms causes trichinosis, a syndrome characterized by acute nausea and vomiting, periorbital edema (a useful

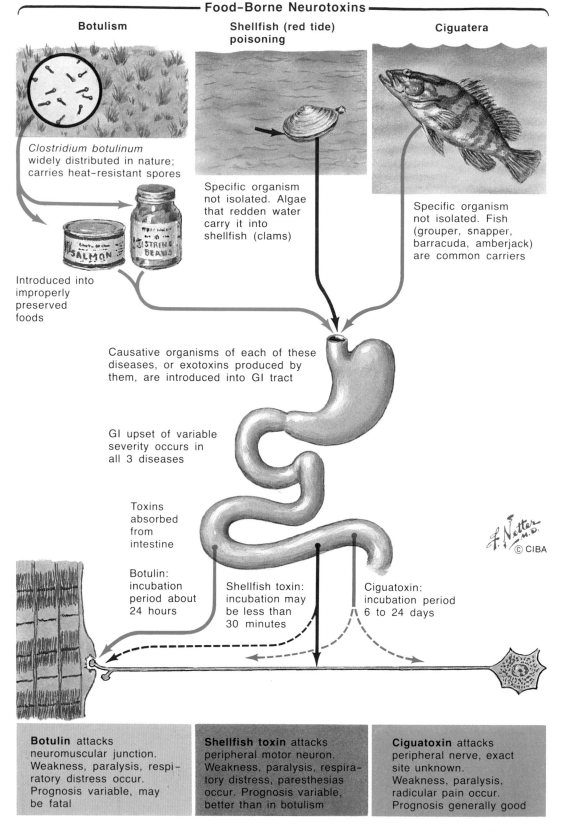

Food-Borne Neurotoxins

Botulism

Clostridium botulinum widely distributed in nature; carries heat-resistant spores

Introduced into improperly preserved foods

Shellfish (red tide) poisoning

Specific organism not isolated. Algae that redden water carry it into shellfish (clams)

Ciguatera

Specific organism not isolated. Fish (grouper, snapper, barracuda, amberjack) are common carriers

Causative organisms of each of these diseases, or exotoxins produced by them, are introduced into GI tract

GI upset of variable severity occurs in all 3 diseases

Toxins absorbed from intestine

Botulin: incubation period about 24 hours

Shellfish toxin: incubation may be less than 30 minutes

Ciguatoxin: incubation period 6 to 24 days

Botulin attacks neuromuscular junction. Weakness, paralysis, respiratory distress occur. Prognosis variable, may be fatal

Shellfish toxin attacks peripheral motor neuron. Weakness, paralysis, respiratory distress, paresthesias occur. Prognosis variable, better than in botulism

Ciguatoxin attacks peripheral nerve, exact site unknown. Weakness, paralysis, radicular pain occur. Prognosis generally good

and important diagnostic clue), muscle pain, weakness and occasionally encephalitis. Laboratory tests show extreme systemic eosinophilia and significant elevations in the serum creatine kinase level (see CIBA COLLECTION, Volume 5, page 247).

Ciguatera. An acute poisoning, ciguatera is caused by ciguatoxin, which is concentrated in the tissues of fish inhabiting the subtropical waters of the Bahamas, Florida and Hawaii. Fish most likely to be contaminated are grouper, red snapper, barracuda and amberjack. Ingestion of these fish produces fulminating gastrointestinal distress followed by muscle aches and pains, which occasionally assume a radicular distribution and sometimes a cerebellar syndrome. There is no

specific treatment for ciguatera, which may be disabling for a few months, but is rarely fatal.

Shellfish Poisoning. Ingestion of clams, mussels, oysters or scallops that have been contaminated by neurotoxin-producing dinoflagellates causes an acute illness, sometimes called "red tide poisoning." Nausea, vomiting and diarrhea are followed by an acute neurologic syndrome characterized by paresthesias of the perioral region and of the extremities. In the most severe cases, bulbar and respiratory paralysis may develop later. Specific diagnostic confirmatory studies are not available. Neurophysiologic studies have suggested that the site of action involves the nerve axon. The course is benign in most patients. □

Selected References

General References

ADAMS RD, VICTOR M: *Principles of Neurology*, ed 2. New York, McGraw-Hill, 1981

BAKER AB, BAKER LH (eds): *Clinical Neurology*. New York, Harper Medical, 1984

ROSENBERG RN (ed): *Clinical Neurosciences, I & III*. New York, Churchill Livingstone, 1983

RUBENSTEIN E, FEDERMAN DD (eds): *Scientific American Medicine*. Vol 7: *Infectious Disease*. Vol 8: *Interdisciplinary Medicine*. Vol 11: *Neurology*. New York, Scientific American, 1985

WALTON JA: *Disorders of Voluntary Muscle*, ed 4. New York, Churchill Livingstone, 1981

WALTON JN (ed): *Brain's Diseases of the Nervous System*, ed 8. New York, Oxford University Press, 1977

Section I

	Plate Number
AMERICAN PSYCHIATRIC ASSOCIATION: *Diagnostic and Statistical Manual of Mental Disorders*, ed 3. Washington DC, APA, 1980	20
BAUMAN ML, KEMPER TL: *The brain in infantile autism: a histoanatomic case report*. Neurology 1984, 34:275	20
BERGEN BJ, CARRY MP, WILSON WB, et al: *Centronuclear myopathy: extraocular- and limb-muscle findings in an adult*. Muscle Nerve 1980, 3:165−171	15
BRETT EM (ed): *Pediatric Neurology*. New York, Churchill Livingstone, 1983	1−5, 10−12, 16, 18, 23
BROOKE MH: *Muscular dystrophies and congenital myopathies*. In SCHEINBERG P (ed): *Neurology and Neurosurgery*, Vol 1. Princeton, Biomedia, 1979	15
BYERS RK, BANKER BQ: *Infantile muscular atrophy*. Arch Neurol 1961, 5:140−164	13
DAUBE JR: *EMG in Motor Neuron Disease*. Minimonograph #18. Rochester MN, American Association of Electromyography and Electrodiagnosis, 1982	13
DAYAN AD: *Peripheral neuropathy of metachromatic leucodystrophy: observations on segmental demyelination and remyelination and the intracellular distribution of sulphatide*. J Neurol Neurosurg Psychiatry 1967, 30:311−318	17
DUBOWITZ V (ed): *The Floppy Infant*, ed 2 (Clinics in Developmental Medicine Ser, Vol 76). London, Spastics Intl England, Lippincott, 1980	11−12
DUBOWITZ V, ROY S: *Central core disease of muscle: clinical histochemical and electron microscopic studies of an affected mother and child*. Brain 1970, 93:133−146	15
FARMER TW (ed): *Pediatric Neurology*, ed 3. Philadelphia, Harper Medical, 1983	1−5, 10−12, 16, 18, 23
GALABURDA AM, KEMPER TL: *Cytoarchitectonic abnormalities in developmental dyslexia: a case study*. Ann Neurol 1979, 6:94−100	19
GESCHWIND N, BEHAN P: *Left-handedness: association with immune disease, migraine, and developmental learning disorders*. Proc Natl Acad Sci 1982, 79:5097−5100	19
GOMEZ MR (ed): *Tuberous Sclerosis*. New York, Raven Press, 1979	23

Section I (*continued*)

	Plate Number
GONATAS NK, SHY GM, GODFREY EH: *Nemaline myopathy: the origin of nemaline structures*. N Engl J Med 1966, 274:535−539	15
KAUFMAN MD, HOPKINS LC, HURWITZ BJ: *Progressive sensory neuropathy in patients without carcinoma: a disorder with distinctive clinical and electrophysiological findings*. Ann Neurol 1981, 9:237−242	14
KEMPER TL: *Asymmetrical lesions in dyslexia*. In GESCHWIND N, GALABURDA AM (eds): *Cerebral Dominance: The Biological Foundations*. Cambridge, Harvard University Press, 1984	19
LOVEJOY FH JR, BRESNAN MJ, LOMBROSO CT, et al: *Anticerebral oedema therapy in Reye's syndrome*. Arch Dis Child 1975, 30:933−937	24
LOVEJOY FH JR, SMITH AL, BRESNAN MJ, et al: *Clinical staging in Reye syndrome*. Am J Dis Child 1974, 128:36−41	24
MATSON DD: *Neurosurgery of Infancy and Childhood*, ed 2. Springfield IL, Charles C Thomas, 1969	21−22
MCLAURIN R, et al (eds): *Pediatric Neurosurgery. Surgery of the Developing Nervous System*. Orlando FL, Grune & Stratton, 1982	21−22
MILLER RG, GUTMANN L, LEWIS RA, et al: *Acquired versus familial demyelinative neuropathies in children*. Muscle Nerve 1985, 8.205−210	17
MISHKIN M, BACHEVALIER J: *Personal communication*	20
MUNSAT TL, WOODS R, FOWLER W, et al: *Neurogenic muscular atrophy of infancy with prolonged survival. The variable course of Werdnig-Hoffmann disease*. Brain 1969, 92:9−24	13
PACKER RJ, BROWN MJ, BERMAN PH: *The diagnostic value of electromyography in infantile hypotonia*. Am J Dis Child 1982, 136:1057−1059	13
PAINE RS: *The future of the "floppy infant": a follow-up study of 33 patients*. Dev Med Child Neurol 1963, 5:115−124	13
PRENSKY AL: *The leukodystrophies, I*. In SCHEINBERG P (ed): *Neurology and Neurosurgery*, Vol 4. Princeton, CPEC, 1983, pp 1−7	17
RINGEL SP, WILSON WB, BARDEN MT: *Extraocular muscle biopsy in chronic progressive external ophthalmoplegia*. Ann Neurol 1979, 6:326−339	15
RUSSMAN BS, MELCHREIT R, DRENNAN JC: *Spinal muscular atrophy: the natural course of disease*. Muscle Nerve 1983, 6:179−181	13
SATRAN R: *Dejerine-Sottas disease revisited*. Arch Neurol 1980, 37:67−68	14
SHERMAN GF, GALABURDA AM, GESCHWIND N: *Ectopic neurons in the brain of the autoimmune mouse: a neuropathological model of dyslexia*. Neurosci Abstr 1983, 9:939	19
STEIMAN GS, RORKE LB, BROWN MJ: *Infantile neuronal degeneration masquerading as Werdnig-Hoffmann disease*. Ann Neurol 1980, 8:317−324	13
TRAUNER DA: *Treatment of Reye syndrome*. Ann Neurol 1980, 7:2−4	24
VOLPE JJ: *Neurology of the Newborn*. Philadelphia, WB Saunders, 1981	1−5, 10, 16

Section I (*continued*)

	Plate Number
WALDMAN RJ, HALL WN, MCGEE H, et al: *Aspirin as a risk factor in Reye's syndrome*. JAMA 1982, 247:3089−3094	24
WINSTON KR: *Craniosynostosis*. In WILKINS RH, RENGACHARY SS (eds): *Neurosurgery*. New York, McGraw-Hill, 1985	1
YUDELL A, GOMEZ MR, LAMBERT EH, et al: *The neuropathy of sulfatide lipidosis (metachromatic leukodystrophy)*. Neurology 1967, 17:103−111	17

Section II

	Plate Number
ANTHONY M, LANCE JW: *Histamine and serotonin in cluster headache*. Arch Neurol 1971, 25:225−231	1−4
BLASS JP, GIBSON GE: *Abnormality of a thiamine-requiring enzyme in patients with Wernicke-Korsakoff syndrome*. N Engl J Med 1977, 297:1367−1370	6
BRANDT T, DAROFF RB: *The multisensory physiological and pathological vertigo syndromes*. Ann Neurol 1980, 7:195−203	5
BRUYN GW: *Complicated migraine*. In VINKEN PJ, BRUYN GW (eds): *Handbook of Clinical Neurology*. Vol 5: *Headaches and Cranial Neuralgias*. Amsterdam, North Holland, 1968, pp 59−95	1−4
CAPLAN LR: *The patient with reduced consciousness or coma*. In SKILLMAN JJ (ed): *Intensive Care*. Boston, Little, Brown, 1975, pp 559−567	15
CARLEN PL, WILKINSON DA, WORTZMAN G: *Cerebral atrophy and functional deficits in alcoholics without clinically apparent liver disease*. Neurology 1981, 31:377−385	6
DALESSIO DJ (ed): *Headache and Other Head Pain*, ed 4. New York, Oxford University Press, 1980	1−4
DELGADO-ESCUETA AV (ed): *Status Epilepticus: Mechanisms of Brain Damage and Treatment* (Advances in Neurology Ser, Vol 34). New York, Raven Press, 1983	14
DELGADO-ESCUETA AV, WASTERLAIN CG, TREIMAN DM, et al: *Current concepts in neurology: management of status epilepticus*. N Engl J Med 1982, 306:1337−1340	14
DRACHMAN DA, HART CW: *An approach to the dizzy patient*. Neurology 1972, 22:323−334	5
FISHER CM: *The neurological examination of the comatose patient*. Acta Neurol (Suppl) Scand 1969, 45:1−56	15
FISHER CM: *Vertigo in cerebrovascular disease*. Arch Otolaryng 1967, 85:529−534	5
FISHER CM, ADAMS R: *Transient global amnesia*. Acta Neurol (Suppl) Scand 1964, 9:1−83	7
FRIEDMAN A: *Nature of headache*. Headache 1979, 19:163−167	1−4
GASTAUT H, et al: *The Physiopathogenesis of the Epilepsies*. Springfield IL, Charles C Thomas, 1969	10−12
GASTAUT H, BROUGHTON R: *Epileptic Seizures: Clinical and Electrographic Features, Diagnosis and Treatment*. Springfield IL, Charles C Thomas, 1972	10−13

Section II (continued)

	Plate Number
GOODWIN J: *Temporal arteritis*. In VINKEN PJ, BRUYN GW (eds): *Handbook of Clinical Neurology. Vol 39: Neurological Manifestations of Systemic Disease, II.* New York, Elsevier North Holland, 1980, pp 313–342	1–4
GUILLEMINAULT C: *Disorders of Sleep and Waking.* Reading MA, Addison-Wesley, 1981	8
LAIDLAW JP, RICHENS A: *A Textbook of Epilepsy*, ed 2. New York, Churchill Livingstone, 1982	9–10, 14
LANCE J: *Headache*. Ann Neurol 1981, 10:1–10	1–4
LANCE J: *Mechanism and Management of Headache*, ed 3. Stoneham MA, Butterworth, 1978	1–4
NIEDERMEYER E: *Compendium of the Epilepsies.* Springfield IL, Charles C Thomas, 1974	11–12
PENFIELD W, JASPER H: *Epilepsy and the Functional Anatomy of the Human Brain.* Boston, Little, Brown, 1954	13
PENMAN J: *Trigeminal neuralgia.* In VINKEN PJ, BRUYN GW (eds): *Handbook of Clinical Neurology. Vol 5: Headaches and Cranial Neuralgias.* Amsterdam, North Holland, 1968, pp 296–322	1–4
PENRY JK: *Perspectives in complex partial seizures.* Adv Neurol 1975, 11:1–14	13
PLUM F, POSNER J: *The Diagnosis of Stupor and Coma*, ed 3. Philadelphia, FA Davis, 1980	15
PRICE RW, POSNER JB: *Chronic paroxysmal hemicrania: a disabling headache syndrome responding to indomethacin.* Ann Neurol 1978, 3:183–184	1–4
SCHMIDT RP, WILDER BJ: *Epilepsy.* Philadelphia, FA Davis, 1968	10–14
SLEEP DISORDERS CLASSIFICATIONS COMMITTEE: *Diagnostic classification of sleep and arousal disorders*, ed 1. Sleep 1979, 2:1–137	8
STOOKEY B, RANSOHOFF J: *Trigeminal Neuralgia.* Springfield IL, Charles C Thomas, 1959	1–4
SYMONDS CP: *Disorders of memory.* Brain 1966, 89:625–644	7
SYMONDS CP: *Particular variety of headache.* Brain 1956, 79:217–232	1–4
VICTOR M: *Treatment of alcoholic intoxication and the withdrawal syndrome.* Psychosom Med 1961, 28:636–650	6
VICTOR M, ADAMS RD: *Effect of alcohol on nervous system.* A Res Nerv & Ment Dis Proc 1953, 32:526–573	6
VICTOR M, ADAMS R, COLLINS G: *The Wernicke-Korsakoff Syndrome.* Philadelphia, FA Davis, 1971	7
VICTOR M, ANGEVINE J, MANCALL E, et al: *Memory loss with lesions of hippocampal formation. Report of a case with some remarks on the anatomical basis of memory.* Arch Neurol 1961, 5:244–263	7
VINKEN PJ, BRUYN GW (eds): *Handbook of Clinical Neurology*, Vol 15. Amsterdam, North Holland, 1974	9–10

Section III

	Plate Number
ACKERMAN RH: *A perspective of noninvasive diagnosis of carotid disease.* Neurology 1979, 29:615–622	20–21
ADAMS HP JR, KASSELL NF, MAZUZ H: *The patient with transient ischemic attacks – is this the time for a new therapeutic approach?* Stroke 1984, 15:371	24

Section III (continued)

	Plate Number
ALVORD EC JR, LOESER JD, BAILEY WL, et al: *Subarachnoid hemorrhage due to ruptured aneurysms. A simple method of estimating prognosis.* Arch Neurol 1972, 27:273	30–36
BARNETT HJM: *Progress towards stroke prevention: Robert Wartenberg lecture.* Neurology 1980, 30:1212	24
BERK ME: *Aneurysms of the middle meningeal artery.* Brit J Radiol 1961, 34:667	30–36
BRATTSTRÖM L, HINDFELT B, NILSSON O: *Transient neurological symptoms associated with mononuclear pleocytosis of the cerebrospinal fluid.* Acta Neurol Scand 1984, 69:104–110	17
BRIERLEY JB, MELDRUM BS, BROWN AW: *The threshold and neuropathology of cerebral "anoxic-ischemic" cell change.* Arch Neurol 1973, 29:367–373	37
CAPLAN L: *Vertebrobasilar occlusive disease.* In BARNETT H, MOHR J, STEIN B, et al (eds): *Stroke: Pathophysiology Diagnosis and Management.* New York, Churchill Livingstone, 1985 (in press)	11
CAPLAN L: *Extracranial vertebral artery: progress in cerebrovascular disease.* Stroke 1984, 19:25–28	12
CAPLAN LR: *Are terms such as completed stroke or RIND of continued usefulness?* Stroke 1983, 14:431–433	4
CAPLAN LR: *Bilateral distal vertebral artery occlusion.* Neurology 1983, 33:552–558	13
CAPLAN LR: *Cerebrovascular diseases.* In TODOROV (illus): *Clinical Neurology.* New York, Thieme-Stratton, 1983, pp 119–136	1
CAPLAN LR: *Vertebrobasilar disease. Time for a new strategy.* Stroke 1981, 12:111–114	11
CAPLAN LR: *"Top of the basilar" syndrome.* Neurology 1980, 30:72–79	15
CAPLAN LR: *Intracerebral hemorrhage.* In TYLER HR, DAWSON D (eds): *Current Neurology, II.* Boston, Houghton Mifflin, 1979, pp 185–205	26–27
CAPLAN LR: *Neurology of the acute cardiac.* In DONOSO E, COHEN S (eds): *Critical Cardiac Care.* New York, Stratton Medical Books, 1979, pp 183–197	37
CAPLAN LR: *Occlusion of the vertebral or basilar artery. Follow up analysis of some patients with benign outcome.* Stroke 1979, 10:277–282	14
CAPLAN LR: *Lacunar infarction: a neglected concept.* Geriatrics 1976, 31:71–75	9
CAPLAN LR, BABIKIAN V, HELGASON C, et al: *Occlusive disease of the middle cerebral artery.* Neurology 1985, 35:975–982	8
CAPLAN LR, HIER DB, BANKS G: *Stroke and drug abuse.* In YATSU FM (ed): *Current Concepts of Cerebrovascular Disease – Stroke.* Dallas, AHA, 1982	17
CAPLAN LR, HIER DB, D'CRUZ I: *Cerebral embolism in the Michael Reese Stroke Registry.* Stroke 1983, 14:530	16
CASTAIGNE P, LHERMITTE F, BUGE A, et al: *Paramedian thalamic and midbrain infarct: clinical and neuropathological study.* Ann Neurol 1981, 10:127–148	15
COME PC, RILEY MF, BIVAS NK: *Roles of echocardiography and arrhythmia monitoring in the evaluation of patients with suspected systemic embolism.* Ann Neurol 1983, 13:527–531	24
CURRIER R, GILES C, DEJONG R: *Some comments on Wallenberg's lateral medullary syndrome.* Neurology 1962, 12:778–791	13
DRAKE CG: *Management of aneurysms of posterior circulation.* In YOUMANS JR (ed): *Neurological Surgery.* Philadelphia, WB Saunders, 1973	30–36

Section III (continued)

	Plate Number
EASTON JD, SHERMAN DG: *Management of cerebral embolism of cardiac origin.* Stroke 1980, 11:433	16
EASTON JD, SHERMAN DG: *Cervical manipulation and stroke.* Stroke 1977, 8:594–597	12
FIELDS WS: *Aortocranial occlusive vascular disease (stroke).* Clin Symp 1974, 26:3–31	3, 6–7, 10
FIELDS WS, BRUETMAN ME, WEIBEL J.: *Collateral circulation of the brain.* Monogr Surg Sci 1965, 2:183–259	3, 6–7, 10
FISHER CM: *Pathological observations in hypertensive cerebral hemorrhage.* J Neuropathol Exp Neurol 1971, 30:536–550	26
FISHER CM: *Occlusion of the vertebral arteries.* Arch Neurol 1970, 22:13–19	12
FISHER CM: *The arterial lesions underlying lacunes.* Acta Neuropathol 1969, 12:1–15	9
FISHER CM: *Lacunes: small deep cerebral infarcts.* Neurology 1965, 15:774–784	9
FISHER CM: *Clinical syndromes in cerebral arterial occlusion.* In FIELDS WS (ed): *Pathogenesis and Treatment of Cerebrovascular Disease.* Springfield IL, Charles C Thomas, 1961, pp 151–181	1, 8
FISHER CM: *Clinical syndromes in cerebral hemorrhages.* In FIELDS WS (ed): *Pathogenesis and Treatment of Cerebrovascular Disease.* Springfield IL, Charles C Thomas, 1961	27
FISHER CM: *The pathology and pathogenesis of intracerebral hemorrhage.* In FIELDS WS (ed): *Pathogenesis and Treatment of Cerebrovascular Disease.* Springfield IL, Charles C Thomas, 1961, pp 295–317	26
FISHER CM: *Observations of the fundus oculi in transient monocular blindness.* Neurology 1959, 9:333–347	3, 6–7, 10, 24
FISHER CM, CAPLAN LR: *Basilar artery branch occlusion: a cause of pontine infarction.* Neurology 1971, 21:900–905	14
FISHER CM, DALAL P, ADAMS RD: *Cerebrovascular diseases.* In HARRISON TR, ADAMS R, BENNETT I, et al (eds): *Principles of Internal Medicine*, ed 5. New York, McGraw-Hill, 1966, pp 1146–1184	1, 11
FISHER CM, KARNES W, KUBIK C: *Lateral medullary infarction: the pattern of vascular occlusion.* J Neuropathol Exp Neurol 1961, 20:323–379	13
FISHER CM, OJEMANN RG, ROBERSON GH: *Spontaneous dissection of cervico-cerebral arteries.* Can J Neurol Sci 1978, 5:9	17
FISHER CM, PICARD E, POLAK A, et al: *Acute hypertensive cerebellar hemorrhage: diagnosis and surgical treatment.* J Nerv Ment Dis 1965, 140:38–57	27
FISHER M: *Occlusion of the internal carotid artery.* Arch Neurol Psychiat 1951, 65:346	3, 6–7, 10
FISHER M, DAVIDSON RI, MARCUS EM: *Transient focal cerebral ischemia as a presenting manifestation of unruptured cerebral aneurysms.* Ann Neurol 1980, 8:367–372	17
FURLAN AJ: *Management of occlusive cerebrovascular disease.* Primary Care 1979, 6:1530	24
FURLAN AJ, CAVALIER SJ, HOBBS RE, et al: *Hemorrhage and anticoagulation after nonseptic embolic brain infarction.* Neurology 1982, 32:280–282	16
GEE W, OLLER DW, WYLIE EJ: *Noninvasive diagnosis of carotid occlusions by ocular pneumoplethysmography.* Stroke 1976, 7:18–21	20–21
GRAUS F, ROGERS LR, POSNER JB: *Cerebrovascular complications in patients with cancer.* Medicine 1985, 64:16	17

Section III (continued)

Plate Number

HARRIS FS, RHOTON AL JR: *Anatomy of the cavernous sinus. A microsurgical study.* J Neurosurg 1976, 45:169 — 30–36

HARVARD MEDICAL SCHOOL AD HOC COMMITTEE: *A definition of irreversible coma: report of the Ad Hoc Committee of Harvard Medical School to examine the definition of brain death.* JAMA 1968, 205:337–340 — 37

HASS WK: *Occlusive cerebrovascular disease.* Med Clin North Am 1972, 56:1281 — 3, 6–7, 10

HAUW J, DER AGOPIAN P, TRELLIS L, et al: *Les infarctus bulbaires. Etude systématique de la topographie lésionnelle dans 49 cas.* J Neurol Sci 1976, 28:83–102 — 13

HIER DB, DAVIS KR, RICHARDSON EP JR: *Hypertensive putaminal hemorrhage.* Ann Neurol 1977, 1:152–159 — 27

HINTON RC, MOHR JP, ACKERMAN RH: *Symptomatic middle cerebral artery stenosis.* Ann Neurol 1979, 5:152–157 — 8

HOLLENHORST RW: *The ocular manifestations of internal carotid arterial thrombosis.* Med Clin N Amer 1960, 44:897–908 — 24

HOLMES MD, BRANT-ZAWADZKI MM, SIMON RP: *Clinical features of meningovascular syphilis.* Neurology 1984, 34:553–556 — 17

HOUSER O, BAKER HL JR, SVIEN H, et al: *Arteriovenous malformations of the parenchyma of the brain. Angiographic aspects.* Radiology 1973, 109:83–90 — 28

HUTTON JT: *Atrial myxoma as a cause of progressive dementia.* Arch Neurol 1981, 38:533 — 17

IGARASHI M, GILMARTIN RC, GERALD B, et al: *Cerebral arteritis and bacterial meningitis.* Arch Neurol 1984, 41:531–535 — 17

JABAILY J, ILAND HJ, LASZLO J, et al: *Neurologic manifestations of essential thrombocythemia.* Ann Int Med 1983, 99:513–518 — 17

JACKSON AC, BOUGHNER DR, BARNETT HJM: *Mitral valve prolapse and cerebral ischemic events in young patients.* Neurology 1984, 34:784–787 — 17

JONES HR, CAPLAN LR, COME PC, et al: *Cerebral emboli of paradoxical origin.* Ann Neurol 1983, 13:314–319 — 17

JONES HR, MILLIKAN CH: *Temporal profile (clinical course) of acute carotid system cerebral infarction.* Stroke 1976, 7:64 — 4

JONES HR, SIEKERT RG, GERACI JE: *Neurologic manifestations of bacterial endocarditis.* Ann Intern Med 1969, 71:21 — 16

KELLY JJ JR, MELLINGER JF, SUNDT TM JR: *Intracranial arteriovenous malformations in childhood.* Ann Neurol 1978, 3:338–343 — 28

KEMPE LG: *Operative Neurosurgery, I: Aneurysm of the Anterior Part of Circle of Willis, chap 2; Aneurysm of the Basilar Artery, chap 20.* New York, Springer-Verlag, 1968 — 30–36

KEMPE LG: *Operative Neurosurgery, II: Aneurysm of the Vertebral Artery.* New York, Springer-Verlag, 1970, chap 7 — 30–36

KOMRAD MS, COFFEY CE, COFFEY KS, et al: *Myocardial infarction and stroke.* Neurology 1984, 34:1403–1409 — 16

KOTT S: *Stroke due to vasculitis.* Primary Care 1979, 6:771–789 — 4

KRUGER RA, MISTRETTA CA, HOUK TL, et al: *Computerized fluoroscopy in real-time for noninvasive visualization of the cardiovascular system.* Radiology 1979, 130:49–57 — 20–21

KUBIK C, ADAMS R: *Occlusion of basilar artery: a clinical and pathological study.* Brain 1946, 69:6–121 — 14

Section III (continued)

Plate Number

KUHN RA, KUGLER H: *False aneurysms of the middle meningeal artery.* J Neurosurg 1964, 21:92 — 30–36

LONGSTRETH WT JR, SWANSON PD: *Oral contraceptives and stroke.* Stroke 1984, 15:747–750 — 17

MAS J-L, GOEAU C, BOUSSER M-G, et al: *Spontaneous dissecting aneurysms of the internal carotid and vertebral arteries – two case reports.* Stroke 1985, 16:125 — 17

MCDOWELL FH, MILLIKAN CH, GOLDSTEIN M: *Treatment of impending stroke.* Stroke 1980, 11:1–3 — 4

MILLIKAN CH, SIEKERT RG, WHISNANT JP: *Intermittent carotid and vertebral-basilar insufficiency associated with polycythemia.* Neurology 1960, 10:188–196 — 17

MOHR JP: *Lacunes.* Stroke 1982, 13:3–11 — 9

MOHR JP, CAPLAN LR, MELSKI JW, et al: *The Harvard Cooperative Registry: a prospective registry.* Neurology 1978, 28:754–762 — 1

MOOSSY J: *Morphology, sites and epidemiology of cerebral atherosclerosis.* Res Publ Assoc Res Nerv Ment Dis 1966, 41:1–22 — 12

OLIVECRONA H, RIIVES J: *Arteriovenous aneurysms of brain; their diagnosis and treatment.* Arch Neurol & Psychiat 1948, 59:567–602 — 28

PERLMUTTER D, RHOTON AL JR: *Microsurgical anatomy of the anterior cerebral-anterior communicating-recurrent artery complex.* J Neurosurg 1976, 45:259 — 30–36

PESSIN MS, DUNCAN GW, MOHR JP, et al: *Clinical and angiographic features of carotid transient ischemic attacks.* N Engl J Med 1977, 296:358–362 — 24

PLUM F, POSNER J: *Delayed neurological deterioration after anoxia.* Arch Intern Med 1962, 110:18–25 — 37

PRUITT AA, RUBIN RH, KARCHMER AW, et al: *Neurologic complications of bacterial endocarditis.* Medicine 1978, 57:329 — 16

RANSOHOFF J, GOODGOLD AL: *Nonoperative management of aneurysms.* In YOUMANS JR (ed): *Neurological Surgery.* Philadelphia, WB Saunders, 1973 — 30–36

RESHEF E, GREENBERG SB, JANKOVIC J: *Herpes zoster ophthalmicus followed by contralateral hemiparesis: report of two cases and review of literature.* J Neurol Neurosurg Psychiatry 1985, 48:122–127 — 17

RHOTON AL, JACKSON FE, GLEAVE J, et al: *Congenital and traumatic intracranial aneurysms.* Clin Symp 1977, 29:2–40 — 30–36

ROSENBLUM WI: *Miliary aneurysms and "fibrinoid" degeneration of cerebral blood vessels.* Hum Pathol 1977, 8:133–139 — 26

SAEKI N, RHOTON AL JR: *Microsurgical anatomy of the upper basilar artery and the posterior circle of Willis.* J Neurosurg 1977, 46:563 — 30–36

SAHS AL, PERRET GE, LOCKSLEY HB, et al: *Intracranial Aneurysms & Subarachnoid Hemorrhage: Cooperative Study.* Philadelphia, JB Lippincott, 1969 — 30–36

SANDOK BA, FURLAN AJ, WHISNANT JP, et al: *Guidelines for the management of transient ischemic attacks.* Mayo Clin Proc 1978, 53:665–674 — 24

SANDOK BA, VON ESTORFF I, GIULIANI ER: *CNS embolism due to atrial myxoma: clinical features and diagnosis.* Arch Neurol 1980, 37:485–488 — 17

Section III (continued)

Plate Number

SCULLY RE, GALDABINI JJ, MCNEELY BU (eds): *Case records of the Massachusetts General Hospital.* N Engl J Med 1976, 295:944–950 — 17

SEGARRA J: *Cerebral vascular disease and behavior. The syndrome of the mesencephalic artery (basilar artery bifurcation).* Arch Neurol 1970, 22:408–418 — 15

SHEEHAN S, BAUER RB, MEYER JS: *Vertebral artery compression in cervical spondylosis, arteriographic demonstration during life of vertebral artery insufficiency due to rotation and extension of the neck.* Neurology 1960, 10:968 — 3, 6–7, 10

STEHBENS WE: *Pathology of the Cerebral Blood Vessels: Intracranial Arterial Aneurysms.* St Louis, CV Mosby, 1972, chap 9 — 30–36

SYMONDS C, MACKENZIE I: *Bilateral loss of vision from cerebral infarction.* Brain 1957, 80:415–454 — 15

TEAL JS, BERGERON RT, RUMBAUGH CL, et al: *Aneurysms of the petrous or cavernous portions of the internal carotid artery associated with nonpenetrating head trauma.* J Neurosurg 1973, 38:568 — 30–36

WEIBEL J, FIELDS WS: *Atlas of Arteriography in Occlusive Cerebrovascular Disease.* Stuttgart, Georg Thieme Verlag, 1969 — 3, 6–7, 10

WEISBERG LA, NICE CN: *Intracranial tumors simulating the presentation of cerebrovascular syndromes: early detection with cerebral computed tomography (CCT).* Am J Med 1977, 63:517–524 — 24

WESTCOTT JL, CHYNN KY, STEINBERG I: *Percutaneous transfemoral selective arteriography of brachiocerebral vessels.* Amer J Roentgen 1963, 90:554 — 3, 6–7, 10

WOOD DH: *Cerebrovascular complications of sickle cell anemia.* In WALTZ AG (ed): *Current Concepts of Cerebrovascular Disease – Stroke.* Dallas, AHA, 1977, pp 73–76 — 17

YASARGIL MG, ANTIC J, LACIGA R, et al: *Microsurgical pterional approach to aneurysms of the basilar bifurcation.* Surg Neurol 1976, 6:83 — 30–36

YASARGIL MG, FOX JL: *The microsurgical approach to intracranial aneurysms.* Surg Neurol 1975, 3:7 — 30–36

Section IV

Plate Number

ALLEN AR: *Surgery of experimental lesions of spinal cord equivalent to crush injury of fracture dislocation of spinal column.* JAMA 1911, 57:878–880 — 17–24

BECKER DP, MILLER JD, WARD JD, et al: *The outcome from severe head injury with early diagnosis and intensive management.* J Neurosurg 1977, 47:491–502 — 1–16

BORS E: *The spinal cord injury center of The Veterans Administration Hospital, Long Beach, California, USA. Facts and thought.* Paraplegia 1967, 5:126–130 — 17–24

BRUCE DA, SCHUT L, BRUNO LA, et al: *Outcome following severe head injuries in children.* J Neurosurg 1978, 48:679–688 — 1–16

CLINE H: Quoted in HOWORTH MB, PETRIE JG (eds): *Injuries of the Spine.* Baltimore, Williams & Wilkins, 1964, p 42 — 17–24

CLOWARD, RB: *Acute cervical spine injuries.* Clin Symp 1980, 32:2–32 — 17–24

Section IV (*continued*) | Plate Number

CLOWARD RB: *The anterior approach for removal of ruptured cervical discs.* J Neurosurg 1958, 15:602 — 17–24

CRUTCHFIELD WG: *Skeletal traction in the treatment of injuries to the cervical spine.* JAMA 1954, 155:29–32 — 17–24

CRUTCHFIELD WG: *Skeletal traction for dislocation of cervical spine. Report of a case.* South Surgeon 1933, 2:156–159 — 17–24

CUTLER RWP: *Head trauma.* Sci Am 1983, 11:3–4 — 1–16

DAY AL: *Aneurysms and arteriovenous fistulae of the intracavernous carotid artery and its branches.* In YOUMANS JR (ed): *Neurological Surgery.* Philadelphia, WB Saunders, 1981 — 1–16

DEBRUN G, LACOUR P, CARON JP, et al: *Detachable balloon and calibrated-leak balloon techniques in the treatment of cerebral vascular lesions.* J Neurosurg 1978, 49:635–649 — 1–16

DONOVAN WH, BEDBROOK G: *Comprehensive management of spinal cord injury.* Clin Symp 1982, 34:2–36 — 17–24

FISHER CM, KISTLER JP, DAVIS JM: *Relation of cerebral vasospasm to subarachnoid hemorrhage visualized by CT scanning.* Neurosurgery 1980, 6:1–9 — 1–16

FLEISCHER AJ, TINDALL GT: *Cerebral vasospasm following aneurysm rupture.* J Neurosurg 1980, 52:149–152 — 1–16

FRIEDMAN WA: *Head injuries.* Clin Symp 1983, 35:2–32 — 1–16

FRIEDMAN WA, DAY AL, QUISLING RG, et al: *Cervical carotid dissecting aneurysms.* Neurosurgery 1980, 7:207–214 — 1–16

FRIEDMAN WA, VRIES JK: *Percutaneous tunnel ventriculostomy: summary of 100 procedures.* J Neurosurg 1980, 53:662–665 — 1–16

FROST EAM: *The physiopathology of respiration in neurosurgical patients.* J Neurosurg 1979, 50:699–714 — 1–16

GIBSON CJ: *Spinal cord injury rehabilitation.* Arch Neurol 1985, 42:113 — 25

GUTTMANN L: *Spinal Cord Injuries – Comprehensive Management and Research*, ed 2. Oxford, Blackwell Scientific Publications, 1976 — 17–24

HARRIS JH JR: *The Radiology of Acute Cervical Spine Trauma.* Baltimore, Williams & Wilkins, 1978 — 17–24

HOOPER R: *Observations on extradural hemorrhage.* Br J Surg 1959, 47:71–87 — 1–16

JEFFERSON G: *Fracture of the atlas vertebra. Report of four cases, and a review of those previously recorded.* Br J Surg 1920, 7:407 — 17–24

KEMPE LG: *Operative Neurosurgery.* New York, Springer-Verlag, 1968 — 1–16

LANGFITT TW: *Measuring the outcome from head injuries.* J Neurosurg 1978, 48:673–678 — 1–16

MARSHALL LF, SMITH RW, SHAPIRO HM: *The outcome with aggressive treatment in severe head injuries.* J Neurosurg 1979, 50:20–30 — 1–16

MARTIN JB, REICHLIN S, BROWN GM: *Neural regulation of water and salt metabolism: physiologic function and disease.* In MARTIN J, et al: *Clinical Neuroendocrinology.* Philadelphia, FA Davis, 1977, pp 63–92 — 1–16

MCKISSOCK W, RICHARDSON A, BLOOM WH: *Subdural haematoma; a review of 389 cases.* Lancet 1960, 1:1365–1369 — 1–16

MCLAURIN RL: *Chronic subdural hematoma in infants.* Contemp Neurosurg 1980, 2:1–6 — 1–16

MUNRO D: *Treatment of Injuries to the Nervous System.* Philadelphia, WB Saunders, 1952 — 17–24

NELSON PB: *Etiology, recognition, and current*

Section IV (*continued*) | Plate Number

management of the syndrome of inappropriate secretion of antidiuretic hormone. Contemp Neurosurg 1980, 2:1–6 — 1–16

OSTERHOLM JL, MATTHEWS GJ: *Altered norepinephrine metabolism following experimental spinal cord injury.* J Neurosurg 1972, 36:386–394 — 17–24

PLUM F, POSNER JB: *The Diagnosis of Stupor and Coma.* Philadelphia, FA Davis, 1972 — 1–16

RHOTON AL JR: *Anatomy of saccular aneurysms.* Surg Neurol 1980, 14:59–66 — 1–16

ROGERS WA: *Treatment of fracture dislocation of the cervical spine.* J Bone Joint Surg 1942, 24:245–258 — 17–24

ROTHMAN RH, SIMEONE FA: *The Spine*, ed 20. Philadelphia, WB Saunders, 1982 — 17–24

SCHNEIDER RC: *Craniocerebral trauma.* In KAHN EA, CROSBY EC, SCHNEIDER RC, et al: *Correlative Neurosurgery.* Springfield IL, Charles C Thomas, 1969, pp 533–596 — 1–16

SCHNEIDER RC, CHERRY GH, PANTEK H: *Syndrome of acute central cervical cord injury with special reference to the mechanisms involved in hyperextension injuries of the cervical spine.* J Neurosurg 1954, 11:546–577 — 17–24

SMITH GW, ROBINSON RA: *The treatment of certain cervical spine disorders by anterior removal of the intervertebral disc and interbody fusion.* J Bone Joint Surg 1958, 40A:607–624 — 17–24

WOOLSEY RM: *Rehabilitation outcome following spinal cord injury.* Arch Neurol 1985, 42:116–119 — 25

YASHON D: *Spinal Injury.* New York, Appleton-Century-Crofts, 1978 — 17–24

Section V

BARONE BM, ELVIDGE AR: *Ependymomas. A clinical survey.* J Neurosurg 1970, 33:428–438 — 3–10, 14–15

BLACK P: *Brain metastasis: current status and recommended guidelines for management.* Neurosurgery 1979, 5:617–631 — 3–10, 14–15

BLACK P: *Spinal metastasis: current status and recommended guidelines for management.* Neurosurgery 1979, 5:726–746 — 3–10, 14–15

BOGGAN JE, TYRRELL JB, WILSON CB: *Transsphenoidal microsurgical management of Cushing's disease. Report of 100 cases.* J Neurosurg 1983, 59:195–200 — 3–10, 14–15

CIRIC I, MIKHAEL M, STAFFORD T, et al: *Transsphenoidal microsurgery of pituitary macroadenomas with long-term follow-up results.* J Neurosurg 1983, 59:395–401 — 3–10, 14–15

CUSHING H, EISENHARDT L: *Meningiomas.* New York, Hafner, 1969 — 3–10, 14–15

DONALDSON JO: *Pathogenesis of pseudotumor cerebri syndromes.* Neurology 1981, 31:877–880 — 2

DRAKE CG: *Total removal of large acoustic neuromas. A modification of the McKenzie operation with special emphasis on saving the facial nerve.* J Neurosurg 1967, 26:554–561 — 11–12

ERIKSSON B, GUNTERBERG B, KINDBLOM LG: *Chordoma: a clinicopathologic and prognostic study of a Swedish National Series.* Acta Orthop Scand 1981, 52:49–58 — 3–10, 14–15

FARIA MA JR, TINDALL GT: *Transsphenoidal microsurgery for prolactin-secreting pituitary adenomas: results in 100 women with the amenorrhea-galactorrhea syndrome.* J Neurosurg 1982, 56:33–43 — 3–10, 14–15

Section V (*continued*) | Plate Number

FISCH U: *Otoneurosurgical approach to acoustic neurinomas.* Prog Neurol Surg 1978, 9:328–336 — 11–12

FREIDBERG SR, HYBELS RL, OLIVER P: *Intranasal approach to the sella turcica.* Surg Neurol 1979, 12:145–146 — 3–10, 14–15

HARDY J: *Transsphenoidal hypophysectomy.* J Neurosurg 1971, 34:582–594 — 3–10, 14–15

HOUSE WF, LUETJE C: *Acoustic Tumors: Diagnosis and Management.* Vol 1: *Diagnosis.* Vol 2: *Management.* Baltimore, University Park Press, 1979. — 11–12

JOHNSTON I, PATERSON A: *Benign intracranial hypertension. II CSF pressure and circulation.* Brain 1974, 97:301–312 — 2

LAWS ER JR, PIEPGRAS DG, RANDALL RV, et al: *Neurosurgical management of acromegaly. Results in 82 patients treated between 1972 and 1977.* J Neurosurg 1979, 50:454–461 — 3–10, 14–15

NEWTON TH, POTTS DG (eds): *Modern Neuroradiology.* Vol 2: *Advanced Imaging Technique.* San Anselmo CA, Clavadel Press, 1983 — 17

PYKETT IL, NEWHOUSE JH, BUONANNO FS, et al: *Principles of nuclear magnetic resonance imaging.* Radiology 1982, 143:157–168 — 17

QUEST DO: *Meningiomas: an update.* Neurosurgery 1978, 3:219–225 — 3–10, 14–15

RAND RW, KURZE TL: *Facial nerve preservation by posterior fossa transmeatal microdissection in total removal of acoustic tumours.* J Neurol Neurosurg Psychiatry 1965, 28:311–316 — 11–12

RHOTON AL JR: *Microsurgery of the internal acoustic meatus.* Surg Neurol 1974, 2:311–318 — 11–12

ROSE A, MATSON DD: *Benign intracranial hypertension in children.* Pediatrics 1967, 39:227–237 — 2

SALCMAN M: *Survival in glioblastoma: historical perspective.* Neurosurgery 1980, 7:435–439 — 3–10, 14–15

STEIN BM: *Supracerebellar-infratentorial approach to pineal tumors.* Surg Neurol 1979, 11:331–337 — 3–10, 14–15

SWEET WH: *Radical surgical treatment of craniopharyngioma.* Clin Neurosurg 1976, 23:52–79 — 3–10, 14–15

TARLOV E: *Total one-stage suboccipital microsurgical removal of acoustic neuromas of all sizes: with emphasis on arachnoid planes and on saving the facial nerve.* Surg Clin North Am 1980, 60:565–591 — 11–12

WALKER MD, ALEXANDER E JR, HUNT WE, et al: *Evaluation of BCNU and/or radiotherapy in the treatment of anaplastic gliomas. A cooperative clinical trial.* J Neurosurg 1978, 49:333–343 — 3–10, 14–15

WEIR B, ELVIDGE AR: *Oligodendrogliomas. An analysis of 63 cases.* J Neurosurg 1968, 29:500–505 — 3–10, 14–15

WOLFSON RJ, SILVERSTEIN H, MARLOWE FI, et al: *Vertigo.* Clin Symp 1981, 33:2–32 — 11–12

YASARGIL MG, FOX JL: *The microsurgical approach to acoustic neurinomas.* Surg Neurol 1974, 2:393–398 — 11–12

Section VI

AMERICAN PSYCHIATRIC ASSOCIATION: *Psychiatry Update, II.* Part V: *Depressive Disorders*, Washington DC, APA, 1983, pp 354–548 — 1

AMERICAN PSYCHIATRIC ASSOCIATION: *Diagnostic and Statistical Manual of Mental Disorders*, ed 3. Washington DC, APA, 1980 — 1–6

Section VI (continued)

	Plate Number
CARR DB, SHEEHAN DV: *Panic anxiety: a new biological model.* J Clin Psychiatry 1984, 45:323–330	4
FALK WE, MAHNKE MW, POSKANZER DC: *Lithium prophylaxis of corticotropin-induced psychosis.* JAMA 1979, 241:1011–1012	3
GERSHON S (ed): *The many faces of anxiety – proceedings from a symposium.* J Clin Psychiatry 1981, 42:3	4
HACKETT, TP: *Disruptive states.* In HACKETT TP, CASSEM NH (eds): *Massachusetts General Hospital Handbook of General Hospital Psychiatry.* St Louis, CV Mosby, 1978	6
HAMILTON JA, PARRY BL, ALAGNA S, et al: *Premenstrual mood changes: a guide to evaluation and treatment.* Psychiatr Ann 1984, 14:426	2
JAMPALA VC, ABRAMS R: *Mania secondary to left and right hemisphere damage.* Am J Psychiatry 1983, 140:1197–1199	3
KAHN RL, ZARIT SH, HILBERT NM, et al: *Memory complaint and impairment in the aged. The effect of depression and altered brain function.* Arch Gen Psychiatry 1975, 32:1569–1573	1
MARSDEN CD, TARSY D, BALDESSARINI RJ: *Spontaneous and drug-induced movement disorders in psychotic patients.* In BENSON DF, BLUMER D (eds): *Psychiatric Aspects of Neurologic Disease.* New York, Grune & Stratton, 1975, pp 219–266	5
SHEEHAN DV: *Current concepts in psychiatry. Panic attacks and phobias.* N Engl J Med 1982, 307:156–158	4
SMITH JW: *Diagnosing alcoholism.* Hosp Community Psychiatry 1983, 34:1017–1026	2
STANTON AH: *Personality disorders.* In NICHOLI AM (ed): *The Harvard Guide to Modern Psychiatry.* Cambridge, Harvard University Press, 1978, pp 283–295	6
STRAUSS JS, CARPENTER WT: *Schizophrenia.* New York, Plenum Medical, 1981	5

Section VII

	Plate Number
ADAMS R, FISHER CM, HAKIM S, et al: *Symptomatic occult hydrocephalus with "normal" cerebrospinal-fluid pressure. A treatable syndrome.* N Engl J Med 1965, 273:117–126	7
ARON AM, FREEMAN JM, CARTER S: *The natural history of Sydenham's chorea. Review of the literature and long-term evaluation with emphasis on cardiac sequelae.* Am J Med 1965, 38:83–95	8
BECK J, BENSON F, SCHEIBEL A, et al: *Dementia in the elderly: the silent epidemic.* Ann Int Med 1982, 97:231–241	1
BERNHEIMER H, BIRKMAYER W, HORNYKIEWICZ O, et al: *Brain dopamine and the syndromes of Parkinson and Huntington: clinical, morphological, and neurochemical correlations.* J Neurol Sci 1973, 20:415–455	9–12
BIRD M, PAULSON G: *The rigid form of Huntington's chorea.* Neurology 1971, 21:271–276	8
CALNE DB: *Developments in the pharmacology and therapeutics of parkinsonism.* Ann Neurol 1977, 1:111–119	9–12
CAPLAN LR: *What can we offer elderly patients with intellectual decline?* Med Times 1980, 108:27–34	6

Section VII (continued)

	Plate Number
DUVOISIN RC: *Parkinson's Disease. A Guide for Patient and Family.* New York, Raven Press, 1978	9–12
FISHER CM: *Hydrocephalus as a cause of disturbances of gait in the elderly.* Neurology 1982, 32:1358–1363	7
FISHER CM: *Left hemiplegia and motor impersistence.* J Nerv Ment Dis 1956, 123:201–218	5
FOSTER N, CHASE T, FEDIO P, et al: *Alzheimer's disease: focal cortical changes shown by positron emission tomography.* Neurology 1983, 33:961–965	1
GAUTIER-SMITH PG: *Clinical aspects of hypoglycemia.* In CUMINGS J, KREMER M (eds): *Biochemical Aspects of Neurological Disorders,* Ser 2. Philadelphia, FA Davis, 1965	6
GESCHWIND N: *Current concepts: aphasia.* N Engl J Med 1971, 284:654–656	4
HIER DB, MONDLOCK J, CAPLAN LR: *Recovery of behavioral abnormalities after right hemisphere stroke.* Neurology 1983, 33:345–350	5
HIER DB, STEIN R, CAPLAN LR: *Cognitive and behavioral deficits after right hemisphere stroke.* Stroke 1985 (in press)	5
HOEHN MM, YAHR MD: *Parkinsonism: onset, progression and mortality.* Neurology 1967, 17:427–442	9–12
JACOBS L, KINKEL W: *Computerized axial transverse tomography in normal pressure hydrocephalus.* Neurology 1976, 26:501–507	7
JOYNT R, GOLDSTEIN M: *Minor cerebral hemisphere.* In FRIEDLANDER WJ (ed): *Current Reviews* (Advances in Neurology Ser, Vol 7). New York, Raven Press, 1975	5
KLEIST K: *Sensory Aphasia and Amusia.* New York, Pergamon Press, 1962	4
LURIA A: *Higher Cortical Functions in Man.* New York, Basic Books, 1966	3
MAGNAES B: *Communicating hydrocephalus in adults. Diagnostic tests and results of treatment with medium pressure shunts.* Neurology 1978, 28:478–484	7
MARTIN JB: *Huntington's disease: new approaches to an old problem. The Robert Wartenberg lecture.* Neurology 1984, 34:1059–1072	8
MCMENEMEY WH: *The dementias and progressive diseases of the basal ganglia.* In BLACKWOOD W, MCMENEMEY WH, MEYER A, et al (eds): *Greenfield's Neuropathology.* Baltimore, Williams & Wilkins, 1963, pp 520–576	2
MOHR JP, PESSIN MS, FINKELSTEIN S, et al: *Broca aphasia: pathologic and clinical.* Neurology 1978, 28:311–324	4
NAUSIEDA PA, KOLLER WC, WEINER W: *Chorea induced by oral contraceptives.* Neurology 1979, 29:1605–1609	8
NIELSEN J: *Agnosia, Apraxia, Aphasia.* New York, Hafner, 1965	4
RINNE UK, KLINGLER M, STAMM G (eds): *Parkinson's Disease: Current Progress, Problems, and Management.* New York, Elsevier North Holland, 1980	9–12
SMITH CM, SWASH M: *Possible biochemical basis of memory disorder in Alzheimer disease.* Ann Neurol 1978, 3:471–473	2
STRUB R, BLACK FW: *The Mental Status Examination in Neurology.* Philadelphia, FA Davis, 1977	3
TERRY R, KATZMAN R: *Senile dementia of the Alzheimer type.* Ann Neurol 1983, 14:497–506	1–2

Section VII (continued)

	Plate Number
TERRY R, PECK A, DETERESA R, et al: *Some morphometric aspects of the brain in senile dementia of the Alzheimer type.* Ann Neurol 1981, 10:184–192	1–2
TOMLINSON BE, BLESSED G, ROTH M: *Observations on the brains of demented old people.* J Neurol Sci 1970, 11:205–242	2
VINKEN P, BRUYN G (eds): *Disorders of Speech, Perception and Symbolic Behavior. Handbook of Clinical Neurology,* Vol 4. Amsterdam, North Holland, 1969	3
WELLS C: *Dementia.* Philadelphia, FA Davis, 1971	6

Section VIII

	Plate Number
APPELBAUM E, KREPS SI, SUNSHINE A: *Herpes zoster encephalitis.* Am J Med 1962, 32:25	11
BAKER AS: *Spinal epidural abscess.* In BRAUDE AI, DAVIS CE, FIERER J (eds): *International Textbook of Medicine. Medical Microbiology and Infectious Disease, II.* Philadelphia, WB Saunders, 1981, pp 1292–1296	3
BAKER AS: *Subdural empyema.* In BRAUDE AI, DAVIS CE, FIERER J (eds): *International Textbook of Medicine. Medical Microbiology and Infectious Disease, II.* Philadelphia, WB Saunders, 1981, pp 1296–1299	3
BAKER AS, OJEMANN RG, SWARTZ MN, et al: *Spinal epidural abscess.* N Engl J Med 1975, 293:463–468	3
BLACKWOOD W, CORSELLIS JAN (eds): *Greenfield's Neuropathology,* ed 3. Chicago, Year Book Medical, 1976	6
CASTLEMAN B, SCULLY RE, MCNEELY BU (eds): *Case records of the Massachusetts General Hospital.* N Engl J Med 1974, 290:1130–1136	7
DAVIDOFF RA: *Tetanus.* In SCHEINBERG P (ed): *Neurology and Neurosurgery, II.* Princeton, Biomedia, 1979	8
DAVIDSON PT, HOROWITZ I: *Skeletal tuberculosis: a review with patient presentations and discussion.* Am J Med 1970, 48:77–84	7
DIAMOND RD: *Cryptococcus neoformans.* In MANDELL GL, DOUGLAS RG JR, BENNETT JE (eds): *Principles and Practice of Infectious Diseases,* ed 2. New York, John Wiley, 1985, pp 1460–1468	5
GAJDUSEK DG: *Unconventional viruses and the origin and disappearance of Kuru.* Science 1977, 197:943–960	12–13
GOFFINET DR, GLATSTEIN EJ, MERIGAN TC: *Herpes zoster-varicella infections and lymphoma.* Ann Intern Med 1972, 76:235–240	11
JOHNSON RT: *Viral Infections of the Nervous System.* New York, Raven Press, 1982	12–13
KERNBAUM S, HAUCHECORNE J: *Administration of levodopa for relief of herpes zoster pain.* JAMA 1981, 246:132–134	11
MEDOFF G: *Cryptococcal meningitis.* In BRAUDE AI, DAVIS CE, FIERER J (eds): *International Textbook of Medicine. Medical Microbiology and Infectious Diseases, II.* Philadelphia, WB Saunders, 1981, pp 1248–1251	5
NASH TE, NEVA FA: *Current concepts. Recent advances in the diagnosis and treatment of cerebral cysticercosis.* N Engl J Med 1984, 311:1492–1496	4
PETERSLUND NA, IPSEN J, SCHONHEYDER H, et al: *Acyclovir in herpes zoster.* Lancet 1981, 8251:827–830	11

REMINGTON JS, McLEOD R: *Toxoplasmosis.* In BRAUDE AI, DAVIS CE, FIERER J (eds): *International Textbook of Medicine. Medical Microbiology and Infectious Diseases, II.* Philadelphia, WB Saunders, 1981, pp 1816–1832   5

RISK WS, BOSCH EP, KIMURA J, et al: *Chronic tetanus: clinical report and histochemistry of muscle.* Muscle Nerve 1981, 4:363–366   8

SABIN AB: *Paralytic poliomyelitis: old dogmas and new perspectives.* Rev Inf Dis 1981, 3:543–564   9–10

SABIN AB: *Vaccination against poliomyelitis in economically underdeveloped countries.* Bull WHO 1980, 58:141–157   9–10

SABIN AB: *Oral poliovirus vaccine. History of its development and prospects for eradication of poliomyelitis.* JAMA 1965, 194:872–876   9–10

SABIN AB: *Pathogenesis of poliomyelitis: reappraisal in the light of new data.* Science 1956, 123:1151–1157   9–10

SABIN AB: *Pathology and pathogenesis of human poliomyelitis.* JAMA 1942, 120:506–511   9–10

SCHELD WM, WINN HR: *Brain abscess.* In MANDELL GL, DOUGLAS RG, BENNETT GE (eds): *Principles and Practice of Infectious Diseases,* ed 2. New York, John Wiley, 1985   3

SCULLY RE, MARK EJ, McNEELY BU (eds): *Case records of the Massachusetts General Hospital.* N Engl J Med 1982, 306:91–97   7

SIMON HB: *Mycobacteria.* In RUBENSTEIN E, FEDERMAN DD (eds): *Scientific American Medicine,* Vol 7, Sec VIII. New York, Scientific American, 1984, pp 1–16   7

SIMON HB, SWARTZ MN, WELLER PF: *Protozoan infections.* In RUBENSTEIN E, FEDERMAN DD (eds): *Scientific American Medicine,* Vol 7, Sec XXXIV. Scientific American, 1985, pp 1–18   4

SOTELLO J, ESCOBEDO F, RODRIGUEZ-CARBAJAL J, et al: *Therapy of parenchymal brain cysticercosis with praziquantel.* N Engl J Med 1984, 310:1001–1007   4

STRUPPLER A, STRUPPLER E, ADAMS RD: *Local tetanus in man: its clinical and neurophysiological characteristics.* Arch Neurol 1963, 8:162–178   8

SWARTZ MN: *Infections.* In RUBENSTEIN E, FEDERMAN DD (eds): *Scientific American Medicine,* Vol 11, Sec VIII. Scientific American, 1982, pp 1–27   1–3

TERMEULEN V, HALL WW: *Slow virus infections of the nervous system: immunological and pathogenetic considerations.* J Gen Virol 1978, 41:1–25   12–13

THOMAS JE, HOWARD FM JR: *Segmental zoster paresis – a disease profile.* Neurology 1972, 22:459   11

WATSON CP, EVANS RJ, REED K, et al: *Amitriptyline versus placebo in postherpetic neuralgia.* Neurology 1982, 32:671–673   11

WHITLEY RJ, SOONG SJ, LINNENAN C JR, et al: *Herpes simplex encephalitis. Clinical assessment.* JAMA 1982, 247:317–320   12–13

Section IX

ADAMS RD, KUBIK CS: *Symposium on multiple sclerosis and demyelinating diseases: morbid anatomy of demyelinative diseases.* Am J Med 1952, 12:510–546   1–4

ANTEL JP (ed): *Multiple Sclerosis. Neurologic Clinics, I.* Philadelphia, WB Saunders, 1983   1, 4

BEHAN PO, MOORE MJ, LAMARCHE JB: *Acute necrotizing hemorrhagic encephalopathy.* Postgrad Med 1973, 54:154–160   5

BERS RK: *Acute hemorrhagic leukoencephalitis: report of three cases and review of the literature.* Pediatrics 1975, 56:727–735   5

LUKES SA, NORMAN D: *Computed tomography in acute disseminated encephalomyelitis.* Ann Neurol 1983, 13:567–572   5

McALPINE D, LUMSDEN C, ACHESON ED: *Multiple Sclerosis, a Reappraisal.* Baltimore, Williams & Wilkins, 1972   1, 4

MOORE MJ, BEHAN PO, KIES MW, et al: *Reaginic antibody in experimental allergic encephalomyelitis. I. Characterization of heat-labile skin-fixing antibody.* Res Commun Chem Pathol Pharmacol 1974, 9:119–132   5

SUCHOWERSKY O, SWEENEY VP, BERRY K, et al: *Acute hemorrhagic leukoencephalopathy: a clinical, pathological, and radiological correlation.* Can J Neurol Sci 1983, 10:63–67   5

Section X

AMERICAN PSYCHIATRIC ASSOCIATION: *Diagnostic and Statistical Manual of Mental Disorders,* ed 3. Washington DC, APA, 1980, pp 241–252, 285–290   16

AMINOFF MJ, LOGUE V: *Clinical features of spinal vascular malformations.* Brain 1974, 97:197–210   3–4

BAKER AS, OJEMANN RG, SWARTZ MN, et al: *Spinal epidural abscess.* N Engl J Med 1975, 293:463–468   3–4

BASTRON JA, THOMAS JE: *Diabetic polyradiculopathy: clinical and electromyographic findings in 105 patients.* Mayo Clin Proc 1981, 56:725–732   18

BERMAN M, FELDMAN S, ALTER M, et al: *Acute transverse myelitis: incidence and etiologic considerations.* Neurology 1981, 31:966–971   3–4

BLACK RG: *The chronic pain syndrome.* Surg Clin North Am 1975, 55:999–1011   16

BLAU JN, LOGUE V: *The natural history of intermittent claudication of the cauda equina: a long term follow-up study.* Brain 1978, 101:211–222   17

BRADLEY WG, CHAD D, VERGHESE JP, et al: *Painful lumbosacral plexopathy with elevated erythrocyte sedimentation rate: a treatable inflammatory syndrome.* Ann Neurol 1984, 15:457–464   19

CASCINO TL, KORI S, KROL G, et al: *CT of the brachial plexus in patients with cancer.* Neurology 1983, 33:1553–1557   19

DEMYER W: *Anatomy and clinical neurology of the spinal cord.* In BAKER AB, BAKER LH: *Clinical Neurology, III.* Philadelphia, Harper Medical, 1984, pp 1–24   1–2

DROSSMAN DA: *The problem patient: evaluation and care of medical patients with psychosocial disturbances.* Ann Intern Med 1978, 88:366–372   16

EMERY S, OCHOA J: *Lumbar plexus neuropathy resulting from retroperitoneal hemorrhage.* Muscle Nerve 1978, 1:330–334   19

EVANS BA, STEVENS JC, DYCK PJ: *Lumbosacral plexus neuropathy.* Neurology 1981, 31:1327–1330   19

FARFAN HF: *A reorientation in the surgical approach to degenerative lumbar intervertebral*

joint disease. Orthop Clin North Am 1977, 8:9–21   14–15

GREENBERG HS, KIM J-H, POSNER JB: *Epidural spinal cord compression from metastatic tumor: results with a new treatment protocol.* Ann Neurol 1980, 8:361–366   3–4

JAECKLE KA, YOUNG DF, FOLEY KM: *The natural history of lumbosacral plexopathy in cancer.* Neurology 1985, 35:8–15   19

KAVANAUGH GJ, SVIEN HJ, HOLMAN CB, et al: *"Pseudoclaudication" syndrome produced by compression of the cauda equina.* JAMA 1968, 206:2477   17

KEIM HA: *Diagnostic problems in the lumbar spine.* Clin Neurosurg 1978, 25:184–192   14–15

KIKTA DG, BREUER AC, WILBOURN AJ: *Thoracic root pain in diabetes: the spectrum of clinical and electromyographic findings.* Ann Neurol 1982, 11:80–85   18

KIRKALDY-WILLIS WH, HILL RJ: *A more precise diagnosis for low-back pain.* Spine 1979, 4:102–109   14–15

KORI SH, FOLEY KM, POSNER JB: *Brachial plexus lesions in patients with cancer: 100 cases.* Neurology 1981, 31:45–50   19

LAST RJ: *Innervation of limbs.* J Bone Joint Surg 1949, 31:452–464   14–15

LEDERMAN RJ, WILBOURN AJ: *Brachial plexopathy: recurrent cancer or radiation?* Neurology 1984, 34:1331–1335   19

MALIS LI: *Intramedullary spinal cord tumors.* Clin Neurosurg 1978, 25:512–540   5–6

MANCALL E: *Combined system disease.* In ROWLAND LP, et al (eds): *Merritt's Textbook of Neurology: Memorial Edition.* Philadelphia, Lea & Febiger, 1984   9

McILROY WJ, RICHARDSON JC: *Syringomyelia: a clinical review of 75 cases.* Can Med Assoc J 1965, 93:731–734   8

McQUARRIE IG: *Recovery from paraplegia caused by spontaneous spinal epidural hematoma.* Neurology 1978, 28:224–228   3–4

MEYER FB, EBERSOLD MJ, REESE DF: *Benign tumors of the foramen magnum.* J Neurosurg 1984, 61:136–142   3–4

RICE EDWARDS JM: *A pathologic study of syringomyelia.* J Neurol Neurosurg Psychiatry 1977, 40:198   8

RODRIGUEZ M, DINAPOLI RP: *Spinal cord compression with special reference to metastatic epidural tumors.* Mayo Clin Proc 1980, 55:442–448   3–4

ROPPER AH, POSKANZER DC: *The prognosis of acute and subacute transverse myelopathy based on early signs and symptons.* Ann Neurol 1978, 4:51–59   3–4

SILVER JR, BUXTON PH: *Spinal stroke.* Brain 1974, 97:539–550   3–4

SIMKIN PA: *Simian stance: a sign of spinal stenosis.* Lancet 1982, 8297:652–653   17

SPANOS NC, ANDREW J: *Intermittent claudication and lateral lumbar disc protrusions.* J Neurol Neurosurg Psychiatry 1966, 29:273   17

STEEGMANN AT: *Syndrome of the anterior spinal artery.* Neurology 1952, 2:15–35   3–4

SUBRAMONY SH, WILBOURN AJ: *Diabetic proximal neuropathy: clinical and electromyographic studies.* J Neurol Sci 1982, 53:293–304   18

THOMAS JE, CASCINO TL, EARLE JD: *Differential diagnosis between radiation and tumor plexopathy of the pelvis.* Neurology 1985, 35:1–7   19

Section X (continued)

	Plate Number
TSAIRIS P, DYCK PJ, MULDER DW: *Natural history of brachial plexus neuropathy. Report on 99 patients.* Arch Neurol 27:109–117	19
WEIR B, DE LEO R: *Lumbar stenosis: analysis of factors affecting outcome in 81 surgical cases.* Can J Neurol Sci 1981, 8:295	17
WILKINSON M: *Cervical Spondylosis.* Philadelphia, WB Saunders, 1971	10

Section XI

	Plate Number
ACCARDO PJ: *An early case report of muscular dystrophy: a footnote to the history of neuromuscular disorders.* Arch Neurol 1981, 38:144	24–25
ADOUR KK: *Current concepts in neurology: diagnosis and management of facial paralysis.* N Engl J Med 1982, 307:348–351	8
ALLSOP KG, ZITER FA: *Loss of strength and functional decline in Duchenne's dystrophy.* Arch Neurol 1981, 38:406–411	24–25
ANGELINI C, FREDDO L, BATTISTELLA P, et al: *Carnitine palmityl transferase deficiency: clinical variability, carrier detection, and autosomal-recessive inheritance.* Neurology 1981, 31:883–886	32
ANGELINI C, GOVONI E, BRAGAGLIA MM, et al: *Carnitine deficiency: acute postpartum crisis.* Neurology 1978, 4:558–561	32
ARCHER AG, WATKINS PJ, THOMAS PK, et al: *Natural history of acute painful neuropathy in diabetes mellitus.* J Neurol Neurosurg Psychiatry 1983, 46:491–499	11
ARGOV Z, MASTAGLIA FL: *Drug-induced peripheral neuropathies.* Br Med J 1979, 1:663–666	11
ARNASON BGW: *Acute inflammatory demyelinating polyradiculoneuropathies.* In DYCK PJ, THOMAS PK, LAMBERT EH, et al (eds): *Peripheral Neuropathy, II,* ed 2. Philadelphia, WB Saunders, 1984, chap 90	15
ASBURY AK: *Diagnostic considerations in Guillain-Barré syndrome.* Ann Neurol (Suppl) 1981, 9:1–5	15
ASBURY AK, ARNASON BG, ADAMS, RD: *The inflammatory lesion in idiopathic polyneuritis: its role in pathogenesis.* Medicine 1969, 48:173	15
ASKARI A, VIGNOS PJ JR, MOSKOWITZ RW: *Steroid myopathy in connective tissue disease.* Am J Med 1976, 61:485	31
AUERBACH SH, DEPIERO TJ, MEJLSZENKIER J: *Familial recurrent peripheral facial palsy: observations of the pediatric population.* Arch Neurol 1981, 38:463–464	8
BARINGER JR, TOWNSEND JJ: *Herpesvirus infection of the peripheral nervous system.* In DYCK PJ, THOMAS PK, LAMBERT EH, et al (eds): *Peripheral Neuropathy, II,* ed 2. Philadelphia, WB Saunders, 1984, chap 83	11
BARNES BE: *Dermatomyositis and malignancy: a review of the literature.* Ann Intern Med 1976, 84:68–76	28–29
BECHELLI LM, MARTÍNEZ DOMÍNGUEZ V: *The leprosy problem in the world.* Bull Wld Hlth Org 1966, 34:811–826	19
BEHSE F, BUCHTHAL F: *Alcoholic neuropathy: clinical, electrophysiological, and biopsy findings.* Ann Neurol 1977, 2:95–110	11
BOHAN A, PETER JB: *Polymyositis and dermatomyositis.* N Engl J Med 1975, 292:344–347, 403–407	28–29

Section XI (continued)

	Plate Number
BOLTON CF: *Electrophysiologic changes in uremic neuropathy after successful renal transplantation.* Neurology 1976, 26:152–161	11
BRADLEY WG, KELEMEN J: *Genetic counseling in Duchenne muscular dystrophy.* Muscle Nerve 1979, 2:325–328	24–25
BROWN MJ, ASBURY AK: *Diabetic neuropathy.* Ann Neurol 1984, 15:2–12	11
BUNCH TW: *Prednisone and azathioprine for polymyositis: long-term follow-up.* Arthritis Rheum 1981, 24:45–48	28–29
CASEY EB, JELLIFE AM, LE QUESNE PM, et al: *Vincristine neuropathy: clinical and electrophysiological observations.* Brain 1973, 96:69–86	11
COCHRANE RG, DAVEY TF (eds): *Leprosy in Theory and Practice,* ed 2. Baltimore, William & Wilkins, 1964	19
COËRS C, TELERMAN-TOPPET N: *Differential diagnosis of limb-girdle muscular dystrophy and spinal muscular atrophy.* Neurology 1979, 29:957–972	26
COMI G, TESTA D, CORNELIO F, et al: *Potassium depletion myopathy: a clinical and morphological study of six cases.* Muscle Nerve 1985, 8:17–21	30
CRISP DE, ZITER FA, BRAY PF: *Diagnostic delay in Duchenne's muscular dystrophy.* JAMA 1982, 247:478–480	24–25
DALAKAS MC, ENGEL WK: *Chronic relapsing (dysimmune) polyneuropathy: pathogenesis and treatment.* Ann Neurol (Suppl) 1981, 9:134–145	15
DALAKAS MC, ENGEL WK: *Polyneuropathy with monoclonal gammopathy. studies of 11 patients.* Ann Neurol 1981, 10:45–52	12
DAU PC: *Response to plasmapheresis and immunosuppressant therapy in sixty myasthenia gravis patients.* Ann NY Acad Sci 1981, 377:700–708	20–22
DAU PC, DENYS EH: *Plasmapheresis and immunosuppressive drug therapy in the Eaton-Lambert syndrome.* Ann Neurol 1982, 11:570–575	23
DEVERE R, BRADLEY WG: *Polymyositis: its presentation, morbidity and mortality.* Brain 1975, 98:637–666	28–29
DIMAURO S: *Metabolic myopathies: disorders of glycogen and lipid metabolism.* In SCHEINBERG P (ed): *Neurology and Neurosurgery, III.* Princeton, CPEC, 1982	32
DIMAURO S, DALAKAS M, MARANDA AF: *Phosphoglycerate kinase deficiency: another cause of recurrent myoglobinuria.* Ann Neurol 1983, 13:11–19	33
DIMAURO S, TREVISAN C, HAYS A: *Disorders of lipid metabolism in muscle.* Muscle Nerve 1980, 3:369–388	32
DRACHMAN DB: *Myasthenia gravis.* N Engl J Med 1978, 298:136–142	20–22
DUBOWITZ V: *The female carrier of Duchenne muscular dystrophy.* Br Med J 1982, 284:1423	24–25
DUBOWITZ V (illus): *Muscle Biopsy: A Practical Approach.* Philadelphia, WB Saunders, 1973, pp 5–33	3–4
DUBOWITZ V, CROME L: *The central nervous system in Duchenne muscular dystrophy.* Brain 1969, 92:805–808	24–25
DYCK PJ: *Neuronal atrophy and degeneration predominantly affecting peripheral sensory and autonomic neurons.* In DYCK PJ, THOMAS PK, LAMBERT EH, et al (eds): *Peripheral Neuropa-*	

Section XI (continued)

	Plate Number
thy, II, ed 2. Philadelphia, WB Saunders, 1984, chap 68	18
DYCK PJ, ARNASON B: *Chronic inflammatory demyelinating polyradiculoneuropathy.* In DYCK PJ, THOMAS PK, LAMBERT EH, et al (eds): *Peripheral Neuropathy, II,* ed 2. Philadelphia, WB Saunders, 1984, chap 91	15
DYCK PJ, JOHNSON WJ, LAMBERT EH, et al: *Comparison of symptoms, chemistry, and nerve function to assess adequacy of hemodialysis.* Neurology 1979, 29:1361–1368	11
DYCK PJ, LAMBERT EH, MULDER DW: *Charcot-Marie-Tooth disease: nerve conduction and clinical studies of a large kinship.* Neurology 1963, 13:1	16–17
DYCK PJ, LOW PA, STEVENS JC: *"Burning feet" as the only manifestation of dominantly inherited sensory neuropathy.* Mayo Clin Proc 1983, 58:426–429	18
DYCK PJ, MELLINGER JF, REAGAN TJ, et al: *Not "indifference to pain" but varieties of hereditary sensory and autonomic neuropathy.* Brain 1983, 106:373–390	18
DYCK PJ, STEVENS JC, O'BRIEN PC, et al: *Neurogenic arthropathy and recurring fractures with subclinical inherited neuropathy.* Neurology 1983, 33:357–367	18
DYCK PJ, THOMAS PK, LAMBERT EH, et al (eds): *Peripheral Neuropathy, I & II,* ed 2. Philadelphia, WB Saunders, 1984	1–34
ENG GD, BECKER MJ, MULDOON SM: *Electrodiagnostic tests in the detection of malignant hyperthermia.* Muscle Nerve 1984, 7:618–625	33
ENGEL AG: *Myasthenia gravis and myasthenic syndromes.* Ann Neurol 1984, 16:519–534	20–22
ENGEL AG: *Metabolic and endocrine myopathies.* In WALTON J (ed): *Disorders of Voluntary Muscle,* ed 4. New York, Churchill Livingstone, 1981	30
ENGEL AG, LAMBERT EH, HOWARD FM JR: *Immune complexes (IgG and C3) at the motor end-plate in myasthenia gravis: ultrastructural and light microscopic localization and electrophysiologic correlations.* Mayo Clin Proc 1977, 52:267–280	20–22
ENGEL AG, LAMBERT EH, ROSEVEAR JW, et al: *Clinical and electromyographic studies in a patient with primary hypokalemic periodic paralysis.* Am J Med 1965, 38:626	30
ENGEL AG, SIEKERT RG: *Lipid storage myopathy responsive to prednisone.* Arch Neurol 1972, 27:174–181	32
FEINGLASS EJ: *Arsenic intoxication from well water in the United States.* N Engl J Med 1973, 288:828–830	13
FELDMAN RG, NILES CA, KELLY-HAYES M, et al: *Peripheral neuropathy in arsenic smelter workers.* Neurology 1979, 29:939–944	13
FINE EJ, HALLETT M: *Neurophysiological study of subacute combined degeneration.* J Neurol Sci 1980, 45:331–336	11
FUKUNAGA H, ENGEL AG, OSAME M, et al: *Paucity and disorganization of presynaptic membrane active zones in the Lambert-Eaton myasthenic syndrome.* Muscle Nerve 1982, 5:686–697	23
GALANT EM, AHERN CP: *Malignant hyperthermia: responses of skeletal muscles to general anesthetics.* Mayo Clin Proc 1983, 58:758–763	33
GIMÉNEZ-ROLDÁN S, ESTEBAN A: *Prognosis in hereditary amyotrophic lateral sclerosis.* Arch Neurol 1977, 34:706–708	5–7

Section XI (*continued*)

	Plate Number
GOODGOLD J, EBERSTEIN A: *Electrodiagnosis of Neuromuscular Diseases*, ed 3. Baltimore, Williams & Wilkins, 1983	24−25
GRIGGS RC: *Periodic paralysis*. In SCHEINBERG P (ed): *Neurology and Neurosurgery, IV*. Princeton, CPEC, 1983	30
GRIGGS RC, ENGEL WK, RESNICK JS: *Acetazolamide treatment of hypokalemic periodic paralysis*. Ann Intern Med 1970, 73:39−48	30
GRIGGS RC, MENDELL JR, BROOKE MH, et al: *Clinical investigation in Duchenne dystrophy: V. use of creatine kinase and pyruvate kinase in carrier detection*. Muscle Nerve 1985, 8:60−67	24−25
GROSSMAN RA, HAMILTON RW, MORSE BM, et al: *Nontraumatic rhabdomyolysis and acute renal failure*. N Engl J Med 1974, 291:807−811	33
HARDING AE, THOMAS PK: *The clinical features of hereditary motor and sensory neuropathy types I and II*. Brain 1980, 103:259−280	16−17
HAUSER WA, KARNES WE, ANNIS J, et al: *Incidence and prognosis of Bell's palsy in the population of Rochester, Minnesota*. Mayo Clin Proc 1971, 46:258−264	8
HAWLEY RJ, KURTZKE JF, ARMBRUSTMACHER VW, et al: *The course of alcoholic-nutritional peripheral neuropathy*. Acta Neurol Scand 1982, 66:582−589	11
HENSON RA, URICH H: *Cancer and the Nervous System: The Neurological Manifestations of Systemic Malignancy*. St Louis, CV Mosby, 1982	11
HEYMAN A, PFEIFFER JB JR, WILLETT RW, et al: *Peripheral neuropathy caused by arsenical intoxication: a study of 41 cases with observations on the effects of BAL (2,3, dimercaptopropanol)*. N Engl J Med 1956, 254:401−409	13
HOHLFELD R, TOYKA KV, BESINGER UA, et al: *Myasthenia gravis: reactivation of clinical disease and of autoimmune factors after discontinuation of long-term azathioprine*. Ann Neurol 1985, 17:238−242	20−22
HUGHES JM, BLUMENTHAL JR, MERSON MH, et al: *Clinical features of types A and B food-borne botulism*. Ann Intern Med 1981, 95:442−445	34
HUGHES JM, MERSON MH: *Current concepts. Fish and shellfish poisoning*. N Engl J Med 1976, 295:1117−1120	34
HUGHES JM, TACKET CO: *"Sausage poisoning" revisited*. Arch Intern Med 1983, 143:425−427	34
HUGHES RAC, KADLUBOWSKI M, HUFSCHMIDT A: *Treatment of acute inflammatory polyneuropathy*. Ann Neurol (Suppl) 1981, 9:125−133	15
HUTTON JT, CHRISTIANS BL, DIPPEL RL: *Arsenic poisoning*. N Engl J Med 1982, 307:1080	13
JABLECKI C: *Lambert-Eaton myasthenic syndrome*. Muscle Nerve 1984, 7:250−257	23
JONES HR JR: *Arsenic and antique copper: a potential source for intoxication and development of peripheral neuropathy*. Ann Neurol 1981, 9:93	13
JONES HR JR: *Acute ataxia associated with ciguatera-type (grouper) tropical fish poisoning*. Ann Neurol 1980, 7:491	34
JUERGENS SM, KURLAND LT, OKAZAKI H, et al: *ALS in Rochester, Minnesota, 1925−1977*. Neurology 1980, 30:463−470	5−7
KAESER HE: *Drug-induced myasthenic syndromes*. Acta Neurol Scand (Suppl) 1984, 70:39−47	20−22

Section XI (*continued*)

	Plate Number
KARNES WE: *Diseases of the seventh cranial nerve*. In DYCK PJ, THOMAS PK, LAMBERT EH, et al (eds): *Peripheral Neuropathy, II*, ed 2. Philadelphia, WB Saunders, 1984, chap 55	8
KARPATI G: *The principles of skeletal muscle histochemistry*. In VINKEN PJ, BRUYN GW (eds): *Handbook of Clinical Neurology*, Vol 40. Amsterdam, North Holland, 1979, pp 1−61	3−4
KATRAK SM, POLLOCK M, O'BRIEN CP, et al: *Clinical and morphological features of gold neuropathy*. Brain 1980, 103:671−693	11
KELLY JJ JR: *Peripheral neuropathies associated with monoclonal proteins: a clinical review*. Muscle Nerve 1985, 8:138−150	12
KELLY JJ JR: *The electrodiagnostic findings in peripheral neuropathy associated with monoclonal gammopathy*. Muscle Nerve 1983, 6:504−509	12
KELLY JJ JR, KYLE RA, MILES JM, et al: *Osteosclerotic myeloma and peripheral neuropathy*. Neurology 1983, 33:202−210	12
KELLY JJ JR, KYLE RA, MILES JM, et al: *The spectrum of peripheral neuropathy in myeloma*. Neurology 1981, 31:24−31	12
KELLY JJ JR, KYLE RA, O'BRIEN PC, et al: *The natural history of peripheral neuropathy in primary systemic amyloidosis*. Ann Neurol 1979, 6:1−7	12
KHALEELI AA, LEVY RD, EDWARDS RHT, et al: *The neuromuscular features of acromegaly: a clinical and pathological study*. J Neurol Neurosurg Psychiatry 1984, 47:1009−1015	31
KIMURA J: *Nerve conduction studies and electromyography*. In DYCK PJ, THOMAS PK, LAMBERT EH, et al (eds): *Peripheral Neuropathy, I*, ed 2. Philadelphia, WB Saunders, 1984, chap 41	2
KNOCHEL JP: *Neuromuscular manifestations of electrolyte disorders*. Am J Med 1982, 72:521	30
KROL TC, MULLEN GM: *Herpes zoster with facial paralysis: an unusual manifestation*. Arch Neurol 1980, 37:391	8
KUHN E, FIEHN W, SEILER D, et al: *The autosomal recessive (Becker) form of myotonia congenita*. Muscle Nerve 1979, 2:109−117	27
LANG B, NEWSOM-DAVIS J, WRAY D, et al: *Autoimmune aetiology for myasthenic (Eaton-Lambert) syndrome*. Lancet 1981, 8240:224−226	23
LE QUESNE PM: *Neurophysiological investigation of subclinical and minimal toxic neuropathies*. Muscle Nerve 1978, 1:392−395	11
LINDSTROM JM, SEYBOLD ME, LENNON VA, et al: *Antibody to acetylcholine receptor in myasthenia gravis. Prevalence, clinical correlates and diagnostic value*. Neurology 1976, 26:1054−1059	20−22
LOVELACE RE: *Mononeuritis multiplex in polyarteritis nodosa*. Neurology 1964, 14:434−442	14
MacDONALD KL, SPENGLER RF, HATHEWAY CL, et al: *Type A botulism from sauteed onions. Clinical and epidemiologic observations*. JAMA 1985, 253:1275−1278	34
MALLETTE LE, PATTEN BM, ENGEL WK: *Neuromuscular disease in secondary hyperparathyroidism*. Ann Intern Med 1975, 82:474−483	31
MASTAGLIA FL, OJEDA VJ: *Inflammatory myopathies: part 1*. Ann Neurol 1985, 17:215−227	28−29
MASTAGLIA FL, OJEDA VJ: *Inflammatory myopathies: part 2*. Ann Neurol 1985, 18:317	28−29
MAYO CLINIC PROCEEDINGS: *Inherited neuropathies*. Mayo Clin Proc 1983, 58:476−480	16−17

Section XI (*continued*)

	Plate Number
MCARDLE B: *Metabolic myopathies: the glycogenoses affecting muscle, and hypo- and hyperkalemic periodic paralysis*. Am J Med 1963, 35:661−672	32
MCCOMBE PA, MCLEOD JG: *The peripheral neuropathy of vitamin B_{12} deficiency*. J Neurol Sci 1984, 66:117−126	11
MERTENS HG, HERTEL G, REUTHER P, et al: *Effect of immunosuppressive drugs (azathioprine)*. Ann NY Acad Sci 1981, 377:691−698	20−22
MILLER RG: *The cubital tunnel syndrome: diagnosis and precise localization*. Ann Neurol 1979, 6:56−59	10
MOORE PM, CUPPS TR: *Neurological complications of vasculitis*. Ann Neurol 1983, 14:155−167	14
MULDER DW: *Motor neuron disease*. In DYCK PJ, THOMAS, PK, LAMBERT EH, et al (eds): *Peripheral Neuropathy, II*, ed 2. Philadelphia, WB Saunders, 1984, chap 66	5−7
MULDER DW, HOWARD FM JR: *Patient resistance and prognosis in amyotrophic lateral sclerosis*. May Clin Proc 1976, 51:537	5−7
MUMENTHALER M, NARAKAS A, GILLIATT RW: *Brachial plexus disorders*. In DYCK PJ, THOMAS PK, LAMBERT EH, et al (eds): *Peripheral Neuropathy, II*, ed 2. Philadelphia, WB Saunders, 1984, chap 60	5−7
MURRAY TJ: *Congenital sensory neuropathy*. Brain 1973, 96:387−394	18
NAKANO KK: *The entrapment neuropathies*. Muscle Nerve 1978, 1:264−279	10
NELSON TE, FLEWELLEN EH: *Current concepts. The malignant hyperthermia syndrome*. N Engl J Med 1983, 309:416−418	33
NUKADA H, POLLOCK M, HAAS LF: *The clinical spectrum and morphology of type II hereditary sensory neuropathy*. Brain 1982, 105:647−665	18
PICKETT JBE III, LAYZER RB, LEVIN SR, et al: *Neuromuscular complications of acromegaly*. Neurology 1975, 25:638−645	31
POLGAR JG, BRADLEY WG, UPTON ARM, et al: *The early detection of dystrophia myotonica*. Brain 1972, 95:761−776	27
POLLARD JD, MCLEOD JG, HONNIBAL TG, et al: *Hypothyroid polyneuropathy. Clinical electrophysiological and nerve biopsy findings in two cases*. J Neurol Sci 1982, 53:461−471	11
RAFF MC, SANGALANG V, ASBURY AK: *Ischemic mononeuropathy multiplex associated with diabetes mellitus*. Arch Neurol 1968, 18:487	14
RAPOPORT S, WATKINS PB: *Descending paralysis resulting from occult wound botulism*. Ann Neurol 1984, 16:359−361	34
RIGGS JE, GRIGGS RC, MOXLEY RT III, et al: *Acute effects of acetazolamide in hyperkalemic periodic paralysis*. Neurology 1981, 31:725−729	30
RINGEL SP, CARROLL JE, SCHOLD SC: *The spectrum of mild X-linked recessive muscular dystrophy*. Arch Neurol 1977, 34:408−416	24−25
RODRIGUEZ M, GOMEZ MR, HOWARD FM JR, et al: *Myasthenia gravis in children: long-term follow-up*. Ann Neurol 1983, 13:504−510	20−22
ROWLAND, LP: *Myoglobinuria, 1984*. Can J Neurol Sci 1984, 11:1−13	33
ROWLAND LP: *Controversies about the treatment of myasthenia gravis*. J Neurol Neurosurg Psychiatry 1980, 43:644−659	20−22
ROWLAND LP, LOVELACE RE, SCHOTLAND DL, et al: *The clinical diagnosis of McArdle's disease: identification of another family with*	

Section XI (continued)

Plate Number

deficiency of muscle phosphorylase. Neurology 1966, 16:93–100 **32**

ROWLAND LP, PENN AS: Myoglobinuria. Med Clin North Am 1972, 56:1233–1256 **33**

SABIN TD, SWIFT TR: Leprosy. In DYCK PJ, THOMAS PK, LAMBERT EH, et al (eds): Peripheral Neuropathy, II, ed 2. Philadelphia, WB Saunders, 1984, pp 1955–1987 **19**

SAID G, BOUDIER L, SELVA J, et al: Different patterns of uremic polyneuropathy: clinicopathologic study. Neurology 1983, 33:567–574 **11**

SARGENT JC, LONG RR, HAMMER K: Serial electromyographic observations in red tide paralysis. Neurology (Suppl) 1981, 31:66–67 **34**

SCHMITT HP, KRAUSE K-H: An autopsy study of a familial oculopharyngeal muscular dystrophy (OPMD) with distal spread and neurogenic involvement. Muscle Nerve 1981, 4:296–305 **26**

SEAY AR, ZITER FA, WU LH, et al: Serum creatine phosphokinase and pyruvate kinase in neuromuscular disorders and Duchenne dystrophy carriers. Neurology 1978, 28:1047–1050 **24–25**

SEYBOLD ME: Myasthenia gravis: a clinical and basic science review. JAMA 1983, 250:2516–2521 **20–22**

SEYBOLD ME, DRACHMAN DB: Gradually increasing doses of prednisone in myasthenia gravis. Reducing the hazards of treatment. N Engl J Med 1974, 290:81–84 **20–22**

SHELBORNE SA: Duchenne's muscular dystrophy. JAMA 1982, 247:496–497 **24–25**

Section XI (continued)

Plate Number

SHIELDS RW JR: Alcoholic polyneuropathy. Muscle Nerve 1985, 8:183–187 **11**

SIMPSON JA: Myasthenia gravis: a personal view of pathogenesis and mechanism, part I. Muscle Nerve 1978, 1:45–56 **20–22**

SINAKI M, MULDER DW: Rehabilitation techniques for patients with amyotrophic lateral sclerosis. Mayo Clin Proc 1978, 53:173–178 **5–7**

SINGH N, BEHSE F, BUCHTHAL F: Electrophysiological study of peroneal palsy. J Neurol Neurosurg Psychiatry 1974, 37:1202–1213 **10**

SMITH RF: Exertional rhabdomyolysis in naval officer candidates. Arch Intern Med 1968, 121:313–319 **33**

STEVENS JC: Lumbosacral plexus lesions. In DYCK PJ, THOMAS PK, LAMBERT EH, et al (eds): Peripheral Neuropathy, II, ed 2. Philadelphia, WB Saunders, 1984, chap 61 **19**

STEWARD JD, AGUAYO AJ: Compression and entrapment neuropathies. In DYCK PJ, THOMAS PK, LAMBERT EH, et al (eds): Peripheral Neuropathy, II, ed 2. Philadelphia, WB Saunders, 1984, chap 62 **10**

SUMNER AJ: The physiological basis for symptoms in Guillain-Barré syndrome. Ann Neurol (Suppl) 1981, 9:28–30 **15**

TAYLOR DA, CARROLL JE, SMITH ME, et al: Facioscapulohumeral dystrophy associated with hearing loss and Coats syndrome. Ann Neurol 1982, 12:395–398 **26**

THOMAS PK: Inherited neuropathies. Clin Proc 1983, 58:476–480 **16–17**

Section XI (continued)

Plate Number

THOMAS PK: Screening for peripheral neuropathy in patients treated by chronic hemodialysis. Muscle Nerve 1978, 1:396–399 **11**

TROJABORG W: Rate of recovery in motor and sensory fibres of the radial nerve: clinical and electrophysiological aspects. J Neurol Neurosurg Psychiatry 1970, 33:625–638 **10**

TYLER KL, MCHENRY LC: Fragments of neurologic history: pseudohypertrophic muscular dystrophy and Gowers' sign. Neurology 1983, 33:88–89 **24–25**

WEES SJ, SUNWOO IN, OH SJ: Sural nerve biopsy in systemic necrotizing vasculitis. Am J Med 1981, 71:525 **14**

WINDEBANK AJ, MCCALL JT, DYCK PJ: Metal neuropathy. In DYCK PJ, THOMAS PK, LAMBERT EH, et al (eds): Peripheral Neuropathy, II, ed 2. Philadelphia, WB Saunders, 1984, chap 93 **13**

WINKELMANN RK, MULDER DW, LAMBERT EH, et al: Course of dermatomyositis-polymyositis: comparison of untreated and cortisone-treated patients. Mayo Clin Proc 1968, 43:545–556 **28–29**

WOLF SM, WAGNER JH JR, DAVIDSON S, et al: Treatment of Bell palsy with prednisone: A prospective, randomized study. Neurology 1978, 28:158–161 **8**

YAMAGUCHI DM, LIPSCOMB PR, SOULE EH: Carpal tunnel syndrome. Minn Med 1965, 48:22–33 **9**

Subject Index

Note: Boldface numbers refer to plates

Alzheimer's disease, 37, 145, 145-146, 146
Amaurosis fugax, 56, 56
Amblyopia, 36
ε-Aminocaproic acid (EACA), 85
Amnesia, 37, 37
Amphotericin B, 162
Ampicillin, 159
Amyloid angiopathy, intracerebral hemorrhage from, 76
Amyloid neuropathy, 215, 215
Amyloidosis, 215, 223
Amyotrophic lateral sclerosis, 208-209, 210
Anatomic classification of pituitary tumors, 122, 122
Anemia, pernicious, 191, 191
Anencephaly, 6, 6
Anesthesia, 190, 198, 198
Aneurysm clips, 86
Aneurysms, intracranial, 80, 80-86, 81, 82, 83, 84, 85, 86
    anatomic sites, 80
    approaches for, 84, 84, 85, 85
    as cerebrovascular lesions, 103-104
    distribution of, 80, 80
    etiology, 80
    manifestations of, 80, 82, 82, 83, 83
    rupture of, 81-84
    therapy for, 84, 84-86, 85, 86
    unruptured, 80
Angiography
    arterial digital subtraction (ADSA), 73, 73
    for brain tumors, 116, 116
    for carotid artery, 55, 75, 75
    cerebrovascular disease and, 72, 73, 73
    for cervical vessels, 72
    for chordomas, 130
    CT and, 73
    for gliomas, 118
    for hematomas, 95
    for intracranial injuries, 95
    intravenous digital subtraction (IDSA), 72, 73, 73
    for meningiomas, 121
    retrograde transfemoral arterial, 72
    of ruptured aneurysm, 84
    stroke and, 67, 74, 74
Angiomas, 10, 78
Angiomatosis, leptomeningeal, 26, 26
Angiopathy, amyloid, 76
Angular gyrus, 148
Anosognosia, 149, 149
Anterior inferior cerebellar artery (AICA), 64, 64
Anticholinesterase, 225, 226
Anticonvulsants, 32
Antidepressant medications, 33, 136
Antiedema therapy, 27
Antifibrinolytic drugs, 85
Antipsychotic medications, 138
Anti-rabies globulin, 170
Antiserotonin compounds, 32
Antitoxin
    for tetanus, 165
    trivalent, 238
Anxiety state, 139, 139
Aortic arch arteritis, 55
Apert's syndrome, 3, 3

Aphasia, 148, 148
Apnea
    head injury and, 101, 102
    hypoxic brain damage and, 87
    mixed, 38
    sleep, 38, 39
Apraxia, 145, 145
Arnold-Chiari malformation, 10, 11, 21, 190
Arrhinencephalia, 6
Arsenical neuropathy, 216, 216
Arterial angiography, 72
Arterial digital subtraction angiography (ADSA), 73, 73
Arterial thrombosis, 52, 52, 53, 53
Arteriography for brain tumors, 24
Arteriosclerotic heart disease, 66, 66
Arteriovenous malformations (AVMs), 76, 78, 78, 79, 79
Arteritis, 33, 33-34, 55, 62
Artery(ies)
    basilar, 60, 64, 64
    carotid. See Carotid artery
    cerebellar, 64, 64
    cerebral, 54, 58, 58, 65, 65
    subclavian, 62, 62
    vertebral, 35, 62, 62, 63, 63
Arthrogryposis multiplex congenita, 15
Arylsulfatase A enzyme deficiency, 20
Asphyxia, 12, 13, 38, 39, 87
Aspirin, 27, 74
Astrocytomas, 24, 25, 133, 187, 188
Asymmetric Moro response, 19
Ataxia, 12, 13
    cerebellar, 36, 174
    cerebral palsy and, 15
    Friedreich's, 17, 17, 21, 21
    hemiparesis and, 59
    spastic, 36
    -telangiectasia, 21
Atheromatous lesions, complicated, 53
Atherosclerosis, 53, 53
    basilar artery as site of, 64
    carotid artery, 55, 55, 75, 75
    subclavian artery occlusion and, 62
Athetosis, 12-13, 13, 152
Atonic (akinetic) seizures, 42, 43
Atonic cerebral palsy, 13
Atonic diplegia, 15
Atresia, choanal, 3
Atrial fibrillation, 66, 66
Atrial myxoma, 67, 67, 217
Atrial shunts, 9
Atrophy, progressive muscular, 208
Audiometry, 35, 126, 126
Auditory seizures, 44, 45
Auscultation in diagnosis of stroke, 74, 74
Autism, infantile, 23, 23
Autonomic disturbances, 82, 183
Autonomic seizures, 44, 45
Autosomal recessive inheritance, metachromatic leukodystrophy and, 20, 20
AVMs. See Arteriovenous malformations
Axon damage, Guillain-Barré syndrome and, 218, 219
Azathioprine, 226, 233

B

Babinski sign, 20, 20, 21, 21
Bacilli, gram-negative, 158, 158
Back pain, 184, 184, 196, 196-197, 198, 198
Bacterial endocarditis, 66, 66, 217
Bacterial meningitis, 158, 158-159, 159
BAER. See Brainstem auditory evoked responses
Ballism in diagnosis of chorea, 152
Barbiturate coma for intracranial injuries, 101
Basilar aneurysms, 80, 80, 85
Basilar artery and branches, 60, 64, 64
Basilar migraine, 32
Basilar skull fractures, 91, 91-92
Basilar trunk aneurysm, 85
Basophilic adenoma, 122
Bassen-Kornzweig syndrome, 21
Becker-type muscular dystrophy, 228
Beevor's sign, 182, 182
Behavior of autistic child, 23, 23
Bell's palsy, 211, 211
Benign congenital hypotonia, 15, 15
Benign intracranial hypertensia. See Pseudotumor cerebri
Benign monoclonal gammopathies, 215
Benign spinal tumors, 186
Benzodiazepine, 139
Beta activity, 40, 40
Beta-adrenergic blocking agents, 32
Bilateral calcarine infarction, 65
Bilateral cerebral hemisphere disease, 47, 48
Bilateral interfacet dislocation, 107, 108
Biopsy, muscle. See under Muscle(s)
Biopsy specimens
    of Reye's syndrome, 27, 27
    of temporal arteritis, 33
Bipolar affective disorder, 138, 138
Bitemporal hemianopsia, 116, 116
Blastoma, pineal, 125, 125
Bleeding diatheses, 76
Blindness, 33, 34, 56, 56
Blocking agents, 32
Blood analysis, in diagnosis of stroke, 74, 74
Blood glucose, elevated, 87
Blood tonicity, head injuries and, 102
Blood vessels, Alzheimer's disease and, 146
Border zone ischemia, 87, 87
Botulism, 16, 225, 238, 238
Braces for cervical spine injury, 110-112, 111, 114
Brachial plexopathy, 19, 19, 201, 201
Brachycephalia, 3, 3
Brain
    abscess, 160, 160
    Alzheimer's disease's effect on, 146, 146
    calcarine area of, 61, 61, 65
    damage, hypoxic, 87, 87

death, 40, 87, 87
developmental dyslexia and, 22, 22
dynamic radioisotope scanning of, 84
infantile autism and, 23, 23
malformations of, 6, 6-7, 7
tuberculosis of, 164, 164
Brainstem
    gliomas, 24, 25
    lesions, 47, 48, 174, 174
    vertebrobasilar ischemia and, 60
Brainstem auditory evoked responses (BAER)
    acoustic neurinomas and, 126, 126
    head injuries and, 105, 105
    multiple sclerosis and, 176, 176-177
Brain tumors, 115-133
    acoustic neurinomas, 35, 126, 126-127, 127
    angiography for, 116, 116
    arteriography for, 24
    chemotherapy for, 25
    in children, 24, 24-25, 25
    chordomas, 130, 130
    common manifestations of, 116, 116
    craniopharyngiomas, 124, 124
    CSF and, 9, 24, 24, 25, 116
    CT for, 24, 24, 25, 116, 116
    differential diagnosis, 131
    equilibrium disorders and, 116, 116
    frontal lobe, 37
    gliomas, 118, 118
    head tilt and, 116, 116
    high-dose steroids and, 24
    intraventricular, 129, 129
    magnetic resonance imaging of, 25, 132-133, 133
    meningiomas, 120, 120-121, 121
    neurofibromatosis, 128, 128
    pineal region tumors, 125, 125
    pituitary tumors, 122, 122-123, 123
    posterior fossa, 21
    pseudotumor cerebri, 117, 117
    seizures and, 41, 41
    temporal lobe, 35
    as treatable dementia, 150, 150
    tumors metastatic to brain, 119, 119
Brain wave activity, EEG and, 40, 40
Breathing, head injuries and, 93, 96
Broca's aphasia, 148
Brooks fusion, 113, 113
Brown-Séquard syndrome, 106, 107, 183
Brudzinski's sign, 158, 159
Bruit analysis of carotid artery blood flow, 71, 71
B-scan imaging system, 71
Bucrylate embolization of cerebral AVM, 79, 79
Bulbar poliomyelitis, 168

C

Calcarine infarction, 61, 61, 65, 65
Calcium channel blocking agents, 32
Caloric stimulation, 35
Caloric testing, 105, 105